AF440453

First Edition

Current

INFECTIOUS DISEASE

Drugs

Vincent T. Andriole

Professor of Medicine
Yale University School of Medicine
Chief, Fitkin Medical Firm
Attending Physician, Yale–New Haven Hospital
New Haven, Connecticut

With 17 contributors

UNIVERSITY OF SUNDERLAND

UNIVERSITY LIBRARY

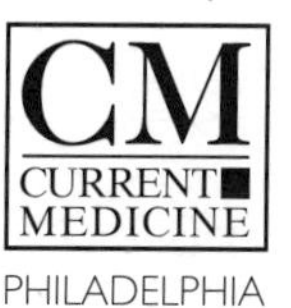

CM

CURRENT
MEDICINE

PHILADELPHIA

Current Medicine
Suite 700
400 Market Street
Philadelphia, PA 19106

Development Editor: *Lee Tevebaugh*
Editorial Assistant: *Danielle Shaw*
Art Director: *Paul Fennessy*
Design and Layout: *Robert LeBrun*
Illustration Director: *Ann Saydlowski*
Illustrator: *Gary Welch*
Typesetting Director: *Colleen Ward*
Production Manager: *David Myers*
Managing Editor: *Lori Bainbridge*

Although every effort has been made to ensure that drug doses and other information are presented accurately in this publication, the ultimate responsibility rests with the prescribing physician. Neither the publishers nor the authors can be held responsible for errors or for any consequences arising from the use of information contained herein. Products mentioned in this publication should be used in accordance with the prescribing information prepared by the manufacturers. No claims or endorsements are made for any drug or compound at present under clinical investigation.

ISBN: 1-878132-71-7
ISSN: 1082-8877
Manufactured in the United States of America
Printed by Princeton Academic Press, Inc.
5 4 3 2 1

© **Copyright 1996 by Current Medicine.** All rights reserved. No part of this publication may be reproduced, stored in a retrieval system, or transmitted in any form by any means electronic, mechanical, photocopying, recording, or otherwise, without prior written permission of the publisher.

Robert H. Alford, MD
Medical Director
Centennial Medical Center
Nashville, Tennessee

Vincent T. Andriole, MD
Professor of Medicine
Yale University School of Medicine
Chief, Fitkin Medical Firm
Attending Physician, Yale–New Haven Hospital
New Haven, Connecticut

Michèle Barry, MD
Professor of Medicine
Yale University School of Medicine
New Haven, Connecticut

Frank J. Bia, MD, MPH
Professor of Medicine and Laboratory Medicine
Director, Yale Affiliated Hospitals Program
Co-director, International Health Program
Department of Internal Medicine
New Haven, Connecticut

Gerald P. Bodey, MD
Professor of Medicine
Chairman, Department of Medical Specialties
Chief, Section of Infectious Diseases
Texas Medical Center
Houston, Texas

Frank M. Calia, MD
Professor of Medicine
Vice Dean, School of Medicine
University of Maryland at Baltimore
Baltimore, Maryland

William A. Craig, MD
Chief of Infectious Disease Section
William S. Middleton Memorial Veterans Hospital
Professor of Medicine
University of Wisconsin School of Medicine
Madison, Wisconsin

Jane M. Farrington, MS, RPh
Clinical Coordinator
Pharmacy Services
Yale–New Haven Hospital
New Haven, Connecticut

Alejandra C. Gurtman, MD
Assistant Professor of Medicine
Assistant Director of AIDS Center
Mount Sinai Medical Center
New York, New York

Catherine Hitt, PharmD
Antibiotic Management/Pharmacoeconomic Fellow
Hartford Hospital
Hartford, Connecticut

Stephen A. Lerner, MD
Professor of Medicine
Vice-Chief and Director of Research
Division of Infectious Diseases
Wayne State University School of Medicine
Detroit, Michigan

Kenneth H. Mayer, MD
Chief, Infectious Disease Division
Memorial Hospital of Rhode Island
Professor of Medicine and Community Health
Brown University School of Medicine
Director, Brown University AIDS Program
Pawtucket, Rhode Island

Burt R. Meyers, MD
Professor of Medicine
Division of Infectious Diseases
Mount Sinai Medical Center
New York, New York

Charles H. Nightingale, PhD
Vice President for Research
Hartford Hospital
Hartford, Connecticut

Harold C. Standiford, MD
Assistant Chief, Medical Service
Baltimore Veterans Medical Center
Professor of Medicine
University of Maryland School of Medicine
Baltimore, Maryland

Richard J. Whitley, MD
Loeb Eminent Scholar Chair in Pediatrics
Professor of Pediatrics, Microbiology, and Medicine
The University of Alabama at Birmingham
Birmingham, Alabama

Stephen H. Zinner, MD
Professor and Interim Chairman
Department of Medicine
Brown University School of Medicine
Providence, Rhode Island

TABLE OF CONTENTS

PREFACE

The development of newer anti-infectives—not only in the field of antibacterial agents but also in the fields of antivirals, antifungals, and newer antiparasitic agents—has occurred and will continue to occur at a rapid pace. These advances have made it difficult, if not impossible, for the health-care professional to easily integrate these new developments into clinical practice.

The purpose of *Current Infectious Disease Drugs* is to aid the health-care professional. With that intent, the authors of this book, who are very knowledgeable in their fields, have written chapters designed to provide current information on all classes and agents used in the care of patients with infectious diseases.

The book is not designed to replace traditional textbooks of infectious diseases. Its purpose it to provide easy accessibility to current data on a particular anti-infective agent. To accomplish this goal, we have utilized a consistent format. Each of the thirteen chapters discusses a particular class of anti-infective agents with an overview of the current and salient points of the agents as a class along with the most recent references from the medical literature.

Each overview is followed by a succinct description of each anti-infective agent in the class, allowing the clinician to compare different agents in a given class, as well as to select an agent for use in clinical practice. Specifically, the antimicrobial activity, resistance, indications, contraindications, dosage, drug interactions, adverse effects, pharmacokinetics and pharmacodynamics, overdosage, patient instructions, and drug availability are described for each agent in a concise, consistent, and user-friendly format.

The expertise and efforts of all contributors to *Current Infectious Disease Drugs* is recognized and greatly appreciated. They are committed to updating *Current Infectious Disease Drugs* frequently to provide the most current information to practicing physicians, nurses, physician assistants, pharmacists, medical students, and others concerned with the treatment of patients with infectious diseases. We hope that this book will be of practical use to all who are engaged in the challenging and rapidly advancing field of current therapy for all infectious diseases.

Vincent T. Andriole, MD

UNIVERSITY OF SUNDERLAND
LIBRARY
Class No. 615.1
Access No.
Order No.
F19764/4   42435
UNIVERSITY OF SUNDERLAND
WITHDRAWN

CLASS DESCRIPTION

Aminoglycoside antibiotics have been available since the isolation and development of streptomycin in the late 1940s. Streptomycin is the only member of the streptidine group. It has been replaced by members of the other group, the 2-deoxystreptamine aminoglycosides, for the treatment of infections caused by aerobic gram-negative bacilli. However, streptomycin still retains utility in the treatment of *Mycobacterium tuberculosis* and enterococcal infections and for other specific infections, such as tularemia, plague, and brucellosis. Kanamycin was used for aerobic gram-negative bacillary infections but was superseded by gentamicin, which had improved activity against many of these species and unique efficacy against systemic infections caused by *Pseudomonas aeruginosa*. Thus, kanamycin is rarely used today for the treatment of systemic infections.

Gentamicin was the first of the modern aminoglycosides, and it has been followed in the United States by tobramycin, amikacin, and netilmicin. The development of these latter aminoglycosides has been directed toward improvement of activity against gram-negative bacilli, especially hospital strains that have acquired resistance to many antibacterial agents (including in some cases aminoglycosides like gentamicin). In addition, developers of newer aminoglycosides also have sought to reduce the potential of nephrotoxicity and ototoxicity, which are properties of all aminoglycoside antibiotics. Although improvement of activity against some strains has been achieved, among the modern aminoglycosides there is no consistent demonstration that one aminoglycoside is less toxic clinically than any others. For systemic therapy, aminoglycosides must be administered parenterally, because they are not absorbed from the gastrointestinal tract. The toxicity of neomycin precludes its systemic use, but it is used topically in the gastrointestinal tract, on the skin, and in the ear and eye. Spectinomycin shares some similarities of structure and site of action with the aminoglycosides and is often classified with them. However, it is not precisely an aminoglycoside because it lacks an aminosugar and has no glycosidic bond.

MECHANISM OF ACTION

Aminoglycosides bind to the smaller subunit of bacterial ribosomes and impair their function in the synthesis of proteins. All aminoglycosides can drastically retard the synthesis of proteins and also can cause mistranslation of messenger RNA into false proteins. Most studies of effects on ribosomal protein synthesis have been carried out with streptomycin, and irreversible cessation of protein synthesis appears to predominate. With the 2-deoxystreptamine aminoglycosides, more extensive mistranslation is seen. In any case, the activity of aminoglycosides is bactericidal, and killing takes place fairly quickly. Furthermore, the cidal effect is concentration-dependent (ie, the higher the concentration of the drug, the more rapid and extensive the killing). The postantibiotic effect is another feature of the activity of aminoglycosides against gram-negative bacilli. Thus, the surviving bacteria continue to be inhibited for hours after the concentration of drug has declined below the minimum inhibitory concentration. The entry of aminoglycosides into the bacterial cell involves active uptake across the plasma membrane. Because this uptake process is diminished under conditions of reduced oxygen or low pH, it is thus clear why anaerobic bacteria are intrinsically resistant to aminoglycosides. Furthermore, even facultative aerobic bacteria are relatively resistant when growing under anaerobic conditions. Because aminoglycosides bind to the nucleic acids in pus, they are poorly active in such an environment. In combination with agents that interfere with cell wall biosynthesis, such as the beta-lactams and vancomycin, aminoglycosides may exhibit synergistic activity against some organisms. As a result of mutual enhancement of penetration into the cell, the activity of an aminoglycoside used together with an anti–cell wall agent is thus greater than the additive sum of the individual activities when used alone.

MECHANISMS OF BACTERIAL RESISTANCE

The most common mechanism of high-level resistance to aminoglycosides in clinical isolates is enzymatic modification of various aminoglycosides that renders them inactive. The diverse array of aminoglycoside-modifying enzymes with different substrate specificities is largely responsible for the variety of aminoglycoside resistance profiles among different clinical strains. Modern aminoglycosides have been developed to circumvent or reduce such inactivation. The principal significant difference among these newer aminoglycosides is in their activity against strains bearing various aminoglycoside-modifying enzymes. Resistance to aminoglycosides arising from alteration of the ribosomal binding site is uncommon among clinical isolates, but such resistance to streptomycin may be seen in *M. tuberculosis*, enterococci, and *Neisseria gonorrhoeae*. The third mechanism of resistance to aminoglycosides is the reduction of penetration into the cell, which may result from impairment of active uptake across the plasma membrane or from changes in the outer membrane of gram-negative bacteria that reduce the permeability of aminoglycosides. Resistance arising from reduced penetration is not well understood, but it is generally relatively modest in degree and relatively nonspecific among the aminoglycosides. Unlike resistance to beta-lactams and the quinolones, which may arise rapidly and sometimes even during therapy of individual patients, resistance to aminoglycosides is generally stable and slow to emerge. One can therefore treat nosocomial infections empirically with aminoglycosides according to susceptibility patterns of organisms in the institution.

ANTIMICROBIAL ACTIVITY

The principal activity of modern aminoglycosides (gentamicin, tobramycin, netilmicin, and amikacin) is against aerobic gram-negative bacilli, including *Escherichia coli*, *Proteus mirabilis*, *Klebsiella* spp, *Serratia marcescens*, *Providencia* spp, *Morganella* spp, *Citrobacter freundii*, *Enterobacter* spp, and *P. aeruginosa*. In the absence of specific resistance to aminoglycosides these drugs are comparably active, except that *P. aeruginosa* is generally less susceptible to gentamicin and may be less susceptible to netilmicin. *S. marcescens* is generally less susceptible to tobramycin.

Because of the patterns of aminoglycoside-modifying enzymes that are present in gram-negative bacteria in the United States, among these organisms the number of strains susceptible to the various aminoglycosides generally is in the increasing order: gentamicin < tobramycin < netilmicin < amikacin. In treating nosocomial infections it is of prime importance to know the resistance patterns of gram-negative bacilli in the institution in order to guide the selection of aminoglycoside. Aminoglycosides also may have activity against *Haemophilus influenzae*, *N. gonorrhoeae*, and *Salmonella* spp and *Shigella* spp, but they are not often used for infections caused by these organisms. Aminoglycosides also have activity against aerobic gram-positive cocci (streptococci, enterococci, and staphylococci). Compared with the other modern amino-

The information here is provided as guidance only. Prescribers should always consult the manufacturer's current prescribing information.

glycosides, gentamicin generally is preferred for the treatment of gram-positive coccal infections, although streptomycin may have activity and may be used against enterococcal strains that are resistant to gentamicin. The activity of aminoglycosides against gram-positive cocci is not sufficient to permit their use alone. Rather, they are used in synergistic combination with beta-lactams, such as ampicillin or penicillin G, or with vancomycin. Systemic enterococcal infections, such as endocarditis, are treated optimally with such combinations. Streptomycin has activity against most strains of *M. tuberculosis*, although amikacin may be used instead. Streptomycin also has activity against *Francisella tularensis*, *Yersinia pestis*, and *Brucella* spp, but may be replaced by gentamicin.

EFFICACY AND USE

The principal uses of aminoglycosides are for the treatment of aerobic, gram-negative, bacillary, and gram-positive coccal infections. Because of the availability of other less toxic agents for gram-negative bacillary infections, the use of aminoglycosides for these infections is generally limited to serious infections, especially when they are nosocomial or the infecting pathogen is known or suspected to be fairly resistant to other classes of antibiotics. Thus, an aminoglycoside generally is included in a treatment regimen with a beta-lactam for initial empiric therapy for patients with a clinical septic state or with suspected gram-negative bacteremia, especially of nosocomial origin. Once the patient's infection is under control and the infecting organism is known, then the aminoglycoside may be dropped from the regimen and the patient may be treated with a single agent. Against organisms such as *P. aeruginosa*, which are generally fairly resistant to antibiotics and have great facility for developing resistance, combination therapy with an aminoglycoside and a beta-lactam usually is preferred. For serious systemic enterococcal infections, gentamicin or streptomycin is used in combination with ampicillin, penicillin G, or vancomycin. Similarly, such combinations also may be used for serious streptococcal infections, such as endocarditis, to shorten therapy. For staphylococcal infections, gentamicin may be used adjunctively with an antistaphylococcal penicillin (*eg*, oxacillin or nafcillin) or with vancomycin.

Other than bacteremia and endocarditis, localized sites of infection that may be treated with aminoglycosides usually include urinary tract (generally not necessary but may be used as a single agent); respiratory tract (aminoglycosides do not penetrate well into pneumonic tissue but may be advisable for organisms resistant to most other classes of antibiotics, such as *P. aeruginosa*); intra-abdominal (generally not necessary but may be used in combination with an agent with antianaerobe activity); bone and joint; skin and soft tissue (especially for an organism for which an aminoglycoside is especially suited); and the eye (topically or by intravitreal injection). Only rarely does one have to resort to an aminoglycoside for the treatment of meningitis. Except in neonates, aminoglycosides penetrate poorly into the cerebrospinal fluid. Therefore, if they are used for meningitis after the neonatal period, they must be instilled directly into the cerebrospinal fluid, as per an Ommaya reservoir into the ventricle. For the empiric treatment of febrile neutropenic patients without a definite infection, most regimens include an aminoglycoside.

TOXICITY

The principal adverse effects of aminoglycosides are nephrotoxicity and ototoxicity; others are quite rare. The clinical manifestation of nephrotoxicity is generally nonoliguric acute renal failure. Although early subclinical effects on renal tubular cells may be detected by measurements of substances released in the urine, the diagnosis of nephrotoxicity usually is reserved for patients who exhibit azotemia. This toxicity is virtually always reversible, but it may complicate the patient's hospital course and requires reduction of dosage of the aminoglycoside (which is renally excreted) if it is to be continued. With careful monitoring of aminoglycoside serum levels and serum creatinine levels and with appropriate dosing that is carried out in many hospitals by pharmacy teams, the incidence and severity of nephrotoxicity have been controlled. Furthermore, toxicity rarely arises in less than 3 days of therapy, so when an aminoglycoside is used only for initial empiric therapy, toxicity is reduced even further.

Ototoxicity may appear as auditory (cochlear) or vestibular dysfunction, and it may affect one or both ears. Clinical symptoms of auditory toxicity may appear as hearing loss (especially at higher frequencies and rarely at lower frequencies than are used in speech), tinnitus, or a feeling of fullness in the ear. Symptoms of severe vestibular toxicity may appear as nausea, vomiting, vertigo, nystagmus, or difficulty with gait. Early auditory deficits may be detected by careful audiometric testing. However, audiometric testing requires patient cooperation, and routing testing is not considered advisable unless the patient is expected to receive an aminoglycoside over many weeks, such as for osteomyelitis. In such a case, audiometry might be carried out every 1 to 2 weeks. Vestibular testing is not standardized, so it is not considered routine for patients receiving an aminoglycoside. Because testing for ototoxicity generally is not performed in patients receiving an aminoglycoside, description of the symptoms of toxicity to any patient who can understand and will receive the drug for more than 5 to 7 days is recommended. In that way, if symptoms arise the patient should tell a nurse or physician so that the possibility of toxicity can be considered further, and the necessity of aminoglycoside therapy can be reexamined. Although careful monitoring of serum levels of aminoglycoside and creatinine can reduce the occurrence of nephro- and ototoxicity, some patients who are treated appropriately still incur toxicity. The contribution of various risk factors for toxicity has not been fully assessed, although renal impairment, either preexisting or from nephrotoxicity, may increase the risk of ototoxicity. Neuromuscular blockade from aminoglycosides is very rare but may occur in special situations, such as with a rapid bolus infusion in a patient receiving a neuromuscular blocking agent or with excess magnesium levels, hypocalcemia, botulism, or myasthenia gravis. It can usually be reversed by prompt administration of calcium gluconate. Hypersensitivity to aminoglycosides is rare, and aminoglycosides are noninflammatory.

PHARMACOKINETICS AND DOSING

Aminoglycosides are absorbed poorly from the gastrointestinal tract, so they must be administered parenterally to achieve adequate concentrations for systemic therapy. Peak serum levels reached between 30 and 90 minutes after intramuscular injection are similar to those determined at 30 minutes after a 30-minute intravenous infusion. Aminoglycosides are completely distributed throughout the extracellular fluid compartment outside the central nervous system. Binding to serum proteins is less than 10%. Aminoglycosides are excreted unchanged by glomerular filtration. Therefore, impairment of renal function results in prolongation of the half-life in serum and tissues and requires alteration of dosage. The goal of aminoglycoside dosing is to adjust the dose and the

The information here is provided as guidance only. Prescribers should always consult the manufacturer's current prescribing information.

interdose interval to achieve serum levels sufficiently high to be efficacious and yet avoid excessive drug exposure that might increase the risk of toxicity. Table 1-1 lists the conventional doses and desired ranges for peak serum levels for the aminoglycosides [1]. The portion of the range of peak serum levels that is targeted depends on the site of infection and the target organisms. It is generally accepted that trough (predose) levels for gentamicin, tobramycin, and netilmicin should be under 2.0 µg/mL, and for amikacin, under 7.5 µg/mL. In patients with normal renal function, the half-life of aminoglycosides is 2 to 2.5 hours, and in the presence of end-stage renal function, the half-life is markedly prolonged, *ie*, up to 60 to 100 hours. Table 1-1 also lists suggested dosage adjustments for reduced renal function [1] according to calculated creatinine clearance estimated by the method of Cockroft and Gault [2].

Because of mutual inactivation of gentamicin and tobramycin by prolonged exposure to high concentrations of penicillins in the serum of patients with renal failure, the half-life of active gentamicin or tobramycin in such patients also treated with a penicillin may be shorter than anticipated. Ultimately, in most clinical situations dosing regimens of aminoglycosides are adjusted according to serum levels, either from peak and trough levels or, more precisely, from individualized pharmacokinetic analysis [3,4]. It should be noted that the desired serum levels (and doses) of amikacin (and kanamycin) are generally three to four times higher than those of gentamicin, tobramycin, and netilmicin to compensate for the lower antibacterial activity of amikacin (and kanamycin) on a molar basis. Fortunately, these higher levels of amikacin are not correlated with an increased risk of toxicity, so they are considered equivalent with the lower levels of the other aminoglycosides. In clinical situations in which rapid attainment of optimal peak serum levels is critical, a roughly one-third higher initial dose, or loading dose, is given. This also may be employed in patients with renal failure because subsequent maintenance doses will be delayed because of slower excretion.

Monitoring of serum creatinine usually is carried out one to three times a week, as long as it seems stable, and more often if renal function is changing. Peak and trough serum levels are checked within the first 24 to 48 hours, and dosage is adjusted as needed. Once the peak and trough serum levels are in the desired ranges, trough levels are rechecked once or twice a week because a rising trough level is a sensitive indicator of declining renal function. Serum levels should be rechecked within 1 or 2 days after any dosage adjustment or in situations of changing renal function.

With extreme renal failure requiring hemodialysis or continuous peritoneal dialysis, dialyzed drug is replaced; two thirds of the usual dose is given after a 4- to 6-hour run of hemodialysis. For peritoneal dialysis, gentamicin, tobramycin, or netilmicin is included at 3 to 4 mg/L dialysate, and for amikacin, 15 to 20 mg/L of dialysate [1].

Other situations also require special considerations, more frequent monitoring of serum levels, and alteration of dosage as indicated. For instance, patients who are cachectic and bedridden may have a serum creatinine value that underestimates impairment of renal function. Obese patients may have a smaller than average volume of distribution on a weight basis. With these patients one may use ideal body weight, based on height and bone structure, or dosage weight, defined as the ideal body weight plus 40% of the actual body weight above that, which is a better measure [5]. The volume of distribution may be larger in patients with ascites or congestive heart failure and may fluctuate, so dosage may have to be adjusted as the serum levels shift. Clearance of aminoglycosides may be increased in patients with burns or cystic fibrosis. The half-life of gentamicin and tobramycin may appear shorter than anticipated in patients with marked renal failure who are also receiving a penicillin because of mutual inactivation of the drugs during prolonged exposure together.

ONCE-DAILY DOSING

Microbiologic considerations, such as concentration-dependent killing and the postantibiotic effect, suggest that administration of the total daily dose of an aminoglycoside once a day, rather than in conventional divided doses, may enhance the antibacterial activity or at least not compromise it. In animal models of infection, once-daily dosing has been at least effective as conventional dosing, either with adjunctive beta-lactam treatment or in the presence of adequate neutrophils. Similarly, in animal models of nephro- and ototoxicity, once-daily dosing of aminoglycosides has been associated with less or equivalent toxicity in comparison with conventional dosing. Studies in humans are limited, either in number of patients or in design. Nonetheless, both efficacy and toxicity appear to be at least

Table 1-1. Conventional Dosing and Desired Peak Serum Concentrations of Aminoglycosides*

Aminoglycoside	Peak serum concentrations, µg/mL	Dose for normal renal function	Adjustment of dosage for renal failure Creatinine clearance, *mL/min*		
			50–80	10–50	< 10
Gentamicin	4–10	1.7 mg/kg every 8 h	60%–90%† every 8–12 h	30%–70% every 12 h	20%–30% every 24–48 h
Tobramycin	4–10	1.7 mg/kg every 8 h	60%–90% every 8–12 h	30%–70% every 12 h	20%–30% every 24–48 h
Netilmicin	6–10	1.7–2.0 mg/kg every 8 h	50%–90% every 8–12 h	20%–60% every 12 h	10%–20% every 24–48 h
Amikacin	15–35	5 mg/kg every 8 h or 7.5 mg/kg every 12 h	60%–90% every 12 h	30%–70% every 12 h	20%–30% every 24–48 h
Kanamycin	15–35	5 mg/kg every 8 h or 7.5 mg/kg every 12 h	60%–90% every 12 h	30%–70% every 12 h	20%–30% every 24–48 h
Streptomycin	15–25	0.5–2.0 g every 24 h (usually 1.0 g)	Every 24 h	—‡	—‡

*Adapted from Sanford et al. [1]; with permission.
†Percent of the individual doses for patients with normal renal function.
‡For tuberculosis in patients with renal failure, one can use amikacin and determine serum levels for dosage adjustment.

The information here is provided as guidance only. Prescribers should always consult the manufacturer's current prescribing information.

as favorable in patients treated with an aminoglycoside once daily, generally with a beta-lactam in the regimen, as in patients treated with conventional dosing.

Until further studies include special populations and infections, it seems prudent to exclude from once-daily dosing patients with baseline impaired renal function (creatinine clearance $\leq$ 40 mL/min), burns, gram-positive coccal infections, and endocarditis [6]. Although one large study [7] of neutropenic patients has shown equivalent efficacy of once-daily and twice-daily amikacin, each with a beta-lactam in the regimen, there were relatively few cases with *P. aeruginosa*. Thus, it would be prudent to continue to use conventional dosing in this population until these results have been verified.

Although desirable peak serum levels have not been standardized for patients treated once daily with an aminoglycoside, one would give the entire daily dose every 24 hours, aiming for a range of 12 to 24 µg/mL (depending on the site of infection and the pathogen) for gentamicin, tobramycin, and netilmicin and 40 to 70 µg/mL for amikacin [1,6]. Actual predose serum levels should be too low for sensitive testing, so one can determine levels at 8 hours (less than 5 µg/mL for gentamicin, tobramycin, and netilmicin and less than 15 µg/mL for amikacin). A rising 8-hour level would indicate probable reduction in renal clearance.

INTERACTIONS

Aminoglycosides, amphotericin B, bacitracin, cisplatin, cyclosporine, loop diuretics (*eg*, ethacrynic acid), methoxyflurane, enflurane, neuromuscular blocking agents, nonsteroidal anti-inflammatory drugs, penicillins (in patients with renal failure), polymyxins, radiographic contrast agents, vancomycin.

OVERDOSAGE

In the presence of impaired renal function, hemodialysis or peritoneal dialysis may aid in removal of excessive amounts of aminoglycosides. The administration of an extended-spectrum penicillin, such as ticarcillin or piperacillin, to accelerate the removal of active gentamicin or tobramycin by inactivation may be considered as an adjunctive measure. In neonates, exchange transfusion may be considered.

REFERENCES

1. Sanford JP, Gilbert DN, Gerberding JL, *et al.*: Guide to Antimicrobial Therapy. Dallas: Antimicrobial Therapy, Inc; 1994.

2. Cockroft DW, Gault MH: Prediction of creatinine clearance from serum creatinine. *Nephron* 1976, 16:31–41.

3. Zaske DE, Cipolle RJ, Rotschafer JC, *et al.*: Gentamicin pharmacokinetics in 1,640 patients: Method for control of serum concentrations. *Antimicrob Agents Chemother* 1982, 21:407–411.

4. Burton ME, Brater DC, Chen PS, *et al.*: A Baylsian feedback method of aminoglycoside dosing. *Clin Pharmacol Ther* 1985, 37:349.

5. Leader WG, Tsubaki T, Chandler MHH: Creatinine-clearance estimates for predicting gentamicin pharmacokinetic values in obese patients. *Am J Hosp Pharm* 1994, 51:2125–2130.

6. Rotschafer JC, Rybak MJ: Single daily dosing of aminoglycosides: A commentary. *Ann Pharmacotherapy* 1994, 28:797–801.

7. EORTC International Antimicrobial Therapy Cooperative Group: Efficacy and toxicity of single daily doses of amikacin and ceftriaxone vs. multiple daily doses of amikacin and ceftazidime for infection in patients with cancer and granulocytopenia. *Ann Intern Med* 1993, 119:584–593.

The information here is provided as guidance only. Prescribers should always consult the manufacturer's current prescribing information.

AMIKACIN (Amikin®)

Amikacin is a semisynthetic aminoglycoside that is derived from kanamycin. Its chemical modification protects it from inactivation by most bacterial enzymes that confer resistance to aminoglycosides. Thus, it is used when resistance to gentamicin and tobramycin is known or suspected. It is also an alternative to streptomycin in regimens for the treatment of tuberculosis.

ANTIMICROBIAL ACTIVITY

Aerobic gram-negative bacilli, including *Pseudomonas* spp, *Escherichia coli*, species of indole-positive and -negative *Proteus*, species of *Providencia*, *Klebsiella-Enterobacter-Serratia*, *Acinetobacter*, *Citrobacter*, *Salmonella*, and *Shigella*, and *Yersinia pestis*.

Other organisms generally susceptible to amikacin include *Mycobacterium tuberculosis* and *Haemophilus influenzae*. Amikacin also may be active against gentamicin- or tobramycin-resistant strains of *Pseudomonas aeruginosa* and other gram-negative bacilli.

Amikacin may be used as part of a regimen for *Mycobacterium avium* complex, an infection common in patients with AIDS.

RESISTANCE

See Mechanisms of Bacterial Resistance and Antimicrobial Activity in introduction.

SPECIAL PRECAUTIONS

See Toxicity and Pharmacokinetics and Dosing in introduction.

SPECIAL GROUPS

Children: Use with caution in premature infants and neonates; prolonged half-life.
Elderly: May have age-related renal impairment; reduced dosage or lengthened intervals may be necessary.
Renal impairment: Increased risk of renal toxicity and ototoxicity; monitor drug levels and renal function closely.
Hepatic impairment: There may be increased risk of nephrotoxicity.

DOSAGE

See Pharmacokinetics and Dosing in introduction.

INDICATIONS

Infections of the following types due to susceptible gram-negative bacteria:

Respiratory tract, urinary tract, bones and joints, central nervous system, skin, soft tissue, intra-abdominal, burn, postoperative, bacterial septicemia (including neonatal sepsis).

Amikacin may be used as an alternative to streptomycin in the treatment of tuberculosis.

Amikacin may be used as part of a regimen for *M. avium* complex, an infection common in patients with AIDS.

CONTRAINDICATIONS

Allergy or hypersensitivity to aminoglycosides (rare)

INTERACTIONS

See Interactions in introduction

ADVERSE EFFECTS

See Toxicity in introduction

PHARMACOKINETICS AND PHARMACODYNAMICS

See Pharmacokinetics and Dosing in introduction

OVERDOSAGE

See Overdosage in introduction

AVAILABILITY

250 mg/mL in 2-mL (500-mg) vials and 4-mL (1-g) vials

The information here is provided as guidance only. Prescribers should always consult the manufacturer's current prescribing information.

GENTAMICIN (Garamycin®, G-myticin®)

Gentamicin is generally the first-line aminoglycoside against susceptible gram-negative bacilli. It is also the preferred aminoglycoside for combined therapy (with a penicillin or vancomycin) against gram-positive coccal infections.

ANTIMICROBIAL ACTIVITY

Gram-negative: Same spectrum as for amikacin.
Gram-positive: Gentamicin is the preferred aminoglycoside for synergistic use with ampicillin or vancomycin in the treatment of systemic enterococcal infections. May also be used adjunctively for staphylococcal infections. (*See* Antimicrobial Activity in introduction.)

RESISTANCE

Strains of gram-negative bacilli that are resistant to gentamicin may be susceptible to tobramycin, netilmicin, and/or amikacin. Enterococcal strains that exhibit high-level resistance to gentamicin may be susceptible to high concentrations of streptomycin, indicating the possibility of synergistic activity between ampicillin or vancomycin plus streptomycin. (*See* Mechanisms of Bacterial Resistance and Antimicrobial Activity in introduction.)

SPECIAL PRECAUTIONS

Contains sodium bisulfite, which can cause allergic reactions and anaphylactic symptoms. (*See* Toxicity and Pharmacokinetics in introduction.)

SPECIAL GROUPS

Children: Use with caution in premature infants and neonates; prolonged half-life.
Elderly: Increased risk for toxicity, may have age-related renal impairment; reduced dosage or lengthened intervals may be necessary.
Renal impairment: Increased risk of renal toxicity and ototoxicity; monitor drug levels and renal function closely.
Hepatic impairment: There may be increased risk of nephrotoxicity.

DOSAGE

See Pharmacokinetics and Dosing in introduction.

INDICATIONS

Infections of the following types due to susceptible gram-negative bacteria:
Respiratory tract, urinary tract, bones and joints, central nervous system, skin, soft tissue, intra-abdominal, burn, postoperative, bacterial septicemia (including neonatal sepsis).
In synergistic combination with ampicillin or vancomycin for systemic infections with enterococcal strains that are susceptible to high concentrations (500–2000 µg/mL) of gentamicin.

CONTRAINDICATIONS

Allergy or hypersensitivity to aminoglycosides (rare)

INTERACTIONS

See Interactions in introduction

ADVERSE EFFECTS

See Toxicity in introduction

PHARMACOKINETICS AND PHARMACODYNAMICS

See Pharmacokinetics and Dosing in introduction

OVERDOSAGE

See Overdosage in introduction

AVAILABILITY

Parenteral injection—40 mg/mL supplied in 2 mL (80-mg) vials and 1.5-mL (60-mg) and 2-mL (80-mg) disposable syringes
Pediatric parenteral injection—10 mg/mL, in 2-mL (20-mg) vials

The information here is provided as guidance only. Prescribers should always consult the manufacturer's current prescribing information.

KANAMYCIN

Prior to the introduction of gentamicin and the other modern aminoglycosides, *kanamycin* was the principal aminoglycoside for gram-negative bacillary infections. Because it lacks activity against *Pseudomonas aeruginosa* and its activity against other gram-negative bacilli is often inferior to that of the modern aminoglycosides, it generally has been replaced by them in the treatment of systemic infections. Like neomycin, kanamycin is used occasionally for irrigation of body cavities, such as the thorax and peritoneal cavity. One must be aware that with prolonged exposure to large mucosal surfaces aminoglycosides may penetrate into the systemic circulation, especially in the presence of inflammation. In a patient with diminished renal excretion, therefore, systemic accumulation may result, thereby enhancing the risk of toxicity. Kanamycin is an alternative to streptomycin in the treatment of tuberculosis. Because kanamycin levels generally are not assayed, however, amikacin may be preferable in patients with renal impairment because amikacin levels can be monitored and the dosage may be altered accordingly.

ANTIMICROBIAL ACTIVITY

Gram-negative: Same as for gentamicin, but excluding *P. aeruginosa*.

RESISTANCE

See Mechanisms of Bacterial Resistance and Antimicrobial Activity in introduction.

SPECIAL PRECAUTIONS

See Toxicity and Pharmacokinetics and Dosing in introduction.

SPECIAL GROUPS

Children: Use with caution in premature infants and neonates; prolonged half-life.
Elderly: May have age-related renal impairment; reduced dosage or lengthened intervals may be necessary.
Renal impairment: Increased risk of renal toxicity and ototoxicity; monitor drug levels and renal function closely.
Hepatic impairment: There may be increased risk of nephrotoxicity.

DOSAGE

INJECTION: See Pharmacokinetics and Dosing in introduction.
ORAL:
Adults: For suppression of intestinal bacteria as an adjunct to mechanical cleansing of the large bowel in short-term therapy, 1 g/h for 4 hours, followed by 1 g every 6 hours for 36 to 72 hours. For hepatic coma, 8 to 12 g/d in divided doses.
Children: No information.
IRRIGATION:
For prophylaxis following peritoneal surgery (*eg*, after fecal spill), 500 mg diluted in 20 mL sterile distilled water instilled through a polyethylene catheter into wound (postpone instillation, if possible, until patient has recovered from anesthesia and muscle relaxants). Concentrations of 0.25% have been used as irrigating solutions in abscess cavities, pleural space, and peritoneal and ventricular cavities.

INDICATIONS

INJECTION:
For short-term treatment of infections due to susceptible gram-negative bacteria, as for other aminoglycosides, but now rarely used.
Kanamycin may be used as an alternative to streptomycin or amikacin in the treatment of tuberculosis.
Also may be used as part of a multiple drug regimen for *Mycobacterium avium* complex, a common infection in patients with AIDS.
ORAL:
For short-term (adjunctive therapy) suppression of intestinal bacteria and hepatic coma.

CONTRAINDICATIONS

Allergy or hypersensitivity to aminoglycosides (rare)

INTERACTIONS

See Interactions in introduction

ADVERSE EFFECTS

See Toxicity in introduction

PHARMACOKINETICS AND PHARMACODYNAMICS

See Pharmacokinetics and Dosing in introduction

OVERDOSAGE

See Overdosage in introduction

AVAILABILITY

Injection—500 mg in 2-mL vials and 1 g in 3-mL vials
Pediatric injection—75 mg in 2-mL vials
Capsules—500 mg

The information here is provided as guidance only. Prescribers should always consult the manufacturer's current prescribing information.

NEOMYCIN (Neosporin®)

Because the potential for nephrotoxicity and ototoxicity of *neomycin* is greater than for other aminoglycosides, its use is restricted to topical therapy on skin and mucosal surfaces and on the surfaces of the eye and external ear. As with kanamycin, which also may be used topically, one must be aware of the potential for toxic systemic accumulation in patients with impaired renal excretion.

ANTIMICROBIAL ACTIVITY

Like gentamicin, principal activity against aerobic gram-negative bacilli, and adjunctive activity against gram-positive cocci.

RESISTANCE

As with other aminoglycosides, resistance can occur.

SPECIAL PRECAUTIONS

TABLETS:
Use with caution in patients with neuromuscular disorders; oral aminoglycosides may aggravate muscle weakness.
Oral neomycin increases fecal bile acid excretion and reduces intestinal lactase activity. Prolonged or repeated use of antibiotics may cause bacterial or fungal overgrowth of nonsusceptible organisms, leading to secondary infection.
GENITOURINARY IRRIGANT:
Prophylactic bladder care with genitourinary irrigant should not be given if there is a possibility of systemic absorption.
Genitourinary irrigant should not be used for irrigation other than the urinary bladder. Use may result in overgrowth of nonsusceptible organisms, including fungi.
OINTMENT, OPHTHALMIC OINTMENT, and *OPHTHALMIC SOLUTION:*
Use may result in overgrowth of nonsusceptible organisms, including fungi.

SPECIAL GROUPS

Children: Use with caution in premature infants and neonates; prolonged half-life.
Elderly: May have age-related renal impairment; reduced dosage or lengthened intervals may be necessary.
Renal impairment: Increased risk of renal toxicity and ototoxicity; monitor drug levels and renal function closely.
Hepatic impairment: There may be increased risk of nephrotoxicity.

INDICATIONS

TABLETS: Preoperative suppression of intestinal bacteria of the bowel, usually concurrently administered with erythromycin.
Reduction of ammonia-forming bacteria in intestinal tract during hepatic coma (reduction in blood ammonia has resulted in neurologic improvement).
GENITOURINARY IRRIGANT: Short-term (up to 10 days) treatment for prevention of bacteriuria and gram-negative rod septicemia in patients with indwelling catheters.
OINTMENT: To aid in prevention of infection in minor cuts, scrapes, and burns.
OPHTHALMIC OINTMENT: Short-term treatment of superficial external ocular infections.
OPHTHALMIC SOLUTION: Short-term treatment of superficial external ocular infections.

CONTRAINDICATIONS

TABLETS: Intestinal obstruction; hypersensitivity to aminoglycosides, polymyxins, or other ingredients contained in the solution.
OINTMENT: Do not use in eyes or external ear canal if ear drum is perforated. Do not use if patient has known hypersensitivity to any components.
OPHTHALMIC OINTMENT and *OPHTHALMIC SOLUTION:* Hypersensitivity

INTERACTIONS

Anticoagulants (oral administration may suppress formation of vitamin K in the intestine)
See Interactions in introduction

ADVERSE EFFECTS

TABLETS: Nausea, vomiting, diarrhea, malabsorption syndrome, colitis (*Clostridium difficile*–associated), nephrotoxicity, ototoxicity
GENITOURINARY IRRIGANT: Irritation of urinary bladder mucosa
OINTMENT: Skin sensitization, ototoxicity, nephrotoxicity
OPHTHALMIC OINTMENT and *OPHTHALMIC SOLUTION:* Cutaneous and conjunctival sensitization, hypersensitivity reactions (skin rash)

PHARMACOKINETICS AND PHARMACODYNAMICS

Bioavailability: generally not absorbed in clinically significant quantities
Metabolism: unabsorbed drug eliminated unchanged in feces
Excretion: renal
Effect of food: oral aminoglycosides are poorly absorbed; the presence of food may further inhibit absorption
Protein binding: no information
Renal impairment: may increase risk for toxicity
Hepatic impairment: no information

The information here is provided as guidance only. Prescribers should always consult the manufacturer's current prescribing information.

NEOMYCIN (CONTINUED)

DOSAGE

TABLETS:

Adults: Hepatic coma: As an adjunct, 4 to 12 g/d in divided doses. Usual duration of treatment, 5 to 6 days (return protein to the diet gradually).

Chronic hepatic impairment: Up to 4 g/d indefinitely.

Elderly: Same as adults.

Child: Hepatic coma: As an adjunct, 50 to 100 mg/kg/d in divided doses. Usual duration of treatment, 5 to 6 days (return protein to the diet gradually).

GENITOURINARY IRRIGATION:

(Designed for use with catheter systems permitting continuous irrigation of the urinary bladder).

Usual dose is one 1-mL ampule/d for up to 10 days.

OINTMENT:

Apply small amount to cleansed affected area one to three times daily.

OPHTHALMIC OINTMENT:

Apply every 3 to 4 hours for 7 to 10 days, according to the severity of infection.

OPHTHALMIC SOLUTION:

One to two drops in affected eye two to four times daily (more frequently if necessary) for 7 to 10 days. In acute infections, initiate therapy with one to two drops every 15 to 30 minutes, reducing frequency as infection becomes controlled.

PATIENT INFORMATION

TABLETS: Finish all medication unless otherwise directed. Increase intake of fluids. May cause nausea, vomiting, and diarrhea. Contact physician if ringing of ears, hearing impairment, dizziness, difficult urination, or rash occurs.

OPHTHALMIC SOLUTION: Discontinue use and contact physician if redness, irritation, swelling, or pain persists or increases. Avoid contaminating applicator tip with material from the eye, fingers, or elsewhere. Drops must remain sterile.

OVERDOSAGE

See Overdosage in introduction

AVAILABILITY

Tablets—500 mg

Oral solution—125 mg in 5 mL

Genitourinary irrigant—1 mL ampules and 20-mL multidose vial

Ointment—0.5- and 1-oz tubes and 0.03-oz foil packets

Ophthalmic ointment—3.5-g tube with ophthalmic tip

Ophthalmic solution—10-mL plastic dispenser bottle

NETILMICIN (Netromycin®)

Netilmicin is a semisynthetic derivative of sisomicin, an aminoglycoside that is not used in the United States. Like amikacin, its chemical modification makes it refractory to inactivation by many bacterial enzymes that confer resistance to aminoglycosides. Therefore, netilmicin generally is used for the treatment of infections caused by aerobic gram-negative bacilli that are known or suspected to be resistant to gentamicin and tobramycin. Amikacin may be active against some bacterial strains that are resistant to netilmicin. Netilmicin generally is administered in slightly higher dosages than gentamicin or tobramycin to achieve slightly higher peak levels in serum.

ANTIMICROBIAL ACTIVITY

Gram-negative: Same spectrum as for amikacin.

RESISTANCE

See Mechanisms of Bacterial Resistance and Antimicrobial Activity in introduction.

SPECIAL PRECAUTIONS

See Toxicity and Pharmacokinetics and Dosing in introduction.

SPECIAL GROUPS

Children: Use with caution in premature infants and neonates; prolonged half-life.

Elderly: May have age-related renal impairment; reduced dosage or lengthened intervals may be necessary.

Renal impairment: Increased risk of renal toxicity and ototoxicity; monitor drug levels and renal function closely.

Hepatic impairment: There may be increased risk of nephrotoxicity.

DOSAGE

See Pharmacokinetics and Dosing in introduction.

INDICATIONS

Infections of the following types due to susceptible gram-negative bacteria:

Respiratory tract, urinary tract, bones and joints, central nervous system, skin, soft tissue, intra-abdominal, burn, postoperative, bacterial septicemia (including neonatal sepsis).

CONTRAINDICATIONS

Allergy or hypersensitivity to aminoglycosides (rare)

INTERACTIONS

See Interactions in introduction

ADVERSE EFFECTS

See Toxicity in introduction

PHARMACOKINETICS AND PHARMACODYNAMICS

See Pharmacokinetics and Dosing in introduction

OVERDOSAGE

See Overdosage in introduction

AVAILABILITY

Injection—100 mg/mL supplied in 1-mL vials

The information here is provided as guidance only. Prescribers should always consult the manufacturer's current prescribing information.

SPECTINOMYCIN (Trobicin®)

Spectinomycin is an aminocyclitol, but it is often considered with the aminoglycoside antibiotics. It is indicated only for the treatment of gonococcal infections, but it has poor efficacy for pharyngeal infection, has no activity for *Chlamydia trachomatis,* and does not treat incubating syphilis.

ANTIMICROBIAL ACTIVITY
Neisseria gonorrhoeae.

RESISTANCE
Occasional resistance has been reported in gonococcal strains.

SPECIAL PRECAUTIONS
Antibiotics used to treat gonorrhea may suppress symptoms of incubating syphilis. Patients with gonorrhea should be serologically tested for syphilis at diagnosis and retested after 3 months because spectinomycin is ineffective in the treatment of syphilis.
Spectinomycin is not effective in the treatment of pharyngeal infections due to *N. gonorrhoeae.*
Monitor for clinical effectiveness and resistance by *N. gonorrhoeae.*
A few cases of anaphylaxis or anaphylactoid reactions have been reported; epinephrine should be readily available.

SPECIAL GROUPS
Children: Safety not established.
Elderly: No information.
Renal impairment: Prolongs half-life.
Hepatic impairment: No information.
Pregnancy: Safety not established.
Breast-feeding: Safety not established.

DOSAGE
Adults: 5 mL for a dose of 2 g, intramuscularly (deep into upper quadrant of gluteal muscle). In cases in which there is known antibiotic resistance, doses of 4 g are preferred for initial treatment; the 10 mL can be divided between two gluteal injection sites.
Gonococcal infections in pregnancy: For patients who are allergic to beta-lactam antibiotics, 2 g intramuscularly followed by erythromycin.
Disseminated gonococcal infections: For patients allergic to beta-lactam antibiotics, 2 g intramuscularly every 12 hours.
Centers for Disease Control and Prevention recommended treatment for gonorrhea*: For patients with uncomplicated urethral, endocervical, or rectal gonococcal infections; an alternative regimen in cases of cephalosporin and quinolone intolerance: 2 g intramuscularly as a single dose followed by doxycycline for possible *Chlamydia trachomatis* infection.
Elderly: No information.
Children: Children weighing 45 kg or above, same as adults. For uncomplicated vulvovaginitis, cervicitis, urethritis, pharyngitis, or proctitis; in cases of ceftriaxone intolerance: 40 mg/kg in a single intramuscular dose.
Impaired renal function: No specific information listed.
*Centers for Disease Control and Prevention: 1993 Sexually transmitted diseases treatment guidelines. MMWR 1993; 42(RR-14):1–102.

INDICATIONS
Treatment of acute gonorrheal urethritis and proctitis in men and acute gonorrheal cervicitis and proctitis in women, when infection is due to susceptible strains of *N. gonorrhoeae.* May also be used for the treatment of disseminated gonococcal infection.

CONTRAINDICATIONS
Hypersensitivity to spectinomycin

INTERACTIONS
See Interactions in introduction

ADVERSE EFFECTS
See Adverse Effects in introduction

PHARMACOKINETICS AND PHARMACODYNAMICS
Peak serum levels: 100 µg/mL at 1 h following a 2-g intramuscular injection
Plasma half-life: normal renal function, 2 h; end-stage renal disease, 100 to 110 h
Bioavailability: no information
Metabolism: not known
Excretion: majority of drug excreted in urine in biologically active form
Effect of food: no information
Protein binding: not significantly bound to plasma protein
Renal impairment: prolongs half-life
Hepatic impairment: no information

OVERDOSAGE
See Overdosage in introduction

AVAILABILITY
Powder—2-g vial supplied with one ampule of Bacteriostatic Water for Injection with Banzyl Alcohol 0.945% w/v added as preservative. For intramuscular use only.

The information here is provided as guidance only. Prescribers should always consult the manufacturer's current prescribing information.

STREPTOMYCIN

Streptomycin has been replaced by newer aminoglycosides for the treatment of gram-negative bacillary infections. It still retains utility in the treatment of tuberculosis, enterococcal infections, and other specific infections, such as tularemia, plague, and brucellosis.

ANTIMICROBIAL ACTIVITY

Yersinia (Pasteurella) pestis, Francisella tularensis, Brucella, Mycobacterium tuberculosis, Enterococcus, and *Streptococci* (in synergistic activity with a penicillin or with vancomycin).

RESISTANCE

Strains of *M. tuberculosis* may be resistant. Strains of enterococci may exhibit high-level resistance, which precludes use in synergistic combination with ampicillin or vancomycin; gentamicin may be an alternative for such strains.

SPECIAL PRECAUTIONS

Vestibulotoxic potential of streptomycin exceeds that of its capacity for cochlear toxicity. Monitor carefully for symptoms and signs.
(*See* Toxicity in introduction.)

SPECIAL GROUPS

Children: Use with caution in premature infants and neonates; prolonged half-life.
Elderly: May have age-related renal impairment; reduced dosage or lengthened intervals may be necessary.
Renal impairment: Increased risk of renal toxicity and ototoxicity; monitor drug levels and renal function closely.
Hepatic impairment: There may be increased risk of nephrotoxicity.

DOSAGE

Adults: Tuberculosis: 15 mg/kg/d (generally 1 g) intramuscularly or intravenously.
Tularemia: 1 to 2 g/d in divided doses for 7 to 14 days, until patient afebrile for 5 to 7 days.
Plague: 2 g/d intramuscularly, in two divided doses (every 12 hours). Minimum of 10 days of treatment.
Bacterial endocarditis *(Streptococcal)*: 500 mg intramuscularly or intravenously twice daily with concomitant penicillin or vancomycin for the first 2 weeks of treatment. *(Enterococcal)*, 500 mg intramuscularly or intravenously twice daily with concomitant penicillin or vancomycin for 6 weeks (ototoxicity may require termination of streptomycin before completion of 6-week course).
Concomitant use of streptomycin with other agents: 1 to 2 g intramuscularly or intravenously in divided doses (every 12 hours). Do not exceed 2 g/d.
Elderly: Same as adults. May have age-related renal impairment and increased risk for toxicity.
Child: Tuberculosis: 20 to 40 mg/kg/d; maximum 1 g intramuscularly or intravenously.
Tularemia, plague, and bacterial endocarditis: Same as adults.
Concomitant use of streptomycin with other agents: 20 to 40 mg/kg/d intramuscularly or intravenously, or 8 to 20 mg/kg/d intramuscularly or intravenously , in divided doses (every 12 hours).
Impaired renal function: Extreme caution must be used when administering streptomycin to patients with renal impairment. In uremic patients, a single dose may produce blood levels for several days, the cumulative effect of which can produce ototoxic sequelae (*See* Table 1-1).

INDICATIONS

Nontuberculous infections in cases where susceptible, causative bacteria are not amenable to agents less potentially toxic, including *P. pestis, F. tularensis* (tularemia), *Brucella, Streptococcus viridans,* and *Enterococcus faecalis* (in endocarditis concomitantly with a penicillin or vancomycin).
The Advisory Council for the elimination of tuberculosis, the American Thoracic Society, and the Centers for Disease Control and Prevention recommend that either streptomycin or ethambutol be added as a fourth drug in a regimen containing isoniazid, rifampin, and pyrazinamide for initial treatment of tuberculosis unless the likelihood of isoniazid or rifampin resistance is very low.

CONTRAINDICATIONS

Hypersensitivity to streptomycin or other aminoglycosides (rare)

INTERACTIONS

See Interactions in introduction

ADVERSE EFFECTS

See Toxicity in introduction

PHARMACOKINETICS AND PHARMACODYNAMICS

Peak serum levels: 25 to 50 µg/mL within 1 h after injection of 1 g
Plasma half-life: normal renal function, 2.5 h; end-stage renal disease, 100 h
Metabolism: none
Excretion: renal, by glomerular filtration; with normal renal function, 29% to 89% in 24 h
Protein binding: negligible
Renal impairment: reduction in glomerular function results in decreased excretion and increased serum and tissue levels
Hepatic impairment: no information

OVERDOSAGE

See Overdosage in introduction

AVAILABILITY

Intramuscular injection—1 g in 2.5-mL ampules (requires refrigeration)

The information here is provided as guidance only. Prescribers should always consult the manufacturer's current prescribing information.

TOBRAMYCIN (Nebcin®, TobraDex®)

Tobramycin is generally more active than gentamicin against strains of *Pseudomonas aeruginosa*, even those that are susceptible to gentamicin. Thus, it is preferred for the treatment of infections caused by this organism. Although susceptibilities to aminoglycosides may vary among institutions, tobramycin may be active against more strains of most non–*Pseudomonas* species of aerobic gram-negative bacilli than gentamicin, although strains of *Serratia marcescens* are generally more susceptible to gentamicin and amikacin than to tobramycin.

ANTIMICROBIAL ACTIVITY

Gram-negative: Same spectrum as for amikacin.

RESISTANCE

See Mechanisms of Bacterial Resistance and Antimicrobial Activity in introduction.

SPECIAL PRECAUTIONS

See Toxicity and Pharmacokinetics and Dosing in introduction.

SPECIAL GROUPS

Children: Use with caution in premature infants and neonates; prolonged half-life.
Elderly: May have age-related renal impairment; reduced dosage or lengthened intervals may be necessary.
Renal impairment: Increased risk of renal toxicity and ototoxicity; monitor drug levels and renal function closely.
Hepatic impairment: There may be increased risk of nephrotoxicity.

DOSAGE

See Pharmacokinetics and Dosing in introduction.

INDICATIONS

Infections of the following types due to susceptible gram-negative bacteria:
Respiratory tract, urinary tract, bones and joints, central nervous system, skin, soft tissue, intra-abdominal, burn, postoperative, bacterial septicemia (including neonatal sepsis).

CONTRAINDICATIONS

Allergy or hypersensitivity to aminoglycosides (rare)

INTERACTIONS

See Interactions in introduction

ADVERSE EFFECTS

See Toxicity in introduction

PHARMACOKINETICS AND PHARMACODYNAMICS

See Pharmacokinetics and Dosing in introduction

OVERDOSAGE

See Overdosage in introduction

AVAILABILITY

Injection—40 mg/mL in 1.5- and 2-mL syringes and 2- and 30-mL vials

The information here is provided as guidance only. Prescribers should always consult the manufacturer's current prescribing information.

CLASS DESCRIPTION

The discovery of cephalosporins was not due to serendipity but rather the careful observations of Dr. G. Brotzu in 1945. He noted that certain waters along the Coast of Sardinia, which were fed from a sewerage outlet, had a decrease in microbial organisms. He thought this was possibly secondary to a compound secreted into these waters by antibiotic-producing microorganisms [1]. His search led him to discover an organism, *ie, Cephalosporium acremonium*; filtrates prepared from this compound were noted to have antimicrobial activity. Further analyses of this organism and its byproducts were carried out at Oxford University. The original compound isolated was called *cephalosporin C*; it had activity against *Staphylococci* that produced an enzyme that destroyed penicillin as well as activity against gram-negative bacilli. Furthermore, it was relatively nontoxic as determined by animal experiments.

STRUCTURE

Cephalosporins are similar in structure to the penicillins in that they contain a four-membered beta-lactam ring but differ from penicillin in that this ring is fused to a six-membered dihydrothiazine ring rather than to the thiazolidine ring (the five-membered structure) of penicillin. The parent structure for cephalosporins is 7-amino cephalosporanic acid. Substitutions of various groups at carbon 3 and at carbon 7 can be performed [2,3]. Substitutions at the carbon 3 site produce compounds with varying degrees of pharmacokinetic properties, including changes in absorption, metabolism, protein binding, and renal excretion. Substitutions at position 7 affect antimicrobial activity, such as enhancing activity against gram-negative bacilli. The introduction of a methoxy group at this position produces compounds with increased stability against beta-lactamases [4]. Most substitutions are beneficial; however, adverse effects in regard to hemostasis have been noted with compounds that contain the methylthiotetrazole moiety in the 3 position, found on some second- and third-generation cephalosporins [5].

MODE OF ACTION

The cephalosporin antibiotics, similar to other beta-lactam antibiotics, interfere with the synthesis of the cell wall by acting on penicillin-sensitive enzymes such as transpeptidases, endopeptidases, and carboxypeptidases found on bacterial cell membranes. Specifically they interfere with the synthesis of the peptidoglycan component of the cell wall. The beta-lactam ring of the cephalosporin is structurally similar to the D-alanine–alanine bond of the pentapeptides, and insertion interrupts the sequence of normal cell wall synthesis. The sites of action of the compounds are enzymes known as *penicillin-binding proteins (PBPs)* that are found on the inner portion of the bacterial cell membrane. These proteins have different physiologic roles, *ie*, septal formation and cell configuration [6]. Inactivation of certain of the PBPs leads to death of the cell. Inactivation of the other PBPs may lead to changes such as cellular swelling among others. Certain bacteria may contain an autolysin that is essential for lysis of bacterial cell walls. Beta-lactams will exert only a bacteriostatic effect in cells that lack this lysin.

MECHANISMS OF RESISTANCE

The most common mechanism of resistance to beta-lactam antibiotics is inactivation by beta-lactamases [7–9]. Changes in porin size [10] and PBPs are other known mechanisms of resistance [11].

Beta-lactamases are enzymes that hydrolyze beta-lactam antibiotics at the nitrogen and carbon bond of the beta-lactam ring, leading to inactive metabolites. Gram-positive bacteria elaborate these enzymes into the milieu. In gram-negative bacteria, these enzymes are found in the periplasmic space. Susceptibility to an antibiotic is related to enzyme binding and rates of hydrolysis. These resistance factors are found either on chromosomes or plasmids; they may be transferred by transposons from one to the other.

Third-generation cephalosporins, as well as cefoxitin and cefotetan, are generally resistant to hydrolysis. However, certain gram-negative bacteria, *eg*, Enterobacter spp and *Pseudomonas aeruginosa*, produce a chromosomal cephalosporinase and, in *Klebsiella pneumoniae*, a plasmid-associated beta-lactamase that may hydrolyze third-generation cephalosporins. It is believed that some antibiotics may induce or derepress chromosomal-mediated beta-lactamase enzymes. This increase in enzyme production may thus act as a barrier to the antibiotic reaching its site of action, in a sense blocking and preventing it from reaching the PBP. However, some antibiotics may be effective against microorganisms that produce these beta-lactamases, although the same compound is susceptible to hydrolysis by cell-free extract: this may be explained by the fact that the antibiotic may "flood the periplasmic space and avoid the beta-lactamase, escaping hydrolysis."

Gram-positive bacteria, *eg, Staphylococcus aureus*, make a potent beta-lactamase; certain cephalosporins are "relatively" more susceptible (*eg*, cefazolin versus cephalothin). Gram-negative organisms have a formidable cell wall consisting of proteins, lipids, and sugars, and antibiotics must enter through channels known as *porins* into the periplasmic space. The channels allow antibiotic passage based on the size, charge, and so forth. Thus, mutation in the porin channel may lead to bacterial resistance because the drug cannot reach its binding site.

The third known mechanism of antibacterial resistance is a change in the PBPs or the decreased affinity of an antibiotic to bind to these proteins. Methicillin-resistant *S. aureus* strains produce a PBP known as PBP2, which has a decreased affinity for cephalosporins and penicillinase-resistant penicillins, rendering them ineffective.

PHARMACOKINETICS

The cephalosporins, both oral and parenteral, are excreted mainly via the kidney [12]. Two agents, ceftriaxone and cefoperazone, have hepatic excretion [13]. Although most of these compounds are not metabolized, cefotaxime and cephalothin are broken down to acetyl derivatives.

All agents diffuse well into pleural, pericardial, peritoneal, and pelvic spaces. Most agents are concentrated in the biliary tract, where they achieve extremely high levels. However, only select cephalosporins penetrate into the cerebrospinal fluid, and these have found a role in treatment of bacterial meningitis, including gram-negative meningitis. These agents include cefotaxime, ceftriaxone, ceftazidime, ceftizoxime, and cefuroxime.

Cephalosporins penetrate well into the aqueous humor but poorly into the vitreous. Penetration by cephalosporins into the prostatic secretions is poor, whereas urinary tract concentrations are extremely high. Studies of tissue spaces in general reveal clinically high levels, and topical administration of these compounds is usually unwarranted.

Dosage adjustment may be necessary for cephalosporins that are excreted in the urinary tract in the presence of renal insufficiency.

The information here is provided as guidance only. Prescribers should always consult the manufacturer's current prescribing information.

Two agents, ceftriaxone and cefoperazone, may require dosage adjustment only in patients with severe liver or renal dysfunction.

The oral cephalosporins in general are well absorbed from the gastrointestinal tract. In some cases food will enhance this absorption. Maximum serum levels are usually obtained within 1 hour following ingestion and then, dependent on the half-time of the compound, gradually decrease. Concomitant administration of probenecid increases the half-life by blocking excretion via the kidney tubule.

ANTIMICROBIAL ACTIVITY

Cephalosporins are active against streptococci and staphylococci but are intrinsically resistant to *enterococcus* spp, including *faecalis* and *faecium*, *Listeria monocytogenes*, and most species of *Legionella*. Although some have *in vitro* activity against moderately penicillin-resistant *Streptococcus pneumoniae*, methicillin-resistant *S. aureus*, and methicillin-resistant *Staphylococcus epidermidis*, other agents should probably be selected.

In terms of antistaphylococcal activity, first-generation agents are more potent than third-generation, and conversely for gram-negative bacteria, including members of the Enterobacteriaceae, third-generation agents are more active. Some cephalosporins, including ceftazidime, cefoperazone, and cefepime (awaiting Food and Drug Administration approval), have activity against *P. aeruginosa;* others have less activity or are inactive. In regard to anaerobic coverage, the cefamycins, *eg,* cefoxitin and cefotetan, (which are really not technically cephalosporins) have enhanced activity against the clinically significant anaerobes, including *Bacteroides fragilis.* Most first- and second-generation and some third-generation cephalosporins are active against oral anaerobic organisms, including anaerobic streptococci. Certain second-generation agents (*eg,* cefuroxime) and third-generation agents are active against *Neisseria* spp and *Haemophilus influenzae* spp, and *Moraxella* spp, including those that produce beta-lactamase.

INDICATIONS

The parenteral cephalosporins have been used to treat a variety of serious infections. In many cases they are employed empirically before the results of cultures and sensitivity have been determined. In general, the first-generation agents are used to treat gram-positive infections, including skin infections secondary to *Streptococci* and *Staphylococci*, as well as respiratory infections due to pneumococci. The oral agents in this class have been used for the treatment of upper respiratory tract infections, including pharyngitis, otitis media, sinusitis, and so forth. These agents also have been used for the treatment of bronchitis and for some patients with pneumonia treated in the outpatient setting. The oral first-generation agents also have been used to treat urinary tract infections [14].

First-generation agents, specifically cefazolin, have become the drugs of choice for surgical prophylaxis; in cases where anaerobic coverage is necessary, cefotetan or cefoxitin have been used. They are generally administered 1 hour prior to a surgical procedure, thus enabling them to attain high tissue levels at the time of surgery.

Second-generation agents, notably cefuroxime, play a major role in the treatment of community-acquired pneumonia secondary to *Pneumococcus* and *Haemophilus* spp, including ampicillin-resistant strains. They also have activity against *Neisseria meningitidis* as well as *Moraxella catarrhalis*, an agent that recently has been implicated as a cause of respiratory tract infections, including bronchitis, otitis media, and in some cases, pneumonia. Cefuroxime has been used to treat meningitis, but third-generation agents appear to have a better therapeutic outcome.

Cefamycins, including cefoxitin and cefotetan, with their expanded activity against anaerobes, have a role in the treatment of mixed aerobic and anaerobic infections such as pelvic, intra-abdominal, and soft-tissue infections. Cefotetan usually has been selected as the agent of choice for prophylaxis because of its prolonged half-life for obstetrical and intra-abdominal infections. These agents have less activity against *Streptococcal* spp.

Third-generation cephalosporins have a broad range of activity, including gram-positive bacteria, but are usually used to treat infections due to gram-negative bacteria; certain agents have activity against *P. aeruginosa* [15]. They penetrate well into the spinal fluid (with the exception of cefoperazone) and have been used to treat meningitis. The main role of third-generation cephalosporins is treatment of hospital-acquired infections, including nosocomial pneumonia, bacteremia, line-related infections, and severe urinary tract infections. Many are active against penicillinase-producing strains of *Neisseria gonorrhoeae* [16]. Recently, organisms such as *K. pneumoniae* and *Enterobacter cloacae* were found to produce a cephalosporinase that hydrolyses both ceftazidime and other third-generation cephalosporins [17,18].

Certain cephalosporins have activity against *Borrelia burgdorferi*, the agent of Lyme disease; both ceftriaxone [19] and the oral agents cefixime and cefuroxime axetil have been used in the treatment of this condition. For the treatment of specific infections such as bacteremia and pneumonia caused by *Pseudomonas*, antipseudomonas cephalosporins used in combination with aminoglycosides are the recommended regimen. Cephalosporins have been used alone (ceftazidime and cefoperazone) in the empiric treatment of the neutropenic patient, in some cases in combination with aminoglycosides or as a double beta-lactam combination. The long half-life of ceftriaxone [20] has made it the drug of choice for outpatient care, including follow-up treatment of nosocomial infection, Lyme disease, osteomyelitis, and endocarditis.

ADVERSE REACTIONS

Like other beta-lactams, the cephalosporins are very safe compounds. With regard to parenteral agents, the earlier first-generation cephalosporin cephalothin produces more thrombophlebitis than cefazolin.

The most common side effects are allergic reactions, which occur in 2% to 20% of patients. In general these reactions are more common in patients who are either allergic to penicillin or who have some underlying allergic diathesis. Most commonly, a rash (macular papular in nature) occurs after 3 to 5 days of therapy. Rarely, associated fever, lymphadenopathy, eosinophilia and eosinophiluria, or serum sickness–like reactions occur.

The immediate hypersensitivity reaction (Type 1) with bronchospasm and hives is the most feared occurrence. For this reason these drugs are usually contraindicated in patients who have already had anaphylactic or immediate reactions to penicillins. In these patients, other agents without the beta-lactam ring structure should be employed. In patients with minor penicillin reactions, cephalosporins have been given, especially when other antimicrobial agents are not available.

Other reactions that have been described with beta-lactam antibiotics [21], including the cephalosporins, are Coombs' positivity and,

The information here is provided as guidance only. Prescribers should always consult the manufacturer's current prescribing information.

on rare occasions, hemolytic anemia. All cephalosporins have the ability to suppress bone marrow function and cause leukopenia, neutropenia, and thrombocytopenia; this is however uncommon. Liver function abnormalities (enzyme elevations) have been reported in 1% to 5% of patients treated with parenteral cephalosporins. Similar to penicillins, interstitial nephritis has been reported.

An older cephalosporin, cephaloridine, given at higher doses (4 g) was associated with nephrotoxicity and acute tubular necrosis. The newer agents have not been associated with these reactions. Earlier studies revealed that cephalosporins, specifically cephalothin, in combination with aminoglycosides were associated with renal dysfunction. Cephalosporins with the methothiotetrazole ring in the 3 position (cefamandole, cefotetan, moxalactam, and cefoperazone) have been associated with disulfiram-like reactions with alcohol ingestion.

Hypoprothrombinemia and in some cases bleeding may occur with these drugs [5]. It is believed that this side chain (*see* preceding paragraph) inhibits conversion of clotting factors 2, 7, 9, and 10 and production of prothrombin. Vitamin K prophylaxis is recommended when they are used, especially in older patients and in those with evidence of renal insufficiency. Certain agents such as ceftriaxone have been reported to cause biliary sludge associated with signs and symptoms of acute cholecystitis, usually in the pediatric population.

The oral agents, like other compounds, have been associated with diarrhea and in some cases with antibiotic-associated diarrhea and colitis secondary to *Clostridium difficile*. Parenteral agents that are excreted in the biliary tree, such as cefoperazone and ceftriaxone, may be associated with a greater incidence of diarrhea. In general there are very few drug–drug interactions with cephalosporins in comparison with other antimicrobial agents.

REFERENCES

1. Abraham EP: Cephalosporins 1945–1986. In *The Cephalosporin Antibiotics*. Edited by Williams JD. Auckland: Adis Press; 1987:1–14.

2. Hou JP, Poole JW: Beta-lactam antibiotics: Their physicochemical properties and biological activities in relation to structure. *J Pharm Sci* 1971, 60:503.

3. O'Callaghan CH, Kirby SM: Some cephalosporins in clinical use and their structure–activity relationship. *Postgrad Med J* 1974, 46:9.

4. Onishi HR, Daoust DR, Zimmerman SB: Cefoxitin, a semisynthetic cephamycin antibiotic: Resistance to beta-lactamase inactivation. *Antimicrob Agents Chemother* 1974, 5:38.

5. Lipsky JJ: *N*-methyl-thiotetrazole inhibition of the gamma carboxylation of glutamic acid: Possible mechanism for antibiotic-associated hypoprothrombinemia. *Lancet* 1983, ii:192–193.

6. Waxman DJ, Strominger JL: Penicillin-binding proteins and the mechanism of action of beta-lactam antibiotics. *Ann Rev Biochem* 1983, 52:825–869.

7. Neu HC: Contributions of beta-lactamases to bacterial resistance and mechanisms to inhibit beta-lactamases. *Am J Med* 1985, 79(Suppl B):2.

8. Richmond MH, Sykes RB: The beta-lactamases of gram-negative bacteria and their possible physiological role. *Adv Microb Physiol* 1973, 9:31–88.

9. Sykes RM, Matthew M: The beta-lactamases of gram-negative bacteria and their role in resistance to beta-lactam antibiotics. *J Antimicrob Chemother* 1976, 2:115–157.

10. Nikaido H, Rosenberg EY, Foulds J: Porin channels in *Escherichia coli*: Studies with beta-lactams in intact cells. *J Bacteriol* 1983, 153:232–240.

11. Georgopapadakou NH: Penicillin-binding proteins and bacterial resistance to beta-lactams. *Antimicrob Agents Chemother* 1993, 37:2045–2053.

12. Bergan T: Pharmacokinetic properties of the cephalosporins. In *The Cephalosporin Antibiotics*. Edited by Williams JD. Auckland: Adis Press; 1987:89–90.

13. Kemmerich B, Lode H, Borner K, *et al.*: Biliary excretion and pharmacokinetics of cefoperazone in humans. *J Antimicrob Chemother* 1983, 12:27–37.

14. Meyers BR: The cephalosporins. *N Y State J Med* 1977, 77:1128–1132.

15. Young LS: Empirical antimicrobial therapy in the neutropenic host. *N Engl J Med* 1986, 315:580.

16. Judson FN, Ehret JM, Handsfield HH: Comparative study of ceftriaxone and spectinomycin for treatment of pharyngeal and anorectal gonorrhea. *JAMA* 1985, 253:1417.

17. Medeiros AA: Nosocomial outbreaks of multiresistant bacteria: Extended-spectrum beta-lactamases have arrived in North America. *Ann Intern Med* 1993, 119:428–430.

18. Jacoby GA, Medeiros AA: More extended-spectrum beta-lactamases. *Antimicrob Agents Chemother* 1991, 35:1697–1704.

19. Dattwyler RJ, Halperin JJ, Volkman DJ, *et al.*: Treatment of late Lyme borreliosis—randomized comparison of ceftriaxone and penicillin. *Lancet* 1988, i:11.

20. Baumgartner JD, Glauser MP: Single daily dose treatment of severe refractory infections with ceftriaxone: Cost savings and possible outpatient treatment. *Arch Intern Med* 1983, 143:1868.

21. Meyers BR: Comparative toxicities of third-generation cephalosporins. *Am J Med* 1985, 79(Suppl 2A):96–103.

The information here is provided as guidance only. Prescribers should always consult the manufacturer's current prescribing information.

CEFACLOR (Ceclor®)

Cefaclor is an oral second-generation cephalosporin. It is more active than cephalexin against gram-positive and gram-negative bacteria such as *Haemophilus influenzae*, *Klebsiella pneumoniae*, *Escherichia coli*, and meningococci.

Although the drug is rapidly absorbed from the gastrointestinal tract, food intake reduces absorption. The kidneys are the main route of elimination. The half-life of cefaclor is 40 to 60 minutes; the drug is administered every 8 hours. The half-life may increase up to 3 hours in anephric patients.

Cefaclor has been used in the treatment of upper respiratory tract infections, including pharyngitis, otitis media, and sinusitis, as well as skin infections.

Adverse effects are similar to those of the other cephalosporins and occur infrequently. A serum sickness–like reaction has been reported (mainly in children), with an incidence ranging from 0.5% to 0.003% according to various reports.

ANTIMICROBIAL ACTIVITY

Gram-positive: Staphylococci (coagulase-positive, coagulase-negative, and penicillinase-producing; some strains resistant), beta-hemolytic streptococci, *Streptococcus pneumoniae*.

Gram-negative: *E. coli*, *H. influenzae* (including some beta-lactamase–producing strains), *Klebsiella* spp, *Moraxella (Branhamella) catarrhalis*, *Proteus mirabilis*. Demonstrated *in vitro* activity against *Neisseria gonorrhoeae*, *Peptococcus*, and *Peptostreptococcus* spp.

RESISTANCE

Generally not effective in the treatment of methicillin-resistant *Staphylococcus aureus* or methicillin-resistant coagulase-negative *Staphylococci*. Generally ineffective in the treatment of highly penicillin-resistant *S. pneumoniae*.

SPECIAL PRECAUTIONS

Use caution in patients with markedly impaired renal function; although half-life of drug is only slightly increased, clinical experience is limited. Careful observation and laboratory studies should be made.

Use caution when administering cephalosporins to patients with sensitivity to penicillin; possible cross-allergenicity and risk of allergic or anaphylactic reaction. If an allergic reaction occurs, discontinue drug. Serious reactions may require epinephrine or other emergency measures (including oxygen, intravenous fluids, intravenous antihistamines, corticosteroids, pressor amines, and airway management).

Use caution when administering broad-spectrum antibiotics to patients with existing or previous gastrointestinal disease. Treatment with broad-spectrum antibiotics alters normal flora of the colon and may permit overgrowth of clostridia, causing antibiotic-associated pseudomembranous colitis. Mild cases usually respond to discontinuation of therapy alone; management of moderate to severe cases should include bacteriologic studies and fluid, electrolyte, and protein supplementation. Positive direct Coomb's tests have been reported with cephalosporin therapy. False-positive reaction for glucose in urine may occur with copper-reduction tests (Benedicts' or Fehling's solution) but not with enzyme-based tests for glycosuria. False-negative results may occur with the ferricyanide test. Glucose oxidase or hexokinase methods are recommended to determine blood plasma glucose levels. Bacterial or fungal overgrowth of nonsusceptible organisms, leading to secondary infection, may occur with prolonged or repeated therapy.

INDICATIONS

Used in the treatment of the following infections due to susceptible strains of designated microorganisms:

Otitis media:
S. pneumoniae, *H. influenzae*, staphylococci, *S. pyogenes* (Group A beta-hemolytic streptococci)

Lower respiratory tract (including pneumonia):
S. pneumoniae, *H. influenzae*, and *Streptococcus pyogenes* (Group A beta-hemolytic streptococci)

Upper respiratory tract (including pharyngitis and tonsillitis):
S. pyogenes (Group A beta-hemolytic streptococci)
(Note: Penicillin is the drug of choice in treatment and prevention of streptococcal infections, including prophylaxis of rheumatic fever.)

Urinary tract (including pyelonephritis and cystitis):
E. coli, *P. mirabilis*, *Klebsiella* spp, coagulase-negative staphylococci

Skin–skin structure infections:
S. aureus and *S. pyogenes* (Group A beta-hemolytic streptococci)

CONTRAINDICATIONS

Allergy to the cephalosporin group of antibiotics

INTERACTIONS

Probenecid may inhibit the renal excretion of cefaclor, resulting in prolonged serum concentrations

ADVERSE EFFECTS

Some of the more common adverse effects include:
Hypersensitivity reactions: *eg*, pruritus, urticaria serum sickness–like reaction
Gastrointestinal distress: nausea, vomiting, diarrhea
Transient hepatitis and cholestatic jaundice have been reported rarely

Listed below are adverse effects reported with the cephalosporin class of antibiotics:
Gastrointestinal distress: nausea, diarrhea, vomiting, anorexia, dysgeusia, glossitis, abdominal pain and cramps, flatulence, heartburn, gallbladder sludge, cholecystitis, dyspepsia, and colitis or pseudomembranous colitis (may appear during or after treatment)
Hypersensitivity: Stevens-Johnson syndrome, erythema multiforme, toxic epidermal necrolysis, renal dysfunction, toxic nephropathy, hepatic dysfunction (cholestasis), aplastic anemia, hemolytic anemia, hemorrhage
Laboratory test changes: transient increase in aspartate aminotransferase (AST), alanine aminotransferase (ALT), alkaline phosphatase, blood urea nitrogen, bilirubin, and lactate dehydrogenase
Hematologic changes: eosinophilia, transient neutropenia, leukocytosis, lymphocytosis, leukopenia, thrombocythemia, thrombocytopenia, agranulocytosis, granulocytopenia, hemolytic anemia, bone marrow depression, pancytopenia, decreased platelet function, bleeding in association with hypoprothrombinemia, anemia, aplastic anemia hemorrhage, transient thrombocytosis, decreases in neutrophil counts, decreased hemoglobin and hematocrit, positive Coomb's test, prolonged prothrombin time
Increases or decreases in glucose, decreases in serum albumin and serum total protein

(Continued on next page)

The information here is provided as guidance only. Prescribers should always consult the manufacturer's current prescribing information.

CEFACLOR (CONTINUED)

SPECIAL GROUPS

Children: Safety and efficacy not established for infants under 1 month of age.
Elderly: May have age-related renal impairment.
Renal impairment: Prolongs half-life only slightly; clinical experience is limited.
Hepatic impairment: No information.
Pregnancy: Adequate human studies not documented. Pregnancy category B, the cephalosporins appear safe in pregnancy, but few controlled studies have been done.
Breast-feeding: Use with caution; small amounts excreted in breast milk.

DOSAGE

Adults: 250 mg every 8 hours; doses may be doubled for more severe infections (*eg*, pneumonia). For treatment of beta-hemolytic streptococcal infections, a 10-day therapy regimen is recommended.
Children: 20 mg/kg/d in divided doses every 8 hours. For more severe infections (*eg*, otitis media or infections caused by less susceptible organisms), 40 mg/kg/d, with a maximum dosage of 1 g/d, is recommended.
Elderly: Same as adults.
Impaired renal function: The half-life of cefaclor in anuria is 2.3 to 2.8 hours. The drug may be administered to patients with moderate to severe renal impairment with no adjustment in normal dosage; however, as clinical experience is limited, caution and careful clinical observation should be used. If creatinine clearance is less than 10 mL/min 50% of the usual dose may be given at the normal dosage interval.

ADVERSE EFFECTS *(CONTINUED)*

Intramuscular administration may result in pain, induration, inflammation, and tenderness
Intravenous or intramuscular administration has caused local swelling, inflammation, burning, cellulitis, paresthesia, phlebitis, and thrombophlebitis
Also, hypotension, headache, fatigue, lethargy, diaphoresis, flushing, generalized tonic–clonic seizures, hemiparesis (mild), fever, interstitial pneumonitis, candidal overgrowth, hyperactivity, nervousness, insomnia, confusion, hypertonia, dizziness, solomnence

PHARMACOKINETICS AND PHARMACODYNAMICS

Peak serum levels: 7, 13, and 23 µg/mL 30 to 60 min after 250-mg, 500-mg, and 1-g doses
Plasma half-life: normal renal function, 0.6 to 0.9 h; end-stage renal disease 2.3 to 2.8 h
Bioavailability: percentage not given; widely distributed
Excretion: renal; 60% to 85% of unchanged drug excreted in urine within 8 h
Effect of food: total absorption does not vary; however, peak concentration with food is 50% to 75% of that observed in fasting patients
Protein binding: 25%
Renal impairment: slightly prolongs half-life
Hepatic impairment: no information

OVERDOSAGE

ORAL:
Symptoms may include nausea, vomiting, epigastric distress, and diarrhea. Unless five times the normal dose has been ingested, gastrointestinal decontamination is not necessary. Always consider possibility of multiple drug overdoses, drug interactions, and unusual drug kinetics. Absorption may be inhibited by administration of activated charcoal. Otherwise, ensure patient's airway and support ventilation, monitor and maintain vital signs, blood gases, serum electrolytes, and so forth. Hemodialysis, peritoneal dialysis, forced diuresis, or charcoal hemoperfusion have not been established as beneficial.

PATIENT INFORMATION

Complete full course of therapy. Take medication with food or milk to prevent gastrointestinal upset. Contact physician if nausea, vomiting, or diarrhea occurs. Refrigerate suspension. Shake the suspension well before use and discard the unused portion after 14 days.

AVAILABILITY

Pulvules—250 mg, and 500 mg
Oral Suspension—125 mg/5 mL, 187 mg/5 mL, 250 mg/5 mL, and 375 mg/5 mL (**refrigeration required after mixing**)

The information here is provided as guidance only. Prescribers should always consult the manufacturer's current prescribing information.

CEFADROXIL (Duricef®)

Cefadroxil is an oral first-generation cephalosporin. It has good activity against gram-positive bacteria, including *Staphylococcus aureus*, *Streptococcus pyogenes*, and *Streptococcus pneumoniae*. Other gram-negative bacteria such as *Haemophilus influenzae*, *Escherichia coli*, *Proteus* spp, and *Klebsiella* may be inhibited by cefadroxil. The compound has a longer half-life (1.6 hours) than other oral cephalosporins in the same group and may be given once or twice daily.

The indications for cefadroxil include skin and soft-tissue infections, urinary tract infection, pharyngitis, and otitis media. Side effects are uncommon and similar to those of other cephalosporins.

ANTIMICROBIAL ACTIVITY

Gram-positive: Staphylococci (coagulase-positive, coagulase-negative, and penicillinase-producing strains), beta-hemolytic streptococci, and *Streptococcus pneumoniae*.
Gram-negative: *E. coli*, *Klebsiella* spp, and *Proteus mirabilis*.

RESISTANCE

Generally ineffective in the treatment of methicillin-resistant *S. aureus* and methicillin-resistant coagulase-negative staphylococci. Generally ineffective in the treatment of highly penicillin-resistant *S. pneumoniae*.

SPECIAL PRECAUTIONS

Use caution when administering cephalosporins to patients with sensitivity to penicillin; possible cross-allergenicity and risk of allergic or anaphylactic reaction. If an allergic reaction occurs, discontinue drug. Serious reactions may require epinephrine or other emergency measures (including oxygen, intravenous fluids, intravenous antihistamines, corticosteroids, pressor amines, and airway management).
Use caution when administering broad-spectrum antibiotics to patients with existing or previous gastrointestinal disease. Treatment with broad-spectrum antibiotics alters normal flora of the colon and may permit overgrowth of clostridia, causing antibiotic-associated pseudomembranous colitis. Mild cases usually respond to discontinuation of therapy alone; management of moderate to severe cases should include bacteriologic studies and fluid, electrolyte, and protein supplementation. Positive direct Coomb's tests have been reported with cephalosporin therapy.
Use caution in patients with impaired renal function. Reduce dosage or prolong dosage intervals. Careful observation and laboratory studies should be made.
Bacterial or fungal overgrowth of nonsusceptible organisms, leading to secondary infection, may occur with prolonged or repeated therapy.
False-positive reaction for glucose in urine may occur with copper-reduction tests (Benedicts' or Fehling's solution) but not with enzyme-based tests for glycosuria. False-negative results may occur with the ferricyanide test. Glucose oxidase or hexokinase methods are recommended to determine blood plasma glucose levels.

SPECIAL GROUPS

Children: Base dosage on body weight.
Elderly: May have age-related renal impairment.
Renal impairment: Use with caution in patients with markedly impaired function.
Hepatic impairment: No information.
Pregnancy: Pregnancy Category B. The cephalosporins appear to be safe for use in pregnancy, but few controlled studies have been done. Adequate human studies not documented.
Breast-feeding: Use with caution.

INDICATIONS

Used in the treatment of the following infections due to susceptible strains of designated microorganisms:
Urinary tract:
E. coli, *P. mirabilis*, and *Klebsiella* spp
Skin–skin structure infections:
Staphylococci or streptococci
Upper respiratory tract (pharyngitis or tonsillitis):
Group A beta-hemolytic streptococci
(Note: Penicillin is the drug of choice in treatment and prevention of streptococcal infections, including prophylaxis of rheumatic fever.)

CONTRAINDICATIONS

Allergy to cephalosporins

INTERACTIONS

Probenecid inhibits the renal excretion of cefadroxil, resulting in prolonged serum concentrations

ADVERSE EFFECTS

Gastrointestinal: nausea, vomiting and diarrhea
Hypersensitivity: rash, urticaria, angioedema, Stevens-Johnson syndrome (rarely)
See the adverse effects reported with the cephalosporin class of antibiotics listed under Adverse Effects of cefaclor.

PHARMACOKINETICS AND PHARMACODYNAMICS

Peak serum levels: 16 and 28 µg/mL following single doses of 500 and 1000 mg, respectively
Plasma half-life: normal renal function, 1.4 h; end-stage renal disease, 20 to 25 h
Bioavailability: percentage not given; rapidly absorbed after oral administration
Metabolism: not metabolized
Excretion: renal; over 90% excreted unchanged in urine in 24 h
Effect of food: may aid in diminishing potential gastrointestinal effects
Protein binding: 20%
Renal impairment: prolongs half-life; reduced dosage required
Hepatic impairment: no information

The information here is provided as guidance only. Prescribers should always consult the manufacturer's current prescribing information.

CEFADROXIL (CONTINUED)

DOSAGE

Adults: Normal renal function, uncomplicated cystitis: 1 to 2 g/d in single or divided doses (twice a day); all other urinary tract infections, 2 g/d in divided doses (twice a day). Skin–skin structure infections, pharyngitis, and tonsillitis: 1 g/d in single or divided doses (twice a day).

Elderly: Monitor for age-related renal impairment; same dosage as adults.

Children: Normal renal function, urinary tract and skin–skin structure infections, 30 mg/kg/d in divided doses (every 12 hours). Pharyngitis, tonsillitis, and impetigo: 30 mg/kg/d in a single daily dose or divided doses (every 12 hours).

In cases of beta-hemolytic streptococcal pharyngitis and tonsillitis infections, therapeutic dosage should be administered for at least 10 days.

Impaired renal function: Adjust dosage according to creatinine clearance rates to prevent drug accumulation. Initial adult dose—1 g; the maintenance dose (based on creatinine clearance rate, mL/min/1.73 m^2) is 500 mg at the following intervals:

Adult Cefadroxil Dosage in Renal Impairment

Creatinine clearance, *mL/min*	Dosage interval, *h*
0–10	36
10–25	24
25–50	12
> 50	No adjustment

OVERDOSAGE

For amounts under 250 mg/kg, no action is required other than general support and observation. For amounts greater than 250 mg/kg, induce gastric emptying.

PATIENT INFORMATION

Complete full course of therapy. Take medication with food or milk to prevent gastrointestinal upset. Contact physician if nausea, vomiting, or diarrhea occurs. Refrigerate the suspension, shake well before use, and discard the unused portion after 14 days.

AVAILABILITY

Capsules—500 mg
Tablets—1 g
Oral Suspension—125 mg/5 mL, 250 mg/5 mL, and 500 mg/5 mL

The information here is provided as guidance only. Prescribers should always consult the manufacturer's current prescribing information.

CEFAMANDOLE (Mandol®)

Cefamandole nafate is a parenteral second-generation cephalosporin with good activity against gram-positive and gram-negative bacteria, including beta-lactamase–producing strains of *Haemophilus influenzae, Proteus* spp, *Escherichia coli*, and *Klebsiella* spp. The serum half-life is approximately 1.3 hours. The drug is not metabolized in the body, and the main route of excretion is via the kidneys.

Cefamandole is used to treat infections of the lower respiratory tract, skin–skin structures, and the urinary tract. It also has been used for prophylaxis in open heart surgery and renal transplant patients.

Because cefamandole has a 3 methylthiotetrazole side chain, disulfiram-like reactions can occur with alcohol ingestion. Hypoprothrombinemia as well as inhibition of vitamin K synthesis may affect hemostasis, causing clinical bleeding. The drug should be used with caution in patients with liver impairment or in patients taking anticoagulants. Vitamin K administration may be necessary.

ANTIMICROBIAL ACTIVITY
Gram-positive: Staphylococci (coagulase-positive, coagulase-negative, and penicillinase-producing), beta-hemolytic streptococci, *S. pneumoniae*.
Gram-negative: *Enterobacter* spp, *E. coli*, *H. influenzae* (including some beta-lactamase–producing strains), *Klebsiella* spp, *Morganella (Proteus) morganii, Proteus mirabilis, Proteus vulgaris* (some strains resistant), *Providencia rettgeri*.
Anaerobic: *Bacteroides* spp, *Clostridium* spp, *Fusobacterium* spp, *Peptococcus* spp, and *Peptostreptococcus* spp.

RESISTANCE
Generally ineffective in the treatment of methicillin-resistant *Staphylococcus aureus* and methicillin-resistant coagulase negative staphylococci. Most strains of *Bacteroides fragilis* are resistant. Inducible resistance has been reported when using the cephalosporins in the treatment of *Enterobacter* infections.

SPECIAL PRECAUTIONS
Accumulation of drug levels and prolongation of half-life have been reported in neonates.
Decreased creatinine clearance and transient elevations in blood urea nitrogen (and in some cases, serum creatinine) have been reported in patients with preexisting renal dysfunction; frequency of these effects increases in patients over 50 years of age.
Use caution when administering cephalosporins to patients with sensitivity to penicillin; possible cross-allergenicity and risk of allergic or anaphylactic reaction. If an allergic reaction occurs, discontinue drug. Serious reactions may require epinephrine or other emergency measures (including oxygen, intravenous fluids, intravenous antihistamines, corticosteroids, pressor amines, and airway management).
Use caution when administering broad-spectrum antibiotics to patients with existing or previous gastrointestinal disease. Treatment with broad-spectrum antibiotics alters normal flora of the colon and may permit overgrowth of clostridia, causing antibiotic-associated pseudomembranous colitis. Mild cases usually respond to discontinuation of therapy alone; management of moderate to severe cases should include bacteriologic studies and fluid, electrolyte, and protein supplementation.
Positive direct Coomb's tests have been reported with cephalosporin therapy.
False-positive reaction for glucose in urine may occur with copper-reduction tests (Benedicts' or Fehling's solution) but not with enzyme-based tests for glycosuria. False-negative results may occur with the ferricyanide test. Glucose oxidase or hexokinase methods are recommended to determine blood plasma glucose levels.
Concomitant administration of aminoglycosides and other cephalosporins has caused nephrotoxicity.

(Continued on next page)

INDICATIONS
Used in the treatment of infections of the following organ systems, due to susceptible strains of designated microorganisms:
Lower respiratory tract (including pneumonia):
S. pneumoniae, H. influenzae, Klebsiella spp, penicillinase- and nonpenicillinase-producing *S. aureus*, beta-hemolytic streptococci, and *P. mirabilis*
Urinary tract:
E. coli, indole-positive and indole-negative *Proteus* spp, *Enterobacter* spp, *Klebsiella* spp, and *Staphylococcus epidermidis*, Group D streptococci (excluding enterococci)
Peritonitis:
E. coli and *Enterobacter* spp
Septicemia:
E. coli, penicillinase- and nonpenicillinase-producing *S. aureus, S. pneumoniae, S. pyogenes* (Group A beta-hemolytic streptococci), *H. influenzae*, and *Klebsiella* spp
Skin–skin structure infections:
Penicillinase- and nonpenicillinase-producing *S. aureus, S. pyogenes* (Group A beta-hemolytic streptococci), *H. influenzae, E. coli, Enterobacter spp*, and *P. mirabilis*
Bone and joint:
Penicillinase- and nonpenicillinase-producing *S. aureus*
Perioperative prophylaxis

CONTRAINDICATIONS
Allergy or hypersensitivity to cephalosporins

INTERACTIONS
Probenecid may inhibit the excretion of cefamandole, resulting in prolonged serum concentrations.
The use of aminoglycosides and cephalosporins concomitantly may potentiate nephrotoxicity.
Alcohol: A disulfiram-like reaction (*eg*, flushing, sweating, tachycardia) has been reported when alcohol has been consumed after cefamandole administration.
Anticoagulants: The hypoprothrombinemic effects of anticoagulants may be potentiated when used concomitantly with cefamandole.

The information here is provided as guidance only. Prescribers should always consult the manufacturer's current prescribing information.

CEFAMANDOLE (CONTINUED)

SPECIAL PRECAUTIONS *(CONTINUED)*

Use caution in patients with impaired renal function. Reduce dosage or prolong dosage intervals. Careful observation and laboratory studies should be made. Bacterial or fungal overgrowth of nonsusceptible organisms, leading to secondary infection, may occur with prolonged or repeated therapy.

Vitamin K deficiency has occurred rarely. Patients at risk include those with poor nutritional status, malabsorption states, alcoholism, or prolonged hyperalimentation regimens. Monitor prothrombin time and administer exogenous vitamin K as clinically indicated.

Use caution in the elderly, debilitated patients, malnourished patients, patients with liver or renal impairment and those taking anticoagulants because they are more likely to experience bleeding abnormalities (prophylactic vitamin K may be necessary in some patients).

SPECIAL GROUPS

Children: Complete laboratory parameters have not been studied extensively in infants aged 1 to 6 months; use with caution in this age group (particularly infants under 1 month).

Elderly: May have age-related renal impairment and subsequent decreased creatinine clearance or transient elevations in blood urea nitrogen.

Renal impairment: Reduced dosage or prolonged dosage intervals may be required.

Hepatic impairment: No information.

Pregnancy: Adequate human studies not performed; pregnancy Category B: the cephalosporins appear safe for use in pregnancy, but few controlled studies have been done.

Breast-feeding: Use with caution.

DOSAGE

Adults: 500 mg to 1 g intravenous or intramuscular every 4 to 8 hours. For skin infections and pneumonia, 500 mg every 6 hours. For uncomplicated urinary tract infections, 500 mg every 8 hours or up to 1 g every 8 hours for more serious infections. For other serious infections, 1 g every 4 to 6 hours. For life-threatening infections or for infections due to less susceptible organisms, doses up to 2 g every 4 hours may be required. For perioperative prophylaxis, 1 to 2 g intravenous or intramuscular 0.5 to 1 hour prior to initial incision (in cesarean section, immediately after cord is clamped) and repeat as necessary dependent on the length and type of surgical procedure.

Elderly: Same as adults.

Children: 50 to 100 mg/kg/d in divided doses every 4 to 8 hours. For severe infections, dose may be increased to a total daily dose of 150 mg/kg. Do not exceed maximum adult dose. For perioperative prophylaxis (children 3 months of age and older) 12.5 to 25 mg/kg given 0.5 to 1 hour prior to the initial incision and repeat as necessary dependent on the length and type of surgical procedure.

Impaired renal function: Administer an initial dose of 1 to 2 g and then as follows:

Adult Cefamandole Dosage in Renal Impairment

Creatinine clearance, mL/min/1.73 m^2	Life-threatening infections	Less severe infections
> 80	2 g every 4 h	1–2 g every 6 h
50–80	1.5 g every 4 h or 2 g every 6 h	0.75–1.5 g every 6 h
25–50	1.5 g every 6 h or 2 g every 8 h	0.75–1.5 g every 8 h
10–25	1 g every 6 h or 1.25 g every 8 h	0.5–1 g every 8 h
2–10	0.67 g every 8 h or 1 g every 12 h	0.5–0.75 g every 12 h
< 2	0.5 g every 8 h or 0.75 g every 12 h	0.25–0.5 g every 12 h

ADVERSE EFFECTS

Decreased creatinine clearance in patients with prior renal function impairment

Hypersensitivity reactions: including urticaria, maculopapular rash, and anaphylaxis

Transient hepatitis and cholestatic jaundice have been rarely reported

See the adverse effects reported with the cephalosporin class of antibiotics listed under Adverse Effects of cefaclor.

PHARMACOKINETICS AND PHARMACODYNAMICS

Peak serum levels: 139 µg/mL after a 1-g intravenous dose

Plasma half-life: normal renal function, 0.5 to 1 h; end-stage renal disease, 8 to 11 h

Bioavailability: percentage not given; reaches therapeutic levels in pleural and joint fluids and in bile and bone

Metabolism: cefamandole nafate is rapidly hydrolyzed in the plasma

Excretion: renal, 65% to 85% recovered unchanged in urine

Protein binding: 70%

Renal impairment: reduced dosage required

Hepatic impairment: no dosage reduction necessary

OVERDOSAGE

PARENTERAL:

Large doses may cause seizures, particularly in patients with renal impairment. Dosage should be reduced when renal function is compromised. If seizures occur, discontinue drug immediately and use anticonvulsant therapy if indicated. In cases of extreme overdosage, hemodialysis may be considered.

AVAILABILITY

Powder—500 mg and 1 g in 10 mL, 1 g in 100 mL, 2 g in 20 mL, 2 g in 100 mL, 10 g in 100 mL (pharmacy bulk package)

The information here is provided as guidance only. Prescribers should always consult the manufacturer's current prescribing information.

CEFAZOLIN (Ancef®, Kefzol®)

Cefazolin is a parenteral first-generation cephalosporin with good activity against gram-positive bacteria, including *Staphylococcus aureus* and streptococci (with the exception of methicillin-resistant staphylococci and penicillin-resistant *Streptococcus pneumoniae*). Cefazolin is more active than cephalothin against gram-negative bacteria. This spectrum against gram-negative bacteria includes *Escherichia coli*, *Klebsiella* spp and *Proteus mirabilis*. The half-life is approximately 2 hours and the drug is eliminated via the kidneys.

Cefazolin is indicated for prophylaxis before open heart and vascular surgery, neurosurgery, orthopedic procedures, gastroduodenal surgery, vaginal–abdominal hysterectomy, and biliary tract surgery in high-risk patients. It also is used for treatment of skin infections due to gram-positive organisms, including *Streptococcus pyogenes* and *S. aureus*, and for treatment of urinary tract infections. Side effects are uncommon and similar to those of other cephalosporins.

ANTIMICROBIAL ACTIVITY

Gram-positive: Staphylococci (coagulase-positive, coagulase-negative, and penicillinase-producing), beta-hemolytic streptococci, *S. pneumoniae*.
Gram-negative: *E. coli*, *Klebsiella* spp, *P. mirabilis*.

RESISTANCE

Generally not effective in the treatment of methicillin-resistant *S. aureus* and methicillin-resistant coagulase-negative staphylococci. Generally ineffective in the treatment of highly penicillin-resistant *S. pneumoniae*.

SPECIAL PRECAUTIONS

Use caution when administering cephalosporins to patients with sensitivity to penicillin; possible cross-allergenicity and risk of allergic or anaphylactic reaction. If an allergic reaction occurs, discontinue drug. Serious reactions may require epinephrine or other emergency measures (including oxygen, intravenous fluids, intravenous antihistamines, corticosteroids, pressor amines, and airway management).
Use caution when administering broad-spectrum antibiotics to patients with existing or previous gastrointestinal disease. Treatment with broad-spectrum antibiotics alters normal flora of the colon and may permit overgrowth of clostridia, causing antibiotic-associated pseudomembranous colitis. Mild cases usually respond to discontinuation of therapy alone; management of moderate to severe cases should include bacteriologic studies and fluid, electrolyte, and protein supplementation.
Positive direct Coomb's tests have been reported with cephalosporin therapy. False-positive reaction for glucose in urine may occur with copper-reduction tests (Benedicts' or Fehling's solution) but not with enzyme-based tests for glycosuria. False-negative results may occur with the ferricyanide test. Glucose oxidase or hexokinase methods are recommended to determine blood plasma glucose levels.
Use caution in patients with impaired renal function. Reduce dosage or prolong dosage intervals. Careful observation and laboratory studies should be made.
Bacterial or fungal overgrowth of nonsusceptible organisms, leading to secondary infection, may occur with prolonged or repeated therapy.

INDICATIONS

Used in the treatment of infections of the following types, due to susceptible strains of designated microorganisms:
Respiratory tract:
S. pneumoniae, *Klebsiella* spp, *S. aureus* (penicillin-sensitive and penicillin-resistant), and Group A beta-hemolytic streptococci (Note: Penicillin is the drug of choice in the treatment and prevention of streptococcal infections, including rheumatic fever.)
Urinary tract:
E. coli, *P. mirabilis*, *Klebsiella* spp
Skin–skin structure infections:
S. aureus (penicillin-sensitive and penicillin-resistant), Group A beta-hemolytic streptococci and other strains of streptococci
Biliary tract:
E. coli, various strains of streptococci, *P. mirabilis*, *Klebsiella* spp, and *S. aureus*
Bone and joint:
S. aureus
Genital (prostatitis and epididymitis):
E. coli, *P. mirabilis*, *Klebsiella* spp
Septicemia:
S. pneumoniae, *S. aureus* (penicillin-sensitive and penicillin-resistant), *P. mirabilis*, *E. coli*, and *Klebsiella* spp
Endocarditis:
S. aureus (penicillin-sensitive and penicillin-resistant) and Group A beta-hemolytic streptococci
Perioperative prophylaxis:
To reduce the incidence of certain postoperative infections in patients undergoing procedures considered potentially contaminated (*eg*, vaginal hysterectomy, cholecystectomy in patients over 70 years of age, acute cholecystitis, obstructive jaundice, common bile duct stones)

CONTRAINDICATIONS

Allergy or hypersensitivity to cephalosporins

INTERACTIONS

Probenecid may inhibit the renal excretion of cefazolin, resulting in prolonged serum concentrations. Cefazolin may provide additive or synergistic antibacterial activity when used in combination with an aminoglycoside for treatment of some organisms.

ADVERSE EFFECTS

Extreme confusion after administration of large doses to patients with renal failure; hypersensitivity reactions (*eg*, rash, urticaria, Stevens-Johnson syndrome).
See the adverse effects reported with the cephalosporin class of antibiotics listed under Adverse Effects of cefaclor.

The information here is provided as guidance only. Prescribers should always consult the manufacturer's current prescribing information.

CEFAZOLIN (CONTINUED)

SPECIAL GROUPS

Children: Safety has not been established for use in infants under 1 month of age or for premature infants.
Elderly: May have age-related renal impairment.
Renal impairment: Reduced dosage required.
Hepatic impairment: No information.
Pregnancy: Adequate human studies not performed; pregnancy Category B. The cephalosporins appear to be safe for use in pregnancy, but few controlled studies have been done.
Breast-feeding: Use with caution; excreted in low concentrations.

DOSAGE

Adults: Moderate to severe infection, 500 mg to 1 g intravenously or intramuscularly every 6 to 8 hours. For mild infection due to gram-positive cocci, 250 to 500 mg every 8 hours. For acute, uncomplicated urinary tract infections, 1 g every 12 hours. For pneumococcal pneumonia, 500 mg every 12 hours. For severe or life-threatening infections (endocarditis or septicemia) 1 to 1.5 g every 6 hours. In general a dosage interval of every 8 hours is appropriate for the treatment of most infections. For perioperative prophylaxis, 1 g intravenously or intramuscularly 0.5 to 1 hour prior to start of surgery and repeat as necessary dependent on length and type of surgical procedure.
Elderly: Same as adults.
Children: 25 to 50 mg/kg/d intravenously or intramuscularly divided in three to four equal doses. For severe infections, dose may be increased up to 100 mg/kg/d.
Impaired renal function: *See* tables below.

Adult Cefazolin Dosage in Renal Impairment

Creatinine clearance, mL/min	Dose
≥ 55	No adjustment necessary
35–54	250 mg–1 g every 8 h
11–34	125–500 mg every 12 h
≤ 10	125–500 mg every 18–24 h

Pediatric Cefazolin Dosage in Renal Impairment

Creatinine clearance, mL/min	Dose
40–70	15–60 mg/kg/d divided in two equal doses
20–40	6.25–25 mg/kg/d divided in two equal doses
5–20	2.5–10 mg/kg/d every 24 h

PHARMACOKINETICS AND PHARMACODYNAMICS

Peak serum levels: 185 to 189 µg/mL after a 1-g intravenous dose
Plasma half-life: normal renal function, 1.5 to 2 h; end-stage renal disease, 3 to 7 h
Bioavailability: no information
Metabolism: not metabolized
Excretion: renal; 60% unchanged in urine after 6 h, increasing to 70% to 80% in 24 h
Protein binding: 80% to 86%
Renal impairment: reduced dosage or prolonged dosage intervals required
Hepatic impairment: in patients with obstructive biliary disease, bile levels are considerably lower than serum levels (< 1.0 µg/mL); patients without obstructive biliary disease may have bile levels that exceed serum levels up to five times

OVERDOSAGE

PARENTERAL:
Large doses may cause seizures, particularly in patients with renal impairment. Dosage should be reduced when renal function is compromised. If seizures occur, discontinue drug immediately and use anti-convulsant therapy if indicated. In cases of extreme overdosage, hemodialysis may be considered.

AVAILABILITY

250 mg, 500 mg, or 1g vials and piggyback vials
5-g, 10-g and 20-g pharmacy bulk vials
500 mg or 1 g in 50-mL (prefrozen) single-dose containers

The information here is provided as guidance only. Prescribers should always consult the manufacturer's current prescribing information.

CEFIXIME (Suprax®)

Cefixime is the first available, oral, third-generation cephalosporin. It is active against streptococci (but not staphylococci), *Neisseria gonorrhoeae, Haemophilus influenzae*, and *Branhamella catarrhalis*, including beta-lactamase–producing strains. Other gram-negative bacilli, including *Escherichia coli, Klebsiella*, and *Serratia*, are sensitive. The half-life is 3 hours, and the drug is administered once a day. It is eliminated mainly by the kidneys, and dose adjustment is necessary in patients with severe renal insufficiency.

The drug may be used once daily in the treatment of pharyngitis, otitis media, bronchitis, and urinary tract infections. Cefixime has no activity against *Pseudomonas* or anaerobes. Gastrointestinal toxicity, mainly diarrhea and nausea, is the most frequent side effect.

ANTIMICROBIAL ACTIVITY

Gram-positive: beta-hemolytic streptococci and *S. pneumoniae*.
Gram-negative: *E. coli, H. influenzae* (including some beta-lactamase–producing strains), *Moraxella (Branhamella) catarrhalis* (including some beta-lactamase–producing strains), *Proteus mirabilis, N. gonorrhoeae* (including penicillinase- and nonpenicillinase-producing strains).
Demonstrated *in vitro* activity against *Citrobacter* spp, *Haemophilus parainfluenzae* (including some beta-lactamase–producing strains), *Klebsiella* spp, *Proteus vulgaris, Providencia* spp (including *P. rettgeri*), and *Salmonella* spp, *Serratia* spp, and *Shigella* spp.

RESISTANCE

Most strains of staphylococci and enterobacter are resistant to cefixime. Ineffective in the treatment of highly penicillin-resistant *S. pneumoniae*.

SPECIAL PRECAUTIONS

False-positive reaction for ketones in urine may occur with tests using nitroprusside but not with those using nitroferricyanide.
Treatment with oral suspension results in higher peak serum concentrations than that with tablet form; therefore, tablet should not be substituted for suspension.
Use caution when administering cephalosporins to patients with sensitivity to penicillin; possible cross-allergenicity and risk of allergic or anaphylactic reaction. If an allergic reaction occurs, discontinue drug. Serious reactions may require epinephrine or other emergency measures (including oxygen, intravenous fluids, intravenous antihistamines, corticosteroids, pressor amines, and airway management).
Use caution when administering broad-spectrum antibiotics to patients with existing or previous gastrointestinal disease. Treatment with broad-spectrum antibiotics alters normal flora of the colon and may permit overgrowth of clostridia, causing antibiotic-associated pseudomembranous colitis. Mild cases usually respond to discontinuation of therapy alone; management of moderate to severe cases should include bacteriologic studies and fluid, electrolyte, and protein supplementation.
Positive direct Coomb's tests have been reported with cephalosporin therapy.
False-positive reaction for glucose in urine may occur with copper-reduction tests (Benedicts' or Fehling's solution) but not with enzyme-based tests for glycosuria.
False-negative results may occur with the ferricyanide test. Glucose oxidase or hexokinase methods are recommended to determine blood plasma glucose levels.
Use caution in patients with impaired renal function. Reduce dosage or prolong dosage intervals. Careful observation and laboratory studies should be made.
Bacterial or fungal overgrowth of nonsusceptible organisms, leading to secondary infection, may occur with prolonged or repeated therapy.

INDICATIONS

Used in the treatment of the following infections, due to susceptible strains of designated microorganisms:
Urinary tract (uncomplicated):
E. coli and *P. mirabilis*
Otitis media:
H. influenzae (beta-lactamase–positive and –negative strains), *M. catarrhalis* (majority of which are beta-lactamase–positive), and *Streptococcus pyogenes**
Pharyngitis or tonsillitis:
S. pyogenes
(Penicillin is the usual drug of choice)
Bronchitis (acute and acute exacerbations of chronic bronchitis):
S. pneumoniae and *H. influenzae* (beta-lactamase–positive and –negative strains)
Gonorrhea (cervical or urethral, uncomplicated):
N. gonorrhoeae (including penicillinase- and nonpenicillinase-producing strains)
**Efficacy for this microorganism in the organ system was studied in fewer than 10 infections.*

CONTRAINDICATIONS

Allergy or hypersensitivity to cephalosporins

INTERACTIONS

Probenecid inhibits the renal excretion of cefixime, resulting in prolonged serum concentrations

ADVERSE EFFECTS

Gastrointestinal effects: nausea, vomiting, diarrhea
Hypersensitivity reactions: headache
See the adverse effects reported with the cephalosporin class of antibiotics listed under Adverse Effects of cefaclor.

PHARMACOKINETICS AND PHARMACODYNAMICS

Peak serum levels: 2 µg/mL following 200 mg and 3.7 µg/mL following 400 mg, 2 to 6 h after administration; oral suspension produces concentrations 25% to 50% higher (not bioequivalent to tablets)
Plasma half-life: normal renal function, 3 to 4 h; end-stage renal disease, 11.5 h
Bioavailability: approximately 40% to 50% absorbed after oral administration
Metabolism: no evidence of metabolism
Excretion: renal and nonrenal mechanisms; 50% unchanged drug excreted in urine in 24 h
Effect of food: time to maximal absorption increased when given with food; otherwise no effect
Protein binding: 65%
Renal impairment: prolongs half-life
Hepatic impairment: animal studies showed excretion of more than 10% in bile

The information here is provided as guidance only. Prescribers should always consult the manufacturer's current prescribing information.

CEFIXIME (CONTINUED)

SPECIAL GROUPS

Children: Safety and efficacy not established in infants younger than 6 months of age.
Elderly: May have age-related renal impairment.
Renal impairment: Dosage adjustment necessary; use with caution.
Hepatic impairment: No information.
Pregnancy: Adequate human studies not performed; pregnancy Category B; the cephalosporins appear to be safe for use in pregnancy, but few controlled trials have been done.
Breast-feeding: Use with caution; not known whether excreted in breast milk.

DOSAGE

Adults: 400 mg/d in single or divided dose (200 mg every 12 hours). Single oral dose of 400 mg recommended for uncomplicated cervical or urethral gonococcal infections.
Elderly: Same as adults.
Children: (oral suspension) 8 mg/kg/d in single or divided dose (4 mg/kg every 12 hours). Children weighing over 50 kg or older than 12 years may be given adult dosage. Safety and efficacy not established for infants under 6 months of age.
Impaired renal function: (adult) Normal dosage may be used in patients whose creatinine clearance is above 60 mL/min. Patients whose clearance is 21 to 60 mL/min or who are undergoing renal hemodialysis may be given 75% of normal dosage (300 mg/d). Patients whose clearance is below 20 mL/min or who are undergoing continuous ambulatory peritoneal dialysis may be given half the normal dosage (200 mg/d).
(Note: Treatment of infections due to *Streptococcus pyogenes* should continue for at least 10 days.)

OVERDOSAGE

Gastric lavage may be indicated. Hemodialysis and peritoneal dialysis are not sufficiently effective.

PATIENT INFORMATION

Complete full course of therapy. Take medication with food or milk to prevent gastrointestinal upset. Contact physician if nausea, vomiting, or diarrhea occurs. Shake suspension well before use. The suspension may be stored in the refrigerator or at room temperature; discard the unused portion after 14 days.

AVAILABILITY

Tablets—200 mg and 400 mg
Powder for Oral Suspension—(100 mg/5 mL after reconstitution) in 50-, 75-, and 100-mL bottles

The information here is provided as guidance only. Prescribers should always consult the manufacturer's current prescribing information.

CEFMETAZOLE (Zefazone®)

Cefmetazole sodium is a cephamycin that is similar to cefoxitin but with less activity against anaerobes, especially *Bacteroides fragilis*. It is active against most Enterobacteriaceae but not *Pseudomonas aeruginosa*. It has some activity against staphylococci and streptococci. *Mycobacterium fortuitum* and *chelonei* are sensitive to cefmetazole.

The serum half-life is 1.3 hours, and it is mainly eliminated by the kidneys. Cefmetazole can be used to treat intra-abdominal infections caused by susceptible organisms and uncomplicated gonorrhea. It has been used for surgical prophylaxis of vaginal hysterectomy, cholecystectomy, and colonorectal surgery in high-risk patients.

Because cefmetazole has a 3 methylthiotetrazole side chain, disulfiram-like reactions can occur with alcohol ingestion. Hypoprothrombinemia as well as inhibition of vitamin K synthesis may affect hemostasis, causing clinical bleeding. The drug should be used with caution in patients with liver impairment or in those taking anticoagulants. Vitamin K administration may be necessary.

ANTIMICROBIAL ACTIVITY

Gram-positive: Staphylococci (coagulase-positive, coagulase-negative, and penicillinase-producing) beta-hemolytic streptococci, *Streptococcus pneumoniae*.
Gram-negative: *Escherichia coli, Haemophilus influenzae* (including some beta-lactamase–producing strains), *Klebsiella* spp, *Morganella morganii, Proteus mirabilis, Proteus vulgaris, Providencia* spp.
Anaerobic: *Bacteroides* spp, *B. fragilis, Clostridium* spp, *Fusobacterium* spp.
Cefmetazole also has shown *in vitro* activity against the following: *Citrobacter* spp, *Enterobacter* spp, *Moraxella (Branhamella) catarrhalis, Providencia rettgeri, Salmonella* spp, *Shigella* spp, *Peptococcus* spp, and *Peptostreptococcus* spp.

RESISTANCE

Generally ineffective in the treatment of methicillin-resistant *Staphylococcus aureus* and methicillin-resistant coagulase-negative staphylococci.

SPECIAL PRECAUTIONS

Use caution when administering cephalosporins to patients with sensitivity to penicillin; possible cross-allergenicity and risk of allergic or anaphylactic reaction. If an allergic reaction occurs, discontinue drug. Serious reactions may require epinephrine or other emergency measures (including oxygen, intravenous fluids, intravenous antihistamines, corticosteroids, pressor amines, and airway management).
Use caution when administering broad-spectrum antibiotics to patients with existing or previous gastrointestinal disease. Treatment with broad-spectrum antibiotics alters normal flora of the colon and may permit overgrowth of clostridia, causing antibiotic-associated pseudomembranous colitis. Mild cases usually respond to discontinuation of therapy alone; management of moderate to severe cases should include bacteriologic studies and fluid, electrolyte, and protein supplementation.
Positive direct Coomb's tests have been reported with cephalosporin therapy.
False-positive reaction for glucose in urine may occur with copper-reduction tests (Benedicts' or Fehling's solution) but not with enzyme-based tests for glycosuria. False-negative results may occur with the ferricyanide test. Glucose oxidase or hexokinase methods are recommended to determine blood plasma glucose levels.
Concomitant administration of aminoglycosides and other cephalosporins has caused nephrotoxicity.
Use caution in patients with impaired renal function. Reduce dosage or prolong dosage intervals. Careful observation and laboratory studies should be made. Bacterial or fungal overgrowth of nonsusceptible organisms, leading to secondary infection, may occur with prolonged or repeated therapy.

(Continued on next page)

INDICATIONS

Treatment of infections of the following types due to designated, susceptible organisms:
Urinary tract (complicated or uncomplicated):
E. coli
Lower respiratory tract (pneumonia and bronchitis):
S. aureus (penicillinase- and nonpenicillinase-producing strains), *E. coli, H. influenzae* (nonpenicillinase-producing strains), *S. pneumoniae*
Skin–skin structure infections:
S. aureus (penicillinase- and nonpenicillinase-producing strains), *S. epidermidis, Streptococcus pyogenes, Streptococcus agalactiae, E. coli, Proteus mirabilis, Proteus vulgaris*, M. morganii*, Providencia stuartii*, Klebsiella pneumoniae*, K. oxytoca*, B. fragilis*, and *Bacteroides melaninogenicus**
Intra-abdominal:
E. coli, K. pneumoniae, K. oxytoca*, B. fragilis, Clostridium perfringens**
Perioperative prophylaxis
**Efficacy for this organism in this organ system was studied in fewer than 20 infections.*

CONTRAINDICATIONS

Documented allergy to cefmetazole or the cephalosporin antibiotics

INTERACTIONS

Probenecid: Inhibits the renal excretion of cefmetazole, resulting in prolonged serum concentrations
Alcohol: A disulfiram-like reaction (*eg*, flushing, sweating, tachycardia) has been reported when alcohol has been consumed after cefmetazole administration
Aminoglycosides: The risk of nephrotoxicity may be potentiated if cefmetazole is used in combination with an aminoglycoside
Anticoagulants: The hypoprothrombinemic effects of anticoagulants may be potentiated when used concomitantly with cefmetazole

ADVERSE EFFECTS

Hypersensitivity reactions: including urticaria and anaphylaxis
Gastrointestinal effects: diarrhea, nausea, vomiting
Coagulation abnormalities: hypoprothrombinemia, platelet dysfunction, thrombocytopenia
See the adverse effects reported with the cephalosporin class of antibiotics listed under Adverse Effects of cefaclor.

The information here is provided as guidance only. Prescribers should always consult the manufacturer's current prescribing information.

CEFMETAZOLE (CONTINUED)

SPECIAL PRECAUTIONS *(CONTINUED)*

Vitamin K deficiency has occurred rarely. Patients at risk include those with poor nutritional status, malabsorption states, alcoholism, or prolonged hyperalimentation regimens. Monitor prothrombin time and administer exogenous vitamin K as clinically indicated.

Use caution in patients with liver impairment and renal impairment and in those taking anticoagulants, the elderly, debilitated or malnourished patients, because they are more likely to experience bleeding abnormalities (prophylactic vitamin K administration may be necessary in some patients).

SPECIAL GROUPS

Children: Safety and efficacy have not been established.
Elderly: May have age-related renal impairment requiring reduced dosage.
Renal impairment: Reduced dosage necessary.
Hepatic impairment: No information.
Pregnancy: Pregnancy Category B; the cephalosporins appear to be safe in pregnancy, but few controlled studies have been done.
Breast-feeding: Excreted in breast milk; use with caution.

DOSAGE

Adults: Generally give 2 g intravenously every 6 to 12 hours for 5 to 14 days.
For perioperative prophylaxis: Administer 1 to 2 g intravenously 30 to 90 minutes prior to surgery and repeat as necessary dependent on the duration and type of procedure.
For a cesarean section, administer 2 g as a single dose after clamping cord.
Elderly: May have age-related renal impairment; otherwise, same as adults.
Children: Not recommended.
Renal impairment: The following guidelines are recommended:

Adult Cefmetazole Dosage in Renal Impairment

Renal function, *degree of impairment*	Creatinine clearance, *mL/min/1.73 m²*	Dose, *g*	Frequency, *h*
Mild	50–90	1–2	Every 12
Moderate	30–49	1–2	Every 16
Severe	10–29	1–2	Every 24
Nonfunctional	< 10	1–2	Every 48 (given after hemodialysis)

PHARMACOKINETICS AND PHARMACODYNAMICS

Peak serum levels: 143 µg/mL after a 2-g intravenous dose infused over 1 h
Serum half-life: 1.2 h (normal renal function)
Bioavailability: widely distributed
Protein binding: 65%
Metabolism: no information
Excretion: 85% unchanged in urine
Renal impairment: reduced dosage necessary
Hepatic impairment: no information

OVERDOSAGE

PARENTERAL:
Large doses may cause seizures, particularly in patients with renal impairment. Dosage should be reduced when renal function is compromised. If seizures occur, discontinue drug immediately and use anticonvulsant therapy if indicated. In cases of extreme overdosage, hemodialysis may be considered.

AVAILABILITY

Powder for Injection—1-g and 2-g vials

The information here is provided as guidance only. Prescribers should always consult the manufacturer's current prescribing information.

CEFONICID (Monocid®)

Cefonicid is a parenteral, second-generation cephalosporin. It is active against gram-positive bacteria, including staphylococci and streptococci but is less active than first-generation cephalosporins. It has good activity against *Escherichia coli, Klebsiella, Proteus* spp, and *Haemophilus influenzae*. It has no activity against anaerobes.

Cefonicid has a prolonged half-life of approximately 4 hours. It can be administered once or twice a day. Most of the drug is excreted in the urine, and dose modification is necessary in patients with renal failure.

The drug may be used to treat urinary tract infections, community-acquired pneumonia, and skin and soft-tissue infections. It has been used as surgical prophylaxis prior to vaginal hysterectomy, cholecystectomy, and colorectal surgery in high-risk patients. Cefonicid is generally well tolerated, and side effects are rare.

ANTIMICROBIAL ACTIVITY

Gram-positive: Staphylococci (coagulase-positive, coagulase-negative, and penicillinase-producing), beta-hemolytic streptococci, and *Streptococcus pneumoniae*.
Gram-negative: *E. coli, H. influenzae* (including some beta-lactamase–producing strains), *Klebsiella pneumoniae, Morganella (Proteus) morganii, Proteus mirabilis, Proteus vulgaris,* and *Providencia rettgeri*.
Demonstrated *in vitro* activity against *Citrobacter* spp, *Enterobacter* spp, *Moraxella catarrhalis, Neisseria gonorrhoeae, Clostridium* spp, *Fusobacterium* spp, *Peptococcus* spp, and *Peptostreptococcus* spp.

RESISTANCE

Generally ineffective in the treatment of methicillin-resistant *Staphylococcus aureus* and methicillin-resistant coagulase-negative staphylococci.

SPECIAL PRECAUTIONS

Use caution when administering cephalosporins to patients with sensitivity to penicillin; possible cross-allergenicity and risk of allergic or anaphylactic reaction. If an allergic reaction occurs, discontinue drug. Serious reactions may require epinephrine or other emergency measures (including oxygen, intravenous fluids, intravenous antihistamines, corticosteroids, pressor amines, and airway management).
Use caution when administering broad-spectrum antibiotics to patients with existing or previous gastrointestinal disease. Treatment with broad-spectrum antibiotics alters normal flora of the colon and may permit overgrowth of clostridia, causing antibiotic-associated pseudomembranous colitis. Mild cases usually respond to discontinuation of therapy alone; management of moderate to severe cases should include bacteriologic studies and fluid, electrolyte, and protein supplementation. Positive direct Coomb's tests have been reported with cephalosporin therapy. False-positive reaction for glucose in urine may occur with copper-reduction tests (Benedicts' or Fehling's solution) but not with enzyme-based tests for glycosuria. False-negative results may occur with the ferricyanide test. Glucose oxidase or hexokinase methods are recommended to determine blood plasma glucose levels. Concomitant administration of aminoglycosides and other cephalosporins has caused nephrotoxicity.
Use caution in patients with impaired renal function. Reduce dosage or prolong dosage intervals. Careful observation and laboratory studies should be made.
Bacterial or fungal overgrowth of nonsusceptible organisms, leading to secondary infection, may occur with prolonged or repeated therapy.

INDICATIONS

Infections of the following type due to the designated organisms
Lower respiratory tract:
S. pneumoniae, K. pneumoniae, E. coli, and *H. influenzae* (ampicillin-resistant and ampicillin-sensitive)
Urinary tract:
E. coli, Proteus spp (may include organisms now called *P. vulgaris, Providencia rettgeri* and *M. morganii*), and *K. pneumoniae*
Skin–skin structure infections:
S. aureus, Staphylococcus epidermidis, S. pyogenes (Group A *Streptococcus*), *Streptococcus agalactiae* (Group B *Streptococcus*)
Septicemia:
S. pneumoniae and *E. coli*
Bone and joint:
S. aureus
Cefonicid also may be used for perioperative prophylaxis

CONTRAINDICATIONS

Allergy or hypersensitivity to cephalosporins

INTERACTIONS

Probenecid inhibits the renal excretion of cefonicid, resulting in prolonged serum concentrations

ADVERSE EFFECTS

Local reactions: pain on injection, thrombophlebitis
Hematologic: increased platelets, eosinophilia
Increased liver function tests
See the adverse effects reported with the cephalosporin class of antibiotics listed under Adverse Effects of cefaclor.

PHARMACOKINETICS AND PHARMACODYNAMICS

Peak serum levels: 221.3 µg/mL after a 1-g intravenous dose
Plasma half-life: normal renal function 4.5 h; end-stage renal disease, 11 h
Bioavailability: well distributed, except to gastrointestinal system
Metabolism: not metabolized
Excretion: 99% excreted unchanged in urine after 24 h
Protein binding: > 90%
Renal impairment: reduced dosage necessary
Hepatic impairment: no information

The information here is provided as guidance only. Prescribers should always consult the manufacturer's current prescribing information.

CEFONICID (CONTINUED)

SPECIAL GROUPS

Children: Safety and efficacy not established.
Elderly: May have age-related renal impairment.
Renal impairment: Reduced dosage necessary.
Hepatic impairment: No information.
Pregnancy: Probably safe; use when clearly indicated.
Breast-feeding: Use with caution; excreted in breast milk.

DOSAGE

Adults: 1 g every 24 hours, intravenously or intramuscularly; although used rarely, doses up to 2 g/d have been well tolerated. For urinary tract infection (uncomplicated), 0.5 g every 24 hours; for mild to moderate infections, 1 g every 24 hours; severe or life-threatening infections, 2 g every 24 hours. For surgical prophylaxis, 1 g administered 1 hour before surgery and repeat as necessary dependent on the type and duration of the surgical procedure.
Elderly: Same as adults.
Impaired renal function: Initial loading dose of 7.5 mg/kg, intravenously or intramuscularly. An individualized dosing schedule should be determined for each patient according to the following maintenance guidelines:

Adult Cefonicid Dosage in Renal Impairment

Creatinine clearance, mL/min/1.73 m^2	Mild to moderate infections	Severe infections
60–79	10 mg/kg every 24 h	25 mg/kg every 24 h
40–59	8 mg/kg every 24 h	20 mg/kg every 24 h
20–39	4 mg/kg every 24 h	15 mg/kg every 24 h
10–19	4 mg/kg every 48 h	15 mg/kg every 48 h
5–9	4 mg/kg every 3 to 5 days	15 mg/kg every 3 to 5 days
< 5	3 mg/kg every 3 to 5 days	4 mg/kg every 3 to 5 days

OVERDOSAGE

PARENTERAL:
Large doses may cause seizures, particularly in patients with renal impairment. Dosage should be reduced when renal function is compromised. If seizures occur, discontinue drug immediately and use anti-convulsant therapy if indicated. In cases of extreme overdosage, hemodialysis may be considered.

AVAILABILITY

Powder for Injection—500-mg and 1-g single-dose vials and 10-g pharmacy bulk vials

The information here is provided as guidance only. Prescribers should always consult the manufacturer's current prescribing information.

CEFOPERAZONE (Cefobid®)

Cefoperazone is a third-generation cephalosporin with good activity against *Pseudomonas aeruginosa* and most gram-negative aerobic bacilli, although it is less stable to beta-lactamases than other antibiotics in the group. It is active against *Staphylococcus aureus* and streptococci but is less so than first- and second-generation cephalosporins.

The half-life is 1.6 hours; high and prolonged serum levels are noted when administered twice daily. Biliary excretion is the primary route of elimination. Dosage adjustment is not usually necessary in patients with renal failure, but caution must be taken in patients with liver disease because the half-life may be prolonged. The cerebrospinal fluid penetration is poor, even in patients with inflamed meninges.

It is used to treat hospital-acquired infections, including those due to *P. aeruginosa*. It is also effective for the treatment of urinary tract and lower respiratory infections due to susceptible gram-negative bacilli.

Changes in intestinal flora and diarrhea appear to be more common with this agent, and this effect is probably secondary to excretion of the compound into the gut via the bile. Like other cephalosporins with the *N*-methylthiotetrazole side chain, this drug can cause hypoprothrombinemia and bleeding, especially in vitamin K–deficient patients. It also may cause a disulfiram-like reaction if alcoholic beverages are ingested. Caution is needed in patients with renal failure, and vitamin K administration is usually necessary.

ANTIMICROBIAL ACTIVITY

Gram-positive: Staphylococci (coagulase-positive, coagulase-negative, and penicillinase-producing), beta-hemolytic streptococci, *Streptococcus pneumoniae.*
Gram-negative: *Acinetobacter* spp (some strains resistant), *Citrobacter* spp, *Enterobacter* spp, *Escherichia coli, Haemophilus influenzae* (including some beta-lactamase–producing strains), *Klebsiella* spp, *Morganella (Proteus) morganii, Neisseria gonorrhoeae* (including some beta-lactamase–producing strains), *Proteus mirabilis, Proteus vulgaris, Providencia rettgeri, P. aeruginosa, Serratia* spp.
Anaerobic: *Bacteroides* spp, *Bacteroides fragilis, Clostridium* spp, *Peptococcus* spp, and *Peptostreptococcus* spp.
Demonstrated *in vitro* activity against *Neisseria meningitidis, Salmonella* spp, *Shigella* spp, *Clostridium difficile, Eubacterium* spp, and *Fusobacterium* spp.

RESISTANCE

Generally ineffective in the treatment of methicillin-resistant *S. aureus* and methicillin-resistant coagulase-negative staphylococci. Inducible resistance has been reported when using the cephalosporins for the treatment of *Enterobacter* infections. Ineffective in the treatment of highly penicillin-resistant *S. pneumoniae.*

INDICATIONS

For treatment of infections of the following, due to the designated susceptible organisms:
Respiratory tract:
S. pneumoniae, penicillinase- and nonpenicillinase-producing *S. aureus, Streptococcus pyogenes** (Group A beta-hemolytic streptococci), *P. aeruginosa, E. coli, Klebsiella pneumoniae, H. influenzae, P. mirabilis,* and *Enterobacter* spp
Urinary tract:
E. coli and *P. aeruginosa*
Gynecologic (pelvic inflammatory disease, endometritis):
N. gonorrhoeae, Staphylococcus epidermidis, S. agalactiae, E. coli, Clostridium* spp*, *Bacteroides* spp (including *Bacteroides fragilis*), and anaerobic gram-positive cocci
Skin–skin structure infections:
Penicillinase- and nonpenicillinase-producing *S. aureus, S. pyogenes**, and *P. aeruginosa*
Intra-abdominal (peritonitis):
*E. coli, P. aeruginosa**, and anaerobic gram-negative bacilli (including *B. fragilis*)
Bacterial septicemia:
S. pneumoniae, S. agalactiae, S. aureus, P. aeruginosa*, E. coli, Klebsiella* spp*, *K. pneumoniae**, indole-positive and indole-negative *Proteus* spp*, *Clostridium* spp*, and anaerobic gram-positive cocci*

Efficacy studied in fewer than 10 infections for this organism in this organ system.

CONTRAINDICATIONS

Allergy or hypersensitivity to cephalosporins

INTERACTIONS

Anticoagulants: The hypoprothrombinemic effects of anticoagulants may be potentiated when used concomitantly with cefoperazone.
Alcohol: A disulfiram-like reaction (*eg*, flushing, sweating, tachycardia) has been reported when alcohol has been consumed after cefoperazone administration.
Aminoglycosides: Concomitant administration of aminoglycosides and cefoperazone may provide synergistic antibacterial activity against certain organisms and may also increase the risk of nephrotoxicity.

ADVERSE EFFECTS

Hepatic: elevated liver enzymes accompanied by clinical signs and symptoms of hepatitis
Gastrointestinal effects: nausea, vomiting, diarrhea
Hypersensitivity reactions
Hematologic: hypoprothrombinemia, neutropenia.
See the adverse effects reported with the cephalosporin class of antibiotics listed under Adverse Effects of cefaclor.

The information here is provided as guidance only. Prescribers should always consult the manufacturer's current prescribing information.

CEFOPERAZONE (CONTINUED)

SPECIAL PRECAUTIONS

Use caution when administering cephalosporins to patients with sensitivity to penicillin; possible cross-allergenicity and risk of allergic or anaphylactic reaction. If an allergic reaction occurs, discontinue drug. Serious reactions may require epinephrine or other emergency measures (including oxygen, intravenous fluids, intravenous antihistamines, corticosteroids, pressor amines, and airway management).

Use caution when administering broad-spectrum antibiotics to patients with existing or previous gastrointestinal disease. Treatment with broad-spectrum antibiotics alters normal flora of the colon and may permit overgrowth of clostridia, causing antibiotic-associated pseudomembranous colitis. Mild cases usually respond to discontinuation of therapy alone; management of moderate to severe cases should include bacteriologic studies and fluid, electrolyte, and protein supplementation.

Positive direct Coomb's tests have been reported with cephalosporin therapy.

False-positive reaction for glucose in urine may occur with copper-reduction tests (Benedicts' or Fehling's solution) but not with enzyme-based tests for glycosuria. False-negative results may occur with the ferricyanide test. Glucose oxidase or hexokinase methods are recommended to determine blood plasma glucose levels.

Concomitant administration of aminoglycosides and other cephalosporins has caused nephrotoxicity.

Bacterial or fungal overgrowth of nonsusceptible organisms, leading to secondary infection, may occur with prolonged or repeated therapy.

Vitamin K deficiency has occurred rarely. Patients at risk include those with poor nutritional status, malabsorption states, alcoholism, or prolonged hyperalimentation regimens. Monitor prothrombin time and administer exogenous vitamin K as clinically indicated.

Use caution in elderly, debilitated patients, malnourished patients, patients with liver or renal impairment and those taking anticoagulants because they are more likely to experience bleeding abnormalities (prophylactic vitamin K may be necessary in some patients).

PHARMACOKINETICS AND PHARMACODYNAMICS

Peak serum levels: 153 µg/mL after a 1-g intravenous dose; (combined renal and hepatic insufficiencies result in accumulation of drug in serum)

Plasma half-life: normal renal function, 1.7 to 2.6 h; end-stage renal disease, 1.3 to 2.9 h

Bioavailability: well distributed

Metabolism: partially metabolized

Excretion: mainly in bile; 20% to 30% recovered unchanged in urine

Protein binding: 82% to 93%

Renal impairment: no effect on clearance

Hepatic impairment: extensively excreted in bile; reduced dosage necessary

OVERDOSAGE

PARENTERAL:

Large doses may cause seizures, particularly in patients with renal impairment. Dosage should be reduced when renal function is compromised. If seizures occur, discontinue drug immediately and use anticonvulsant therapy if indicated. In cases of extreme overdosage, hemodialysis may be considered.

AVAILABILITY

Powder—1-g and 2-g vials and 1-g and 2-g piggyback units

Premixed injection—1 g and 2 g in 50-mL single-dose containers (frozen)

SPECIAL GROUPS

Children: Safety and efficacy not established.

Elderly: May have age-related renal impairment.

Renal impairment: No dosage adjustment necessary with impaired renal function alone; however, in patients with both renal and hepatic impairment, do not exceed 1 to 2 g/d.

Hepatic impairment: Serum half-life increased two to four times. Do not exceed 4 g/d.

Pregnancy: Use with caution; adequate human studies not performed.

Breast-feeding: Use with caution; excreted in breast milk.

DOSAGE

Adults: 2 to 4 g/d intramuscularly or intravenously divided every 12 hours. Dosage may be increased in cases of severe infection or infection due to less susceptible organisms (doses of 6 to 12 g/d divided every 6 to 12 hours).

Elderly: Same as adults.

Children: Safety and efficacy not established.

Impaired renal function: Renal excretion is not the main route of elimination of cefoperazone. Patients with renal failure require no adjustment in normal dosage. If high doses are used, serum concentrations should be monitored, and the dosage should be reduced if evidence of accumulation exists. *In patients with both renal and hepatic dysfunction, the total daily dose should not exceed 1 to 2 g* unless appropriate monitoring is done.

The information here is provided as guidance only. Prescribers should always consult the manufacturer's current prescribing information.

CEFOTAXIME (Claforan®)

Cefotaxime is an extended-spectrum third-generation cephalosporin. It has good activity against gram-positive cocci and most Enterobacteriaceae. It also is active against anaerobic gram-positive bacteria, such as *Peptostreptococcus*, *Actinomyces*, *Peptococcus*, and *Propionibacterium*, as well as *Clostridium perfringens*. It is stable in the presence of most beta-lactamases.

The major metabolite of cefotaxime is desacetylcefotaxime, which has independent antibacterial activity; *in vitro* it has synergistic activity with the parent compound. Cefotaxime and its metabolites are excreted in the urine. The drug has very good penetration into inflamed meninges and is one of the drugs of choice for the treatment of community-acquired meningitis in children and adults. In geographic areas where highly penicillin-resistant pneumococci have been encountered, it is prudent to administer cefotaxime with vancomycin or rifampin.

Cefotaxime is indicated for treating gram-positive infections, including respiratory tract, skin and soft-tissue, and gram-negative nosocomial infections, such as pneumonia, complicated urinary tract infection, and wound infections. The lack of potent antipseudomonas activity limits its use as an empiric agent in many tertiary care centers. It is probably one of the safest antimicrobial agents. The side effects are similar to those of other cephalosporins.

ANTIMICROBIAL ACTIVITY

Gram-positive: Staphylococci (coagulase-positive, coagulase-negative, and penicillinase-producing strains; beta-hemolytic streptococci, *Streptococcus pneumoniae*.
Gram-negative: *Escherichia coli, Haemophilus influenzae* (including some beta-lactamase–producing strains), *Haemophilus parainfluenzae, Morganella (Proteus) morganii, Neisseria gonorrhoeae* (including penicillinase- and nonpenicillinase-producing strains), *Neisseria meningitis, Proteus mirabilis, Proteus vulgaris, Acinetobacter* spp, *Citrobacter* spp, *Enterobacter* spp, *Klebsiella* spp, *Providencia rettgeri*, and *Serratia* spp.
Anaerobic: *Peptococcus* spp, *Peptostreptococcus* spp, *Bacteroides* (including some strains of *B. fragilis*), *Fusobacterium* spp, and *Clostridium* spp (excluding *C. difficile*). Demonstrated *in vitro* activity against *Shigella* spp, *Salmonella* spp (and *Salmonella typhi*), and *Providencia* spp.

RESISTANCE

Generally ineffective in the treatment of methicillin-resistant *Staphylococcus aureus* and methicillin-resistant coagulase-negative staphylococci. Inducible resistance has been reported when using the cephalosporins for the treatment of *Enterobacter* infections. Ineffective in the treatment of highly penicillin-resistant *S. pneumoniae*.

INDICATIONS

For treatment of infections of the following, due to the designated susceptible organisms:
Lower respiratory tract (including pneumonia):
S. pneumoniae (formerly *Diplococcus pneumoniae*), *Streptococcus pyogenes* (Group A streptococci)*, and other streptococci excluding enterococci (eg, *Enterococcus faecalis*), penicillinase- and nonpenicillinase-producing *S. aureus, E. coli, Klebsiella* spp, *H. influenzae* (including ampicillin-resistant strains), *H. parainfluenzae, P. mirabilis, Serratia marcescens*, *Enterobacter* spp, indole-positive *Proteus* spp.
Genitourinary:
Staphylococcus epidermidis, penicillinase- and nonpenicillinase-producing *S. aureus*, *Citrobacter* spp, *Enterobacter* spp, *E. coli, Klebsiella* spp, *P. mirabilis, P. vulgaris*, *Proteus inconstans* Group B, *M. morganii*, *P. rettgeri*, *S. marcescens*. Also used for uncomplicated gonorrhea due to *N. gonorrhoeae*, including penicillinase-producing strains.
Gynecologic (including pelvic inflammatory disease, endometritis, and pelvic cellulitis):
S. epidermidis, Streptococcus spp, *Enterobacter* spp*, *Klebsiella* spp*, *E. coli, P. mirabilis, Bacteroides* spp (including *B. fragilis*), *Clostridium* spp, and anaerobic cocci (including *Peptostreptococcus* spp and *Peptococcus* spp)
Bacteremia or septicemia:
E. coli, Klebsiella spp, *S. marcescens, S. aureus*, and *Streptococcus* spp (including *S. pneumoniae*)
Skin–skin structure infections:
Penicillinase- and nonpenicillinase-producing *S. aureus, S. epidermidis, S. pyogenes* (Group A streptococci) and other streptococci, *Acinetobacter* spp*, *E. coli, Citrobacter* spp (including *C. freundii*), *Enterobacter* spp, *Klebsiella* spp, *P. mirabilis, P. vulgaris*, *M. morganii, P. rettgeri*, *S. marcescens, Bacteroides* spp, and anaerobic cocci (including *Peptostreptococcus* spp, and *Peptococcus* spp)
Intra-abdominal (including peritonitis):
Streptococcus spp*, *E. coli, Klebsiella* spp, *Bacteroides* spp, *P. mirabilis*, *Clostridium* spp*, and anaerobic cocci (including *Peptostreptococcus* spp*, and *Peptococcus* spp*)
Bone and joint:
Penicillinase- and nonpenicillinase-producing *S. aureus, Streptococcus* spp (including *S. pyogenes*), and *P. mirabilis*
Central nervous system (meningitis and ventriculitis):
N. meningitidis, H. influenzae, S. pneumoniae, K. pneumoniae, and *E. coli**
Perioperative prophylaxis
*Efficacy studied in fewer than 10 infections for this organism in this organ system.

CONTRAINDICATIONS

Allergy or hypersensitivity to cephalosporin antibiotics

The information here is provided as guidance only. Prescribers should always consult the manufacturer's current prescribing information.

CEFOTAXIME (CONTINUED)

SPECIAL PRECAUTIONS

Use caution when administering cephalosporins to patients with sensitivity to penicillin; possible cross-allergenicity and risk of allergic or anaphylactic reaction. If an allergic reaction occurs, discontinue drug. Serious reactions may require epinephrine or other emergency measures (including oxygen, intravenous fluids, intravenous antihistamines, corticosteroids, pressor amines, and airway management).

Use caution when administering broad-spectrum antibiotics to patients with existing or previous gastrointestinal disease. Treatment with broad-spectrum antibiotics alters normal flora of the colon and may permit overgrowth of clostridia, causing antibiotic-associated pseudomembranous colitis. Mild cases usually respond to discontinuation of therapy alone; management of moderate to severe cases should include bacteriologic studies and fluid, electrolyte, and protein supplementation. Positive direct Coomb's tests have been reported with cephalosporin therapy. False-positive reaction for glucose in urine may occur with copper-reduction tests (Benedicts' or Fehling's solution) but not with enzyme-based tests for glycosuria. False-negative results may occur with the ferricyanide test. Glucose oxidase or hexokinase methods are recommended to determine blood plasma glucose levels. Concomitant administration of aminoglycosides and other cephalosporins has caused nephrotoxicity.

Use caution in patients with impaired renal function. Reduce dosage or prolong dosage intervals. Careful observation and laboratory studies should be made. Bacterial or fungal overgrowth of nonsusceptible organisms, leading to secondary infection, may occur with prolonged or repeated therapy.

SPECIAL GROUPS

Children: Dosage based on age and weight.
Elderly: May have age-related renal impairment.
Renal impairment: Reduce dosage.
Hepatic impairment: No dosage reduction necessary.
Pregnancy: Adequate human studies not performed; pregnancy Category B; the cephalosporins appear safe for use in pregnancy, but few controlled trials have been done.
Breast-feeding: Caution; excreted in breast milk in low concentrations.

DOSAGE

Adults: Uncomplicated infections, 2 g/d intramuscularly or intravenously every 12 hours; gonorrhea, 1 g as a single dose; moderate to severe infections, 3 to 6 g/d intramuscularly or intravenously (1–2 g every 8 hours); septicemia and other infections requiring higher dosage, 6 to 8 g/d intravenously (2 g every 6–8 hours); life-threatening infections, up to 12 g/d intravenously (2 g every 4 hours); perioperative prophylaxis, 1 g intravenously or intramuscularly 30 to 60 minutes before surgery and repeat as necessary dependent on length and type of surgical procedure. Cesarean section, 1 g intravenously after umbilical cord is clamped.
Elderly: Same as adults.
Children: Neonates 0 to 1 week of age, 50 mg/kg intravenously every 12 hours; 1 to 4 weeks of age, 50 mg/kg intravenously every 8 hours. It is not necessary to differentiate between premature and normal gestational age infants. Infants and children aged 1 month to 12 years, 50 to 180 mg/kg/d intravenously or intramuscularly every 4 to 6 hours. Higher doses should be used for more serious infections. For children over 50 kg, use adult dosage. Do not exceed 12 g/d.
Impaired renal function: Patients with creatinine clearance of less than 20 mL/min/1.73 m² should receive half the usual dose of cefotaxime at the usual time interval.

INTERACTIONS

Probenecid inhibits the renal excretion of cefotaxime and its metabolites, resulting in prolonged serum concentrations.
The use of aminoglycosides and cephalosporins concomitantly may potentiate nephrotoxicity.

ADVERSE EFFECTS

Local reactions: pain, thrombophlebitis
Hypersensitivity reactions
See the adverse effects reported with the cephalosporin class of antibiotics listed under Adverse Effects of cefaclor.

PHARMACOKINETICS AND PHARMACODYNAMICS

Peak serum levels: 11.7 and 20.5 µg/mL within 30 minutes of single 500-mg and 1-g intramuscular doses, respectively; 102 µg/mL after a 1-g intravenous dose
Plasma half-life: 1 h; end-stage renal disease 3 to 11 h
Bioavailability: widely distributed
Metabolism: 20% to 36% excreted as unchanged drug; 15% to 25% excreted as the desacetyl derivative, the major metabolite
Excretion: renal, 60% in urine after 6 h
Protein binding: 30% to 40%
Renal impairment: half-life may be increased
Hepatic impairment: no dosage adjustment is necessary

OVERDOSAGE

PARENTERAL:
Large doses may cause seizures, particularly in patients with renal impairment. Dosage should be reduced when renal function is compromised. If seizures occur, discontinue drug immediately and use anticonvulsant therapy if indicated. In cases of extreme overdosage, hemodialysis may be considered.

AVAILABILITY

Crystalline powder—1-g, 2-g, and 10-g vials
Premixed injection—1 g and 2 g in 50-mL single-dose containers (frozen)

The information here is provided as guidance only. Prescribers should always consult the manufacturer's current prescribing information.

CEFOTETAN (Cefotan®)

Cefotetan disodium is a second-generation cephalosporin with extensive anaerobic coverage that includes *Bacteroides fragilis* but excludes the *B. fragilis* group (ie, *B. ovatus, B. distasonis,* and *B. thetaiotaomicron*). It is active against aerobic gram-positive and gram-negative bacteria, including *Escherichia coli* and *Klebsiella* spp.

Cefotetan is somewhat less potent than cefoxitin but has a longer half-life, allowing twice-a-day administration. It may be used as a single agent to treat community-acquired intra-abdominal infections. The drug has less *in vitro* activity against *Streptococcus* than other cephalosporins and may be less effective in the treatment of skin and soft-tissue infections. Cefotetan has been used preferentially as a prophylactic agent prior to intra-abdominal and pelvic surgery.

Because cefotetan has a 3 methylthiotetrazole side chain, disulfiram-like reactions can occur with alcohol ingestion. Hypoprothrombinemia as well as inhibition of vitamin K synthesis may affect hemostasis, causing clinical bleeding. The drug should be used with caution in patients with liver impairment or in patients taking anticoagulants. Vitamin K administration may be necessary.

ANTIMICROBIAL ACTIVITY

Gram-positive: Staphylococci (coagulase-positive, coagulase-negative, and penicillinase-producing strains), beta-hemolytic streptococci, *Streptococcus pneumoniae.*
Gram-negative: *E. coli, Haemophilus influenzae* (including some beta-lactamase–producing strains), *Klebsiella* spp, *Morganella (Proteus) morganii, Neisseria gonorrhoeae* (nonpenicillinase-producing strains), *Proteus mirabilis, Proteus vulgaris, Providencia* spp (including *P. rettgeri*), *Serratia marcescens.*
Anaerobic: *Bacteroides* spp (some strains resistant), *B. fragilis, Clostridium* spp, *Fusobacterium* spp, *Peptococcus* spp, and *Peptostreptococcus* spp.
Demonstrated *in vitro* activity against *Citrobacter* spp, *Neisseria meningitidis, Salmonella* spp, *Serratia* spp, and *Shigella* spp.

RESISTANCE

Generally ineffective in the treatment of methicillin-resistant *Staphylococcus aureus* and methicillin-resistant coagulase-negative staphylococci. A significant number of *Enterobacter* spp are resistant to cefotetan.

SPECIAL PRECAUTIONS

High concentrations may interfere with determination of creatinine levels by the Jaffé reaction, producing false results. Serum samples obtained within 2 hours of administration should not be analyzed for creatinine.
Use caution when administering cephalosporins to patients with sensitivity to penicillin; possible cross-allergenicity and risk of allergic or anaphylactic reaction. If an allergic reaction occurs, discontinue drug. Serious reactions may require epinephrine or other emergency measures (including oxygen, intravenous fluids, intravenous antihistamines, corticosteroids, pressor amines, and airway management).
Use caution when administering broad-spectrum antibiotics to patients with existing or previous gastrointestinal disease. Treatment with broad-spectrum antibiotics alters normal flora of the colon and may permit overgrowth of clostridia, causing antibiotic-associated pseudomembranous colitis. Mild cases usually respond to discontinuation of therapy alone; management of moderate to severe cases should include bacteriologic studies and fluid, electrolyte, and protein supplementation. Positive direct Coomb's tests have been reported with cephalosporin therapy.

(Continued on next page)

INDICATIONS

For treatment of infections of the following, due to the designated susceptible organisms:
Lower respiratory tract (including pneumonia):
S. pneumoniae, penicillinase- and nonpenicillinase-producing *S. aureus, E. coli, Klebsiella* spp, *H. influenzae* (including ampicillin-resistant strains)
Urinary tract:
E. coli, Klebsiella spp, *P. mirabilis, P. vulgaris, M. morganii, P. rettgeri*
Gynecologic:
Penicillinase- and nonpenicillinase-producing strains of *S. aureus*, *Staphylococcus epidermidis, Streptococcus* spp (excluding enterococci), *N. gonorrhoeae, E. coli, P. mirabilis, Bacteroides* spp (excluding *B. distasonis, B. ovatus, B. thetaiotaomicron*), *Fusobacterium* spp*, and gram-positive anaerobic cocci (including *Peptostreptococcus* spp and *Peptococcus spp).* (Note: If *Chlamydia trachomatis* is suspected for gynecologic infection, additional antichlamydial coverage should be added because cefotetan has no activity against this organism.)
Skin–skin structure infections:
Penicillinase- and nonpenicillinase-producing strains of *S. aureus, S. epidermidis, S. pyogenes, Streptococcus* spp (excluding enterococci), *E. coli*
Intra-abdominal (including peritonitis):
E. coli, Klebsiella spp (including *K. pneumoniae**), *Streptococcus* spp (excluding enterococci), *Bacteroides* spp (excluding *B. distasonis, B. ovatus, B. thetaiotaomicron*), and *Clostridium* spp*
Bone and joint:
*S. aureus**
Perioperative prophylaxis
**Efficacy studied in fewer than 10 infections for this organism in this organ system.*

CONTRAINDICATIONS

Allergy or hypersensitivity to cephalosporins

INTERACTIONS

Aminoglycosides: Concomitant use of cefotetan and the aminoglycosides may provide additive or synergistic antibacterial activity against certain organisms.
Alcohol: A disulfiram-like reaction (*eg,* flushing, sweating, tachycardia) has been reported when alcohol is consumed after cefotetan administration.
Anticoagulants: The hypoprothrombinemic effects of anticoagulants may be potentiated when used concomitantly with cefotetan.

ADVERSE EFFECTS

Hematologic: eosinophilia, thrombocytopenia, hypothrombinemia
Gastrointestinal effects: nausea, vomiting, diarrhea
Hypersensitivity reactions
See the adverse effects reported with the cephalosporin class of antibiotics listed under Adverse Effects of cefaclor.

The information here is provided as guidance only. Prescribers should always consult the manufacturer's current prescribing information.

CEFOTETAN (CONTINUED)

SPECIAL PRECAUTIONS *(CONTINUED)*

False-positive reaction for glucose in urine may occur with copper-reduction tests (Benedicts' or Fehling's solution) but not with enzyme-based tests for glycosuria. False-negative results may occur with the ferricyanide test. Glucose oxidase or hexokinase methods are recommended to determine blood plasma glucose levels. Concomitant administration of aminoglycosides and other cephalosporins has caused nephrotoxicity.

Use caution in patients with impaired renal function. Reduce dosage or prolong dosage intervals. Careful observation and laboratory studies should be made. Bacterial or fungal overgrowth of nonsusceptible organisms, leading to secondary infection, may occur with prolonged or repeated therapy.

Vitamin K deficiency has occurred rarely. Patients at risk include those with poor nutritional status, malabsorption states, alcoholism, or prolonged hyperalimentation regimens. Monitor prothrombin time and administer exogenous vitamin K as clinically indicated.

Use caution in the elderly, debilitated patients, malnourished patients, patients with liver or renal impairment and those taking anticoagulants because they are more likely to experience bleeding abnormalities (prophylactic vitamin K may be necessary in some patients).

SPECIAL GROUPS

Children: Safety and efficacy not established.
Elderly: May have age-related renal impairment.
Renal impairment: Caution; reduced dosage or prolonged intervals required.
Hepatic impairment: No information.
Pregnancy: Adequate human studies not performed; pregnancy Category B; the cephalosporins appear safe for use in pregnancy, but few controlled trials have been done.
Breast-feeding: Use caution; excreted in breast milk.

DOSAGE

Adults: 1 to 2 g intravenously or intramuscularly every 12 hours for 5 to 10 days. To prevent postoperative infection, give 1 to 2 g intravenously in a single dose 30 to 60 minutes before surgery (in cesarean section, administer only after umbilical cord is clamped).
Urinary tract infection, 1 to 4 g/day intravenously or intramuscularly divided every 12 hours. Skin–skin structure infections (mild to moderate) 2 g intravenously every 24 hours or 1 g every 12 hours; (severe) 2 g intravenously every 12 hours. Other infections, 1 to 2 g intravenously every 12 hours; (severe) 2 g intravenously every 12 hours; (life-threatening) 3 g intravenously every 12 hours. Daily dosage should not exceed 6 g.
Elderly: May have age-related renal impairment. Same as adults.
Children: Safety and efficacy not established.
Impaired renal function: *See* table below.

Adult Cefotetan Dosage in Renal Impairment

Creatinine clearance, *mL/min*	Recommended dosage
10–30	Usual dose every 24 h
< 10	Usual dose every 48 h

PHARMACOKINETICS AND PHARMACODYNAMICS

Peak serum levels: 158 µg/mL 30 minutes after a 1-g intravenous dose
Plasma half-life: normal renal function, 3 to 4.5 h; end-stage renal disease, 13 to 35 h
Bioavailability: widely distributed
Metabolism: no active metabolites found; < 7% in plasma and urine may be converted to its tautomer, with antimicrobial activity similar to the parent drug
Excretion: renal; 51% to 81% recovered unchanged in urine over 24 h
Protein binding: 88% to 90%
Renal impairment: prolongs half-life
Hepatic impairment: no information

OVERDOSAGE

PARENTERAL:
Large doses may cause seizures, particularly in patients with renal impairment. Dosage should be reduced when renal function is compromised. If seizures occur, discontinue drug immediately and use anticonvulsant therapy if indicated. In cases of extreme overdosage, hemodialysis may be considered.

AVAILABILITY

1-g and 2-g vials
1-g and 2-g piggyback vials
10 g in 100-mL vial
1 and 2 g in 50 mL plastic container

The information here is provided as guidance only. Prescribers should always consult the manufacturer's current prescribing information.

CEFOXITIN (Mefoxin®)

Cefoxitin is a cephamycin with more activity than the other first- and third-generation cephalosporins against anaerobes, especially *Bacteroides fragilis*, *Bacteroides melaninogenicus*, and *Fusobacterium* spp. Aerobic gram-positive cocci are less sensitive. It is also highly resistant to beta-lactamases produced by gram-negative rods (*ie, Escherichia coli, Klebsiella,* and *Proteus* spp). Some strains of *Mycobacterium chelonei* and *fortuitum* are sensitive to cefoxitin.

The half-life is 45 minutes, and the drug is excreted almost entirely by the kidneys in an unchanged form. Cefoxitin has very good penetration into the peritoneal fluid and pelvic tissue.

The drug is used in the treatment of intra-abdominal and other anaerobic infections of the female genital tract including pelvic inflammatory disease, pleuropulmonary infections, sacral decubitus, and infected diabetic feet. It may be less effective for treatment of skin or soft-tissue infections caused by *Staphylococcus aureus* or *Streptococcus pyogenes*. It also is used for prophylaxis in large bowel surgery. Side effects are similar to those of the other cephalosporins.

ANTIMICROBIAL ACTIVITY

Gram-positive: Staphylococci (coagulase-positive, coagulase-negative, and penicillinase-producing strains), beta-hemolytic streptococci, *Streptococcus pneumoniae.*
Gram-negative: *E. coli, Haemophilus influenzae* (including some beta-lactamase–producing strains), *Klebsiella* spp, *Morganella (Proteus) morganii, Neisseria gonorrhoeae,* (including penicillinase- and nonpenicillinase-producing strains) *Proteus mirabilis, Proteus vulgaris, Providenica* spp, *Providencia rettgeri.*
Anaerobic: *Bacteroides* spp, *Bacteroides fragilis, Clostridium* spp, *Peptococcus* spp, and *Peptostreptococcus* spp.

RESISTANCE

Generally ineffective in the treatment of methicillin-resistant *S. aureus* and methicillin-resistant coagulase-negative Staphylococci. Generally ineffective in the treatment of highly penicillin-resistant *S. pneumoniae.*

SPECIAL PRECAUTIONS

High concentrations may interfere with determination of creatinine levels by the Jaffé reaction, producing false results. Serum samples obtained within 2 hours of administration should not be analyzed for creatinine.

Use caution when administering cephalosporins to patients with sensitivity to penicillin; possible cross-allergenicity and risk of allergic or anaphylactic reaction. If an allergic reaction occurs, discontinue drug. Serious reactions may require epinephrine or other emergency measures (including oxygen, intravenous fluids, intravenous antihistamines, corticosteroids, pressor amines, and airway management).

Use caution when administering broad-spectrum antibiotics to patients with existing or previous gastrointestinal disease. Treatment with broad-spectrum antibiotics alters normal flora of the colon and may permit overgrowth of clostridia, causing antibiotic-associated pseudomembranous colitis. Mild cases usually respond to discontinuation of therapy alone; management of moderate to severe cases should include bacteriologic studies and fluid, electrolyte, and protein supplementation. Positive direct Coomb's tests have been reported with cephalosporin therapy. False-positive reaction for glucose in urine may occur with copper-reduction tests (Benedicts' or Fehling's solution) but not with enzyme-based tests for glycosuria. False-negative results may occur with the ferricyanide test. Glucose oxidase or hexokinase methods are recommended to determine blood plasma glucose levels. Concomitant administration of aminoglycosides and other cephalosporins has caused nephrotoxicity.

(Continued on next page)

INDICATIONS

For treatment of infections of the following, due to the designated susceptible organisms:
Lower respiratory tract (including pneumonia and lung abscess):
S. pneumoniae and other streptococci, penicillinase- and nonpenicillinase-producing *S. aureus, E. coli, Klebsiella* spp, *H. influenzae,* and *Bacteroides* spp
Genitourinary or urinary tract:
E. coli, Klebsiella spp, *P. mirabilis,* indole-positive *Proteus* (including *Proteus vulgaris* and *Morganella morganii*), and *Providenica* spp (including *P. rettgeri*). Also used for uncomplicated gonorrhea due to *N. gonorrhoeae,* including penicillinase- and nonpenicillinase-producing strains
Gynecologic (including pelvic inflammatory disease, endometritis, and pelvic cellulitis):
E. coli, N. gonorrhoeae (including penicillinase- and nonpenicillinase-producing strains), *Bacteroides* spp (including *B. fragilis* group*), *Clostridium* spp, *Peptostreptococcus* spp and *Peptococcus* spp, and Group B streptococci
Bacteremia or septicemia:
E. coli, Klebsiella spp, *S. aureus* (penicillinase- and nonpenicillinase-producing), *S. pneumoniae,* and the *B. fragilis* group*
Skin–skin structure infections:
Penicillinase- and nonpenicillinase producing *S. aureus, Staphylococcus epidermidis,* streptococci *E. coli, P. mirabilis, Klebsiella* spp, *Bacteroides* spp, including the *B. fragilis* group*, *Clostridium* spp, *Peptostreptococcus* spp and *Peptococcus* spp
Intra-abdominal (including peritonitis and intra-abdominal abscess):
E. coli, Klebsiella spp, *Bacteroides* spp, including the *B. fragilis* group*, and *Clostridium* spp
Bone and joint:
Penicillinase- and nonpenicillinase-producing *S. aureus*
Perioperative prophylaxis
B. fragilis, B. distasonis, B. ovatus, B. thetaiotaomicron, B. vulgatus

CONTRAINDICATIONS

Allergy or hypersensitivity to cefoxitin or the cephalosporins

The information here is provided as guidance only. Prescribers should always consult the manufacturer's current prescribing information.

CEFOXITIN (CONTINUED)

SPECIAL PRECAUTIONS *(CONTINUED)*

Use caution in patients with impaired renal function. Reduce dosage or prolong dosage intervals. Careful observation and laboratory studies should be made. Bacterial or fungal overgrowth of nonsusceptible organisms, leading to secondary infection, may occur with prolonged or repeated therapy.

SPECIAL GROUPS

Children: Safety and efficacy not established in infants younger than 3 months of age.
Elderly: May have age-related renal impairment.
Renal impairment: Reduced dosage or prolonged dosage intervals required.
Hepatic impairment: No dosage reduction necessary.
Pregnancy: Adequate human studies not performed; pregnancy Category B; the cephalosporins appear safe in pregnancy, but few controlled trials have been done.
Breast-feeding: Use caution; excreted in breast milk.

DOSAGE

Adults: 1 to 2 g intravenously or intramuscularly every 6 to 8 hours. For uncomplicated infections, administer 1 g every 6 to 8 hours; for moderately severe or severe, administer 1 g every 4 hours or 2 g every 6 to 8 hours. Maximum dose is 2 g every 4 hours or 3 g every 6 hours. Acute pelvic inflammatory disease, the recommended dose is 2 g every 6 hours. In the treatment of gonorrhea (uncomplicated) a 2-g intramuscular dose is recommended in conjunction with oral probenecid. For surgical prophylaxis, administer 2 g and repeat as necessary dependent on length and type of surgical procedure.
Elderly: May have age-related renal impairment. Same as adults.
Children: For those aged 3 months and older, 80 to 160 mg/kg/d divided every 4 to 6 hours. Do not exceed 12 g/d. For surgical antibiotic prophylaxis administer 30 to 40 mg/kg/dose and repeat as necessary dependent on length and type of surgical procedure
Impaired renal function: Adults: administer an initial 1- to 2-g dose followed by:

Adult Cefoxitin Dosage in Renal Impairment

Creatinine clearance, mL/min/1.73m^2	Dose, g	Frequency, h
30–50	1–2	8–12
10–29	1–2	12–24
5–9	0.5–1	12–24
< 5	0.5–1	24–48

INTERACTIONS

Probenecid inhibits the renal excretion of cefoxitin, resulting in prolonged serum concentrations

ADVERSE EFFECTS

Local reactions: pain on injection, thrombophlebitis
See the adverse effects reported with the cephalosporin class of antibiotics listed under Adverse Effects of cefaclor.

PHARMACOKINETICS AND PHARMACODYNAMICS

Peak serum levels: 64 to 110 µg/mL at 5 min after a 1-g intravenous dose
Plasma half-life: normal renal function, 0.7 to 1 h; end-stage renal disease, 20 h
Bioavailability: well-distributed
Metabolism: 2% or less
Excretion: renal; 85% to 99% recovered unchanged in urine in 6 h
Protein binding: 73%
Renal impairment: prolongs half-life
Hepatic impairment: no dosage adjustment necessary

OVERDOSAGE

PARENTERAL:
Large doses may cause seizures, particularly in patients with renal impairment. Dosage should be reduced when renal function is compromised. If seizures occur, discontinue drug immediately and use anticonvulsant therapy if indicated. In cases of extreme overdosage, hemodialysis may be considered.

AVAILABILITY

Premixed solution—1 g and 2 g in 50 mL
Dry powder—1-g and 2-g vials and infusion bottles
10-g pharmacy bulk vials

The information here is provided as guidance only. Prescribers should always consult the manufacturer's current prescribing information.

CEFPODOXIME PROXETIL (Vantin®)

Cefpodoxime proxetil is a third-generation cephalosporin available for oral administration only. It is active against *Streptococcus pneumoniae* and beta-hemolytic streptococci. The activity against gram-negative bacilli includes *Escherichia coli*, *Klebsiella* spp, *Proteus* spp, and *Haemophilus influenzae*. It has more activity against *Staphylococcus aureus* than cefixime.

Cefpodoxime proxetil is an ester product that, after deesterification, produces the active metabolite cefpodoxime, which has a half-life of 2 to 3 hours. Food increases the bioavailability of cefpodoxime.

The drug is indicated in the treatment of community-acquired respiratory tract infections caused by non–beta-lactamase–producing strains of *H. influenzae* and *S. pneumoniae*; gonorrhea, including penicillinase-producing strains; and uncomplicated skin–skin structure infections. Uncomplicated urinary tract infections also may be treated. Gastrointestinal disturbances, usually dose related, and diarrhea may occur.

ANTIMICROBIAL ACTIVITY

Gram-positive: *S. aureus* (including penicillinase-producing; some strains resistant), beta-hemolytic streptococci, *S. pneumoniae*, *S. saprophyticus*.
Gram-negative: *E. coli*, *H. influenzae* (including some beta-lactamase–producing strains), *Klebsiella pneumoniae*, *Moraxella (Branhamella) catarrhalis*, *Neisseria gonorrhoeae* (including penicillinase-producing strains), *Proteus mirabilis*. Demonstrated *in vitro* activity against *Citrobacter diversus*, *Haemophilus parainfluenzae*, *Proteus vulgaris*, *Providencia rettgeri*, and *Peptostreptococcus* spp.

RESISTANCE

Generally inactive against methicillin-resistant *S. aureus* and most strains of *Pseudomonas* and *Enterobacter*. Generally ineffective against highly penicillin-resistant *S. pneumoniae*.

SPECIAL PRECAUTIONS

Extreme caution should be used when administering this agent to patients at increased risk for antibiotic-induced pseudomembranous colitis due to exposure to institutional settings with endemic *Clostridium difficile*.
Use caution when administering cephalosporins to patients with sensitivity to penicillin; possible cross-allergenicity and risk of allergic or anaphylactic reaction. If an allergic reaction occurs, discontinue drug. Serious reactions may require epinephrine or other emergency measures (including oxygen, intravenous fluids, intravenous antihistamines, corticosteroids, pressor amines, and airway management).
Positive direct Coomb's tests have been reported with cephalosporin therapy.
False-positive reaction for glucose in urine may occur with copper-reduction tests (Benedicts' or Fehling's solution) but not with enzyme-based tests for glycosuria. False-negative results may occur with the ferricyanide test. Glucose oxidase or hexokinase methods are recommended to determine blood plasma glucose levels.
Use caution in patients with impaired renal function. Reduce dosage or prolong dosage intervals. Careful observation and laboratory studies should be made.
Bacterial or fungal overgrowth of nonsusceptible organisms, leading to secondary infection, may occur with prolonged or repeated therapy.

INDICATIONS

Used in the treatment of infections of the following organ systems caused by designated organisms:
Lower respiratory tract:
Chronic bronchitis: *S. pneumoniae*, *H. influenzae* (non–beta-lactamase–producing strains) or *M. catarrhalis*
S. pneumoniae or *H. influenzae* (non–beta-lactamase–producing strains only)
Community-acquired pneumoniae
Sexually transmitted diseases (acute, uncomplicated urethral and cervical gonorrhea and rectal infections):
N. gonorrhoeae, including penicillinase- and nonpenicillinase-producing strains (Note: Efficacy of cefpodoxime in male patients with rectal infections caused by *N. gonorrhoeae* has not been established.)
Skin–skin structure infections:
Penicillinase- and nonpenicillinase-producing *S. aureus* or *Streptococcus pyogenes*
Upper respiratory tract:
Acute otitis media—*S. pneumoniae*, *H. influenzae* (including beta-lactamase–producing strains), or *M. catarrhalis*
Pharyngitis/tonsillitis, *S. pyogenes*
Urinary tract (uncomplicated):
E. coli, *K. pneumoniae*, *P. mirabilis*, or *S. saprophyticus*

CONTRAINDICATIONS

Allergy or hypersensitivity to cephalosporin antibiotics

INTERACTIONS

Probenecid inhibits the renal excretion of cefpodoxime, resulting in prolonged serum concentrations.
Antacids and H_2 blockers: The peak plasma and extent of absorption of cefpodoxime decreases when given concomitantly

ADVERSE EFFECTS

Gastrointestinal effects: diarrhea (appears to be dose related), nausea, vomiting, abdominal pain
Other: vaginal fungal infections, rash, headache
See the adverse effects reported with the cephalosporin class of antibiotics listed under Adverse Effects of cefaclor.

The information here is provided as guidance only. Prescribers should always consult the manufacturer's current prescribing information.

CEFPODOXIME PROXETIL (CONTINUED)

SPECIAL GROUPS

Children: Safety and efficacy in infants younger than 6 months of age not established.
Elderly: No overall differences with normal renal function.
Renal impairment: Reduced dosage necessary.
Hepatic impairment: No dosage adjustment is necessary.
Pregnancy: Adequate human studies not performed; pregnancy Category B; the cephalosporins appear safe for use in pregnancy, but few controlled trials have been done.
Breast-feeding: Excreted in human milk.

DOSAGE

Adults: Pharyngitis or tonsillitis or urinary tract infection (uncomplicated), 200 mg/d divided every 12 hours for 10 days and 7 days, respectively. Gonorrhea (rectal, uncomplicated), 200 mg as a single dose. Pneumonia (acute community-acquired), or acute bacterial exacerbation of chronic bronchitis, 400 mg/d divided every 12 hours for 14 days and 10 days, respectively. Skin–skin structure infections, 800 mg/d divided every 12 hours for 7 to 14 days.
Elderly: Same as adults.
Children: For patients aged 6 months to 12 years, for otitis media (acute), 10 mg/kg/d divided (maximum 200 mg dose) every 12 hours for 10 days. Do not exceed 400 mg/d. Pharyngitis or tonsillitis, 10 mg/kg/d divided (maximum 100 mg dose) every 12 hours for 10 days.
Impaired renal function: For patients with severe impairment, dosing intervals should be increased to every 24 hours. In patients undergoing hemodialysis, frequency should be three times per week after hemodialysis.

PHARMACOKINETICS AND PHARMACODYNAMICS

Peak serum levels: (tablet) 1.4 µg/mL, 2.3 µg/mL, and 3.9 µg/mL after 100-mg, 200-mg, and 400-mg doses, respectively; (oral suspension) 1.5 µg/mL after 100-mg dose
Plasma half-life: normal renal function, 2 to 3 h; end-stage renal disease, 9.8 h
Bioavailability: 50%
Metabolism: de-esterified to active metabolite, cefpodoxime
Excretion: renal; 29% to 33% recovered unchanged in urine
Effect of food: increases mean peak plasma concentration; inhibits gastrointestinal effects
Protein binding: 21% to 29%
Renal impairment: elimination is reduced
Hepatic impairment: absorption is reduced; elimination unchanged

OVERDOSAGE

ORAL:

Symptoms may include nausea, vomiting, epigastric distress, and diarrhea. Unless five times the normal dose has been ingested, gastrointestinal decontamination is not necessary. Always consider possibility of multiple drug overdoses, drug interactions, and unusual drug kinetics. Absorption may be inhibited by administration of activated charcoal. Otherwise, ensure patient's airway and support ventilation, monitor and maintain vital signs, blood gases, serum electrolytes, and so forth. Hemodialysis, peritoneal dialysis, forced diuresis, or charcoal hemoperfusion have not been established as beneficial.

PATIENT INFORMATION

Complete full course of therapy. Take medication with food to enhance absorption. Contact physician if nausea, vomiting, or diarrhea occurs. Shake suspension well before using. Refrigerate the suspension and discard the unused portion after 14 days.

AVAILABILITY

Tablets—100 mg and 200 mg
Oral suspension—50 mg/mL and 100 mg/mL in 100-mL bottles

The information here is provided as guidance only. Prescribers should always consult the manufacturer's current prescribing information.

CEFPROZIL (Cefzil®)

Cefprozil is a second-generation cephalosporin available for oral administration only. It has good activity against *Streptococcus pyogenes*, *Staphylococcus aureus*, *Moraxella catarrhalis*, and *Haemophilus influenzae*, including beta-lactamase–producing strains.

The half-life is 1.3 hours and is prolonged to 5.9 hours with oliguria. The drug is well absorbed (95%). It is indicated in the treatment of pharyngitis, tonsillitis, otitis media, chronic bronchitis, and skin and soft-tissue infections caused by susceptible organisms. The adverse reactions are similar to those of the other cephalosporins.

ANTIMICROBIAL ACTIVITY

Gram-positive: Staphylococci (coagulase-positive, coagulase-negative, and penicillinase-producing), beta-hemolytic streptococci, *Streptococcus pneumoniae*.
Gram-negative: *H. influenzae* (including some beta-lactamase–producing strains), *M. (Branhamella) catarrhalis*.
Cefprozil also has shown *in vitro* activity against the following: *Escherichia coli*, *Klebsiella* spp, *Neisseria gonorrhoeae*, *Proteus mirabilis*, *Salmonella* spp, *Shigella* spp, *Bacteroides* spp, *Clostridium* spp, *Citrobacter* spp, *Clostridium difficile*, *Fusobacterium* spp, and *Peptostreptococcus* spp.

RESISTANCE

Generally ineffective in the treatment of methicillin-resistant *S. aureus* and methicillin-resistant coagulase-negative staphylococci. Generally ineffective in the treatment of highly penicillin-resistant *S. pneumoniae*.

SPECIAL PRECAUTIONS

Use caution when administering cephalosporins to patients with sensitivity to penicillin; possible cross-allergenicity and risk of allergic or anaphylactic reaction. If an allergic reaction occurs, discontinue drug. Serious reactions may require epinephrine or other emergency measures (including oxygen, intravenous fluids, intravenous antihistamines, corticosteroids, pressor amines, and airway management).
Use caution when administering broad-spectrum antibiotics to patients with existing or previous gastrointestinal disease. Treatment with broad-spectrum antibiotics alters normal flora of the colon and may permit overgrowth of clostridia, causing antibiotic-associated pseudomembranous colitis. Mild cases usually respond to discontinuation of therapy alone; management of moderate to severe cases should include bacteriologic studies and fluid, electrolyte, and protein supplementation.
Positive direct Coomb's tests have been reported with cephalosporin therapy.
False-positive reaction for glucose in urine may occur with copper-reduction tests (Benedicts' or Fehling's solution) but not with enzyme-based tests for glycosuria. False-negative results may occur with the ferricyanide test. Glucose oxidase or hexokinase methods are recommended to determine blood plasma glucose levels.
Use caution in patients with impaired renal function. Reduce dosage or prolong dosage intervals. Careful observation and laboratory studies should be made.
Bacterial or fungal overgrowth of nonsusceptible organisms, leading to secondary infection, may occur with prolonged or repeated therapy.

INDICATIONS

Treatment of infections of the following types due to designated, susceptible organisms:
Pharyngitis or tonsillitis:
S. pyogenes
(Note: Usual drug of choice is penicillin.)
Otitis media:
S. pneumoniae, *H. influenzae*, *M. catarrhalis*
Secondary bacterial infection of acute bronchitis or acute bacterial exacerbation of chronic bronchitis:
S. pneumoniae, *H. influenzae* (beta-lactamase–positive and negative strains), *M. catarrhalis*
Skin–skin structure infections (uncomplicated):
S. aureus (including penicillinase- and nonpenicillinase-producing strains), *S. pyogenes*

CONTRAINDICATIONS

Allergy or hypersensitivity to cephalosporins

INTERACTIONS

Probenecid inhibits the renal excretion of cefprozil, resulting in prolonged serum concentrations

ADVERSE EFFECTS

Gastrointestinal effects: nausea, diarrhea and vomiting
Hepatobiliary: elevation of AST, ALT, alkaline phosphates, and bilirubin
Hypersensitivity reaction: rash, urticaria
Other: dizziness, eosinophilia, vaginitis
See the adverse effects reported with the cephalosporin class of antibiotics listed under Adverse Effects of cefaclor.

PHARMACOKINETICS AND PHARMACODYNAMICS

Peak serum levels: 6.1, 10.5, and 18.3 µg/mL 1.5 hours after 250-mg, 500-mg, and 1-g doses
Serum half-life: 1.3 h (normal renal function); 5.2 to 5.9 h (end-stage renal disease)
Bioavailability: widely distributed
Protein binding: 36%
Metabolism: not appreciably metabolized
Excretion: 60% recovered unchanged in urine
Renal impairment: reduced dosage necessary
Hepatic impairment: no dosage adjustment necessary

The information here is provided as guidance only. Prescribers should always consult the manufacturer's current prescribing information.

CEFPROZIL (CONTINUED)

SPECIAL GROUPS

Children: Safe for use in children older than 6 months of age.
Elderly: May have age-related renal impairment.
Renal impairment: Reduced dosage necessary.
Hepatic impairment: No dosage adjustment is necessary.
Pregnancy: Pregnancy Category B; the cephalosporins appear safe for use in pregnancy, but few controlled trials have been done.
Breast-feeding: Excreted in breast milk; use with caution.

DOSAGE

Adults: For upper respiratory tract infection (pharyngitis or tonsillitis), 500 mg every 24 hours for 10 days. For lower respiratory tract infection (secondary bacterial infection of acute bronchitis, acute bacterial exacerbation of chronic bronchitis), 500 mg every 12 hours for 10 days. For skin–skin structure infections (uncomplicated), 250 mg every 12 hours or 500 mg every 24 hours; in severe infections 500 mg every 12 hours.
(Note: For treatment of infection due to *S. pyogenes*, therapy should continue for at least 10 days.)
Elderly: May have age-related renal impairment; otherwise, same as adults.
Children: For otitis media (children aged 6 months to 12 years), 15 mg/kg every 12 hours for 10 days. For pharyngitis or tonsillitis (children aged 2 to 12 years), 7.5 mg/kg every 12 hours.
Renal impairment: Usual dosage for patients with creatinine clearance 30 to 120 mL/min is standard. For patients with creatinine clearance 0 to 30 mL/min, use 50% of standard dose at normal intervals. (If the patient is being hemodialyzed, administer the dose after the completion of hemodialysis.)

OVERDOSAGE

ORAL:
Symptoms may include nausea, vomiting, epigastric distress, and diarrhea. Unless five times the normal dose has been ingested, gastrointestinal decontamination is not necessary. Always consider possibility of multiple drug overdoses, drug interactions, and unusual drug kinetics. Absorption may be inhibited by administration of activated charcoal. Otherwise, ensure patient's airway and support ventilation, monitor and maintain vital signs, blood gases, serum electrolytes, and so forth. Hemodialysis, peritoneal dialysis, forced diuresis, or charcoal hemoperfusion have not been established as beneficial.

PATIENT INFORMATION

Complete full course of therapy. Contact a physician if nausea, vomiting, or diarrhea occurs. Refrigerate suspension, shake well before use, and discard unused portion after 14 days.

AVAILABILITY

Tablets—250 mg and 500 mg
Powder for Suspension—125 mg and 250 mg per 5 mL (as anhydrous, with aspartame and sucrose)

The information here is provided as guidance only. Prescribers should always consult the manufacturer's current prescribing information.

CEFTAZIDIME (Ceptaz®, Fortaz®, Tazicef®, Tazidime®)

Ceftazidime is a third-generation cephalosporin with potent activity against *Pseudomonas aeruginosa* strains compared with other cephalosporins. Most strains of *Pseudomonas maltophilia* are resistant to ceftazidime. The drug is also highly active against the Enterobacteriaceae, including *Escherichia coli, Serratia, Citrobacter, Enterobacter, Haemophilus influenzae, Neisseria meningitidis,* and *Neisseria gonorrhoeae.* The *in vitro* activity against gram-positive bacteria is less than first- and second-generation cephalosporins. The activity against anaerobic organisms is less than other third-generation agents. Recently, some strains of *Klebsiella pneumoniae* and *Enterobacter cloacae* have become resistant to ceftazidime because they develop beta-lactamases that hydrolyze the compound.

The half-life is 2 hours, and excretion is via the kidneys. Dose reduction is needed in patients with renal failure. Ceftazidime has good penetration into peritoneal and pleural fluid as well as cerebrospinal fluid, especially in patients with bacterial meningitis.

Ceftazidime is indicated in the treatment of hospital-acquired infections, including those caused by *P. aeruginosa.* It has been used as monotherapy in neutropenic patients and to treat nosocomial-acquired pneumonia and cystic fibrosis. It is used to treat malignant external otitis. Rash, eosinophilia, and reversible abnormalities in liver function and leukocyte count may occur with this drug.

ANTIMICROBIAL ACTIVITY

Gram-positive: *Staphylococcus aureus* (including penicillinase-producing strains), beta-hemolytic streptococci, *Streptococcus pneumoniae.*
Gram-negative: *Citrobacter* spp, *Enterobacter* spp, *E. coli, H. influenzae* (including some beta-lactamase–producing strains), *Klebsiella* spp, *N. meningitidis, Proteus mirabilis, Proteus vulgaris, P. aeruginosa,* and *Serratia* spp.
Demonstrated *in vitro* activity against *Acinetobacter* spp, *Haemophilus parainfluenzae, Morganella (Proteus) morganii, N. gonorrhoeae, Providencia* spp, *Providencia rettgeri, Salmonella* spp, *Shigella* spp, *Clostridium* spp, and *Peptococcus* spp, and *Peptostreptococcus* spp, and *Staphylococcus epidermidis.*

RESISTANCE

Generally ineffective in the treatment of methicillin-resistant *S. aureus.* Inducible resistance has been reported when using the cephalosporins for the treatment of *Enterobacter* infections. Some strains of *K. pneumoniae* may be resistant. Generally ineffective in the treatment of highly penicillin-resistant *S. pneumoniae.*

SPECIAL PRECAUTIONS

Use caution when administering cephalosporins to patients with sensitivity to penicillin; possible cross-allergenicity and risk of allergic or anaphylactic reaction. If an allergic reaction occurs, discontinue drug. Serious reactions may require epinephrine or other emergency measures (including oxygen, intravenous fluids, intravenous antihistamines, corticosteroids, pressor amines, and airway management).
Use caution when administering broad-spectrum antibiotics to patients with existing or previous gastrointestinal disease. Treatment with broad-spectrum antibiotics alters normal flora of the colon and may permit overgrowth of clostridia, causing antibiotic-associated pseudomembranous colitis. Mild cases usually respond to discontinuation of therapy alone; management of moderate to severe cases should include bacteriologic studies and fluid, electrolyte, and protein supplementation. Positive direct Coomb's tests have been reported with cephalosporin therapy. False-positive reaction for glucose in urine may occur with copper-reduction tests (Benedicts' or Fehling's solution) but not with enzyme-based tests for glycosuria.

(Continued on next page)

INDICATIONS

Used for treatment of infections of the following organ systems, due to the designated organisms:
Lower respiratory tract (including pneumonia):
P. aeruginosa and other *Pseudomonas* spp, *H. influenzae* (including ampicillin-resistant strains), *Klebsiella* spp, *Enterobacter* spp, *P. mirabilis, E. coli, Serratia* spp, *Citrobacter* spp, *S. pneumoniae,* and methicillin-susceptible strains of *S. aureus*
Skin–skin structure infections:
P. aeruginosa, Klebsiella spp, *E. coli, Proteus* spp (including *P. mirabilis* and indole-positive *Proteus*) *Enterobacter* spp; *Serratia* spp, methicillin-susceptible strains of *S. aureus,* and *Streptococcus pyogenes* (Group A beta-hemolytic streptococci)
Urinary tract (complicated and uncomplicated):
P. aeruginosa, Enterobacter spp, *Proteus* spp (including *P. mirabilis* and indole-positive *Proteus*), *Klebsiella* spp, and *E. coli*
Bacterial septicemia:
P. aeruginosa, Klebsiella spp, *H. influenzae, E. coli, Serratia* spp, *S. pneumoniae,* and methicillin-susceptible strains of *S. aureus*
Bone and joint:
P. aeruginosa, Klebsiella spp, *Enterobacter* spp, and methicillin-susceptible strains of *S. aureus*
Gynecologic (endometritis, pelvic cellulitis):
E. coli
Intra-abdominal (including peritonitis):
E. coli, Klebsiella spp, methicillin-susceptible strains of *S. aureus,* and polymicrobial infections caused by aerobic and anaerobic organisms, and *Bacteroides* spp (many strains of *B. fragilis* are resistant)
Central nervous system (including meningitis):
H. influenzae and *N. meningitidis*; also used successfully in a limited number of patients with meningitis due to *P. aeruginosa* and *S. pneumoniae*

CONTRAINDICATIONS

Allergy or hypersensitivity to cephalosporins

INTERACTIONS

The use of aminoglycosides and ceftazidime concomitantly may provide additive or synergistic antibacterial activity against certain organisms. Concomitant use may also increase the risk of nephrotoxicity.

ADVERSE EFFECTS

Local effects: phlebitis
Hypersensitivity reactions: rash, pruritus, fever
Other: eosinophilia, reversible elevations in hepatic enzymes
See the adverse effects reported with the cephalosporin class of antibiotics listed under Adverse Effects of cefaclor.

The information here is provided as guidance only. Prescribers should always consult the manufacturer's current prescribing information.

CEFTAZIDIME (CONTINUED)

SPECIAL PRECAUTIONS *(CONTINUED)*

False-negative results may occur with the ferricyanide test. Glucose oxidase or hexokinase methods are recommended to determine blood plasma glucose levels. Concomitant administration of aminoglycosides and other cephalosporins has caused nephrotoxicity.

Use caution in patients with impaired renal function. Reduce dosage or prolong dosage intervals. Careful observation and laboratory studies should be made. Bacterial or fungal overgrowth of nonsusceptible organisms, leading to secondary infection, may occur with prolonged or repeated therapy.

SPECIAL GROUPS

Children: Safety and efficacy not established for the ceftazidime L-arginine formulation. If ceftazidime therapy is required for a pediatric patient (younger than 12 years of age) use a sodium carbonate formulation.
Elderly: No differences in effectiveness with normal renal function.
Renal impairment: Reduced dosage required.
Hepatic impairment: No dosage adjustment required.
Pregnancy: Adequate human studies not performed; pregnancy Category B; the cephalosporins appear safe for use in pregnancy, but few controlled trials have been done.
Breast-feeding: Use caution. Excreted in breast milk in low concentration. Do not use the ceftazidime L-arginine formulation in nursing mothers.

DOSAGE

Adults: 1 g intravenously or intramuscularly every 8 to 12 hours. *See* table below.

Adult Dosage of Ceftazidime in Patients With Normal Renal Function

Uncomplicated urinary tract infection	250 mg intravenously or intramuscularly every 12 h
Complicated urinary tract infection	500 mg intravenously or intramuscularly every 8 to 12 h
Uncomplicated pneumonia; mild skin and skin structure infections	500 mg to 1 g intravenously or intramuscularly every 8 h
Bone and joint infections	2 g intravenously every 12 h
Serious gynecologic and intra-abdominal infections; meningitis; life-threatening infections	2 g intravenously every 8 h
Cystic fibrosis	30 to 50 mg/kg intravenously every 8 h (maximum = 6 g/d)

Elderly: Same as adults.
Children: *See* table below.

Pediatric Dosage of Ceftazidime in Patients With Normal Renal Function

Neonates (0 to 4 weeks)	30 mg/kg intravenously every 12 h
Infants and children (1 month to 12 years)	30 to 50 mg/kg intravenously every 8 h (maximum = 6 g/day)

Impaired renal function: In adult patients with suspected renal insufficiency, an initial loading dose of 1 g may be administered. Maintenance dosage as follows:

Adult Ceftazidime Dosage in Renal Impairment

Creatinine clearance, *mL/min*	Recommended dosage
31–50	1 g every 12 h
16–30	1 g every 24 h
6–15	500 mg every 24 h
≤ 5	500 mg every 48 h

For severe infections, the above dosage may be increased by 50%, or the dosing frequency may be appropriately increased.

Hemodialysis patients: Administer a 1-g intravenous initial dose followed by 1 g intravenously after each dialysis session.
Continuous ambulatory peritoneal dialysis. Administer a 1-g intravenous initial dose followed by 500 mg intravenous every 24 hours (ceftazidime also may be added to the peritoneal dialysis fluid, 250 mg/2L of dialysate).

PHARMACOKINETICS AND PHARMACODYNAMICS

Peak serum levels: 45 µg/mL and 90 µg/mL after 500-mg and 1-g intravenous doses, respectively after 5 min
Plasma half-life: normal renal function, 1.9 to 2 h; end-stage renal disease, 14 to 30 h
Bioavailability: percentage not given; widely distributed
Metabolism: not metabolized
Excretion: renal; almost entirely by glomerular filtration; 80% to 90% recovered unchanged in urine
Protein binding: <10% to 17%
Renal impairment: half-life significantly prolonged
Hepatic impairment: no effect on pharmacokinetics

OVERDOSAGE

PARENTERAL:

Large doses may cause seizures, particularly in patients with renal impairment. Dosage should be reduced when renal function is compromised. If seizures occur, discontinue drug immediately and use anticonvulsant therapy if indicated. In cases of extreme overdosage, hemodialysis may be considered.

AVAILABILITY

Injection—500-mg vials, 1-g and 2-g vials, and piggyback injection
Pharmacy bulk vials of 6 g and 10 g

The information here is provided as guidance only. Prescribers should always consult the manufacturer's current prescribing information.

CEFTIZOXIME (Cefizox®)

Ceftizoxime sodium is a third-generation cephalosporin that is similar to cefotaxime and has good activity against gram-positive bacteria, gram-negative cocci, including beta-lactamase–producing strains of gonorrhea, as well as most anaerobic bacteria. The drug has less activity than cephamycins. It has a high degree of stability to beta-lactamases produced by gram-negative aerobic bacilli, *Haemophilus influenzae*, and *Acinetobacter* spp. The activity against *Pseudomonas aeruginosa* is poor.

The half-life is approximately 1.7 hours. The drug is not metabolized in the body and is mainly excreted via the kidneys. Therefore, dose reduction is necessary in patients with impaired renal function. The drug has good penetration into inflamed meninges. It has been effective in treatment of nosocomially acquired infections, such as pyelonephritis, pneumonia, and sepsis secondary to infection with gram-negative organisms. Adverse reactions are mild, infrequent, and similar to those of other cephalosporins.

ANTIMICROBIAL ACTIVITY

Gram-positive: Staphylococci (coagulase-positive, coagulase-negative, and penicillinase-producing), beta-hemolytic streptococci, *Streptococcus pneumoniae.*
Gram-negative: *Acinetobacter* spp, *Enterobacter* spp, *Escherichia coli*, *H. influenzae* (including some beta-lactamase–producing strains), *Klebsiella* spp, *Morganella (Proteus) morganii*, *Neisseria gonorrhoeae*, *Proteus mirabilis*, *Proteus vulgaris*, *Providencia rettgeri*, *Serratia* spp.
Anaerobic: *Bacteroides fragilis*, *Peptococcus* spp, and *Peptostreptococcus* spp. Demonstrated *in vitro* activity against *Citrobacter* spp, *Moraxella (Branhamella) catarrhalis*, *Neisseria meningitidis*, *Providencia* spp, *Salmonella* spp, *Shigella* spp, *Bacteroides* spp, *Clostridium* spp, *Eubacterium* spp, and *Fusobacterium* spp.

RESISTANCE

Inducible resistance has been reported when using the cephalosporins in the treatment of *Enterobacter* infections. Generally ineffective in the treatment of methicillin-resistant *Staphylococcus aureus* and methicillin-resistant coagulase-negative staphylococci. Generally ineffective in the treatment of highly penicillin-resistant *S. pneumoniae.*

SPECIAL PRECAUTIONS

High concentrations may interfere with determination of creatinine by the Jaffé reaction, producing false results.
Use caution when administering cephalosporins to patients with sensitivity to penicillin; possible cross-allergenicity and risk of allergic or anaphylactic reaction. If an allergic reaction occurs, discontinue drug. Serious reactions may require epinephrine or other emergency measures (including oxygen, intravenous fluids, intravenous antihistamines, corticosteroids, pressor amines, and airway management).
Use caution when administering broad-spectrum antibiotics to patients with existing or previous gastrointestinal disease. Treatment with broad-spectrum antibiotics alters normal flora of the colon and may permit overgrowth of clostridia, causing antibiotic-associated pseudomembranous colitis. Mild cases usually respond to discontinuation of therapy alone; management of moderate to severe cases should include bacteriologic studies and fluid, electrolyte, and protein supplementation.
Positive direct Coomb's tests have been reported with cephalosporin therapy.
False-positive reaction for glucose in urine may occur with copper-reduction tests (Benedicts' or Fehling's solution) but not with enzyme-based tests for glycosuria.

(Continued on next page)

INDICATIONS

Used in the treatment of infections of the following organ systems, due to susceptible strains of designated microorganisms:
Lower respiratory tract:
Klebsiella spp, *P. mirabilis*, *E. coli*, *H. influenzae* (including ampicillin-resistant strains), penicillinase- and nonpenicillinase-producing *S. aureus*, *Serratia* spp, *Enterobacter* spp, *Bacteroides* spp, and *Streptococcus* spp (including *S. pneumoniae*)
Urinary tract:
Penicillinase- and nonpenicillinase-producing *S. aureus*, *E. coli*, *Pseudomonas* spp, *P. mirabilis*, *P. vulgaris*, *P. rettgeri*, *M. morganii* (formerly *Proteus morganii*), *Klebsiella* spp, *Serratia* spp (including *S. marcescens*), and *Enterobacter* spp
Gonorrhea:
(including uncomplicated urethral and cervical) due to *N. gonorrhoeae*
Genitourinary (pelvic inflammatory disease):
N. gonorrhoeae, *E. coli*, and *Streptococcus agalactiae*
Intra-abdominal:
E. coli, *Staphylococcus epidermidis*, *Streptococcus* spp, *Enterobacter* spp, *Klebsiella* spp, *Bacteroides* spp (including *B. fragilis*), and anaerobic cocci (including *Peptococcus* and *Peptostreptococcus* spp)
Septicemia:
Streptococcus spp (including *S. pneumoniae*) penicillinase- and nonpenicillinase-producing *S. aureus*, *E. coli*, *Bacteroides* spp (including *B. fragilis*), *Klebsiella* spp, and *Serratia* spp
Skin–skin structure infections:
Penicillinase- and nonpenicillinase-producing *S. aureus*, *S. epidermidis*, *E. coli*, *Klebsiella* spp, *Streptococcus* spp (including *Streptococcus pyogenes*) *P, mirabilis*, *Serratia* spp, *Enterobacter* spp, *Bacteroides* spp (including *B. fragilis*), and anaerobic cocci (including *Peptococcus* and *Peptostreptococcus* spp)
Bone and joint:
Penicillinase- and nonpenicillinase-producing *S. aureus*, *Streptococcus* spp, *P. mirabilis*, *Bacteroides* spp, and anaerobic cocci (including *Peptococcus* and *Peptostreptococcus* spp)
Meningitis:
H. influenzae. Also used successfully in a limited number of adult and pediatric patients with meningitis caused by *S. pneumoniae.*

CONTRAINDICATIONS

Allergy or hypersensitivity to ceftizoxime or other cephalosporins

INTERACTIONS

Probenecid inhibits the renal excretion of ceftizoxime, resulting in prolonged serum concentrations.
The use of aminoglycosides and cephalosporins concomitantly may potentiate nephrotoxicity.

The information here is provided as guidance only. Prescribers should always consult the manufacturer's current prescribing information.

CEFTIZOXIME (CONTINUED)

SPECIAL PRECAUTIONS (CONTINUED)

False-negative results may occur with the ferricyanide test. Glucose oxidase or hexokinase methods are recommended to determine blood plasma glucose levels. Concomitant administration of aminoglycosides and other cephalosporins has caused nephrotoxicity.

Use caution in patients with impaired renal function. Reduce dosage or prolong dosage intervals. Careful observation and laboratory studies should be made. Bacterial or fungal overgrowth of nonsusceptible organisms, leading to secondary infection, may occur with prolonged or repeated therapy.

SPECIAL GROUPS

Children: Safety and efficacy not established in infants younger than 6 months of age.
Elderly: May have age-related renal impairment requiring reduced dosage.
Renal impairment: Reduced dosage and prolonged dosage intervals necessary.
Hepatic impairment: No information.
Pregnancy: Adequate human studies not performed; pregnancy Category B; the cephalosporins appear safe for use in pregnancy, but few controlled trials have been done.
Breast-feeding: Use caution; excreted in breast milk in low concentrations.

DOSAGE

Adults: 1 to 2 g intravenously or intramuscularly every 8 to 12 hours. Uncomplicated gonorrhea, single 1 g intramuscularly injection. Uncomplicated urinary tract infection, 500 mg every 12 hours. Severe or refractory infections, 3 to 6 g/d intravenously or intramuscularly in doses of 1 g every 8 hours or 2 g every 8 to 12 hours (with 2-g intramuscular doses, dose should be divided and administered in different sites of large muscle mass). Pelvic inflammatory disease, 6 g/d intravenously in doses of 2 g every 8 hours. In life-threatening infections, 9 to 12 g/d intravenously in doses of 3 to 4 g every 8 hours.
Elderly: Same as adults.
Children: (6 months and older) 50 mg/kg every 6 to 8 hours; may be increased to 200 mg/kg/d but do not exceed maximum adult dose for serious infection.
Impaired renal function: Following an initial dose of 500 mg to 1 g, give a maintenance dose as follows:

Adult Ceftizoxime Dosage in Renal Impairment

Creatinine clearance, mL/min	Less severe infections	Life-threatening infections
50–79	500 mg every 8 h	750 mg to 1.5 g every 8 h
5–49	250 mg to 500 mg every 12 h	500 mg to 1 g every 12 h
0–4	500 mg every 48 hours or 250 mg every 24 h	500 mg to 1 g every 48 h or 500 mg every 24 h

Schedule dose at the end of dialysis in hemodialysis patients.

ADVERSE EFFECTS

Hypersensitivity: rash, pruritus, fever
Hepatic: elevation in AST, ALT and alkaline phosphatase
Hematologic: eosinophilia, thrombocytosis
Local reactions: pain, thrombophlebitis
See the adverse effects reported with the cephalosporin class of antibiotics listed under Adverse Effects of cefaclor.

PHARMACOKINETICS AND PHARMACODYNAMICS

Peak serum levels: 39 µg/mL after a 1-g intramuscular dose; 60–87 µg/mL after a 1-g intravenous dose
Plasma half-life: normal renal function, 1.4 to 1.9 h; end-stage renal disease, 25 to 30 h
Bioavailability: percentage not given; achieves therapeutic levels in most body fluids
Metabolism: not metabolized
Excretion: renal; 80% recovered unchanged in urine
Protein binding: 30%
Renal impairment: prolongs half-life and increases serum levels; reduced dosage necessary
Hepatic impairment: no information

OVERDOSAGE

PARENTERAL:
Large doses may cause seizures, particularly in patients with renal impairment. Dosage should be reduced when renal function is compromised. If seizures occur, discontinue drug immediately and use anticonvulsant therapy if indicated. In cases of extreme overdosage, hemodialysis may be considered.

AVAILABILITY

500 mg in 10-mL (single-dose) vials
1 g and 2 g in 20-mL (single-dose) vials
1 g and 2 g in 50-mL and 100-mL (single-dose, piggyback) vials
10 g in 100-mL vial (pharmacy bulk package)

The information here is provided as guidance only. Prescribers should always consult the manufacturer's current prescribing information.

CEFTRIAXONE (Rocephin®)

Ceftriaxone is a third-generation cephalosporin with a prolonged half-life that allows once or twice daily dosing. Ceftriaxone is active against gram-positive bacteria, including *Staphylococcus aureus*, streptococci, and anaerobic gram-positive bacteria. It is very active against *Neisseria meningitidis* and beta-lactamase–producing strains of *Neisseria gonorrhoeae*, *Haemophilus influenzae*, and gram-negative aerobic bacilli with less activity against *Pseudomonas aeruginosa*.

The half-life is 6 to 8 hours, and dose adjustment is usually unnecessary in patients with renal failure because it is mainly excreted in the bile. Ceftriaxone is the drug of choice to treat bacterial meningitis in children and adults. In geographic areas where highly penicillin-resistant pneumococci have been encountered, it is prudent to administer ceftriaxone with vancomycin or rifampin. The drug is useful in treating hospital-acquired infections where pseudomonas infections are unlikely. It has been used to treat a variety of infections in the outpatient setting, including skin and soft-tissue infections, Lyme disease, endocarditis, and osteomyelitis. It is the drug of choice for the treatment of urethral, anorectal, and pharyngeal gonorrhea.

A cholecystitis-like syndrome has been observed infrequently and is believed to be caused by formation of biliary sludge. Other side effects are similar to those of other cephalosporins.

ANTIMICROBIAL ACTIVITY

Gram-positive: Staphylococci (coagulase-positive, coagulase-negative, and penicillinase-producing), beta-hemolytic streptococci, *Streptococcus pneumoniae*, viridans group streptococci.
Gram-negative: *Enterobacter* spp, *Escherichia coli*, *H. influenzae* (including some beta-lactamase–producing strains), *Haemophilus parainfluenzae*, *Klebsiella* spp, *Morganella (Proteus) morganii*, *N. gonorrhoeae* (including penicillinase- and non-penicillinase-producing strains), *N. meningitidis*, *Proteus mirabilis*, *Proteus vulgaris*, *Serratia marcescens*, *Acinetobacter calcoaceticus*.
Anaerobic: *Bacteroides* spp, *Peptostreptococcus*.
Demonstrated *in vitro* activity against *Citrobacter* spp, *Providencia* spp, *Providencia rettgeri*, *Salmonella* spp, *Salmonella typhi*, *Shigella* spp, *Fusobacterium* spp, *Peptococcus* spp, *Peptostreptococcus* spp, *Bacteroides fragilis*, *Clostridium* spp.

RESISTANCE

Inducible resistance has been reported when using the cephalosporins in the treatment of *Enterobacter* infections. Generally ineffective in the treatment of methicillin-resistant *S. aureus* and methicillin-resistant coagulase-negative staphylococci.
Generally ineffective in the treatment of highly penicillin-resistant *S. pneumoniae*.

SPECIAL PRECAUTIONS

Use caution in patients with both renal and hepatic impairment. Careful observation and laboratory studies should be made; if evidence of accumulation exists, reduce dosage or prolong dosage intervals accordingly.
There have been rare cases in which sonographic abnormalities have been seen in the gallbladder of patients treated with ceftriaxone; such patients also may have evidence of gallbladder disease. Therapy should be discontinued in patients who develop signs suggestive of gallbladder disease or who demonstrate abnormal sonographic material.

(Continued on next page)

INDICATIONS

Used in the treatment of infections of the following organ systems, due to susceptible strains of designated microorganisms:
Lower respiratory tract:
S. pneumoniae, *S. aureus*, *H. influenzae*, *H. parainfluenzae*, *Klebsiella pneumoniae*, *E. coli*, *Enterobacter aerogenes*, *P. mirabilis* or *Serratia marcescens*
Skin–skin structure infections:
S. aureus, *Staphylococcus epidermidis*, *Streptococcus pyogenes*, viridans group streptococci, *E. coli*, *Enterobacter cloacae*, *Klebsiella oxytoca*, *Klebsiella pneumoniae*, *P. mirabilis*, *M. morganii**, *S. marcescens*, *Acinetobacter calcoaceticus*, *B. fragilis**, or *Peptostreptococcus* spp
Urinary tract (complicated and uncomplicated):
E. coli, *P. mirabilis*, *P. vulgaris*, *M. morganii* or *K. pneumoniae*
Gonorrhea (cervical, urethral, or rectal, uncomplicated):
N. gonorrhoeae (including both penicillinase- and nonpenicillinase-producing strains). Also effective in treating pharyngeal gonorrhea caused by nonpenicillinase-producing strains of *N. gonorrhoeae*
Bone and joint:
S. aureus, *S. pneumoniae*, *E. coli*, *P. mirabilis*, *K. pneumoniae* or *Enterobacter* spp
Intra-abdominal infections:
E. coli, *K. pneumoniae*, *B. fragilis*, *Clostridium* spp (Note: Most strains of *Clostridium difficile* are resistant), or *Peptostreptococcus* spp
Pelvic inflammatory disease:
caused by *N. gonorrhoeae*
Bacterial septicemia:
S. aureus, *S. pneumoniae*, *E. coli*, *H. influenzae*, or *K. pneumoniae*
Meningitis:
H. influenzae, *N. meningitidis*, or *S. pneumoniae*. Also used successfully in a limited number of patients with meningitis and shunt infection due to *S. epidermidis** and *E. coli**
Perioperative prophylaxis:
Lyme disease—in patients that have failed to respond to standard treatment (unlabeled use)
*Efficacy for this organism in this organ system studied in fewer than 10 cases.

CONTRAINDICATIONS

Allergy or hypersensitivity to cephalosporins

INTERACTIONS

Ceftriaxone and the aminoglycosides may have synergistic antibacterial activity against certain organisms

ADVERSE EFFECTS

Hematologic: eosinophilia, thrombocytosis, leukopenia
Hepatic: elevation of AST, ALT
Other: diarrhea, local reactions
Hypersensitivity: rash
See the adverse effects reported with the cephalosporin class of antibiotics listed under Adverse Effects of cefaclor.

The information here is provided as guidance only. Prescribers should always consult the manufacturer's current prescribing information.

CEFTRIAXONE (CONTINUED)

SPECIAL PRECAUTIONS *(CONTINUED)*

Use caution when administering cephalosporins to patients with sensitivity to penicillin; possible cross-allergenicity and risk of allergic or anaphylactic reaction. If an allergic reaction occurs, discontinue drug. Serious reactions may require epinephrine or other emergency measures (including oxygen, intravenous fluids, intravenous antihistamines, corticosteroids, pressor amines, and airway management).

Use caution when administering broad-spectrum antibiotics to patients with existing or previous gastrointestinal disease. Treatment with broad-spectrum antibiotics alters normal flora of the colon and may permit overgrowth of clostridia, causing antibiotic-associated pseudomembranous colitis. Mild cases usually respond to discontinuation of therapy alone; management of moderate to severe cases should include bacteriologic studies and fluid, electrolyte, and protein supplementation.

False-positive reaction for glucose in urine may occur with copper-reduction tests (Benedicts' or Fehling's solution) but not with enzyme-based tests for glycosuria. False-negative results may occur with the ferricyanide test. Glucose oxidase or hexokinase methods are recommended to determine blood plasma glucose levels. Concomitant administration of aminoglycosides and other cephalosporins has caused nephrotoxicity.

Bacterial or fungal overgrowth of nonsusceptible organisms, leading to secondary infection, may occur with prolonged or repeated therapy.

SPECIAL GROUPS

Children: Do not administer to hyperbilirubinemic neonates, especially premature infants.

Elderly: No specific restrictions.

Renal impairment: Dosage reduction necessary only in cases of concurrent hepatic impairment.

Hepatic impairment: Dosage reduction necessary only in cases of concurrent renal impairment.

Pregnancy: Adequate human studies not performed; pregnancy Category B; the cephalosporins appear safe for use in pregnancy, but few controlled trials have been done.

Breast-feeding: Use caution; low concentrations excreted in breast milk.

DOSAGE

Adults: 1 to 2 g/d intravenously or intramuscularly, in single or divided doses. Do not exceed 4 g/d. For uncomplicated gonococcal infections, a single 250-mg intramuscular dose is recommended. For surgical prophylaxis, a single 1-g intravenous or intramuscular dose is recommended 0.5 to 1 hour prior to surgery.

Elderly: Same as adults.

Children: Serious infections other than meningitis, 50 to 75 mg/kg/d in divided doses every 12 hours. For skin–skin structure infections, 50 to 75 mg/kg/d in single or divided doses. Do not exceed 2 g/d.

In therapeutic treatment of meningitis, initial recommended dose is 100 mg/kg intravenously or intramuscularly; thereafter, a total daily dose of 100 mg/kg intravenously or intramuscularly may be given in single or divided doses. Do not exceed 4 g/d. Usual duration of therapy is 7 to 14 days; in cases of infection due to *Streptococcus pyogenes*, continue therapy for at least 10 days.

Impaired renal function: Dosage reduction is not necessary with impaired renal function alone; however, careful monitoring of blood levels is recommended in patients with severe renal impairment and in those with both renal and hepatic impairment.

PHARMACOKINETICS AND PHARMACODYNAMICS

Peak serum levels: 151 µg/mL 1 h after a 1-g intravenous dose

Plasma half-life: normal renal function, 5.8 to 8.7 h; end-stage renal disease, 15.7 h

Bioavailability: widely distributed

Metabolism: metabolized to inactive metabolites (small extent)

Excretion: renal and nonrenal mechanisms, 33% to 67% excreted unchanged in urine; remainder excreted in bile

Protein binding: 85% to 95%

Renal impairment: no adjustment necessary*

Hepatic impairment: no dosage adjustment necessary*

*In patients with both renal and hepatic failure, dosage should not exceed 2 g/d without careful monitoring of serum concentrations.

OVERDOSAGE

PARENTERAL:

Large doses may cause seizures, particularly in patients with renal impairment. Dosage should be reduced when renal function is compromised. If seizures occur, discontinue drug immediately and use anticonvulsant therapy if indicated. In cases of extreme overdosage, hemodialysis may be considered.

AVAILABILITY

250-mg, 500-mg, 1-g, and 2-g vials
1-g and 2-g piggyback bottles
10-g bulk pharmacy containers
Premixed solution (frozen)
1 g and 2 g in 50-mL containers (with 1.9 g and 1.2 Dextrose Hydrous USP, respectively)

The information here is provided as guidance only. Prescribers should always consult the manufacturer's current prescribing information.

CEFUROXIME (Kefurox®, Zinacef®)

Cefuroxime is a second-generation cephalosporin with increased stability to beta-lactamases. It has good activity against gram-positive bacteria, including *Staphylococcus aureus, Streptococcus pyogenes, Streptococcus pneumoniae*, and Group B streptococci. It is active against *Neisseria meningitidis* and *Neisseria gonorrhoeae* including many beta-lactamase–producing strains, as well as gram-negative bacilli, such as *Haemophilus influenzae, Escherichia coli*, and *Proteus mirabilis*.

Cefuroxime is available for parenteral administration, and *cefuroxime-axetil*, an ester of the drug, is suitable for oral administration. The half-life is approximately 1.5 hours, and the drug is excreted via the kidneys in an unchanged form. Good levels are achieved in the cerebrospinal fluid in patients with bacterial meningitis following parenteral administration, and cefuroxime also has good penetration into pleural fluid and into middle ear effusions.

Parenteral cefuroxime is indicated in the treatment of community-acquired respiratory tract infections of unknown etiology in children with epiglottitis, *H. influenzae* Type B bacteremia, pneumonia, and meningitis. It is also effective for the treatment of skin and soft-tissue infections, septic arthritis, osteomyelitis, and urinary tract infections caused by susceptible gram-negative aerobic bacilli. Side effects are low in frequency and similar to those of other cephalosporins.

ANTIMICROBIAL ACTIVITY

Gram-positive: Staphylococci (coagulase-positive, coagulase-negative, and penicillinase-producing), beta-hemolytic streptococci, *S. pneumoniae*.
Gram-negative: *Citrobacter* spp (some strains resistant), *Enterobacter* spp (some strains resistant), *E. coli, H. influenzae* (including some beta-lactamase–producing strains), *Klebsiella* spp, *Morganella (Proteus) morganii* (some strains resistant), *N. gonorrhoeae, N. meningitidis, P. mirabilis, Providencia* spp, *Providencia rettgeri, Salmonella* spp, *Shigella* spp.
Anaerobic: *Bacteroides* spp, *Clostridium* spp, *Fusobacterium* spp, *Peptococcus* spp, and *Peptostreptococcus* spp.
Demonstrated *in vitro* activity against *Haemophilus parainfluenzae*, and *Moraxella (Branhamella) catarrhalis*.

RESISTANCE

Generally ineffective against highly penicillin-resistant *S. pneumoniae*. Generally ineffective in the treatment of methicillin-resistant *S. aureus* and methicillin-resistant coagulase-negative staphyloccci. Most strains of *Bacteroides fragilis* and *Clostridium difficile* are resistant to cefuroxime.

SPECIAL PRECAUTIONS

Cefuroxime rarely causes changes in renal function; however, in seriously ill patients (especially those receiving maximum dosage) evaluation of renal status during therapy is recommended.
Use caution when administering cephalosporins to patients with sensitivity to penicillin; possible cross-allergenicity and risk of allergic or anaphylactic reaction. If an allergic reaction occurs, discontinue drug. Serious reactions may require epinephrine or other emergency measures (including oxygen, intravenous fluids, intravenous antihistamines, corticosteroids, pressor amines, and airway management).
Use caution when administering broad-spectrum antibiotics to patients with existing or previous gastrointestinal disease. Treatment with broad-spectrum antibiotics alters normal flora of the colon and may permit overgrowth of clostridia, causing antibiotic-associated pseudomembranous colitis. Mild cases usually respond to discontinuation of therapy alone; management of moderate to severe cases should include bacteriologic studies and fluid, electrolyte, and protein supplementation.

(Continued on next page)

INDICATIONS

Used in the treatment of infections of the following types and organ systems, due to susceptible strains of designated microorganisms:
Lower respiratory tract (including pneumonia):
S. pneumoniae, H. influenzae, (including ampicillin-resistant strains), *Klebsiella* spp, penicillinase- and nonpenicillinase-producing *S. aureus, S. pyogenes*, and *E. coli*
Urinary tract:
E. coli and *Klebsiella* spp
Skin–skin structures infections:
Penicillinase- and nonpenicillinase-producing *S. aureus, S. pyogenes, E. coli, Klebsiella* spp, and *Enterobacter* spp
Septicemia:
Penicillinase- and nonpenicillinase-producing *S. aureus, S. pneumoniae, E. coli, H. influenzae* (including ampicillin-resistant strains), and *Klebsiella* spp
Meningitis:
S. pneumoniae, H. influenzae (including ampicillin-resistant strains), *N. meningitidis*, and penicillinase- and nonpenicillinase-producing *S. aureus*
Gonorrhea (uncomplicated and disseminated):
Penicillinase- and nonpenicillinase-producing *N. gonorrhoeae*
Bone and joint:
Penicillinase- and nonpenicillinase-producing *S. aureus*
Perioperative prophylaxis

CONTRAINDICATIONS

Allergy or hypersensitivity to cephalosporins

INTERACTIONS

Probenecid inhibits the renal excretion of cefuroxime, resulting in prolonged serum concentrations.
Cefuroxime and the aminoglycoside antibiotics may provide additive additive or synergistic antibacterial activity against some organisms.

ADVERSE EFFECTS

Local reactions: thrombophlebitis
Hypersensitivity reactions
See the adverse effects reported with the cephalosporin class of antibiotics listed under Adverse Effects of cefaclor.

PHARMACOKINETICS AND PHARMACODYNAMICS

Peak serum levels: 50 µg/mL and 100 µg/mL after 750-mg and 1.5-g intravenous doses, respectively
Plasma half-life: normal renal function, 1.3 h; end-stage renal disease, 16 to 22 h (after injection only)
Bioavailability: widely distributed (including the cerebrospinal fluid in patients with meningitis)
Metabolism: not significantly metabolized
Excretion: renal; approximately 90% recovered unchanged in the urine over 24 h
Protein binding: 33% to 50%
Renal impairment: reduced dosage necessary
Hepatic impairment: dosage adjustment not necessary

The information here is provided as guidance only. Prescribers should always consult the manufacturer's current prescribing information.

CEFUROXIME (CONTINUED)

SPECIAL PRECAUTIONS *(CONTINUED)*

Positive direct Coomb's tests have been reported with cephalosporin therapy. False-positive reaction for glucose in urine may occur with copper-reduction tests (Benedicts' or Fehling's solution) but not with enzyme-based tests for glycosuria. False-negative results may occur with the ferricyanide test. Glucose oxidase or hexokinase methods are recommended to determine blood plasma glucose levels. Concomitant administration of aminoglycosides and other cephalosporins has caused nephrotoxicity.

Use caution in patients with impaired renal function. Reduce dosage or prolong dosage intervals. Careful observation and laboratory studies should be made. Accumulation of drug levels and prolongation of half-life have been reported in neonates.

SPECIAL GROUPS

Children: Safety and efficacy not established for infants younger than 3 months of age.
Elderly: May have age-related renal impairment.
Renal impairment: Reduced dosage necessary.
Hepatic impairment: Dose reduction is not necessary.
Pregnancy: Adequate human studies not performed; pregnancy Category B; the cephalosporins appear safe in pregnancy, but few controlled trials have been done.
Breast-feeding: Use caution; excreted in breast milk.

DOSAGE

Adults: 750 mg to 1.5 g intravenously or intramuscularly every 8 hours, for 5 to 10 days. In life-threatening infections or infections due to less susceptible organisms, 1.5 g every 6 hours may be necessary. In bacterial meningitis, do not exceed 3 g every 8 hours. For uncomplicated gonorrhea, 1.5 g intramuscularly in a single dose (administered at two separate sites) concomitant with 1 g of oral probenecid. As prophylaxis for surgery, 1.5 g intravenously given 0.5 to 1 hour prior to the procedure, and repeat as necessary dependent on the length and type of surgical procedure.
Elderly: Same as adults.
Children: (over 3 months of age) 50 to 100 mg/kg/d in divided doses every 6 to 8 hours. For bone and joint infections, 150 mg/kg/d in divided doses every 8 hours. For bacterial meningitis, initially 200 to 240 mg/kg/d intravenously in divided doses every 6 to 8 hours. In all cases, do not exceed maximum adult dosage.
Impaired renal function: *See* table below.

Adult Cefuroxime Dosage in Renal Impairment

Creatinine clearance, mL/min	Dose and frequency
> 20	Give standard dose
10–20	750 mg every 12 h
< 10	750 mg every 24 h*

Administer dose after dialysis in hemodialysis patients.

OVERDOSAGE

Experience with cefuroxime overdose is limited. Inappropriately large doses of parenteral cephalosporins may cause seizures, especially in the renally impaired. Reduce dosage in patients with impaired renal function. If seizures occur, discontinue drug immediately and administer anticonvulsant therapy. Hemodialysis should be considered in severe cases of overdose.

AVAILABILITY

750 mg in 10-mL vials
1.5 g in 20-mL vials
750 mg and 1.5 g in 100-ml vials
750 mg and 1.5 g in 50-mL piggyback
7.5 g pharmacy bulk vial

The information here is provided as guidance only. Prescribers should always consult the manufacturer's current prescribing information.

CEFUROXIME AXETIL (Ceftin®)

Cefuroxime is a second-generation cephalosporin with increased stability to beta-lactamases. It has good activity against gram-positive bacteria, including *Staphylococcus aureus*, *Streptococcus pyogenes*, *Streptococcus pneumoniae*, and group B streptococci. It is active against *Neisseria meningitidis* and *Neisseria gonorrhoeae* including many beta-lactamase–producing strains, as well as gram-negative bacilli, such as *Haemophilus influenzae*, *Escherichia coli*, and *Proteus mirabilis*.

Cefuroxime is available for parenteral administration, and *cefuroxime-axetil*, an ester of the drug, is suitable for oral administration. The half-life is approximately 1.5 hours, and the drug is excreted via the kidneys in an unchanged form. Good levels are achieved in the cerebrospinal fluid in patients with bacterial meningitis following parenteral administration, and cefuroxime also has good penetration into pleural fluid and into middle ear effusions.

Parenteral cefuroxime is indicated in the treatment of community-acquired respiratory tract infections of unknown etiology in children with epiglottitis, *H. influenzae* Type B bacteremia, pneumonia, and meningitis. It is also effective for the treatment of skin and soft-tissue infections, septic arthritis, osteomyelitis, and urinary tract infections caused by susceptible gram-negative aerobic bacilli. Side effects are low in frequency and similar to those of other cephalosporins.

ANTIMICROBIAL ACTIVITY

Gram-positive: *S. aureus* (including penicillinase-producing), beta-hemolytic streptococci, *S. pneumoniae*.
Gram-negative: *E. coli*, *H. influenzae* (including some beta-lactamase–producing strains), *Klebsiella* spp, *Morganella (Proteus) morganii* (some strains resistant), *N. gonorrhoeae*, *N. meningitidis*, *P. mirabilis*, *Providencia* spp, *Providencia rettgeri*, *Salmonella* spp, *Shigella* spp, *Moraxella catarrhalis*, and *Haemophilus parainfluenzae*. Demonstrated *in vitro* activity against *Citrobacter* spp (some strains resistant), *Enterobacter* spp (some strains resistant), *Bacteroides* spp, *Clostridium* spp, *Fusobacterium* spp, *Peptococcus* spp, and *Peptostreptococcus* spp.

RESISTANCE

Generally ineffective in the treatment of infections caused by methicillin-resistant *S. aureus* and methicillin-resistant coagulase-negative staphylococci. Generally ineffective in the treatment of highly penicillin-resistant *S. pneumoniae*.

SPECIAL PRECAUTIONS

Use caution when administering cephalosporins to patients with sensitivity to penicillin; possible cross-allergenicity and risk of allergic or anaphylactic reaction. If an allergic reaction occurs, discontinue drug. Serious reactions may require epinephrine or other emergency measures (including oxygen, intravenous fluids, intravenous antihistamines, corticosteroids, pressor amines, and airway management).
Use caution when administering broad-spectrum antibiotics to patients with existing or previous gastrointestinal disease. Treatment with broad-spectrum antibiotics alters normal flora of the colon and may permit overgrowth of clostridia, causing antibiotic-associated pseudomembranous colitis. Mild cases usually respond to discontinuation of therapy alone; management of moderate to severe cases should include bacteriologic studies and fluid, electrolyte, and protein supplementation. Positive direct Coomb's tests have been reported with cephalosporin therapy. False-positive reaction for glucose in urine may occur with copper-reduction tests (Benedicts' or Fehling's solution) but not with enzyme-based tests for glycosuria. False-negative results may occur with the ferricyanide test. Glucose oxidase or hexokinase methods are recommended to determine blood plasma glucose levels. Bacterial or fungal overgrowth of nonsusceptible organisms, leading to secondary infection, may occur with prolonged or repeated therapy.

INDICATIONS

Used in the treatment of infections of the following organ systems, due to susceptible strains of designated microorganisms:
Pharyngitis or tonsillitis:
S. pyogenes (Note: Penicillin is the usual drug of choice in the treatment of streptococcal infections, including the prophylaxis of rheumatic fever.)
Otitis media:
S. pneumoniae, *H. influenzae* (ampicillin-susceptible and ampicillin-resistant strains), *M. catarrhalis*, and *S. pyogenes*.
Lower respiratory tract (bronchitis):
S. pneumoniae, *H. influenzae* (ampicillin-susceptible strains), and *H. parainfluenzae* (ampicillin-susceptible strains)
Urinary tract (uncomplicated):
E. coli and *Klebsiella pneumoniae*
Skin–skin structures infections:
S. aureus (including beta-lactamase–producing strains) and *S. pyogenes*
Gonorrhea (urethral and endocervical, uncomplicated):
Nonpenicillinase-producing strains of *N. gonorrhoeae*

CONTRAINDICATIONS

Allergy or hypersensitivity to cephalosporins

INTERACTIONS

Probenecid inhibits the renal excretion of cefuroxime, resulting in prolonged serum concentrations

ADVERSE EFFECTS

Gastrointestinal effects: nausea, vomiting, and diarrhea
Hypersensitivity reactions
See the adverse effects reported with the cephalosporin class of antibiotics listed under Adverse Effects of cefaclor.

PHARMACOKINETICS AND PHARMACODYNAMICS

Peak serum levels: 2.1, 4.1, 7.0, and 13.6 µg/mL after 125-mg, 250-mg, 500-mg, and 1000 doses, respectively (administered after a meal)
Plasma half-life: normal renal function, 1.2 h; elderly with creatinine clearance of 34.9 mL/min, 3.5 h
Bioavailability: 52% when administered with food; widely distributed to extracellular fluids
Metabolism: hydrolyzed by nonspecific esterases to cefuroxime
Excretion: in urine, unchanged
Effect of food: increases absorption
Protein binding: 50%
Renal impairment: no specific recommendations available
Hepatic impairment: no dosage adjustment necessary

The information here is provided as guidance only. Prescribers should always consult the manufacturer's current prescribing information.

CEFUROXIME AXETIL (CONTINUED)

SPECIAL GROUPS

Children: Tablets generally well tolerated if swallowed whole (crushed tablet has strong, persistently bitter taste).
Elderly: No clinically important differences observed.
Renal impairment: Half-life prolonged.
Hepatic impairment: Dose reduction not necessary.
Pregnancy: Adequate human studies not performed; pregnancy Category B; the cephalosporins appear safe in pregnancy, but few controlled trials have been done.
Breast-feeding: Excreted in breast milk; use caution.

DOSAGE

Adults: 250 mg twice a day; dosage may be increased up to 500 mg twice a day in more severe infections or infections due to less susceptible organisms. For gonorrhea (uncomplicated urethral or endocervical), 1 g in a single oral dose. For uncomplicated urinary tract infections, 125 mg twice a day is the recommended dose.
Elderly: Same as adults.
Children: Tablets (children who can swallow whole tabelts): For acute otitis media, 250 mg twice a day. For pharyngitis or tonsillitis, 125 mg twice a day. Suspension (3 months to 12 years): For otitis media and impetigo the dose is 30 mg/kg/d every 12 hours. For pharyngitis or tonsillitis, the dose 20 mg/kg/d divided every 12 hours.
Impaired renal function: No specific dosage reduction is recommended; the half-life of cefuroxime is prolonged in patients with renal failure.

OVERDOSAGE

ORAL:
Symptoms may include nausea, vomiting, epigastric distress, and diarrhea. Unless five times the normal dose has been ingested, gastrointestinal decontamination is not necessary. Always consider possibility of multiple drug overdoses, drug interactions, and unusual drug kinetics. Absorption may be inhibited by administration of activated charcoal. Otherwise, ensure patient's airway and support ventilation, monitor and maintain vital signs, blood gases, serum electrolytes, and so forth. Hemodialysis, peritoneal dialysis, forced diuresis, or charcoal hemoperfusion have not been established as beneficial.

PATIENT INFORMATION

Complete full course of therapy. Contact physician if nausea, vomiting, or diarrhea occurs. The tablet should be swallowed whole; if crushed the tablet has a strong persistent bitter taste. Absorption of the tablet is enhanced if administered with food. The suspension should be administered with food. Shake the suspension well before use; may be stored in the refrigerator or at room temperature. Discard the unused portion of the suspension after 10 days.

AVAILABILITY

Tablets—125 mg, 250 mg, and 500 mg
Suspension—125 mg/5 mL

The information here is provided as guidance only. Prescribers should always consult the manufacturer's current prescribing information.

CEPHALEXIN (Biocef®, Keflet®, Keflex®, Keftab®)

Cephalexin is a first-generation cephalosporin available for oral administration. It has good activity against *Staphylococcus aureus, Streptococcus pyogenes, Streptococcus viridans* and *Streptococcus pneumoniae*. Some strains of *Klebsiella, Proteus* spp, and *Escherichia coli* are inhibited by cephalexin. Gram-negative and gram-positive anaerobic bacteria from the oropharynx (*Peptococcus, Peptostreptococcus, Fusobacterium*) are usually sensitive.

Cephalexin is almost completely absorbed. Food delays absorption but the drug is not absorbed in patients with achlorhydria. The half-life is 0.9 hours. The drug is mainly excreted in the urine, but some is excreted in the bile. Dose adjustment is necessary, in particular in patients with renal failure.

Cephalexin has been used in patients with upper respiratory infections, including otitis media, pharyngitis, bronchitis, and pneumonia secondary to *S. pneumoniae* infection but not to *Haemophilus influenzae* infection. Other uses include skin, soft-tissue, and urinary tract infections. Hypersensitivity reactions and gastrointestinal side effects can occur.

ANTIMICROBIAL ACTIVITY

Gram-positive: Staphylococci (coagulase-positive, coagulase-negative, and penicillinase-producing; some strains resistant), beta-hemolytic streptococci, *S. pneumoniae*.
Gram-negative: *E. coli, Klebsiella* spp, *Proteus mirabilis*.
Demonstrated *in vitro* activity against *Moraxella (Branhamella) catarrhalis; Peptococcus, Peptostreptococcus*, and *Fusobacterium* are usually sensitive.

RESISTANCE

Generally ineffective in the treatment of methicillin-resistant *S. aureus* and methicillin-resistant coagulase-negative staphylococci. Generally ineffective in the treatment of highly penicillin-resistant *S. pneumoniae*.

SPECIAL PRECAUTIONS

Use caution when administering cephalosporins to patients with sensitivity to penicillin; possible cross-allergenicity and risk of allergic or anaphylactic reaction. If an allergic reaction occurs, discontinue drug. Serious reactions may require epinephrine or other emergency measures (including oxygen, intravenous fluids, intravenous antihistamines, corticosteroids, pressor amines, and airway management).
Use caution when administering broad-spectrum antibiotics to patients with existing or previous gastrointestinal disease. Treatment with broad-spectrum antibiotics alters normal flora of the colon and may permit overgrowth of clostridia, causing antibiotic-associated pseudomembranous colitis. Mild cases usually respond to discontinuation of therapy alone; management of moderate to severe cases should include bacteriologic studies and fluid, electrolyte, and protein supplementation.
Positive direct Coomb's tests have been reported with cephalosporin therapy.
Use caution in patients with impaired renal function. Reduce dosage or prolong dosage intervals. Careful observation and laboratory studies should be made.
Bacterial or fungal overgrowth of nonsusceptible organisms, leading to secondary infection, may occur with prolonged or repeated therapy.
False-positive reaction for glucose in urine may occur with copper-reduction tests (Benedicts' or Fehling's solution) but not with enzyme-based tests for glycosuria. False-negative results may occur with the ferricyanide test. Glucose oxidase or hexokinase methods are recommended to determine blood plasma glucose levels.

INDICATIONS

Used in the treatment of infections of the following organ systems, due to susceptible strains of designated microorganisms:
Respiratory tract:
S. pneumoniae and *S. pyogenes* (Note: Penicillin is the usual drug of choice for treatment of streptococcal infections, including the prophylaxis of rheumatic fever.)
Otitis media:
S. pneumoniae, staphylococci, streptococci, and *M. catarrhalis*
Skin–skin structure infections:
Staphylococci or streptococci
Bone and joint:
Staphylococci or *P. mirabilis*
Genitourinary (including acute prostatitis):
E. coli, P. mirabilis, Klebsiella pneumoniae

CONTRAINDICATIONS

Allergy or hypersensitivity to cephalosporins

INTERACTIONS

Probenecid may inhibit the renal excretion of cephalexin, resulting in prolonged serum concentrations

ADVERSE EFFECTS

Diarrhea is the most frequently reported adverse effect; cholestatic jaundice and transient hepatitis have been reported rarely
Hypersensitivity reactions such as rash, urticaria, and angioedema have been reported
See the adverse effects reported with the cephalosporin class of antibiotics listed under Adverse Effects of cefaclor.

PHARMACOKINETICS AND PHARMACODYNAMICS

Peak serum levels: 9 µg/mL, 18 µg/mL, and 32 µg/mL following 250-, 500-mg, and 1-g doses, respectively
Plasma half-life: normal renal function, 0.8 to 1.3 h; end-stage renal disease, 19 to 22 h
Bioavailability: rapidly absorbed after oral administration
Metabolism: not metabolized
Excretion: renal, more than 90% recovered unchanged in the urine
Effect of food: may be given without regard to meals
Protein binding: 10%
Renal impairment: reduced dosage or prolonged dosage intervals may be necessary
Hepatic impairment: no information

The information here is provided as guidance only. Prescribers should always consult the manufacturer's current prescribing information.

CEPHALEXIN (CONTINUED)

SPECIAL GROUPS

Children: Cephalexin monohydrate is safe for use in children; safety of the cephalexin HCl monohydrate formulation has not been established in children.
Elderly: May have age-related renal impairment requiring reduced dosage.
Renal impairment: Reduced dosage or prolonged dosage intervals may be necessary.
Hepatic impairment: No information.
Pregnancy: Pregnancy Category B; the cephalosporins appear to be safe for use in pregnancy, but few controlled studies have been done.
Breast-feeding: Use caution; excreted in breast milk.

DOSAGE

Adults: 1 to 4 g/d in divided doses; usually 250 mg every 6 hours. For streptococcal pharyngitis, skin–skin structure infections, and uncomplicated cystitis in patients over 15 years of age, 500 mg every 12 hours may be used. (Note: Therapy for cystitis should continue for 7 to 14 days.) For more severe infections, larger doses may be necessary; however, if more than 4 g/d of cephalexin is required, an alternative, parenteral cephalosporin antibiotic is indicated.
Elderly: Same as adults.
Children: 25 to 50 mg/kg/d in divided doses. For severe infections, the dose may be doubled. For streptococcal pharyngitis in patients over 1 year of age or skin–skin structure infections, total daily dose may be divided and administered every 12 hours. For otitis media, clinical studies demonstrate that 75 to 100 mg/kg/d in four divided doses is required.
Therapy for beta-hemolytic streptococcal infections should continue for a minimum of 10 days.
Impaired renal function: Administer an initial loading dose of 250 mg to 1 g and then a maintenance dosage as follows:

Adult Cephalexin Dosage in Renal Impairment

Creatinine clearance, *mL/min*	Dosage
0–10	250 mg every 12 to 24 h
11–40	500 mg every 8 to 12 h
> 40	No adjustment

OVERDOSAGE

ORAL:
Symptoms may include nausea, vomiting, epigastric distress, and diarrhea. Unless five times the normal dose has been ingested, gastrointestinal decontamination is not necessary. Always consider possibility of multiple drug overdoses, drug interactions, and unusual drug kinetics. Absorption may be inhibited by administration of activated charcoal. Otherwise, ensure patient's airway and support ventilation, monitor and maintain vital signs, blood gases, serum electrolytes, and so forth. Hemodialysis, peritoneal dialysis, forced diuresis, or charcoal hemoperfusion have not been established as beneficial.

PATIENT INFORMATION

Complete full course of therapy. Contact physician if nausea, vomiting, or diarrhea occurs. Refrigerate the suspension, shake well before use, and discard the unused portion after 14 days.

AVAILABILITY

Cephalexin monohydrate Oral Suspension—125 mg in 5 mL, 250 mg in 5 mL and 100 mg/mL
Capsules—250 mg and 500 mg
Tablets—250 mg, 500 mg, and 1 g
Cephalexin HCl monohydrate tablets—250 mg and 500 mg

The information here is provided as guidance only. Prescribers should always consult the manufacturer's current prescribing information.

CEPHALOTHIN (Keflin®)

Cephalothin sodium is a first-generation, semisynthetic cephalosporin antibiotic for parenteral use.

ANTIMICROBIAL ACTIVITY

Gram-positive: Staphylococci (coagulase-positive, coagulase-negative, and penicillinase-producing), beta-hemolytic streptococci, *Streptococcus pneumoniae*.
Gram-negative: *Escherichia coli, Klebsiella* spp, *Proteus mirabilis, Salmonella* spp, *Shigella* spp.

RESISTANCE

Generally not effective in the treatment of methicillin-resistant *Staphylococcus aureus* and methicillin-resistant coagulase-negative staphylococci. Generally ineffective in the treatment of highly penicillin-resistant *S. pneumoniae*.

SPECIAL PRECAUTIONS

High concentrations may interfere with determination of creatinine levels by the Jaffé reaction, producing false results. Serum samples obtained within 2 hours of administration should not be analyzed for creatinine.
Use caution when administering cephalosporins to patients with sensitivity to penicillin; possible cross-allergenicity and risk of allergic or anaphylactic reaction. If an allergic reaction occurs, discontinue drug. Serious reactions may require epinephrine or other emergency measures (including oxygen, intravenous fluids, intravenous antihistamines, corticosteroids, pressor amines, and airway management).
Use caution when administering broad-spectrum antibiotics to patients with existing or previous gastrointestinal disease. Treatment with broad-spectrum antibiotics alters normal flora of the colon and may permit overgrowth of clostridia, causing antibiotic-associated pseudomembranous colitis. Mild cases usually respond to discontinuation of therapy alone; management of moderate to severe cases should include bacteriologic studies and fluid, electrolyte, and protein supplementation.
Positive direct Coomb's tests have been reported with cephalosporin therapy.
False-positive reaction for glucose in urine may occur with copper-reduction tests (Benedicts' or Fehling's solution) but not with enzyme-based tests for glycosuria. False-negative results may occur with the ferricyanide test. Glucose oxidase or hexokinase methods are recommended to determine blood plasma glucose levels.
Use caution in patients with impaired renal function. Reduce dosage or prolong dosage intervals. Careful observation and laboratory studies should be made.
Bacterial or fungal overgrowth of nonsusceptible organisms, leading to secondary infection, may occur with prolonged or repeated therapy.

SPECIAL GROUPS

Children: Safe for use in children.
Elderly: Same as adults.
Renal impairment: Reduced dosage necessary.
Hepatic impairment: No information.
Pregnancy: Pregnancy Category B; cephalosporins appear to be safe for use in pregnancy, but few controlled trials have been done.
Breast-feeding: Use caution; excreted in low concentration.

INDICATIONS

Used in the treatment of infections of the following organ systems, due to susceptible strains of designated microorganisms:
Respiratory tract:
S. pneumoniae, staphylococci (penicillinase- and nonpenicillinase-producing strains), Group A beta-hemolytic streptococci, *Klebsiella* spp
Skin and soft tissue (including peritonitis):
Staphylococci (penicillinase- and nonpenicillinase-producing strains), Group A beta-hemolytic streptococci, *E. coli, P. mirabilis*, and *Klebsiella* spp
Genitourinary tract:
E. coli, P. mirabilis, and *Klebsiella* spp
Septicemia (including endocarditis):
S. pneumoniae, Staphylococcus aureus (penicillinase- and nonpenicillinase-producing strains), Group A beta-hemolytic streptococci, *Streptococcus viridans, E. coli, P. mirabilis*, and *Klebsiella* spp.
Gastrointestinal:
Salmonella and *Shigella* spp
Meningitis:
S. pneumoniae, staphylococci (penicillinase- and nonpenicillinase-producing strains), Group A beta-hemolytic streptococci (Note: Due to the fact that only low drug levels are found in cerebrospinal fluid, cephalothin is not reliable for treatment of meningitis. Cephalothin has been effective in limited cases of meningitis, however, and may be considered for use in unusual situations, in which more effective antibiotics cannot be used.)
Bone and joint:
Staphylococci (penicillinase- and nonpenicillinase-producing)
Perioperative prophylaxis:
To minimize the incidence of postoperative infections in patients undergoing contaminated or potentially contaminated surgeries or in patients undergoing procedures in which infection at the surgical site would present serious danger

CONTRAINDICATIONS

Allergy or hypersensitivity to cephalosporins

INTERACTIONS

Probenecid inhibits the renal excretion of cephalothin, resulting in prolonged serum concentrations.
Cephalothin may provide additive or synergistic antibacterial activity when used in combination with an aminoglycoside for some organisms.

The information here is provided as guidance only. Prescribers should always consult the manufacturer's current prescribing information.

CEPHALOTHIN (CONTINUED)

DOSAGE

Adults: 500 mg to 1 g intravenously or intramuscularly every 4 to 6 hours. For severe infections, 500 mg to 1 g every 4 hours. For life-threatening infections, up to 2 g every 4 hours.

For bacteremia or septicemia or other severe or life-threatening infections, 4 to 12 g/d intravenously (for septicemia, 6 to 8 g/d intravenously for first several days, then decrease gradually). For perioperative prophylaxis, 1 to 2 g 0.5 to 1 hour prior to initial incision, and repeat as necessary, dependent on the length and type of surgical procedure.

Elderly: Same as adults.

Children: 80 to 160 mg/kg/d in divided doses. For perioperative prophylaxis, 20 to 30 mg/kg 0.5 to 1 hour prior to initial incision, and repeat as necessary dependent on the length and type of surgical procedure.

Impaired renal function: After an initial dose of 1 to 2 g, administer a maintenance dose as follows:

Adult Cephalothin Dosage in Renal Impairment

Creatinine clearance, mL/min	Adult dosage
50–80	Up to 2 g every 6 h
25–50	Up to 1.5 g every 6 h
10–25	Up to 1 g every 6 h
2–10	Up to 0.5 g every 6 h
< 2	Up to 0.5 g every 8 h

ADVERSE EFFECTS

Hypersensitivity reactions (*eg*, rash, urticaria, Stevens-Johnson syndrome)

See the adverse effects reported with the cephalosporin class of antibiotics listed under Adverse Effects of cefaclor.

PHARMACOKINETICS AND PHARMACODYNAMICS

Peak serum levels: 30 µg/mL after a 1-g intravenous dose

Plasma half-life: normal renal function, 30 to 50 m; end-stage renal disease, 3 to 15 h

Bioavailability: widely distributed

Metabolism: partially metabolized in the liver and kidneys

Excretion: renal, approximately 70% recovered unchanged in the urine

Protein binding: 70%

Renal impairment: reduced dosage necessary

Hepatic impairment: no information

OVERDOSAGE

PARENTERAL:

Large doses may cause seizures, particularly in patients with renal impairment. Dosage should be reduced when renal function is compromised. If seizures occur, discontinue drug immediately and use anti-convulsant therapy if indicated. In cases of extreme overdosage, hemodialysis may be considered.

AVAILABILITY

Injection—1 g and 2 g in 50-mL single-dose containers (premixed, frozen)

Powder for injection—1-g and 2-g vials and piggy-back vials

Powder for injection—20-g bulk pharmacy vial

The information here is provided as guidance only. Prescribers should always consult the manufacturer's current prescribing information.

CEPHAPIRIN (Cefadyl®)

Cephapirin is a parenteral first-generation cephalosporin with good activity against *Staphylococcus aureus*, streptococci, and gram-positive bacilli, including anaerobes (such as *Clostridium perfringens, Clostridium tetani*, and other *Clostridium*). It is not active against beta-lactamase–producing strains of gonorrhea or other Enterobacteriaceae. *Haemophilus influenzae* strains also are sensitive.

The serum half-life is 0.3 hours. The drug is metabolized in the liver by deacetylation and is rapidly excreted by the kidneys. The drug is inactivated in the body, and dose adjustments are needed only in patients with severe renal impairment. Cephapirin has very poor penetration into the cerebrospinal fluid, even in patients with bacterial meningitis. The drug has been used for the treatment of skin infections due to *Streptococcus pyogenes* and *Staphylococcus aureus* and urinary tract infections. Eosinophilia and serum sickness–like reactions have occurred.

ANTIMICROBIAL ACTIVITY

Gram-positive: Staphylococci (coagulase-positive, coagulase-negative, and penicillinase-producing), beta-hemolytic streptococci, *Streptococcus pneumoniae*.
Gram-negative: *Escherichia coli, H. influenzae, Klebsiella* spp, *Proteus mirabilis*.

RESISTANCE

Generally not effective in the treatment of methicillin-resistant *S. aureus* and methicillin-resistant coagulase-negative staphylococci. Generally ineffective in the treatment of highly penicillin-resistant *S. pneumoniae*.

SPECIAL PRECAUTIONS

Use caution when administering cephalosporins to patients with sensitivity to penicillin; possible cross-allergenicity and risk of allergic or anaphylactic reaction. If an allergic reaction occurs, discontinue drug. Serious reactions may require epinephrine or other emergency measures (including oxygen, intravenous fluids, intravenous antihistamines, corticosteroids, pressor amines, and airway management).
Use caution when administering broad-spectrum antibiotics to patients with existing or previous gastrointestinal disease. Treatment with broad-spectrum antibiotics alters normal flora of the colon and may permit overgrowth of clostridia, causing antibiotic-associated pseudomembranous colitis. Mild cases usually respond to discontinuation of therapy alone; management of moderate to severe cases should include bacteriologic studies and fluid, electrolyte, and protein supplementation. Positive direct Coomb's tests have been reported with cephalosporin therapy. False-positive reaction for glucose in urine may occur with copper-reduction tests (Benedicts' or Fehling's solution) but not with enzyme-based tests for glycosuria. False-negative results may occur with the ferricyanide test. Glucose oxidase or hexokinase methods are recommended to determine blood plasma glucose levels. Use caution in patients with impaired renal function. Reduce dosage or prolong dosage intervals. Careful observation and laboratory studies should be made. Bacterial or fungal overgrowth of nonsusceptible organisms, leading to secondary infection, may occur with prolonged or repeated therapy.

SPECIAL GROUPS

Children: Safety and efficacy in children under 3 months of age have not been established.
Elderly: May have age-related renal impairment.
Renal impairment: Reduced dosage recommended.
Hepatic impairment: No information.
Pregnancy: Probably safe; use only when clearly indicated; pregnancy Category B.
Breast-feeding: Use caution; excreted in breast milk.

INDICATIONS

Infections of the following types due to designated organisms:
Respiratory tract:
S. pneumoniae, S. aureus (penicillinase- and nonpenicillinase-producing), *Klebsiella* spp, *H. influenzae*, and Group A beta-hemolytic streptococci
Skin–skin structure infections:
S. aureus (penicillinase- and nonpenicillinase-producing), *Staphylococcus epidermidis* (methicillin-susceptible strains), *E. coli, P. mirabilis, Klebsiella* spp, and Group A beta-hemolytic streptococci
Urinary tract:
S. aureus (penicillinase- and nonpenicillinase-producing), *E. coli, P. mirabilis*, and *Klebsiella* spp
Septicemia:
S. aureus (penicillinase- and nonpenicillinase-producing), *Streptococcus viridans, E. coli, Klebsiella* spp, and Group A beta-hemolytic streptococci
Endocarditis:
S. viridans and *S. aureus* (penicillinase- and nonpenicillinase-producing)
Osteomyelitis:
S. aureus (penicillinase- and nonpenicillinase-producing), *Klebsiella* spp, *P. mirabilis*, and Group A beta-hemolytic streptococci
Perioperative prophylaxis

CONTRAINDICATIONS

Allergy or hypersensitivity to cephalosporins

INTERACTIONS

Probenecid inhibits the renal excretion of cephaprin, resulting in prolonged serum concentrations

ADVERSE EFFECTS

Eosinophilia and serum sickness–like reactions have occurred
See the adverse effects reported with the cephalosporin class of antibiotics listed under Adverse Effects of cefaclor.

PHARMACOKINETICS AND PHARMACODYNAMICS

Peak serum levels: 73 µg/mL after a 1-g intravenous dose
Plasma half-life: normal renal function, 24 to 36 min; end-stage renal disease, 1.8 to 4 h
Bioavailability: widely distributed
Metabolism: partially metabolized in the liver
Excretion: renal, 68% to 70% recovered unchanged in the urine
Protein binding: 54%
Renal impairment: reduced dosage necessary
Hepatic impairment: no information

The information here is provided as guidance only. Prescribers should always consult the manufacturer's current prescribing information.

CEPHAPIRIN (CONTINUED)

DOSAGE

Adults: 500 mg to 1 g every 4 to 6 hours, intravenously or intramuscularly. Use lower doses for most urinary tract infections and skin–skin structure infections and higher doses for more severe infections. For serious or life-threatening infections up to 12 g/d may be used. Intravenous administration is recommended for higher doses. For peri-operative prophylaxis, 1 to 2 g intramuscularly or intravenously given 0.5 to 1 hour before surgery and repeat as necessary, dependent on the length and type of surgical procedure.

Elderly: Same as adults.

Children: Dosage depends on age, weight, and degree of infection. Total daily dose is 40 to 80 mg/kg given in four divided doses.

Impaired renal function: Relative to causative organisms and degree of infection, doses of 7.5 to 15 mg/kg every 12 hours may be given. Patients undergoing dialysis should receive the same dose immediately before dialysis and every 12 hours thereafter.

OVERDOSAGE

PARENTERAL:

Large doses may cause seizures, particularly in patients with renal impairment. Dosage should be reduced when renal function is compromised. If seizures occur, discontinue drug immediately and use anti-convulsant therapy if indicated. In cases of extreme overdosage, hemodialysis may be considered.

AVAILABILITY

Powder for injection: 500 mg, 1 g, 2 g in 10 mL vials
1 g in 100-mL vials and piggyback vials
2 g in 100-mL vials and piggyback vials
4 g in 100-mL vials and piggyback vials
20 g in 100-mL vials and pharmacy bulk packages

The information here is provided as guidance only. Prescribers should always consult the manufacturer's current prescribing information.

CEPHRADINE

Cephradine is a first-generation cephalosporin available for oral and parenteral administration. It has good activity against gram-positive bacteria, and it is less active against *Escherichia coli*, *Klebsiella*, and *Proteus* spp. The drug is inactive against *Haemophilus influenzae*, but the intrinsic antibacterial activity is less than cefazolin and cephalothin.

The serum half-life is 1 hour. The drug is mainly eliminated by the kidneys, and some is excreted in the bile. Dose reduction is necessary in patients with renal insufficiency. It has a very poor penetration into the cerebrospinal fluid, even with inflamed meninges.

Cephradine has been used in the treatment of skin, soft-tissue, pharyngeal, respiratory, and urinary tract infections. Toxicity due to cephradine is uncommon, but gastrointestinal symptoms can occur.

ANTIMICROBIAL ACTIVITY

Gram-positive: Staphylococci (coagulase-positive, coagulase-negative, and penicillinase-producing), beta-hemolytic streptococci, *Streptococcus pneumoniae*.
Gram-negative: *E. coli*, *Klebsiella* spp, *Proteus mirabilis*.

RESISTANCE

Generally ineffective in the treatment of methicillin-resistant *Staphylococcus aureus* and methicillin-resistant coagulase-negative staphylococci. Generally ineffective in the treatment of highly penicillin-resistant *S. pneumoniae*.

SPECIAL PRECAUTIONS

May cause false-positive reaction in urinary protein tests that use sulfosalicylic acid. Use caution when administering cephalosporins to patients with sensitivity to penicillin; possible cross-allergenicity and risk of allergic or anaphylactic reaction. If an allergic reaction occurs, discontinue drug. Serious reactions may require epinephrine or other emergency measures (including oxygen, intravenous fluids, intravenous antihistamines, corticosteroids, pressor amines, and airway management).
Use caution when administering broad-spectrum antibiotics to patients with existing or previous gastrointestinal disease. Treatment with broad-spectrum antibiotics alters normal flora of the colon and may permit overgrowth of clostridia, causing antibiotic-associated pseudomembranous colitis. Mild cases usually respond to discontinuation of therapy alone; management of moderate to severe cases should include bacteriologic studies and fluid, electrolyte, and protein supplementation. Positive direct Coomb's tests have been reported with cephalosporin therapy. False-positive reaction for glucose in urine may occur with copper-reduction tests (Benedicts' or Fehling's solution) but not with enzyme-based tests for glycosuria. False-negative results may occur with the ferricyanide test. Glucose oxidase or hexokinase methods are recommended to determine blood plasma glucose levels. Use caution in patients with impaired renal function. Reduce dosage or prolong dosage intervals. Careful observation and laboratory studies should be made. Bacterial or fungal overgrowth of nonsusceptible organisms, leading to secondary infection, may occur with prolonged or repeated therapy.

INDICATIONS

Used in the treatment of infections of the following types, due to susceptible strains of designated microorganisms:
ORAL:
Respiratory tract (tonsillitis, pharyngitis, lobar pneumonia):
Group A beta-hemolytic streptococci and *S. pneumoniae*
Otitis media:
Group A beta-hemolytic streptococci, *S. pneumoniae*, and staphylococci
Skin–skin structure infections:
Staphylococci (penicillinase- and nonpenicillinase-producing), and beta-hemolytic streptococci
Urinary tract (including prostatitis):
E. coli, *P. mirabilis*, and *Klebsiella* spp
PARENTERAL:
Respiratory tract:
S. pneumoniae, *Klebsiella* spp, penicillinase- and nonpenicillinase-producing *S. aureus*, and Group A beta-hemolytic streptococci
Urinary tract:
E. coli, *P. mirabilis*, and *Klebsiella* spp
Skin–skin structure infections:
Penicillinase- and nonpenicillinase-producing *S. aureus* and Group A beta-hemolytic streptococci
Bone and joint:
Penicillinase- and nonpenicillinase-producing *S. aureus*
Septicemia:
S. pneumoniae, penicillinase- and nonpenicillinase-producing *S. aureus*, *P. mirabilis*, and *E. coli*
Perioperative prophylaxis:
To reduce the incidence of certain postoperative infections in patients undergoing surgical procedures that are considered to be potentially contaminated

CONTRAINDICATIONS

Allergy or hypersensitivity to cephalosporins

INTERACTIONS

Probenecid inhibits the renal excretion of cephradine, resulting in prolonged serum concentrations

ADVERSE EFFECTS

Gastrointestinal effects: nausea, vomiting, diarrhea
Hypersensitivity reactions:
See the adverse effects reported with the cephalosporin class of antibiotics listed under Adverse Effects of cefaclor.

The information here is provided as guidance only. Prescribers should always consult the manufacturer's current prescribing information.

CEPHRADINE (CONTINUED)

SPECIAL GROUPS

Children: Safety not established for use in children under 1 month of age. Safety for use of oral form not established for children under 9 months of age.
Elderly: May have age-related renal impairment.
Renal impairment: Reduced dosage necessary.
Hepatic impairment: No information.
Pregnancy: Adequate human studies not performed; pregnancy Category B, the cephalosporins appear to be safe for use in pregnancy, but few controlled trials have been done.
Breast-feeding: Use caution; excreted in breast milk.

DOSAGE

Adults: *ORAL:* Skin–skin structure and respiratory tract infections (except lobar pneumonia), 250 mg every 6 hours or 500 mg every 12 hours. For lobar pneumonia, 500 mg every 6 hours or 1 g every 12 hours. For uncomplicated urinary tract infections, 500 mg every 12 hours. For more severe infections or for prostatitis, 500 mg every 6 hours or 1 g every 12 hours. Severe or chronic infections also may require larger doses, up to 1 g every 6 hours.
PARENTERAL: 2 to 4 g/d intravenously or intramuscularly divided equally every 6 hours. For bone infections, 1 g intravenously every 6 hours. For skin–skin structure, uncomplicated pneumonia, and most urinary tract infections, 500 mg intravenously or intramuscularly every 6 hours. For more severe infections, the dose may be increased to every 4 hours or to a maximum of 8 g/d. For cesarean section, administer 1 g intravenously immediately after umbilical cord is clamped. For perioperative prophylaxis, administer 1 g intravenously or intramuscularly 0.5 to 1.5 hours prior to start of surgery and repeat as necessary depending on length and type of surgical procedure.
Elderly: Same as adults; may have age-related renal impairment.
Children: (Note: There are insufficient data on the efficacy of twice-daily regimens in children under 9 months of age.) *ORAL:* For children over 9 months of age, 25 to 50 mg/kg/d divided in equal doses every 6 hours or every 12 hours. Do not exceed 4 gm/d. *PARENTERAL:* 50 to 100 mg/kg/d divided in equal doses every 6 hours. Do not exceed adult dose.
Impaired renal function: *See* table below.

Adult Cephradine Dosage in Renal Impairment

Creatinine clearance, mL/min	Dosage
>20	500 mg every 6 h
5–20	250 mg every 6 h
< 5	250 mg every 12 h

Chronic or intermittent hemodialysis: Initial dose 250 mg, repeat at 12 hours and after 36 to 48 hours.

PHARMACOKINETICS AND PHARMACODYNAMICS

Peak serum levels: 86 µg/mL after a 1-g intravenous dose
Plasma half-life: normal renal function, 0.8 to 1.3 h; end-stage renal disease, 8 to 15 h
Bioavailability: rapidly and almost completely absorbed after oral administration
Metabolism: not metabolized
Excretion: renal, > 90% recovered unchanged in urine
Effect of food: oral therapy may be given without regard to meals
Protein binding: 8% to 17%
Renal impairment: reduced dosage required
Hepatic impairment: no information

OVERDOSAGE

ORAL:
Symptoms may include nausea, vomiting, epigastric distress, and diarrhea. Unless five times the normal dose has been ingested, gastrointestinal decontamination is not necessary. Always consider possibility of multiple drug overdoses, drug interactions, and unusual drug kinetics. Absorption may be inhibited by administration of activated charcoal. Otherwise, ensure patient's airway and support ventilation, monitor and maintain vital signs, blood gases, serum electrolytes, and so forth. Hemodialysis, peritoneal dialysis, forced diuresis, or charcoal hemoperfusion have not been established as beneficial.
PARENTERAL:
Large doses may cause seizures, particularly in patients with renal impairment. Dosage should be reduced when renal function is compromised. If seizures occur, discontinue drug immediately and use anticonvulsant therapy if indicated. In cases of extreme overdosage, hemodialysis may be considered.

PATIENT INFORMATION

Complete full course of therapy. Take medication with food or milk to prevent gastrointestinal upset. Contact physician if nausea, vomiting, or diarrhea occurs. Diabetics should not change diet or dosage of diabetes medication without consent of physician. Shake the suspension well before use. The suspension may be stored at room temperature; discard the unused portion after 14 days.

AVAILABILITY

Capsules—250 mg and 500 mg
Oral suspension—125 mg/5 mL and 250 mg/5mL
Powder for Injection—250-mg, 500-mg, and 1-g vials; and 2 g in 100-mL infusion bottles

The information here is provided as guidance only. Prescribers should always consult the manufacturer's current prescribing information.

LORACARBEF (Lorabid®)

Loracarbef is a carbacephem with antimicrobial activity similar to that of second-generation cephalosporins available for oral administration. It is active against most gram-positive bacteria, including pneumonococci, Group A streptococci, and *Staphylococcus aureus*. It also is active against *Haemophilus influenzae* and *Moraxella catarrhalis*, including most beta-lactamase–producing strains, and most strains of *Escherichia coli*, *Klebsiella*, and *Proteus* spp.

Most of the drug is absorbed from the gastrointestinal tract, and the half-life is approximately 1 hour. It is excreted unchanged in the urine. Loracarbef is used in the treatment of lower respiratory tract infections, including those secondary to beta-lactamase–producing strains of *H. influenzae* and *Bacteroides catarrhalis*, as well as upper respiratory tract infections, otitis media, sinusitis, pharyngitis, tonsillitis, skin and skin structure infections caused by *S. aureus*, and uncomplicated urinary tract infections. Adverse reactions are infrequent.

ANTIMICROBIAL ACTIVITY

Gram-positive: Staphylococci (coagulase-positive, coagulase-negative, and penicillinase-producing), beta-hemolytic streptococci, *Streptococcus pneumoniae*.
Gram-negative: *E. coli*, *H. influenzae* (including some beta-lactamase–producing strains), *M. (Branhamella) catarrhalis* (including some beta-lactamase–producing strains).
Loracarbef also has shown *in vitro* activity against the following: *Haemophilus parainfluenzae*, *Klebsiella* spp, *Neisseria gonorrhoeae* (including penicillinase-producing), *P. mirabilis*, *Salmonella* spp, *Clostridium* spp, *Citrobacter* spp, *Shigella* spp, *Fusobacterium* spp, *Peptococcus* spp, and *Peptostreptococcus* spp.

RESISTANCE

Generally ineffective in the treatment of highly penicillin-resistant *S. pneumoniae*. Generally ineffective in the treatment of methicillin-resistant *S. aureus* and methicillin-resistant coagulase-negative staphylococci.

SPECIAL PRECAUTIONS

Use caution when administering cephalosporins to patients with sensitivity to penicillin; possible cross-allergenicity and risk of allergic or anaphylactic reaction. If an allergic reaction occurs, discontinue drug. Serious reactions may require epinephrine or other emergency measures (including oxygen, intravenous fluids, intravenous antihistamines, corticosteroids, pressor amines, and airway management).
Use caution when administering broad-spectrum antibiotics to patients with existing or previous gastrointestinal disease. Treatment with broad-spectrum antibiotics alters normal flora of the colon and may permit overgrowth of clostridia, causing antibiotic-associated pseudomembranous colitis. Mild cases usually respond to discontinuation of therapy alone; management of moderate to severe cases should include bacteriologic studies and fluid, electrolyte, and protein supplementation.
Use caution in patients with impaired renal function. Reduce dosage or prolong dosage intervals. Careful observation and laboratory studies should be made.
Bacterial or fungal overgrowth of nonsusceptible organisms, leading to secondary infection, may occur with prolonged or repeated therapy.

INDICATIONS

Treatment of infections of the following types due to designated, susceptible organisms:
Lower respiratory tract:
(Secondary bacterial infection of acute bronchitis and acute bacterial infection of chronic bronchitis):
S. pneumoniae, *H. influenzae*, (including beta-lactamase–producing strains), *M. catarrhalis* (including beta-lactamase–producing strains)
(Pneumonia):
S. pneumoniae, *H. influenzae* (non–beta-lactamase–producing strains only)
Upper respiratory tract
(Otitis media):
S. pneumoniae, *H. influenzae* (including beta-lactamase–producing strains), *M. catarrhalis* (including beta-lactamase–producing strains), *S. pyogenes*
(Acute maxillary sinusitis):
S. pneumoniae, *H. influenzae* (non–beta-lactamase–producing strains only), *M. catarrhalis* (including beta-lactamase–producing strains)
(Pharyngitis/tonsillitis):
S. pyogenes
(Note: Intramuscular penicillin is the usual drug of choice.)
Skin–skin structure infections (uncomplicated):
S. aureus (including penicillinase-producing strains), *S. pyogenes*
Urinary tract
(Uncomplicated cystitis):
E. coli, *Staphylococcus saprophyticus* (efficacy in this organ system for this infection studied in less than 10 cases).
(Uncomplicated pyelonephritis):
E. coli

CONTRAINDICATIONS

Allergy or hypersensitivity to loracarbef or cephalosporin class antibiotics

INTERACTIONS

Probenecid inhibits the renal excretion of loracarbef, resulting in prolonged serum concentrations

ADVERSE EFFECTS

Gastrointestinal: diarrhea, nausea, vomiting
Hypersensitivity reactions: skin rashes, urticaria, pruritus
Other: headache
See the adverse effects reported with the cephalosporin class of antibiotics listed under Adverse Effects of cefaclor.

The information here is provided as guidance only. Prescribers should always consult the manufacturer's current prescribing information.

LORACARBEF (CONTINUED)

SPECIAL GROUPS

Children: Safety and efficacy in infants less than 6 months of age have not been established.
Elderly: May have age-related renal impairment requiring dosage adjustment.
Renal impairment: Reduced dosage or prolonged dosage intervals necessary.
Hepatic impairment: No information.
Pregnancy: Pregnancy Category B; the cephalosporins appear safe in pregnancy, but few controlled trials have been done.
Breast-feeding: Unknown whether loracarbef is excreted in human milk; use with caution.

DOSAGE

Adults: (≥ 13 years of age) *See* table below.

Adult Dosage of Loracarbef

Infection	Dosage, *mg*	Duration, *d*
Lower respiratory		
Secondary bacterial infection of acute bronchitis	200–400 every 12 h	7
Acute bacterial exacerbation of chronic bronchitis	400 every 12 h	7
Pneumonia	400 every 12 h	14
Upper respiratory		
Pharyngitis or tonsillitis	200 every 12 h	10*
Sinusitis	400 every 12 h	10
Skin–skin structure infections		
Uncomplicated	200 every 12 h	7
Urinary tract		
Uncomplicated cystitis	200 every 24 h	7
Uncomplicated pyelonephritis	400 every 12 h	14

Continue treatment for minimum of 10 days in infections due to Streptococcus pyogenes.

Elderly: May have age-related renal impairment; otherwise, same as adults.
Children: (For ages 6 months to 12 years) For acute otitis media[†], 30 mg/kg/d in divided doses every 12 hours for 10 days. For pharyngitis or tonsillitis, 15 mg/kg/d in divided doses every 12 hours for 10 days (continue treatment for minimum of 10 days in infections due to *S. pyogenes*). For impetigo, 15 mg/kg/d in divided doses every 12 hours for 7 days.
Renal impairment: Normal dosing may be used in patients with creatinine clearance of 50 mL/min or higher. Patients with clearance between 10 to 49 mL/min should be given half the normal dose at the usual intervals. Patients with clearance below 10 mL/min may receive the usual dose every 3 to 5 days; those on hemodialysis should receive another dose after completing hemodialysis.

[†]Use of suspension is recommended over capsules because of more rapid absorption and subsequent higher peak plasma levels for equal doses.

PHARMACOKINETICS AND PHARMACODYNAMICS

Peak serum levels: 8 and 14 µg/mL 1.2 h after 200-mg and 400-mg doses (capsules), 17 µg/mL 48 min after a 400-mg dose of suspension
Serum half-life: 1 h (normal renal function), 32 h (end-stage renal disease)
Bioavailability: 90% absorbed (approximately)
Protein binding: 25%
Metabolism: no information
Excretion: > 90% unchanged in urine
Renal impairment: reduced dosage or prolonged intervals necessary
Hepatic impairment: no information

OVERDOSAGE

ORAL:
Symptoms may include nausea, vomiting, epigastric distress, and diarrhea. Unless five times the normal dose has been ingested, gastrointestinal decontamination is not necessary. Always consider possibility of multiple drug overdoses, drug interactions, and unusual drug kinetics. Absorption may be inhibited by administration of activated charcoal. Otherwise, ensure patient's airway and support ventilation, monitor and maintain vital signs, blood gases, serum electrolytes, and so forth. Hemodialysis, peritoneal dialysis, forced diuresis, or charcoal hemoperfusion have not been established as beneficial.

PATIENT INFORMATION

Complete full course of therapy. Take loracarbef at least 1 hour before or 2 hours after a meal. Contact physician if nausea, vomiting, or diarrhea occurs. Shake the suspension well before use; may be stored at room temperature; discard the unused portion after 14 days.

AVAILABILITY

Pulvules or capsules—200 mg
Powder for Suspension—100 mg/5 mL

The information here is provided as guidance only. Prescribers should always consult the manufacturer's current prescribing information.

CLASS DESCRIPTION

Penicillins are a class of beta-lactam antibiotics that are structurally similar and highly effective in the treatment of a variety of bacterial infections. The first member of this class, penicillin G, was isolated from the mold *Penicillium notatum* in 1929 [1]. However, commercial production was not feasible until 1941. Analogues of penicillin G initially were obtained by adding different precursors during the fermentation process. The isolation of the penicillin nucleus, 6-aminopenicillanic acid, led to the successful development of a variety of semisynthetic penicillins with different spectrums of activity and pharmacokinetic characteristics [2]. The popularity of the penicillins is due to their high potency and bactericidal capability, broad spectrum of activity, excellent distribution throughout the body, low incidence of adverse reactions (even at high doses), low cost, and proven effectiveness.

CHEMISTRY AND CLASSIFICATION

All penicillins consist of a thiazolidine ring, a beta-lactam ring, and a side chain (Fig. 3-1). An intact beta-lactam ring is essential for activity. However, it is the side chain that determines the distinguishing antimicrobial and pharmacologic properties of a particular penicillin [3]. In penicillin G, the side chain consists of a benzyl group. The penicillin nucleus, 6-aminopenicillanic acid, can be obtained by removal of the side chain by treatment with an amidase enzyme. Subsequent chemical attachment of other side chains to the penicillin nucleus has led to a variety of useful semisynthetic agents.

The penicillins are classified according to their mode of production, their chemical structure, and their spectrum of activity (Table 3-1). The natural penicillins consist of penicillin G and V. The semisynthetic penicillins are divided into the penicillinase-resistant penicillins and the broad-spectrum penicillins. The broad-spectrum penicillins are further divided into the aminopenicillins, the carboxypenicillins, and the ureidopenicillins.

Clavulanic acid, sulbactam, and tazobactam were developed as beta-lactamase inhibitors [4]. They differ slightly from the penicillins in that they have no side chain on the beta-lactam ring. Clavulanic acid has an oxygen in place of the sulfur atom in the thiazolidine ring. Sulbactam and tazobactam are sulfone derivatives and have a SO_2 in place of the sulfur atom in the thiazolidine ring. These agents are marketed in combination with several broad-spectrum penicillins to expand activity against some beta-lactamase–producing strains.

MECHANISM OF ACTION

The penicillins inhibit bacterial cell growth by interfering with the synthesis of the bacterial cell wall [5]. The penicillins inhibit the final stage in cell wall synthesis, in which strands of peptidoglycan are cross-linked via peptide side chains. The penicillins bind covalently to the active site of the enzyme that produces the transpeptidation reaction. Although this is the major site of action of the penicillins, these drugs also bind to other cell membrane proteins [6]. These membrane components are referred to as the *penicillin-binding proteins* (PBPs). Some PBPs are enzymes, such as transpeptidases and carboxypeptidases, that are involved in cell wall synthesis; the functions of others have not been fully identified. PBPs are numbered in the order of decreasing molecular weight.

Inhibition of cell wall synthesis indirectly activates bacterial enzymes (murein hydrolases) that cause bacterial cell lysis [6]. This is the mechanism of bactericidal activity for most organisms. Killing of *Streptococcus pyogenes* occurs in the absence of lysis and results from penicillin-induced hydrolysis of cellular RNA [3]. The rate of bacterial killing by penicillins exhibits minimal dependence on drug concentration [7]. Maximum killing rates are usually observed at concentrations that are four to five times the minimum inhibitory concentration.

ANTIMICROBIAL ACTIVITY

The penicillins have a broad spectrum of activity against both aerobic and anaerobic bacteria [3,8]. Because the penicillins must first pass across the outer lipid membrane of gram-negative bacilli before they can reach their site of action, these drugs are more active against gram-positive than gram-negative bacteria. The natural penicillins are highly active against non–beta-lactamase–producing strains of staphylococci, streptococci, meningococci, gonococci, anaerobic cocci, and spirochetes. The penicillinase-resistant penicillins are active against penicillinase-producing staphylococci. The broad-spectrum penicillins have increased activity against gram-negative bacilli. Table 3-2 gives the *in vitro* activity of selected penicillins.

MECHANISMS OF BACTERIAL RESISTANCE

The major mechanism for resistance to the penicillins is inactivation of the beta-lactam ring by beta-lactamases [9]. There are a variety of beta-lactamases generated by different bacteria. The genes for production of these beta-lactamases may be chromosomal or plasmid-mediated. The spread of plasmid-mediated beta-lactamases (*eg*, TEM-1) among the Enterobacteriaceae and to *Haemophilus* and

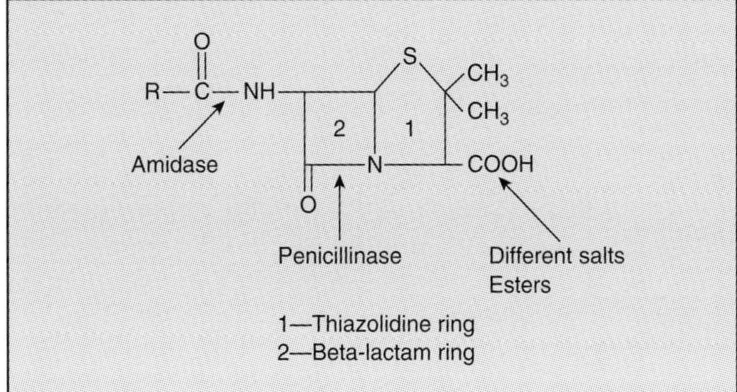

FIGURE 3-1.

Chemical structure of penicillins.

Table 3-1. Classification of the Penicillins

I. Natural penicillins: penicillin G, penicillin V

II. Semisynthetic penicillins

    A. Penicillinase-resistant penicillins: methicillin, nafcillin, oxacillin, cloxacillin, dicloxacillin

    B. Broad-spectrum penicillins

        1. Aminopenicillins: ampicillin, amoxicillin

        2. Carboxypenicillins: carbenicillin, ticarcillin

        3. Ureidopenicillins: mezlocillin, piperacillin

III. Beta-lactamase inhibitors: clavulanic acid, sulbactam, tazobactam

The information here is provided as guidance only. Prescribers should always consult the manufacturer's current prescribing information.

Neisseria species has markedly altered susceptibility to the penicillins. Resistance to the penicillins also can occur by alteration of the penicillin-binding protein [10]. Amino acid substitutions or insertions in the PBPs can result from mutations of the PBP genes or by replacement of part of the gene with corresponding genes from other bacterial species. Penicillin resistance in pneumococci and methicillin resistance in staphylococci are important forms of resistance caused by alteration of the site of action. Mutations that change the outer membrane porins of gram-negative bacilli and decrease permeability provide a final mechanism for resistance to the penicillins [11].

PHARMACOKINETICS

Many of the penicillins are unstable in the acidic milieu of the stomach and are restricted to parenteral administration. Penicillin V, the aminopenicillins, the isoxazolyl penicillins, nafcillin, and ester formulations are sufficiently stable in acid to allow for oral absorption. The penicillins distribute widely in the extracellular compartment and will penetrate the cerebrospinal fluid and humors of the eye in the presence of inflammation. The penicillins are eliminated via the kidneys, primarily by tubular secretion. From 25% to 40% of nafcillin, the isoxazolyl penicillins, and the ureidopenicillins also are eliminated by biliary secretion. Because of their rapid half-lives (30–60 minutes), the penicillins usually are administered three to six times a day. Procaine and benzathine penicillin G are relatively insoluble formulations for intramuscular administration, designed to provide more sustained drug concentrations. The pharmacokinetic properties of selected penicillins are shown in Table 3-3 [3,8].

Table 3-2. *In-vitro* Activity of Selected Penicillins as Measured by Mean Minimum Inhibitory Concentration in mg/L

Organism	Penicillin G	Oxacillin	Ampicillin	Ticarcillin	Piperacillin	Ampicillin sulbactam	Ticarcillin clavulanate
Gram-positive aerobes							
Staphylococcus aureus	0.02 (> 32)*	0.2 (0.4)	0.1 (> 32)	1 (16)	1 (16)	0.1 (2)	1 (2)
Staphylococcus epidermidis	0.02 (> 32)	0.2 (0.4)	0.1 (> 32)	2 (16)	0.2 (16)	0.1 (2)	2 (4)
Staphylococcus pyogenes	0.005	0.02	0.01	0.2	0.02	0.01	0.2
Staphylococcus agalactiae	0.05	0.1	0.2	1	0.2	0.2	1
Streptococcus pneumoniae	0.01	0.05	0.02	0.4	0.02	0.02	0.4
Enterococcus	2	16	1	32	1	1	32
Listeria monocytogenes	0.4	4	0.2	2	1	0.2	2
Gram-positive anaerobes							
Peptococcus	0.1	0.5	0.1	0.1	0.1	0.1	0.1
Peptostreptococcus	0.1	0.4	0.2	0.5	0.5	0.2	0.5
Clostridium spp	0.1	0.5	0.1	0.5	0.5	0.1	0.5
Gram-negative aerobes							
Neisseria meningitidis	0.05	4	0.05	0.05	0.01	0.05	0.05
Neisseria gonorrhoeae	0.05 (> 32)	1 (2)	0.05 (> 32)	0.1 (8)	0.05 (2)	0.05 (1)	0.1 (0.5)
Moraxella catarrhalis	0.1 (2)	4	0.1 (2)	0.1 (4)	0.1 (0.5)	0.1 (0.2)	0.1 (0.5)
Haemophilus influenzae	0.4 (> 16)	16	0.4 (> 16)	0.4 (4)	0.1 (0.5)	0.4 (1)	0.4 (1)
Escherichia coli	64	> 128	4 (> 128)	4 (> 128)	8 (128)	2 (16)	4 (32)
Proteus mirabilis	32	> 128	4	2	0.5	1	1
Klebsiella pneumoniae	> 128	> 128	> 128	> 128	8	16	4
Enterobacter spp	> 128	> 128	128	8	4	16	8
Citrobacter spp	> 128	> 128	32	8	4	> 128	8
Serratia spp	> 128	> 128	> 128	128	32	> 128	64
Salmonella spp	8	> 128	2	4	2	1	2
Shigella spp	16	> 128	2	2	4	1	2
Morganella spp	> 128	> 128	128	16	8	128	16
Providencia spp	> 128	> 128	> 128	16	8	> 128	16
Proteus vulgaris	> 128	> 128	64	8	16	64	1
Acinetobacter spp	> 128	> 128	32	16	8	1	16
Pseudomonas aeruginosa	> 128	> 128	> 128	32	8	> 128	32
Gram-negative anaerobes							
Bacteroides fragilis	16	> 128	16	32	32	2	2
Prevotella melaninogenicus	0.2	32	0.2	0.5	0.5	0.2	0.5
Fusobacterium spp	0.1	>128	0.1	0.5	0.1	0.1	0.5

*Numbers in parentheses represent minimum inhibitory concentrations for beta-lactamase–positive strains.

The information here is provided as guidance only. Prescribers should always consult the manufacturer's current prescribing information.

DOSAGE ADJUSTMENTS FOR RENAL AND HEPATIC INSUFFICIENCY

Because most penicillins are eliminated primarily by the kidneys, dosage adjustments are required in the presence of renal insufficiency [12]. The dosing interval of most penicillins in patients with normal renal function is 4 to 6 hours. The suggested adjustment for penicillin G, penicillin V, ampicillin, ampicillin-sulbactam, amoxicillin, amoxicillin-clavulanate, and methicillin is to give a standard dose every 6 to 8 hours in patients with creatinine clearances of 10 to 50 mL/min and every 12 hours in patients with creatinine clearances below 10 mL/min. Similar dosing frequencies are recommended for ticarcillin and ticarcillin-clavulanate, but the usual dose is reduced to 2 g. Mezlocillin and piperacillin also are eliminated by biliary excretion and require less modification in renal insufficiency. Doses of 2 g every 8 hours are recommended in patients with creatinine clearances below 10 mL/min. Nafcillin and the isoxazolyl penicillins have sufficient biliary elimination to require no dose adjustments in renal insufficiency.

No dosage adjustment of the penicillins is needed for patients with hepatic diseases alone. However, in patients with concomitant hepatic and renal insufficiency, the dose is further reduced by one half [3,8].

INDICATIONS

The penicillins are highly efficacious in a large variety of infections, including upper and lower respiratory tract infections; endocarditis; meningitis; urinary tract infections; skin and soft-tissue infections; bone and joint infections; intra-abdominal infections; gynecologic infections; and some sexually transmitted diseases. The penicillins are still the drugs of choice for most staphylococcal, streptococcal, enterococcal, meningococcal, clostridial, listerial, and spirochetal infections. The carboxy- and ureidopenicillins are major agents for the treatment of *Pseudomonas* infections. The penicillin and beta-lactamase inhibitor combinations are useful in mixed aerobic–anaerobic infections.

ADVERSE REACTIONS

Penicillins are associated with a low incidence of adverse reactions. Hypersensitivity reactions are the most common untoward effects produced by the penicillins [3,13]. The frequency of reactions is 0.004% to 0.015% for anaphylaxis, 1% to 5% for urticaria, and 2% to 9% for rashes. Interstitial nephritis, which is a cellular hypersensitivity reaction, is most common with methicillin (1%–2%). Hemolytic anemia due to antipenicillin antibodies is rare, whereas neutropenia occurs in 1% to 4% of patients receiving high doses. Platelet dysfunction can also result from high doses, especially with the carboxypenicillins, but clinical bleeding is uncommon. Central nervous system toxicities, such as myoclonic jerks and seizures, are associated with high-dose therapy, primarily in patients with renal insufficiency. Sodium overload and hypokalemia also can be observed with high doses of penicillins, especially the carboxypenicillins. Gastrointestinal reactions, such as nausea, vomiting, and diarrhea, occur in 1% to 5% of patients receiving oral penicillins.

DRUG INTERACTIONS

Drug interactions are uncommon with the penicillins [3]. Probenecid inhibits the tubular secretion of the penicillins and increases drug half-life approximately twofold. Penicillins, especially the carboxy- and ureidopenicillins, can inactivate aminoglycosides [3]. These two drug classes should not be mixed in the same intravenous solution. The inactivation of aminoglycosides by penicillins also can shorten aminoglycoside half-lives in patients with renal impairment.

PATIENT INFORMATION

Patients should be advised to 1) take oral penicillins with liberal amounts of fluid on an empty stomach 1 hour before or 2 hours following a meal; 2) take penicillins at regular intervals, around the clock, and

Table 3-3. Pharmacokinetic Characteristics of the Penicillins

Drug	Oral bioavailability, %	Dose	C max, *mg/L*	Half-life, *h*	Protein binding, %	Route of excretion
Penicillin G	< 20	2 g intravenous	120	0.5	60	Renal
Penicillin V	60	0.5 g oral	5	0.5	78	Renal
Methicillin	< 5	2 g intravenous	100	0.5	37	Renal
Oxacillin	30	2 g intravenous	200	0.4	93	Renal plus hepatic
Cloxacillin	50	0.5 g oral	12	0.4	94	Renal plus hepatic
Dicloxacillin	50	0.5 g oral	15	0.7	97	Renal plus hepatic
Nafcillin	25	2 g intravenous	160	0.5	89	Renal plus hepatic
Ampicillin	40	2 g intravenous	100	1.0	18	Renal
Amoxicillin	80	0.5 g oral	8	0.9	17	Renal
Ticarcillin	< 5	2 g intravenous	170	1.2	45	Renal
Mezlocillin	< 5	2 g intravenous	200	1.0	35	Renal plus hepatic
Piperacillin	< 5	2 g intravenous	200	1.0	50	Renal plus hepatic
Clavulanic acid	70	0.125 g oral	3	0.8	< 15	Renal
Sulbactam	< 10	1 g intravenous	50	1.0	< 15	Renal

The information here is provided as guidance only. Prescribers should always consult the manufacturer's current prescribing information.

complete all medication unless otherwise directed by the physician; 3) throw away any unused liquid forms of penicillin after 7 days when stored at room temperature and after 14 days when stored in a refriger- ator; and 4) discontinue the penicillin and contact the physician if rash, itching, hives, shortness of breath, wheezing, severe diarrhea, fever, swelling of joints, or unusual bleeding and bruising develops.

REFERENCES

1. Fleming A: On antibacterial action of cultures of a penicillium, with special reference to their use in isolation of *B. influenzae*. *Br J Exp Pathol* 1929, 10:226.

2. Batchelor FR, Doyle FP, Naylor JHC, *et al.*: Synthesis of penicillin: 6-Aminopenicillanic acid in penicillin fermentations. *Nature* 1959, 183:257.

3. Craig WA: Penicillin. In *Infectious Diseases*. Edited by Gorbach SL, Bartlet JG, Blacklow NR. Philadelphia: WB Saunders Co; 1992:160–171.

4. Bush K: Beta-lactamase inhibitors from laboratory to clinic. *Clin Microbiol Rev* 1988, 1:109.

5. Tipper DJ, Strominger JL: Mechanism of action of penicillins: A proposal based on their structural similarity to acyl-Dalanyl-Dalanine. *Proc Natl Acad Sci U S A* 1965, 54:1133.

6. Tomasz A: From penicillin-binding proteins to the lysis and death of bacteria: A 1979 view. *Rev Infect Dis* 1979, 1:434.

7. Vogelman B, Craig WA: Kinetics of antimicrobial activity. *J Pediatr* 1986, 108:835.

8. Neu HC: Beta-lactam antibiotics: Structural relationships affecting *in vitro* activity and pharmacologic properties. *Rev Infect Dis* 1986, 8(Suppl 3):237.

9. Medeiros AA, Jacoby GA: Beta-lactamase–mediated resistance. In *Beta-Lactam Antibiotics for Clinical Use*. Edited by Queener SW. New York: Marcel Dekker; 1986:49–84.

10. Malouin F, Bryan LE: Modification of penicillin-binding proteins as mechanisms of beta-lactam resistance. *Antimicrob Agents Chemother* 1986, 30:1.

11. Hancock RE, Woodruff WA: Roles of porin and beta-lactamase in beta-lactam resistance in *Pseudomonas aeruginosa*. *Rev Infect Dis* 1988, 10:770.

12. Bennett WM, Muther RS, Parker RA, *et al.*: Drug therapy in renal failure: Dosing guidelines for adults. *Ann Intern Med* 1980, 93(Part 1):62.

13. Faxon A, Beall GN, Rohr AF, *et al.*: Immediate hypersensitivity reactions to beta-lactam antibiotics. *Ann Intern Med* 1987, 107:204.

The information here is provided as guidance only. Prescribers should always consult the manufacturer's current prescribing information.

AMOXICILLIN (Amoxil®, Trimox®, Wymox®)

Amoxicillin is a semisynthetic penicillin that closely resembles ampicillin both structurally and pharmacologically. However, amoxicillin is more completely absorbed than ampicillin: this results in blood levels that are two to two and a half times higher than those obtained with similar doses of ampicillin. It has a broad spectrum of antimicrobial activity against many gram-positive and gram-negative organisms. It is useful in the treatment of otitis media, bronchitis, pneumonia, urinary tract infections, and gonococcal infections. It is not as effective as ampicillin in the treatment of shigellosis. Because amoxicillin is almost completely absorbed, the incidence of gastrointestinal side effects is lower than with ampicillin.

ANTIMICROBIAL ACTIVITY

Gram positive: Staphylococci (nonpenicillinase-producing), *Streptococcus pneumoniae*, beta-hemolytic streptococci, *Enterococcus faecalis*, *viridans* streptococci.
Gram negative: *Escherichia coli*, *Haemophilus influenzae*, *Neisseria gonorrhoeae*, *Proteus mirabilis*.
Anaerobic: *Clostridium* spp, *Peptococcus* spp, *Peptostreptococcus* spp.

RESISTANCE

Many strains of *E. coli*, *H. influenzae* and *N. gonorrhoeae* produce beta-lactamase enzymes that inactivate amoxicillin.

SPECIAL PRECAUTIONS

A large percentage of patients with mononucleosis who received amoxicillin develops a skinrash. An alternative to ampicillin class antibiotics should be used in such cases. Estimated incidence of hypersensitivity is 1% to 10%; serious and occasionally fatal immediate reactions have occurred. Although anaphylaxis is more frequent after parenteral administration, it can occur with oral forms as well. Accelerated reactions (*eg*, urticaria, laryngeal edema) and delayed reactions (serum sickness–like syndrome) may occur. Reactions are most likely to be immediate and severe in patients with penicillin sensitivity and a history of atopic conditions.
Cross-allergenicity with cephalosporins is common in patients with penicillin hypersensitivity.
Desensitization may be considered in patients who have positive skin test results to a penicillin determinant and who have need where no alternative to penicillin exists (*eg*, neurosyphilis, congenital syphilis, or syphilis in pregnancy).
Skin rashes, urticaria, and serum sickness–like reactions may be controlled by antihistamines or corticosteroids if necessary. Unless condition being treated is life-threatening or only amenable to penicillin therapy, discontinuation is recommended.
Bacteriologic studies should be performed to determine causative organisms and their susceptibility.
Use caution in administering broad-spectrum antibiotics to patients with existing or previous gastrointestinal disease. Treatment with broad-spectrum antibiotics alters normal flora of the colon and may permit overgrowth of *Clostridium difficile*, causing antibiotic-associated pseudomembranous colitis. Mild cases usually respond to discontinuation of therapy alone; management of moderate to severe cases should include bacteriologic studies and fluid, electrolyte, and protein supplementation.
White blood and differential cell counts should be performed prior to initiation of therapy and every week during therapy with penicillinase-resistant penicillins.
Monitor AST and ALT to observe for liver function abnormalities during therapy; this is especially important in newborns and infants receiving higher doses.
Prolonged or repeated antibiotic therapy may result in bacterial or fungal overgrowth of nonsusceptible organisms, leading to secondary infection.
The number of strains of staphylococci resistant to penicillinase-resistant penicillins has been growing. Interpret resistance to any penicillinase-resistant penicillin as evidence of clinical resistance to all. Cross-resistance to cephalosporin derivatives also occurs often.

(Continued on next page)

INDICATIONS

For treatment of infections of the following types due to susceptible strains of designated organisms:
Ear, nose and throat:
Streptococci, pneumococci, nonpenicillinase-producing staphylococci, and *H. influenzae*
Genitourinary tract:
E. coli, *P. mirabilis*, and *E. faecalis*
Skin–soft tissue:
Streptococci, staphylococci, and *E. coli*

CONTRAINDICATIONS

Patients with a history of immediate hypersensitivity reactions to any of the penicillins

INTERACTIONS

Probenecid
ORAL: Beta-blockers
PARENTERAL: Aminoglycosides (parenteral) anticoagulants heparin
BOTH: Chloramphenicol, erythromycin, tetracyclines, oral contraceptives

ADVERSE EFFECTS

Moderate increase in AST (significance unknown), dizziness (rare), behavioral changes (rare)

PHARMACOKINETICS AND PHARMACODYNAMICS

Peak serum levels: 12 h after oral use; 3.5 to 5 µg/mL and 5.5 to 7.5 µg/mL (for 250-mg and 500-mg doses, respectively)
Plasma half-life: 0.7 to 1.5 h
Bioavailability: diffuses into most body tissues, except brain and spinal fluid (unless meninges are inflamed)
Metabolism: approximately 20% is partially metabolized to penicilloic acids
Elimination: glomerular filtration and active tubular secretion
Excretion: in 6 h, approximately 60% is excreted largely unchanged in urine
Effect of food: may be taken with meals
Protein binding: 20%
Renal impairment: half-life is 5.2 to 1.5 h in patients with creatinine clearances less than than 30 mL/min
Hepatic impairment: half-life is 1.2 to 3 h

OVERDOSAGE

Excessive doses may cause neuromuscular hyperexcitability or convulsive seizures. Dose-related toxicity can arise with the use of large doses of intravenous penicillin (40–100 MU/d), especially in patients with severe renal impairment. Symptoms include agitation, confusion, asterixis, hallucinations, stupor, coma, multifocal myoclonus, seizures, and encephalopathy. Hypokalemia also has occurred.
In case of overdose, discontinue drug therapy and treat patient symptomatically, using supportive care as required. Hemodialysis may be used if necessary to reduce blood levels of penicillin, although effectiveness is uncertain.

The information here is provided as guidance only. Prescribers should always consult the manufacturer's current prescribing information.

AMOXICILLIN (CONTINUED)

SPECIAL PRECAUTIONS (CONTINUED)

In streptococcal infections, therapy must be completed to eliminate the organism (*ie*, minimum of 10 days) to prevent sequelae, such as rheumatic fever, from occurring.

In gonococcal infections in which primary or secondary syphilis may be suspected, proper diagnostic procedures, including darkfield examinations and monthly serologic tests for a minimum of 4 months, are indicated. Continuation of clinical and serologic examinations every 6 months for 2 to 3 years is recommended for all cases.

Patients with cystic fibrosis have a higher incidence of adverse effects with extended-spectrum penicillins.

Care should be taken with intravenous administration due to the possibility of thrombophlebitis. Intravenous doses higher than recommended for most penicillins may cause neuromuscular excitability and convulsions.

Avoid subcutaneous and fat layer injections; pain and induration may occur.

Inadvertent intravascular administration, including direct arterial injection (or injection immediately adjacent to arteries) has resulted in severe neurovascular damage, including transverse myelitis with permanent paralysis; gangrene, requiring amputation of digits and more proximal portions of extremities; and necrosis and sloughing at the injection site and surrounding area. Other complications include immediate pallor, mottling, or cyanosis of the extremity (both distal and proximal to the injection site), ensuing bleb formation, and severe edema requiring anterior–posterior compartment fasciotomy in the lower extremities. These effects have occurred most frequently in infants and young children. Immediate consultation with a specialist is recommended if any evidence of compromise of blood supply occurs at, proximal to, or distal to the site of injection.

Quadriceps femoris fibrosis and atrophy have occurred after repeated intramuscular injections of penicillin preparations to the anterolateral thigh.

False-positive urine glucose reactions may occur with Clinitest (Ames, Elkhart, IN), Benedicts' solution, or Fehling's solution.

Positive Coombs' test results have occurred.

SPECIAL GROUPS

Children: Safe for use in children.
Elderly: Serum levels slightly higher and half-lives slightly longer.
Renal impairment: Dosage modification needed with creatinine clearances less than 30 mL/min.
Hepatic impairment: Half-lives slightly prolonged, but dosage modification not required.
Pregnancy: Use only if clearly needed; controlled human studies not performed.
Breast-feeding: Use caution; excreted in breast milk.

DOSAGE

Adults: For infections of ear, nose, and throat due to streptococci, pneumococci, nonpenicillinase-producing staphylococci, and *H. influenzae*; infections of genitourinary tract due to *E. coli*, *P. mirabilis*, and *E. faecalis*; and infections of skin or soft tissue due to streptococci, susceptible staphylococci, and *E. coli*: 250 to 500 mg every 8 hours. For infections of lower respiratory tract due to streptococci, pneumonococci, nonpenicillinase-producing staphylococci, and *H. influenzae*: 500 mg every 8 hours. As an alternative regimen* for gonococcal infections (uncomplicated, urethral, endocervical, or rectal): once source of infection is proved not to have penicillin-resistant gonorrhea, 3 g amoxicillin with 1 g probenecid followed by doxycycline. For prevention of bacterial endocarditis: 3 g 1 hour prior to procedure and 1.5 g 6 hours after initial dose.
Elderly: Same as adults.
Children: For children under 20 kg. For infections of ear, nose, and throat due to streptococci, pneumococci, nonpenicillinase-producing staphylococci, and *H. influenzae*; infections of genitourinary tract due to *E. coli*, *P. mirabilis*, and *E. faecalis*; and infections of skin or soft tissue due to streptococci, susceptible staphylococci, and *E. coli*: 20 to 40 mg/kg/d in divided doses every 8 hours. For children over 20 kg, use adult dosage (not to exceed maximal daily adults dose). For infections of lower respiratory tract due to streptococci, pneumococci, nonpenicillinase-producing staphylococci, and *H. influenzae*: 40 mg/kg/d in divided doses every 8 hours.

Centers for Disease Control and Prevention: 1989 Sexually transmitted diseases treatment guidelines. MMWR 1989 Sept 1;38(No. S-8):1–43.

PATIENT INFORMATION

Complete all medication unless otherwise directed by physician. Take medication with a full glass of water on an empty stomach 1 hour before or 2 hours following a meal. Take at regular intervals around the clock. Contact physician if rash, itching, hives, severe diarrhea, shortness of breath or wheezing, black tongue, sore throat, nausea, vomiting, fever, swelling of joints, or unusual bleeding or bruising occurs. Throw away any unused liquid form of penicillin after 7 days when stored in room temperature and after 14 days when stored in refrigerator.

AVAILABILITY

Chewable tables—125 mg and 250 mg
Capsules—250 mg and 500 mg
Powder for oral suspension—50 mg/mL, 125 mg/mL, and 250 mg/5 mL (as trihydrate, when reconstituted)

The information here is provided as guidance only. Prescribers should always consult the manufacturer's current prescribing information.

AMOXICILLIN–CLAVULANIC ACID (Augmentin®)

Amoxicillin-clavulanic acid is a fixed combination of an aminopenicillin with a beta-lactamase inhibitor for oral administration. Clavulanic acid has little antimicrobial activity of its own but inhibits the inactivation of amoxicillin by beta-lactamase–producing strains of staphylococci, gonococci, *Haemophilus influenzae*, *Moraxella catarrhalis*, *Escherichia coli*, *Klebsiella pneumoniae*, and *Bacteroides fragilis*. It has been used to treat upper and lower respiratory tract infections and skin and soft-tissue infections. It is especially useful in the treatment of human and animal bite wounds. Two separate combinations are available for three-times-a-day dosing—one with 125 mg of clavulanic acid and 250 mg of amoxicillin and one with 125 mg of clavulanic acid and 500 mg of amoxicillin. Administration of more than 375 mg of clavulanic acid per day is associated with a high frequency of diarrhea.

ANTIMICROBIAL ACTIVITY

Gram-positive: Staphylococci, *Staphylococcus aureus*, *Streptococcus pneumoniae*, beta-hemolytic streptococci, *Enterococcus faecalis*, *viridans* streptococci.
Gram-negative: *E. coli*, *H. influenzae*, *Klebsiella* spp, *Neisseria gonorrhoeae*, *Neisseria meningitidis*, *Proteus mirabilis*, *Enterobacter* species, *Moraxella (Branhamella) catarrhalis*.
Anaerobic: *Clostridium* spp, *Peptococcus* spp, *Peptostreptococcus* spp.

RESISTANCE

Organisms with new extended-spectrum beta-lactamases that inactivate clavulanic acid have been reported but are extremely rare.

SPECIAL PRECAUTIONS

A large percentage of patients with mononucleosis who receive amoxicillin develop a skin rash. An alternative to ampicillin class antibiotics should be used in such cases.
See Special Precautions for amoxicillin.

SPECIAL GROUPS

Children: Safe for use in children.
Elderly: *See* amoxicillin.
Renal impairment: *See* amoxicillin.
Hepatic impairment: *See* amoxicillin.
Pregnancy: Use only if clearly indicated; no controlled human studies performed.
Breast-feeding: Use caution; excreted in breast milk.

INDICATIONS

For treatment of infections of the following types due to susceptible strains of designated organisms:
Lower respiratory tract:
  Beta-lactamase–producing strains of *H. influenzae*
Otitis media and sinusitis:
  Beta-lactamase–producing strains of *H. influenzae* and *M. (Branhamella) catarrhalis*
Skin–skin structure:
  Beta-lactamase–producing strains of *S. aureus*, *E. coli*, and *Klebsiella* spp
Urinary tract:
  Beta-lactamase–producing strains of *E. coli*, *Klebsiella* spp, and *Enterobacter* spp

CONTRAINDICATIONS

Patients with a history of immediate hypersensitivity reactions to any of the penicillins

INTERACTIONS

Probenecid
ORAL: Beta-blockers
PARENTERAL: Aminoglycosides (parenteral), anticoagulants, heparin
BOTH: Chloramphenicol, erythromycin, tetracyclines, oral contraceptives

ADVERSE EFFECTS

Hypersensitivity: urticaria, maculopapular–exfoliative dermatitis, vesicular eruptions, angioneurotic edema, laryngospasm, bronchospasm, hypotension, vascular collapse, death, erythema multiforme, Stevens-Johnson syndrome (rare), serum sickness–like reactions, laryngeal edema, and prostration. Drug fever also can occur.
Gastrointestinal: (most common with oral forms) glossitis, stomatitis, gastritis, sore or dry mouth or tongue, "furry" tongue, black "hairy" tongue, abnormal taste, nausea, vomiting, abdominal pain, epigastric distress, diarrhea, bloody diarrhea, rectal bleeding, flatulence, enterocolitis, and pseudomembranous colitis
Hematologic or lymphatic: anemia, thrombocytopenia, thrombocytopenic purpura, eosinophilia, leukopenia, granulocytopenia, neutropenia, bone marrow depression, agranulocytosis, decreased hemoglobin or hematocrit, prolonged bleeding or prothrombin time (associated hemorrhagic manifestations have occurred), decreased leukocyte and lymphocyte counts, and increased lymphocytes, monocytes, basophils, and platelets (all effects reversible and believed to be hypersensitivity phenomena)
Renal: such as interstitial nephritis and nephropathy, are not frequent and usually are associated with parenteral forms (have occurred with all forms); elevations in creatinine or blood urea nitrogen also may occur
Central nervous system: neurotoxicity with large doses (especially in patients with renal failure), anxiety, confusion, agitation, depression, hallucinations, convulsions and seizures, dizziness, insomnia, fatigue, hyperactivity (reversible), and prolonged muscle relaxation. Sciatic neuritis has been reported with intramuscular injection of penicillin.
Hepatic: such as transient hepatitis and cholestatic jaundice, are very uncommon and observed primarily with oxacillin
Local reactions at injection site: such as pain accompanied by induration, ecchymosis, deep vein thrombosis, hematoma, vein irritation, and phlebitis, have occurred

(Continued on next page)

AMOXICILLIN–CLAVULANIC ACID (CONTINUED)

DOSAGE

Adults: (Note: Because both the 250-mg and 500-mg tablets have equal amounts of clavulanic acid [125 mg potassium salt], two 250-mg tablets are not equivalent to one 500-mg tablet.)

Usual dose is one 250-mg tablet every 8 hours. For serious infections or infections of the respiratory tract, one 500-mg tablet every 8 hours. For chancroid (*Haemophilus ducreyi* infection)*, one 500-mg tablet every 8 hours for 7 days as an alternative to erythromycin or ceftriaxone (not evaluated in the United States).

For disseminated gonococcal infection* (after appropriate parenteral therapy with ceftriaxone, ceftrizoxime, or cefotaxime; to complete therapy at home), one 500-mg tablet every 8 hours for 1 week.

Elderly: Same as adults.

Children: Dosages based on amoxicillin content. Usual dose for children under 40 kg is 20 mg/kg/d in divided doses every 8 hours. For serious infections or respiratory tract infections, 40 mg/kg/d in divided doses every 8 hours. For otitis media, sinusitis, or lower respiratory tract infections, 40 mg/kg/d in divided doses every 8 hours.

Centers for Disease Control and Prevention: 1989 Sexually transmitted diseases treatment guidelines. MMWR 1989 Sept 1;38(No. S-8):1–43.

ADVERSE EFFECTS *(CONTINUED)*

Test abnormalities: increases in serum alkaline phosphatase and hypernatremia and decreases in serum potassium, albumin, total proteins, and uric acid

Jarisch-Herxheimer: reactions have occurred in the treatment of syphilis

Miscellaneous: vaginitis and itchy eyes

PHARMACOKINETICS AND PHARMACODYNAMICS

Peak serum levels: 1 to 2 h after oral use; 3.5 to 5 µg/mL and 5.5 to 7.5 µg/mL (for 250-mg and 500-mg doses, respectively) for amoxicillin and 2 to 4 µg/mL for 125 mg clavulanic acid

Plasma half-life: 0.9 to 1.3 h for amoxicillin and 0.8 to 1.2 hours for clavulanic acid

Bioavailability: 74% to 92% for amoxicillin; diffuses into most body tissues, except brain and spinal fluid (unless meninges are inflamed)

Metabolism: approximately 20% is partially metabolized to penicilloic acids

Elimination: glomerular filtration

Excretion: in 6 h, 60% of amoxicillin and 35% of clavulanic acid excreted largely unchanged in urine

Effect of food: may take with meals

Protein binding: 20%

Renal impairment: mean half-life was 7.5 h for amoxicillin and 4.3 hours for clavulanic acid in patients with creatinine clearances less than 10 mL/min

Hepatic impairment: half-life of amoxicillin is 1.2 to 3 h

OVERDOSAGE

Excessive doses may cause neuromuscular hyperexcitability or convulsive seizures. Dose-related toxicity can arise with the use of large doses of intravenous penicillin (40–100 MU/d), especially in patients with severe renal impairment. Symptoms include agitation, confusion, asterixis, hallucinations, stupor, coma, multifocal myoclonus, seizures, and encephalopathy. Hypokalemia also has occurred.

In case of overdose, discontinue drug therapy and treat patient symptomatically, using supportive care as required. Hemodialysis may be used if necessary to reduce blood levels of penicillin, although effectiveness is uncertain.

PATIENT INFORMATION

Complete all medication unless otherwise directed by physician. Take medication with a full glass of water on an empty stomach 1 hour before or 2 hours following a meal. Take at regular intervals around the clock. Contact physician if rash, itching, hives, severe diarrhea, shortness of breath or wheezing, black tongue, sore throat, nausea, vomiting, fever, swelling of joints, or unusual bleeding or bruising occurs. Throw away any unused liquid form of penicillin after 7 days when stored at room temperature and after 14 days when stored in refrigerator.

AVAILABILITY

Chewable tablets—125 mg and 250 mg (31.25 mg and 62.5 mg clavulanic acid, respectively)

Tablets—250 mg and 500 mg (both with 125 mg clavulanic acid)

Powder for oral suspension—125 mg and 250 mg (31.25 and 62.5 mg clavulanic acid, respectively)

The information here is provided as guidance only. Prescribers should always consult the manufacturer's current prescribing information.

AMPICILLIN (Omnipen®, Totacillin®)

Ampicillin is a semisynthetic penicillin that is the alpha-aminobenzyl derivative of penicillin G. It has a broad spectrum of antimicrobial activity against many gram-positive and gram-negative organisms. Ampicillin is preferred over penicillin G for enterococcal and *Listeria* infections. Ampicillin is only partially absorbed from the gastrointestinal tract. It is well distributed throughout the body and produces therapeutic concentrations in the cerebrospinal fluid for treatment of meningitis. It also has been used to treat respiratory tract infections, urinary tract infections, skin and soft-tissue infections, and gonococcal infections.

ANTIMICROBIAL ACTIVITY

Gram-positive: Staphylococci (nonpenicillinase-producing), Streptococci, *Streptococcus pneumoniae*, beta-hemolytic streptococci, *Enterococcus faecalis*, viridans streptococci, *Bacillus anthracis*, *Listeria monocytogenes*.
Gram-negative: *Escherichia coli*, *Haemophilus influenzae*, *Neisseria gonorrhoeae*, *Neisseria meningitidis*, *Proteus mirabilis*, *Salmonella* spp, *Shigella* spp.
Anaerobic: *Clostridium* spp, *Peptococcus* spp.

RESISTANCE

Many strains of *E. coli*, *H. influenzae*, and *N. gonorrhoeae* produce beta-lactamase enzymes that inactivate ampicillin.

SPECIAL PRECAUTIONS

Direct intravenous administration should be given slowly over at least 10 to 15 minutes. More rapid administration can result in convulsive seizures.
See Special Precautions for amoxicillin.

SPECIAL GROUPS

Children: Safety not established for use in neonates and premature infants.
Elderly: May have age-related renal impairment.
Renal impairment: Increased dosage interval necessary with creatinine clearances less than 30 mL/min.
Hepatic impairment: Dosage modification not required.
Pregnancy: Use only if clearly indicated; no human studies performed.
Breast-feeding: Use caution; excreted in breast milk.

INDICATIONS

Treatment of infections due to susceptible strains of *Shigella*, *Salmonella* (including *S. typhosa*), *E. coli*, *H. influenzae*, *P. mirabilis*, N. gonorrhoeae, and enterococci
Also used for treatment of meningitis due to *N. meningitidis* and in infections due to susceptible gram-positive organisms, such as penicillin G–penicillin G–sensitive staphylococci, streptococci, and pneumococci

CONTRAINDICATIONS

Patients with a history of immediate hypersensitivity reactions to any of the penicillins

INTERACTIONS

Allopurinol, bacteriostatic antibiotics (chloramphenicol, erythromycins, sulfonamides, tetracyclines), probenecid
ORAL: beta-blockers
PARENTERAL: aminoglycosides (parenteral), anticoagulants, heparin
BOTH: chloramphenicol, erythromycin, tetracyclines, oral contraceptives

ADVERSE EFFECTS

Laryngeal stridor (rare), high fever
See Adverse Effects for amoxicillin-clavulanic acid.

PHARMACOKINETICS AND PHARMACODYNAMICS

Peak serum levels: 2 µg/mL 1 to 2 h after a 250-mg dose (fasting patient)
Plasma half-life: 0.0 to 1.2 h
Bioavailability: 30% to 55% of an oral dose diffuse, except in brain and cerebrospinal fluid (unless meninges are inflamed)
Metabolism: approximately 10% is partially metabolized to penicilloic acids
Elimination: glomerular filtration
Excretion: approximately 40% of oral dose and 70% of a parenteral dose excreted unchanged in urine in 6 h
Effect of food: inhibits absorption
Protein binding: 20%
Renal impairment: half-lives 7.4 to 21 h in patients with creatinine clearance less than 10 mL/min
Hepatic impairment: half-life 1.9 h in patients with cirrhosis

The information here is provided as guidance only. Prescribers should always consult the manufacturer's current prescribing information.

AMPICILLIN (CONTINUED)

DOSAGE

(Note: Parenteral form should be reserved for moderately severe and severe infections or for patients unable to take oral form. Change to oral form as soon as appropriate.)

Adults: (Note: Adults are usually over 40 kg.) In general, 1 to 2 g/d in divided doses every 4 to 6 hours.

For respiratory tract or soft-tissue infections *PARENTERAL*: 250 to 500 mg every 6 hours; *ORAL*: 250 to 500 mg every 6 hours, For bacterial meningitis due to *H. influenzae, S. pneumoniae,* or *N. meningitis* treatment is usually by intravenous drip 8 to 14 g/d in divided doses every 4 to 6 hours. For septicemia *PARENTERAL:* 150 to 200 mg/kg/d intravenously in divided doses every 4 to 6 hours. For disseminated gonococcal infections (after source of infection is proved to be penicillin-sensitive parenteral therapy may be changed to ampicillin 1 g every 6 hours. For prevention of bacterial endocarditis, 1 to 2 g ampicillin with gentamicin 1.5 mg/kg both intramuscularly and intravenously 0.5 hours before the procedure (not to exceed 80 mg), followed by 1.5 g amoxicillin 6 hours after initial dose or repeat parenteral dose 8 hours after initial dose. For genitourinary or gastrointestinal procedures, 2 g ampicillin with gentamicin 1.5 mg/kg, both intramuscularly and intravenously 0.5 hours before the procedure (not to exceed 80 mg), followed by 1.5 g amoxicillin 6 hours after initial dose or repeat parenteral dose 8 hours after initial dose. For rape victims (prophylaxis of infection) as an alternative when tetracycline is contraindicated in pregnant women, 3.5 g orally with 1 g probenecid.

Elderly: Same as adults.

Children: In general, 50 to 200 mg/kg/d in divided doses every 4 to 6 hours. For infants over 7 days and over 2000 g, 100 mg/kg/d in divided doses every 6 hours.

For infants over 7 days and under 2000 g, 75 mg/kg/d in divided doses every 8 hours.

For infants under 7 days and over 2000 g, 75 mg/kg/d in divided doses every 8 hours.

For infants under 7 days and under 2000 g, 50 mg/kg/d in divided doses every 12 hours.

(Note: For meningitis, double dosage [*ie*, 200 mg/kg, 150 mg/kg, 150 mg/kg, and 200 mg/kg, respectively] and administer in divided doses every 4 to 6 hours.) For respiratory tract or soft-tissue infections, *see* adult dosage. For prevention of bacterial endocarditis, 50 mg/kg ampicillin with 2 mg/kg gentamicin both intramuscularly and intravenously 0.5 hours before surgery, followed by 25 mg/kg amoxicillin 6 hours after initial dose or repeat parenteral therapy 8 hours after initial dose. For genitourinary or gastrointestinal procedures, 50 mg/kg with gentamicin 2 mg/kg 0.5 hours before surgery, followed by 25 mg/kg amoxicillin 6 hours after initial dose or repeat parenteral therapy 8 hours after initial dose.

Impaired renal function: Prolong dosage interval to 12 hours for patients with severe impairment (creatinine clearance below 10 mL/min).

OVERDOSAGE

Excessive doses may cause neuromuscular hyperexcitability or convulsive seizures. Dose-related toxicity can arise with the use of large doses of intravenous penicillin (40–100 MU/d), especially in patients with severe renal impairment. Symptoms include agitation, confusion, asterixis, hallucinations, stupor, coma, multifocal myoclonus, seizures, and encephalopathy. Hypokalemia also has occurred.

In case of overdose, discontinue drug therapy and treat patient symptomatically, using supportive care as required. Hemodialysis may be used if necessary to reduce blood levels of penicillin, although effectiveness is uncertain.

PATIENT INFORMATION

Complete all medication unless otherwise directed by physician. Take medication with a full glass of water on an empty stomach 1 hour before or 2 hours following a meal. Take at regular intervals around the clock. Contact physician if rash, itching, hives, severe diarrhea, shortness of breath or wheezing, black tongue, sore throat, nausea, vomiting, fever, swelling of joints, or unusual bleeding or bruising occurs. Throw away any unused liquid form of penicillin after 7 days when stored at room temperature and after 14 days when stored in refrigerator.

AVAILABILITY

Capsules—250 mg and 500 mg
Powder for oral suspension—125 mg/5 mL and 250 mg/5 mL (to make 100, 150, or 200 mL of suspension)

The information here is provided as guidance only. Prescribers should always consult the manufacturer's current prescribing information.

AMPICILLIN–SULBACTAM (Unasyn®)

Ampicillin-sulbactam is a fixed combination of an aminopenicillin and a beta-lactamase inhibitor for parenteral use. Sulbactam has little antimicrobial activity of its own (except with *Acinetobacter* species) but inhibits the inactivation of ampicillin by beta-lactamase–producing strains of staphylococci, gonococci, *Haemophilus influenzae*, *Moraxella catarrhalis*, *Escherichia coli*, *Klebsiella pneumoniae*, and *Bacteroides fragilis*. It has been used to treat upper and lower respiratory tract infections, skin and soft-tissue infections, and intra-abdominal infections. It is especially useful in the parenteral treatment of human and animal bite wounds. The pharmacokinetics of sulbactam are similar to those of ampicillin. Ampicillin and sulbactam are combined in a 2:1 ratio.

ANTIMICROBIAL ACTIVITY

Gram positive: *Staphylococcus aureus**, *Staphylococcus epidermidis**, S. *saprophyticus**, *Enterococcus faecalis*†, *Streptococcus pneumoniae**, *Streptococcus pyogenes*†, *Streptococcus viridans*†.
Gram-negative: *H. influenzae**, *Moraxella (Branhamella) catarrhalis**, *E. coli**, *Klebsiella* spp, *Proteus mirabilis**, *Proteus vulgaris*, *Providencia rettgeri*, *Providencia stuartii*, *Morganella morganii*, and *Neisseria gonorrhoeae**.
Anaerobic: *Clostridium* spp†, *Peptococcus* spp*, *Peptostreptococcus* spp, *Bacteroides* spp (including *B. fragilis*)*.
**Beta-lactamase and non–beta-lactamase–producing.*
†These are not beta-lactamase–producing strains and therefore are susceptible to ampicillin alone.

RESISTANCE

Organisms with new extended-spectrum beta-lactamases that inactivate clavulanic acid have been reported but are extremely rare.

SPECIAL PRECAUTIONS

Direct intravenous administration should be given slowly over at least 10 to 15 minutes. More rapid administration can result in convulsive seizures.
A large percentage of patients with mononucleosis who receive ampicillin develop a skin rash. An alternative should be used in such cases.
Estimated incidence of hypersensitivity is 1% to 10%; serious and occasionally fatal immediate reactions have occurred. Although anaphylaxis is more frequent after parenteral administration, it can occur with oral forms as well. Accelerated reactions (*eg*, urticaria, laryngeal edema) and delayed reactions (serum sickness–like syndrome) may occur. Reactions are most likely to be immediate and severe in patients with penicillin sensitivity and a history of atopic conditions.
Cross-allergenicity with cephalosporins is common in patients with penicillin hypersensitivity.
Desensitization may be considered in patients who have positive skin test results to a penicillin determinant and who have need where no alternative to penicillin exists (*eg*, neurosyphilis, congenital syphilis, or syphilis in pregnancy).
Skin rashes, urticaria, and serum sickness–like reactions may be controlled by antihistamines or corticosteroids if necessary. Unless condition being treated is life-threatening or only amenable to penicillin therapy, discontinuation is recommended.
Bacteriologic studies should be performed to determine causative organisms and their susceptibility.
Use caution in administering broad-spectrum antibiotics to patients with existing or previous gastrointestinal disease. Treatment with broad-spectrum antibiotics alters normal flora of the colon and may permit overgrowth of *Clostridium difficile*, causing antibiotic-associated pseudomembranous colitis. Mild cases usually respond to discontinuation of therapy alone; management of moderate to severe cases should include bacteriologic studies and fluid, electrolyte, and protein supplementation.
White blood and differential cell counts should be performed prior to initiation of therapy and every week during therapy with penicillinase-resistant penicillins.
Monitor AST and ALT to observe for liver function abnormalities during therapy; this is especially important in newborns and infants receiving higher doses.

(Continued on next page)

INDICATIONS

Treatment of infections of the following types due to designated susceptible organisms:
Skin–skin structure:
  Beta-lactamase–producing strains of *S. aureus*, *E. coli*,* *Klebsiella* spp (including *K. pneumoniae*)*, *P. mirabilis**, *B. fragilis**, *Enterobacter* spp*, and *Acinetobacter calcoaceticus**
Intra-abdominal:
  Beta-lactamase–producing strains of *E. coli*, *Klebsiella* spp (including *K. pneumoniae*),* *Bacteroides* spp (including *B. fragilis*)*, and *Enterobacter* spp*
Gynecologic:
  Beta-lactamase–producing strains of *E. coli** and *Bacteroides* spp (including *B. fragilis*)*
**Efficacy for this organism in this type of infection has been studied in less than 10 cases.*

CONTRAINDICATIONS

Patients with a history of immediate hypersensitivity reactions to any of the penicillins

INTERACTIONS

ORAL: beta-blockers
PARENTERAL: aminoglycosides (parenteral), anticoagulants, heparin
BOTH: chloramphenicol, erythromycin, tetracyclines, oral contraceptives

ADVERSE EFFECTS

Pain at intramuscular injection site, mucosal bleeding, substernal pain
See Adverse Effects for amoxicillin-clavulanic acid.

PHARMACOKINETICS AND PHARMACODYNAMICS

Peak serum levels: 109 to 150 µg/mL and 40 to 71 µg/mL for ampicillin after 2-g and 1-g dose, respectively; 48 to 88 and 21 to 40 µg/mL for sulbactam after 1- and 0.5-g dose, respectively.
Plasma half-life: 0.8 to 1.2 h for both ampicillin and sulbactam
Bioavailability: not given orally; diffuses to most body tissues, except brain and cerebrospinal fluid (unless meninges are inflamed)
Metabolism: approximately 10% at ampicillin partially metabolized to penicilloic acids
Elimination: glomerular filtration
Excretion: 75% to 85% of both drugs excreted unchanged in urine after 8 h
Protein binding: ampicillin 28%; sulbactam 38%
Renal impairment: elimination of ampicillin and sulbactam is similarly affected; reduced dosage and prolonged dosage intervals are necessary
Hepatic impairment: ampicillin half-life 1.9 h in patients with cirrhosis

The information here is provided as guidance only. Prescribers should always consult the manufacturer's current prescribing information.

AMPICILLIN–SULBACTAM (CONTINUED)

SPECIAL PRECAUTIONS (CONTINUED)

Prolonged or repeated antibiotic therapy may result in bacterial or fungal overgrowth of nonsusceptible organisms, leading to secondary infection.

The number of strains of staphylococci resistant to penicillinase-resistant penicillins has been growing. Interpret resistance to any penicillinase-resistant penicillin as evidence of clinical resistance to all. Cross-resistance to cephalosporin derivatives also occurs often.

In streptococcal infections, therapy must be completed to eliminate the organism (*ie*, minimum of 10 days) to prevent sequelae, such as rheumatic fever, from occurring.

In gonococcal infections in which primary or secondary syphilis may be suspected, proper diagnostic procedures, including darkfield examinations and monthly serologic tests for a minimum of 4 months, are indicated. Continuation of clinical and serologic examinations every 6 months for 2 to 3 years is recommended for all cases.

Patients with cystic fibrosis have a higher incidence of adverse effects with extended-spectrum penicillins.

Care should be taken with intravenous administration due to the possibility of thrombophlebitis.

Intravenous doses higher than recommended for most penicillins may cause neuromuscular excitability and convulsions.

Avoid subcutaneous and fat layer injections; pain and induration may occur. Inadvertent intravascular administration, including direct arterial injection (or injection immediately adjacent to arteries) has resulted in severe neurovascular damage, including transverse myelitis with permanent paralysis; gangrene, requiring amputation of digits and more proximal portions of extremities; and necrosis and sloughing at the injection site and surrounding area. Other complications include immediate pallor, mottling, or cyanosis of the extremity (both distal and proximal to the injection site), ensuing bleb formation, and severe edema requiring anterior–posterior compartment fasciotomy in the lower extremities. These effects have occurred most frequently in infants and young children. Immediate consultation with a specialist is recommended if any evidence of compromise of blood supply occurs at, proximal to, or distal to the site of injection.

Quadriceps femoris fibrosis and atrophy have occurred after repeated intramuscular injections of penicillin preparations to the anterolateral thigh.

False-positive urine glucose reactions may occur with Clinitest (Ames, Elkhart, IN), Benedicts' solution, or Fehling's solution.

Positive Coombs' test results have occurred.

SPECIAL GROUPS

Children: Safety and efficacy not established for infants and children under 12 years.
Elderly: May have age-related renal impairment.
Renal impairment: Reduced dosage and prolonged dosage intervals necessary in patients with creatinine clearances less than 30 mL/min.
Hepatic impairment: Dosage modification not required.
Pregnancy: Use only if clearly indicated; human studies not performed.
Breast-feeding: Use caution; excreted in breast milk.

DOSAGE

Adults: 1.5 g (1 g ampicillin and 0.5 g sulbactam) to 3 g (2 g ampicillin and 1 g sulbactam) every 6 hours by slow intravenous drip or deep intramuscular injection. Total dose or sulbactam should not exceed 4 g/d.
Elderly: Same as adults.
Children: Safety and efficacy not established for infants and children under 12 years. Prolong dosage interval to 12 hours for patients with creatinine clearances between 10 to 30 mL/min and to 24 hours for patients not on dialysis with creatinine clearances less than 10 mL/min.

OVERDOSAGE

Excessive doses may cause neuromuscular hyperexcitability or convulsive seizures. Dose-related toxicity can arise with the use of large doses of intravenous penicillin (40–100 MU/d), especially with severe renal impairment. Symptoms include agitation, confusion, asterixis, hallucinations, stupor, coma, multifocal myoclonus, seizures, and encephalopathy. Hypokalemia also has occurred.

In case of overdose, discontinue drug therapy and treat patient symptomatically, using supportive care as required. Hemodialysis may be used if necessary to reduce blood levels of penicillin, although effectiveness is uncertain.

AVAILABILITY

Powder for injection
1.5-g vials and bottles (consisting of 1 g ampicillin and 0.5 g sulbactam)
3-g vials and bottles (consisting of 2 g ampicillin and 1 g sulbactam)

The information here is provided as guidance only. Prescribers should always consult the manufacturer's current prescribing information.

BACAMPICILLIN (Spectrobid®)

Bacampicillin is the 1-ethoxycarboxyloxyethyl ester of ampicillin. Ester formulations are inactive until hydrolyzed to ampicillin by esterase enzymes present in the gastrointestinal tract and serum. Four-hundred milligrams of bacampicillin contain the equivalent of 280 mg of ampicillin. Bacampicillin is more stable to acid inactivation and better absorbed from the gastrointestinal tract than ampicillin. Bacampicillin produces blood levels of ampicillin that are two or three times higher than those obtained with oral ampicillin. The indications for use are the same as for amoxicillin.

ANTIMICROBIAL ACTIVITY

Bacampicillin has no *in vitro* activity per se; its *in vivo* activity is due to its parent compound, ampicillin. The ampicillin class of antibiotics has a broad spectrum of activity against many gram-negative and gram-positive organisms. (*See* ampicillin.)

RESISTANCE

Many strains of *Escherichia coli; Haemophilus influenzae*, and *Neisseria gonorrhoeae* produce beta-lactamase enzymes that inactivate bacampicillin.

SPECIAL PRECAUTIONS

A large percentage of patients with mononucleosis who received bacampicillin develop a skin rash. An alternative should be used in such cases. Antibiotics used in high doses for short periods to treat gonococcal infection may mask signs of syphilis. Evaluate patients with gonorrhea for syphilis prior to treatment.
See Special Precautions for amoxicillin.

SPECIAL GROUPS

Children: Safe in children weighing 25 kg or more.
Elderly: No medications required.
Renal impairment: Dosage modification required in patients with creatinine clearances less than 10 mL/min.
Hepatic impairment: No modification required.
Pregnancy: Use only if clearly indicated; controlled human studies not performed.
Breast-feeding: Use caution; excreted in breast milk.

INDICATIONS

Treatment of infections of the following types due to designated susceptible organisms:
Upper and lower respiratory tract (including acute exacerbations of chronic bronchitis):
Streptococci (beta-hemolytic streptococci, *Streptococcus pyogenes*), pneumococci (*Streptococcus pneumoniae*), nonpenicillinase-producing staphylococci, *H. influenzae*
Urinary tract:
E. coli, Proteus mirabilis, Streptococcus faecalis (enterococci)
Skin–skin structure:
Streptococci and susceptible staphylococci
Gonorrhea (acute, uncomplicated urogenital infections):
N. gonorrhoeae

CONTRAINDICATIONS

Patients with a history of immediate hypersensitivity reactions to any of the penicillins

INTERACTIONS

ORAL: beta-blockers
PARENTERAL: aminoglycosides (parenteral), anticoagulants, heparin
BOTH: chloramphenicol, erythromycin, tetracyclines, oral contraceptives

ADVERSE EFFECTS

See Adverse Effects for amoxicillin-clavulanic acid.

PHARMACOKINETICS AND PHARMACODYNAMICS

Peak serum levels: 7.9, 12.9, and 20.1 µg/mL after 400-, 800-, and 1600-mg doses, respectively
Plasma half-life: 0.8 to 1.2 h
Bioavailability: 83% widely distributed
Metabolism: approximately 10% of ampicillin is partially metabolized to penicilloic acids rapidly converted to ampicillin by hydrolysis of the ester linkage
Elimination: glomerular filtration and tubular secretion
Excretion: 75% unchanged in urine
Effect of food: no significant effect
Protein binding: 20%
Renal impairment: half-life of ampicillin 7.4 to 21 h in patients with creatinine clearance less than 10 mL/min
Hepatic impairment: half-life of ampicillin 1.9 h in patients with cirrhosis

The information here is provided as guidance only. Prescribers should always consult the manufacturer's current prescribing information.

BACAMPICILLIN (CONTINUED)

DOSAGE

Adults: For infections of upper respiratory tract (including otitis media), urinary tract, or skin–skin structure, one 400-mg table every 12 hours. For severe infections or those due to less susceptible organisms, two 400-mg tablets every 12 hours. For infections of the lower respiratory tract, two 400-mg tables every 12 hours. For acute, uncomplicated gonorrhea, 1.6 g (four 400-mg tablets) with 1 g probenecid, as a single oral dose.

Elderly: Same as adults.

Children: Safety not established for children weighing less than 25 kg. For infections of the upper respiratory tract (including otitis media), urinary tract, or skin–skin structure, 25 mg/kg/d in equally divided doses every 12 hours. For severe infections or those due to less susceptible organisms, 50 mg/kg/d in equally divided doses every 12 hours. For infections of the lower respiratory tract, 50 mg/kg/d in equally divided doses every 12 hours. (Note: For infections due to hemolytic streptococci, it is recommended that duration of treatment continue a minimum of 10 days to prevent the occurrence of rheumatic fever or glomerulonephritis.)

OVERDOSAGE

Excessive doses may cause neuromuscular hyperexcitability or convulsive seizures. Dose-related toxicity can arise with the use of large doses of intravenous penicillin (40–100 MU/d), especially in patients with severe renal impairment. Symptoms include agitation, confusion, asterixis, hallucinations, stupor, coma, multifocal myoclonus, seizures, and encephalopathy. Hypokalemia also has occurred.

In case of overdose, discontinue drug therapy and treat patient symptomatically, using supportive care as required. Hemodialysis may be used if necessary to reduce blood levels of penicillin, although effectiveness is uncertain.

PATIENT INFORMATION

Complete all medication unless otherwise directed by physician. Take medication with a full glass of water on an empty stomach 1 hour before or 2 hours following a meal. Take at regular intervals around the clock. Contact physician if rash, itching, hives, severe diarrhea, shortness of breath or wheezing, black tongue, sore throat, nausea, vomiting, fever, swelling of joints, or unusual bleeding or bruising occurs. Throw away any unused liquid form of penicillin after 7 days when stored at room temperature and after 14 days when stored in refrigerator.

AVAILABILITY

Tablets—400 mg

The information here is provided as guidance only. Prescribers should always consult the manufacturer's current prescribing information.

CARBENICILLIN INDANYL SODIUM (Geocillin®)

Indanyl carbenicillin is the alpha-carboxyl ester of carbenicillin. It has no antimicrobial activity until hydrolyzed to carbenicillin by esterase enzymes present in the gastrointestinal tract and serum. The ester is highly stable to acid inactivation and well absorbed from the gastrointestinal tract. Carbenicillin is a broad-spectrum penicillin with enhanced activity against *Pseudomonas aeruginosa*. The drug was available in parenteral form for many years, but its use was replaced by ticarcillin. The oral ester formulation provides therapeutic concentrations in the urinary tract only. It is especially useful in the oral treatment of *Pseudomonas* infections of the urinary tract in pediatric patients in whom other agents, such as the quinolones, are not recommended.

ANTIMICROBIAL ACTIVITY

Demonstrated clinical efficacy for urinary tract infections due to susceptible strains of the following:
Escherichia coli, Proteus mirabilis, Proteus vulgaris, Morganella morganii, Pseudomonas spp, *Providencia rettgeri, Enterobacter* spp, *Enterococcus faecalis.*
In vitro data indicate the following pathogens to be generally susceptible, although this is not substantiated by clinical data:
Staphylococcus spp (nonpenicillinase-producing) and *Streptococcus* spp.

RESISTANCE

Some strains of *Pseudomonas* have developed resistance.

SPECIAL PRECAUTIONS

Estimated incidence of hypersensitivity is 1% to 10%; serious and occasionally fatal immediate reactions have occurred. Although anaphylaxis is more frequent after parenteral administration, it can occur with oral forms as well. Accelerated reactions (*eg*, urticaria, laryngeal edema) and delayed reactions (serum sickness–like syndrome) may occur. Reactions are most likely to be immediate and severe in patients with penicillin sensitivity and a history of atopic conditions.
Cross-allergenicity with cephalosporins is common in patients with penicillin hypersensitivity.
Desensitization may be considered in patients who have positive skin test results to a penicillin determinant and who have need where no alternative to penicillin exists (*eg*, neurosyphilis, congenital syphilis, or syphilis in pregnancy).
Skin rashes, urticaria, and serum sickness–like reactions may be controlled by antihistamines or corticosteroids if necessary. Unless condition being treated is life-threatening or only amenable to penicillin therapy, discontinuation is recommended.
Bacteriologic studies should be performed to determine causative organisms and their susceptibility.
Use caution in administering broad-spectrum antibiotics to patients with existing or previous gastrointestinal disease. Treatment with broad-spectrum antibiotics alters normal flora of the colon and may permit overgrowth of *Clostridium difficile*, causing antibiotic-associated pseudomembranous colitis. Mild cases usually respond to discontinuation of therapy alone; management of moderate to severe cases should include bacteriologic studies and fluid, electrolyte, and protein supplementation.
White blood and differential cell counts should be performed prior to initiation of therapy and every week during therapy with penicillinase-resistant penicillins.
Monitor AST and ALT to observe for liver function abnormalities during therapy; this is especially important in newborns and infants receiving higher doses.
Prolonged or repeated antibiotic therapy may result in bacterial or fungal overgrowth of nonsusceptible organisms, leading to secondary infection.

(Continued on next page)

INDICATIONS

Treatment of infections of the following types due to susceptible strains of designated organisms:
Acute and chronic upper or lower urinary tract infection or asymptomatic bacteriuria:
E. coli, P. mirabilis, M. morganii, P. rettgeri, P. vulgaris, Pseudomonas, Enterobacter, enterococci
Prostatitis:
E. coli, Enterococcus (*S. faecalis*), *P. mirabilis, Enterobacter*

CONTRAINDICATIONS

Patients with a history of immediate hypersensitivity reactions to any of the penicillins

INTERACTIONS

ORAL: beta-blockers
PARENTERAL: aminoglycosides (parenteral), anticoagulants, heparin
BOTH: chloramphenicol, erythromycin, tetracyclines, oral contraceptives

ADVERSE EFFECTS

Hyperthermia, headache, itchy eyes, vaginitis
See Adverse Effects for amoxicillin-clavulanic acid.

PHARMACOKINETICS AND PHARMACODYNAMICS

Peak serum levels: 6.5 µg/mL 1 hour after 500-mg dose
Plasma half-life: 1 to 1.3 h
Bioavailability: 30% to 40% of oral dose
Metabolism: rapidly converted to carbenicillin by hydrolysis of the ester linkage
Elimination: glomerular filtration and tubular secretion
Excretion: in urine, approximately 30% unchanged within 12 h
Effect of food: no significant effect
Protein binding: 45%
Renal impairment: half-life of carbenicillin is 9.4 to 23 h in patients with creatinine clearance less than 30 mL/min

OVERDOSAGE

Excessive doses may cause neuromuscular hyperexcitability or convulsive seizures. Dose-related toxicity can arise with the use of large doses of intravenous penicillin (40–100 MU/d), especially in patients with severe renal impairment. Symptoms include agitation, confusion, asterixis, hallucinations, stupor, coma, multifocal myoclonus, seizures, and encephalopathy. Hypokalemia also has occurred.
In case of overdose, discontinue drug therapy and treat patient symptomatically, using supportive care as required. Hemodialysis may be used if necessary to reduce blood levels of penicillin, although effectiveness is uncertain

The information here is provided as guidance only. Prescribers should always consult the manufacturer's current prescribing information.

CARBENICILLIN INDANYL SODIUM (CONTINUED)

SPECIAL PRECAUTIONS (CONTINUED)

The number of strains of staphylococci resistant to penicillinase-resistant penicillins has been growing. Interpret resistance to any penicillinase-resistant penicillin as evidence of clinical resistance to all. Cross-resistance to cephalosporin derivatives also occurs often.

In streptococcal infections, therapy must be completed to eliminate the organism (*ie*, minimum of 10 days) to prevent sequelae, such as rheumatic fever, from occurring.

In gonococcal infections in which primary or secondary syphilis may be suspected, proper diagnostic procedures, including darkfield examinations and monthly serologic tests for a minimum of 4 months, are indicated. Continuation of clinical and serologic examinations every 6 months for 2 to 3 years is recommended for all cases.

Patients with cystic fibrosis have a higher incidence of adverse effects with extended-spectrum penicillins.

Care should be taken with intravenous administration due to the possibility of thrombophlebitis. Intravenous doses higher than recommended for most penicillins may cause neuromuscular excitability and convulsions.

Avoid subcutaneous and fat layer injections; pain and induration may occur. Inadvertent intravascular administration, including direct arterial injection (or injection immediately adjacent to arteries) has resulted in severe neurovascular damage, including transverse myelitis with permanent paralysis; gangrene, requiring amputation of digits and more proximal portions of extremities; and necrosis and sloughing at the injection site and surrounding area. Other complications include immediate pallor, mottling, or cyanosis of the extremity (both distal and proximal to the injection site), ensuing bleb formation, and severe edema requiring anterior–posterior compartment fasciotomy in the lower extremities. These effects have occurred most frequently in infants and young children. Immediate consultation with a specialist is recommended if any evidence of compromise of blood supply occurs at, proximal to, or distal to the site of injection.

Quadriceps femoris fibrosis and atrophy have occurred after repeated intramuscular injections of penicillin preparations to the anterolateral thigh.

False-positive urine glucose reactions may occur with Clinitest (Ames, Elkhart, IN), Benedicts' solution, or Fehling's solution.

Positive Coombs' test results have occurred.

SPECIAL GROUPS

Children: Safety and efficacy not established.
Elderly: May have age-related renal impairment.
Renal impairment: Patients with creatinine clearance less than 30 mL/min may require dosage adjustment to prevent accumulation of drug.
Hepatic impairment: No modification required.
Pregnancy: Use only when clearly indicated; controlled human studies not performed.
Breast-feeding: Use caution; excreted in breast milk.

DOSAGE

Adults: For urinary tract infections due to *E. coli*, *Proteus* spp, and *Enterobacter*: one to two tablets every 6 hours; due to *Pseudomonas* and *Enterococcus*, two tablets every 6 hours. For prostatitis, two tablets every 6 hours.
Elderly: Same as adults.
Children: Safety not established.

PATIENT INFORMATION

Complete all medication unless otherwise directed by physician. Take medication with a full glass of water on an empty stomach 1 hour before or 2 hours following a meal. Take at regular intervals around the clock. Contact physician if rash, itching, hives, severe diarrhea, shortness of breath or wheezing, black tongue, sore throat, nausea, vomiting, fever, swelling of joints, or unusual bleeding or bruising occurs. Throw away any unused liquid form of penicillin after 7 days when stored at room temperature and after 14 days when stored in refrigerator.

AVAILABILITY

Tablets—each contains carbenicillin indanyl sodium equivalent to 382 mg carbenicillin

The information here is provided as guidance only. Prescribers should always consult the manufacturer's current prescribing information.

CLOXACILLIN (Cloxipen®, Tegopen®)

Cloxacillin is one of the isoxazolyl class of penicillinase-resistant penicillins. It differs in structure from oxacillin only by the addition of a chloride atom on the phenyl ring of the side chain. This modification accounts for the increased gastrointestinal absorption and decreased hepatic clearance of cloxacillin compared with oxacillin. The drug is used for oral treatment of staphylococcal infections, including osteomyelitis.

ANTIMICROBIAL ACTIVITY

Gram-positive: *Staphylococcus aureus* of the staphylococci spp and *Streptococcus pneumoniae.*

RESISTANCE

See dicloxacillin.

SPECIAL PRECAUTIONS

Elevations of AST, ALT, bilirubin, and LDH have been particularly noted with cloxacillin.

Estimated incidence of hypersensitivity is 1% to 10%; serious and occasionally fatal immediate reactions have occurred. Although anaphylaxis is more frequent after parenteral administration, it can occur with oral forms as well. Accelerated reactions (eg, urticaria, laryngeal edema) and delayed reactions (serum sickness–like syndrome) may occur. Reactions are most likely to be immediate and severe in patients with penicillin sensitivity and a history of atopic conditions.

Cross-allergenicity with cephalosporins is common in patients with penicillin hypersensitivity.

Desensitization may be considered in patients who have positive skin test results to a penicillin determinant and who have need where no alternative to penicillin exists (*eg*, neurosyphilis, congenital syphilis, or syphilis in pregnancy).

Skin rashes, urticaria, and serum sickness–like reactions may be controlled by antihistamines or corticosteroids if necessary. Unless condition being treated is life-threatening or only amenable to penicillin therapy, discontinuation is recommended.

Bacteriologic studies should be performed to determine causative organisms and their susceptibility.

Use caution in administering broad-spectrum antibiotics to patients with existing or previous gastrointestinal disease. Treatment with broad-spectrum antibiotics alters normal flora of the colon and may permit overgrowth of *Clostridium difficile*, causing antibiotic-associated pseudomembranous colitis. Mild cases usually respond to discontinuation of therapy alone; management of moderate to severe cases should include bacteriologic studies and fluid, electrolyte, and protein supplementation.

White blood and differential cell counts should be performed prior to initiation of therapy and every week during therapy with penicillinase-resistant penicillins.

Monitor AST and ALT to observe for liver function abnormalities during therapy; this is especially important in newborns and infants receiving higher doses.

Prolonged or repeated antibiotic therapy may result in bacterial or fungal overgrowth of nonsusceptible organisms, leading to secondary infection.

The number of strains of staphylococci resistant to penicillinase-resistant penicillins has been growing. Interpret resistance to any penicillinase-resistant penicillin as evidence of clinical resistance to all. Cross-resistance to cephalosporin derivatives also occurs often.

In streptococcal infections, therapy must be completed to eliminate the organism (*ie*, minimum of 10 days) to prevent sequelae, such as rheumatic fever, from occurring.

(Continued on next page)

INDICATIONS

Treatment of infections due to penicillinase-producing staphylococci. Cloxacillin may be used to initiate therapy when staphylococcal infection is suspected because of the high frequency of penicillinase-producing staphylococci in the community as well as in the hospital.

Also effective in infections due to pneumococci group A beta-hemolytic streptococci.

CONTRAINDICATIONS

Patients with a history of immediate hypersensitivity reactions to any of the penicillins

INTERACTIONS

ORAL: beta-blockers
PARENTERAL: aminoglycosides (parenteral), anticoagulants, heparin
BOTH: chloramphenicol, erythromycin, tetracyclines, oral contraceptives

ADVERSE EFFECTS

See Adverse Effects for amoxicillin-clavulanic acid.

PHARMACOKINETICS AND PHARMACODYNAMICS

Peak serum levels: 1 to 2 h, 6.9 to 15 µg/mL for 500-mg dose
Plasma half-life: 0.4 to 0.8 h
Bioavailability: 37% to 60%
Metabolism: approximately 35% metabolized to active and inactive metabolites
Excretion: approximately 40% is excreted unchanged in urine in 6 to 8 h
Elimination: glomerular filtration and tubular secretion
Effect of food: food inhibits absorption
Protein binding: 95%
Renal impairment: half-life 0.8 to 2.3 h in patients with severe renal impairment
Hepatic impairment: no information

OVERDOSAGE

Excessive doses may cause neuromuscular hyperexcitability or convulsive seizures. Dose-related toxicity can arise with the use of large doses of intravenous penicillin (40 –100 MU/d), especially in patients with severe renal impairment. Symptoms include agitation, confusion, asterixis, hallucinations, stupor, coma, multifocal myoclonus, seizures, and encephalopathy. Hypokalemia also has occurred.

In case of overdose, discontinue drug therapy and treat patient symptomatically, using supportive care as required. Hemodialysis may be used if necessary to reduce blood levels of penicillin, although effectiveness is uncertain.

The information here is provided as guidance only. Prescribers should always consult the manufacturer's current prescribing information.

CLOXACILLIN (CONTINUED)

SPECIAL PRECAUTIONS (CONTINUED)

In gonococcal infections in which primary or secondary syphilis may be suspected, proper diagnostic procedures, including darkfield examinations and monthly serologic tests for a minimum of 4 months, are indicated. Continuation of clinical and serologic examinations every 6 months for 2 to 3 years is recommended for all cases.

Patients with cystic fibrosis have a higher incidence of adverse effects with extended-spectrum penicillins.

Care should be taken with intravenous administration due to the possibility of thrombophlebitis.

Intravenous dosage higher than recommended for most penicillins may cause neuromuscular excitability and convulsions.

Avoid subcutaneous and fat layer injections; pain and induration may occur. Inadvertent intravascular administration, including direct arterial injection (or injection immediately adjacent to arteries) has resulted in severe neurovascular damage, including transverse myelitis and permanent paralysis; gangrene, requiring amputation of digits and more proximal portions of extremities; and necrosis and sloughing at the injection site and surrounding area. Other complications include immediate pallor, mottling, or cyanosis of the extremity (both distal and proximal to the injection site), ensuing bleb formation, and severe edema requiring anterior–posterior compartment fasciotomy in the lower extremities. These effects have occurred most frequently in infants and young children. Immediate consultation with a specialist is recommended if any evidence of compromise of blood supply occurs at, proximal to, or distal to the site of injection.

Quadriceps femoris fibrosis and atrophy have occurred after repeated intramuscular injections of penicillin preparations to the anterolateral thigh.

False-positive urine glucose reactions may occur with Clinitest (Ames, Elkhart, IN), Benedicts' solution, or Fehling's solution.

Positive Coombs' test results have occurred.

SPECIAL GROUPS

Children: Dosage is based on body weight.
Elderly: No modification required.
Renal impairment: No modification required.
Hepatic impairment: No modification required.
Pregnancy: Use only when clearly indicated; human studies not performed.
Breast-feeding: Use caution; excreted in breast milk.

DOSAGE

Adults: For mild to moderate upper respiratory infections and localized skin or soft-tissue infections, 250 mg every 6 hours. For severe infections, lower respiratory tract, or disseminated infections, 500 mg every 6 hours.
Elderly: Same as adults.
Children: (Children weighing under 20 kg) For mild to moderate upper respiratory infections and localized skin or soft-tissue infections, 50 mg/kg/d in equally divided doses every 6 hours. For severe infections, lower respiratory tract, or disseminated infections, 100 mg/kg/d in equal doses every 6 hours. (Children weighing over 20 kg, use adult dosage.)

PATIENT INFORMATION

Complete all medication unless otherwise directed by physician. Take medication with a full glass of water on an empty stomach 1 hour before or 2 hours following a meal. Take at regular intervals around the clock. Contact physician if rash, itching, hives, severe diarrhea, shortness of breath or wheezing, black tongue, sore throat, nausea, vomiting, fever, swelling of joints, or unusual bleeding or bruising occurs. Throw away any unused liquid form of penicillin after 7 days when stored at room temperature and after 14 days when stored in refrigerator.

AVAILABILITY

Capsules—250 mg and 500 mg
Powder for oral suspension—125 mg/5 mL (when reconstituted)

The information here is provided as guidance only. Prescribers should always consult the manufacturer's current prescribing information.

DICLOXACILLIN (Dycill®, Dynapen®, Pathocil®)

Dicloxacillin is one of the isoxazolyl class of penicillinase-resistant penicillins. It differs in structure from oxacillin by the addition of two chloride atoms to the phenyl ring of the side chain. Dicloxacillin has the best gastrointestinal absorption of all the penicillinase-resistant penicillins. The drug is used for oral treatment of staphylococcal infections, including osteomyelitis.

ANTIMICROBIAL ACTIVITY

Gram-positive: beta-hemolytic streptococci, pneumococci, penicillin G–sensitive staphylococci, penicillin G–resistant staphylococci.

RESISTANCE

Strains resistant to methicillin are usually resistant to all other penicillinase-resistant penicillins (cross-resistance with cephalosporin derivatives also is frequent). Resistance to any penicillinase-resistant penicillin should be interpreted as clinical evidence of resistance to all, regardless of the fact that minor variations in *in vitro* sensitivity may be encountered when more than one penicillinase-resistant penicillin is tested against the same strain of *Staphylococcus*.

SPECIAL PRECAUTIONS

Estimated incidence of hypersensitivity is 1% to 10%; serious and occasionally fatal immediate reactions have occurred. Although anaphylaxis is more frequent after parenteral administration, it can occur with oral forms as well. Accelerated reactions (*eg*, urticaria, laryngeal edema) and delayed reactions (serum sickness–like syndrome) may occur. Reactions are most likely to be immediate and severe in patients with penicillin sensitivity and a history of atopic conditions.
Cross-allergenicity with cephalosporins is common in patients with penicillin hypersensitivity.
Desensitization may be considered in patients who have positive skin test results to a penicillin determinant and who have need where no alternative to penicillin exists (*eg*, neurosyphilis, congenital syphilis, or syphilis in pregnancy).
Skin rashes, urticaria, and serum sickness–like reactions may be controlled by antihistamines or corticosteroids if necessary. Unless condition being treated is life-threatening or only amenable to penicillin therapy, discontinuation is recommended. Bacteriologic studies should be performed to determine causative organisms and their susceptibility.
Use caution in administering broad-spectrum antibiotics to patients with existing or previous gastrointestinal disease. Treatment with broad-spectrum antibiotics alters normal flora of the colon and may permit overgrowth of *Clostridium difficile*, causing antibiotic-associated pseudomembranous colitis. Mild cases usually respond to discontinuation of therapy alone; management of moderate to severe cases should include bacteriologic studies and fluid, electrolyte, and protein supplementation. White blood and differential cell counts should be performed prior to initiation of therapy and every week during therapy with penicillinase-resistant penicillins. Monitor AST and ALT to observe for liver function abnormalities during therapy; this is especially important in newborns and infants receiving higher doses. Prolonged or repeated antibiotic therapy may result in bacterial or fungal overgrowth of nonsusceptible organisms, leading to secondary infection.
The number of strains of staphylococci resistant to penicillinase-resistant penicillins has been growing. Interpret resistance to any penicillinase-resistant penicillin as evidence of clinical resistance to all. Cross-resistance to cephalosporin derivatives also occurs often.
In streptococcal infections, therapy must be completed to eliminate the organism (*ie*, minimum of 10 days) to prevent sequelae, such as rheumatic fever, from occurring.

(Continued on next page)

INDICATIONS

Treatment of infections due to penicillinase-producing staphylococci. Cloxacillin may be used to initiate therapy when staphylococcal infection is suspected because of the high frequency of penicillinase-producing staphylococci in the community as well as in the hospital.
Also effective in infections due to pneumococci group A beta-hemolytic streptococci.
See Indications for cloxacillin.

CONTRAINDICATIONS

Patients with a history of immediate hypersensitivity reactions to any of the penicillins

ADVERSE EFFECTS

See Adverse Effects for amoxicillin-clavulanic acid.

PHARMACOKINETICS AND PHARMACODYNAMICS

Peak serum levels: 1 to 2 h, 10 to 18 µg/mL for 500-mg dose
Plasma half-life: 0.6 to 0.8 h
Bioavailability: 35% to 76%
Metabolism: approximately 25% metabolized to active and inactive metabolites
Elimination: glomerular filtration and tubular generation
Excretion: approximately 40% is excreted unchanged in urine in 6 to 8 h
Effect of food: food inhibits absorption
Protein binding: 98%
Renal impairment: half-life is 1.0 to 2.2 h in patients with severe renal impairment
Hepatic impairment: no information

The information here is provided as guidance only. Prescribers should always consult the manufacturer's current prescribing information.

DICLOXACILLIN (CONTINUED)

SPECIAL PRECAUTIONS (CONTINUED)

In gonococcal infections in which primary or secondary syphilis may be suspected, proper diagnostic procedures, including darkfield examinations and monthly serologic tests for a minimum of 4 months, are indicated. Continuation of clinical and serologic examinations every 6 months for 2 to 3 years is recommended for all cases.

Patients with cystic fibrosis have a higher incidence of adverse effects with extended-spectrum penicillins.

Care should be taken with intravenous administration due to the possibility of thrombophlebitis.

Intravenous doses higher than recommended for most penicillins may cause neuromuscular excitability and convulsions.

Avoid subcutaneous and fat layer injections; pain and induration may occur.

Inadvertent intravascular administration, including direct arterial injection (or injection immediately adjacent to arteries) has resulted in severe neurovascular damage, including transverse myelitis with permanent paralysis; gangrene, requiring amputation of digits and more proximal portions of extremities; and necrosis and sloughing at the injection site and surrounding area. Other complications include immediate pallor, mottling, or cyanosis of the extremity (both distal and proximal to the injection site), ensuing bleb formation, and severe edema requiring anterior–posterior compartment fasciotomy in the lower extremities. These effects have occurred most frequently in infants and young children. Immediate consultation with a specialist is recommended if any evidence of compromise of blood supply occurs at, proximal to, or distal to the site of injection.

Quadriceps femoris fibrosis and atrophy have occurred after repeated intramuscular injections of penicillin preparations to the anterolateral thigh.

False-positive urine glucose reactions may occur with Clinitest (Ames, Elkhart, IN), Benedicts' solution, or Fehling's solution.

Positive Coombs' test results have occurred.

SPECIAL GROUPS

Children: Safety not established for use in neonates or premature infants.
Elderly: No modification required.
Renal impairment: No modification required.
Hepatic impairment: No modification required.
Pregnancy: Use only when clearly indicated; controlled human studies not performed.
Breast-feeding: Use caution; excreted in breast milk.

DOSAGE

Adults: For mild to moderate upper respiratory infection and localized skin or soft-tissue infections, 125 mg every 6 hours. For more severe infections (lower respiratory tract or disseminated infections), 250 to 500 mg every 6 hours.
Elderly: Same as adults.
Children: (Children weighing under 40 kg) For mild to moderate upper respiratory infection and localized skin or soft-tissue infections, 12.5 mg/kg/d in equally divided doses every 6 hours. For more severe infections (lower respiratory tract or disseminated infections), 25 mg/kg/d or more in equally divided doses every 6 hours. (Children weighing over 40 kg, *see* adult dosage.)
Safety and efficacy not established for use in neonates and premature infants.
(Note: Treatment of infections due to Group A beta-hemolytic streptococci should continue for a minimum of 10 days to prevent the occurrence of rheumatic fever or acute glomerulonephritis.)

OVERDOSAGE

Excessive doses may cause neuromuscular hyperexcitability or convulsive seizures. Dose-related toxicity can arise with the use of large doses of intravenous penicillin (40–100 MU/d), especially in patients with severe renal impairment. Symptoms include agitation, confusion, asterixis, hallucinations, stupor, coma, multifocal myoclonus, seizures, and encephalopathy. Hypokalemia also has occurred.

In case of overdose, discontinue drug therapy and treat patient symptomatically, using supportive care as required. Hemodialysis may be used if necessary to reduce blood levels of penicillin, although effectiveness is uncertain.

AVAILABILITY

Capsules—250 mg and 500 mg
Powder for oral suspension—bottles containing 62.5 mg/5 mL (when reconstituted)

The information here is provided as guidance only. Prescribers should always consult the manufacturer's current prescribing information.

METHICILLIN (Staphcillin®)

Methicillin was the first penicillinase-resistant penicillin available for clinical use. It is rapidly destroyed by gastric acid and is available for parenteral administration only. The drug is used for the treatment of serious staphylococcal infections. Methicillin does not provide adequate cerebrospinal fluid concentrations for the treatment of staphylococcal meningitis. Methicillin also has been associated with a higher incidence of interstitial nephritis than other penicillins.

ANTIMICROBIAL ACTIVITY

Gram-positive: *Staphylococcus aureus,* other staphylococci, streptococci, *Streptococcus pneumoniae.*

RESISTANCE

See Resistance for dicloxacillin.

SPECIAL PRECAUTIONS

Interstitial nephritis (oliguria, proteinuria, hematuria, hyaline casts, pyuria) and nephropathy are associated with high doses of parenteral penicillins, most frequently methicillin.

Estimated incidence of hypersensitivity 1% to 10%; serious and occasionally fatal immediate reactions have occurred. Although anaphylaxis is more frequent after parenteral administration, it can occur with oral forms as well. Accelerated reactions (*eg*, urticaria, laryngeal edema) and delayed reactions (serum sickness–like syndrome) may occur. Reactions are most likely to be immediate and severe in patients with penicillin sensitivity and a history of atopic conditions.

Cross-allergenicity with cephalosporins is common in patients with penicillin hypersensitivity.

Desensitization may be considered in patients who have positive skin test results to a penicillin determinant and who have need where no alternative to penicillin exists (*eg*, neurosyphilis, congenital syphilis, or syphilis in pregnancy).

Skin rashes, urticaria, and serum sickness–like reactions may be controlled by antihistamines or corticosteroids if necessary. Unless condition being treated is life-threatening or only amenable to penicillin therapy, discontinuation is recommended. Bacteriologic studies should be performed to determine causative organisms and their susceptibility.

Use caution in administering broad-spectrum antibiotics to patients with existing or previous gastrointestinal disease. Treatment with broad-spectrum antibiotics alters normal flora of the colon and may permit overgrowth of *Clostridium difficile*, causing antibiotic-associated pseudomembranous colitis. Mild cases usually respond to discontinuation of therapy alone; management of moderate to severe cases should include bacteriologic studies and fluid, electrolyte, and protein supplementation. White blood and differential cell counts should be performed prior to initiation of therapy and every week during therapy with penicillinase-resistant penicillins. Monitor AST and ALT to observe for liver function abnormalities during therapy; this is especially important in newborns and infants receiving higher doses.

Prolonged or repeated antibiotic therapy may result in bacterial or fungal overgrowth of nonsusceptible organisms, leading to secondary infection.

The number of strains of staphylococci resistant to penicillinase-resistant penicillins has been growing. Interpret resistance to any penicillinase-resistant penicillin as evidence of clinical resistance to all. Cross-resistance to cephalosporin derivatives also occurs often.

In streptococcal infections, therapy must be completed to eliminate the organism (*ie*, minimum of 10 days) to prevent sequelae, such as rheumatic fever, from occurring.

(Continued on next page)

INDICATIONS

Treatment of infection due to penicillinase-producing staphylococci. Methicillin may be used to initiate therapy when staphylococcal infection is suspected because of the high frequency of penicillinase-producing staphylococci in the community as well as the hospital.

CONTRAINDICATIONS

Patients with a history of immediate hypersensitivity reactions to any of the penicillins

INTERACTIONS

ORAL: beta-blockers
PARENTERAL: aminoglycosides (parenteral), anticoagulants, heparin
BOTH: chloramphenicol, erythromycin, tetracyclines, oral contraceptives

ADVERSE EFFECTS

See Adverse Effects for amoxicillin-clavulanic acid.

PHARMACOKINETICS AND PHARMACODYNAMICS

Peak serum levels: 109 and 60µg/mL for doses of 1 and 2 g, respectively
Plasma half-life: 0.4 to 0.5 h
Bioavailability: not used orally; diffuses into most body tissues, except brain and spinal fluid (unless meninges inflamed)
Metabolism: minimal
Elimination: glomerular filtration and tubular secretion
Excretion: approximately 70% of dose excreted unchanged in urine in 12 h
Effect of food: methicillin is for parenteral use only
Protein binding: 40%
Renal impairment: half-life 4 to 6 h in patients with creatinine clearance less than 10 mL/min
Hepatic impairment: no information

OVERDOSAGE

Excessive doses may cause neuromuscular hyperexcitability or convulsive seizures. Dose-related toxicity can arise with the use of large doses of intravenous penicillin (40–100 MU/d), especially in patients with severe renal impairment. Symptoms include agitation, confusion, asterixis, hallucinations, stupor, coma, multifocal myoclonus, seizures, and encephalopathy. Hypokalemia also has occurred.

In case of overdose, discontinue drug therapy and treat patient symptomatically, using supportive care as required. Hemodialysis may be used if necessary to reduce blood levels of penicillin, although effectiveness is uncertain.

The information here is provided as guidance only. Prescribers should always consult the manufacturer's current prescribing information.

METHICILLIN (CONTINUED)

SPECIAL PRECAUTIONS (CONTINUED)

In gonococcal infections in which primary or secondary syphilis may be suspected, proper diagnostic procedures, including darkfield examinations and monthly serologic tests for a minimum of 4 months, are indicated. Continuation of clinical and serologic examinations every 6 months for 2 to 3 years is recommended for all cases. Patients with cystic fibrosis have a higher incidence of adverse effects with extended-spectrum penicillins.

Care should be taken with intravenous administration due to the possibility of thrombophlebitis. Intravenous doses higher than recommended for most penicillins may cause neuromuscular excitability and convulsions.

Avoid subcutaneous and fat layer injections; pain and induration may occur. Inadvertent intravascular administration, including direct arterial injection (or injection immediately adjacent to arteries) has resulted in severe neurovascular damage, including transverse myelitis with permanent paralysis; gangrene, requiring amputation of digits and more proximal portions of extremities; and necrosis and sloughing at the injection site and surrounding area. Other complications include immediate pallor, mottling, or cyanosis of the extremity (both distal and proximal to the injection site), ensuing bleb formation, and severe edema requiring anterior–posterior compartment fasciotomy in the lower extremities. These effects have occurred most frequently in infants and young children. Immediate consultation with a specialist is recommended if any evidence of compromise of blood supply occurs at, proximal to, or distal to the site of injection.

Quadriceps femoris fibrosis and atrophy have occurred after repeated intramuscular injections of penicillin preparations to the anterolateral thigh.

False-positive urine glucose reactions may occur with Clinitest (Ames, Elkhart, IN), Benedicts' solution, or Fehling's solution.

Positive Coombs' test results have occurred.

SPECIAL GROUPS

Children: Safe for use.
Elderly: No modification required.
Renal impairment: Dosage modification required in patients with creatinine clearance less than 10 mL/min.
Hepatic impairment: No modification required.
Pregnancy: Use only if clearly indicated; controlled human studies not performed.
Breast-feeding: Use caution; excreted in breast milk.

DOSAGE

Adults: 4 to 12 g/d in divided doses every 4 to 6 hours.*
Elderly: May have age-related renal impairment.
Children: 100 to 400 mg/kg/d in divided doses every 4 to 6 hours.
For infants over 7 days and over 2000 g, 100 mg/kg/d in divided doses every 6 hours.*
For infants over 7 days and under 2000 g, 75 mg/kg/d in divided doses every 8 hours.*
For infants under 7 days and over 2000 g, 75 mg/kg/d in divided doses every 8 hours.*
For infants under 7 days and under 2000 g, 50 mg/kg/d in divided doses every 12 hours.*
Double dosage for meningitis (eg, normal dose = 100 mg/kg/d; meningitis dose = 200 mg/kg/d).

Impaired renal function: In severe renal impairment (creatinine clearance below 10 mL/min) do not exceed 2 g every 12 hours.

PATIENT INFORMATION

Complete all medication unless otherwise directed by physician. Take medication with a full glass of water on an empty stomach 1 hour before or 2 hours following a meal. Take at regular intervals around the clock. Contact physician if rash, itching, hives, severe diarrhea, shortness of breath or wheezing, black tongue, sore throat, nausea, vomiting, fever, swelling of joints, or unusual bleeding or bruising occurs. Throw away any unused liquid form of penicillin after 7 days when stored at room temperature and after 14 days when stored in refrigerator.

AVAILABILITY

Powder for injection
1 g in vials and piggyback vials
4-g vials
6-g vials
10-g bulk vials

The information here is provided as guidance only. Prescribers should always consult the manufacturer's current prescribing information.

MEZLOCILLIN (Mezlin®)

Mezlocillin is a semisynthetic, broad-spectrum ureidopenicillin. It has a broad spectrum of antimicrobial activity against many gram-positive and gram-negative organisms, including *Pseudomonas aeruginosa*. The drug also is active against many isolates of *Klebsiella*. Mezlocillin is not orally absorbed and must be given parenterally. The drug's pharmacology is similar to the carboxypenicillins, except that about a third of the drug is eliminated by biliary excretion. Mezlocillin contains less sodium than the carboxypenicillins; it is also less likely to cause platelet dysfunction. It has been used to treat lower respiratory tract infections, skin and soft-tissue infections, intra-abdominal infections, and gynecologic infections.

ANTIMICROBIAL ACTIVITY

Gram-positive: *Staphylococcus aureus* (nonpenicillinase-producing strains), beta-hemolytic streptococci (groups A and B), *Streptococcus pneumoniae, Enterococcus faecalis*.
Gram-negative: *Escherichia coli, Proteus mirabilis, Proteus vulgaris, Morganella morganii, Providencia rettgeri, Providencia stuartii, Citrobacter* spp*, *Klebsiella* spp (including *K. pneumoniae*), *Enterobacter* spp, *Shigella* spp*, *Pseudomonas aeruginosa* (and other species), *Haemophilus influenzae, Haemophilus parainfluenzae, Neisseria* spp; many strains of *Serratia, Salmonella*, and *Acinetobacter** are also susceptible to mezlocillin.
Anaerobic: *Peptococcus* spp, *Peptostreptococcus* spp, *Clostridium* spp*, *Fusobacterium* spp*, *Veillonella* spp*, *Eubacterium* spp*, and *Bacteroides* spp (including *B. fragilis*).
Mezlocillin has demonstrated in vitro activity against these organisms, but clinical efficacy has yet to be established.

RESISTANCE

In vitro resistance to mezlocillin develops slowly (involving multiple step mutation), although some strains of *P. aeruginosa* have developed resistance rather rapidly. Some strains of *E. coli* and *Klebsiella* produce high quantities of beta-lactamase and are resistant to mezlocillin. Mezlocillin is not stable in the presence of penicillinase, and strains of *S. aureus* that are resistant to penicillin are likewise resistant to mezlocillin.

SPECIAL PRECAUTIONS

Hypokalemia has been reported in rare cases; this should be kept in mind particularly when treating patients with electrolyte imbalances. Periodic monitoring of serum potassium is recommended for patients undergoing prolonged therapy.
Mezlocillin is a monosodium salt containing 42.6 mg of sodium per gram of mezlocillin; this should be kept in mind when treating patients requiring restricted salt intake.
Ureidopenicillins have been reported to cause neuromuscular blockage of vecuronium. Therefore, use caution when using mezlocillin preoperatively.
Antibiotics used in high doses for short periods to treat gonococcal infection may mask signs of syphilis. Evaluate patients with gonorrhea for syphilis prior to treatment.
May cause hemorrhagic manifestations associated with abnormalities of coagulation tests; withdrawal of drug should stop bleeding and enable coagulation to return to normal.

INDICATIONS

Treatment of infections of the following types due to designated susceptible organisms:
Lower respiratory tract (including pneumonia and lung abscess):
  H. influenzae, Klebsiella spp (including *K. pneumoniae*), *P. mirabilis, Pseudomonas* spp (including *P. aeruginosa*), *E. coli*, and *Bacteroides* spp (including *B. fragilis*)
Intra-abdominal (including acute cholecystitis, cholangitis, peritonitis, hepatic abscess):
  E. coli, P. mirabilis, Klebsiella spp, *Pseudomonas* spp, *S. faecalis* (enterococcus), *Bacteroides* spp, *Peptococcus* spp, and *Peptostreptococcus* spp
Urinary tract:
  E. coli, Proteus mirabilis, indole-positive *Proteus* spp, *M. morganii, Klebsiella* spp, *E. faecalis*
Uncomplicated gonorrhea:
  N. gonorrhoeae
Gynecologic (including endometritis, pelvic cellulitis, and pelvic inflammatory disease):
  N. gonorrhoeae, Peptococcus spp, *Peptostreptococcus* spp, *E. coli, P. mirabilis, Klebsiella* spp, and *Enterobacter* spp
Skin–skin structure:
  S. faecalis (enterococcus), *E. coli, P. mirabilis, P. rettgeri, Klebsiella* spp, *Enterobacter* spp, *Pseudomonas* spp, *Peptococcus* spp, and *Bacteroides* spp
Septicemia (including bacteremia):
  E. coli, Klebsiella spp, *Enterobacter* spp, *Pseudomonas* spp, *Bacteroides* spp, and *Peptococcus* spp
Mezlocillin also may be used as perioperative prophylaxis

CONTRAINDICATIONS

Patients with a history of immediate hypersensitivity reactions to any of the penicillins

INTERACTIONS

Probenecid
ORAL: beta-blockers
PARENTERAL: aminoglycosides (parenteral), anticoagulants, heparin
BOTH: chloramphenicol, erythromycin, tetracyclines, oral contraceptives

The information here is provided as guidance only. Prescribers should always consult the manufacturer's current prescribing information.

MEZLOCILLIN (CONTINUED)

SPECIAL GROUPS

Children: Limited safety and efficacy data available. Dosages exist for cases of serious infection where mezlocillin is considered the appropriate agent.
Elderly: May have age-related renal impairment.
Renal impairment: Reduced dosage necessary in patients with creatinine clearance less than 10 mL/min.
Hepatic impairment: Dosage modification required in severe hepatic impairment.
Pregnancy: Use only when clearly indicated; controlled human studies not performed.
Breast-feeding: Use caution; excreted in breast milk.

DOSAGE

Adults: (Note: For serious infection, use intravenous route. When using intramuscular route, do not exceed 2 g per injection.) For serious infection, 200 to 300 mg/kg/d in four to six divided doses (usually 3 g every 4 hours, or 4 g every 6 hours). For life-threatening infections, up to 350 mg/kg/d may be used, using care not to exceed 24 g/d (4 g every 4 hours). Maximum dosage (3–4 g every 4 hours) required for serious *Pseudomonas* infections. For acute, uncomplicated gonococcal urethritis, 1 to 2 g administered once intravenously or intramuscularly, along with 1 g oral probenecid concurrently or 0.5 hours before. For surgical prophylaxis, 4 g intravenously given 0.5 to 1.5 hours before surgery, followed by 4 g intravenously given 6 and 12 hours after surgery. For cesarean section, give first 4-g dose as soon as umbilical cord is clamped; second and third doses should be given intravenously at 4 and 8 hours after first dose, respectively.
Elderly: May have age-related renal impairment.
Children: For infants over 1 month of age and children up to 12 years of age, 50 mg/kg may be given every 4 hours (300 mg/kg/d), infused intravenously over 30 minutes or by intramuscular injection.
For infants over 7 days and over 2000 g, 75 mg/kg every 6 hours.
For infants over 7 days and under 2000 g, 75 mg/kg every 8 hours.
For infants under 7 days and over 2000 g, 75 mg/kg every 12 hours.
For infants under 7 days and under 2000 g, 75 mg/kg every 12 hours.
Impaired renal function: 1.5 to 3 g every 8 hours and 1.5 to 2 g every 8 hours in patients with creatinine clearances of 10 to 30 mL/min and less than 10 mL/min, respectively.
Severe hepatic impairment: Reduce dose by half or double dosing interval.

ADVERSE EFFECTS

Thrombophlebitis
See Adverse Effect for amoxicillin-clavulanic acid.

PHARMACOKINETICS AND PHARMACODYNAMICS

Peak serum levels: 22 to 83 and 55 to 112 µg/mL at 30 min after 1- and 2-g intravenous doses, respectively; 15 to 25 µg/mL after a 1-g intramuscular dose
Plasma half-life: 0.7 to 1.3 h
Bioavailability: Used parenterally only; widely distributed in body tissues, except to cerebrospinal fluid (unless meninges are inflamed)
Metabolism: slight, only 10% excreted in urine as penicilloic and penilloic acids
Elimination: glomerular filtration, tubular secretion, and biliary excretion
Excretion: approximately 55% recovered unchanged in urine within 6 h; 20% to 30% excreted in bile
Effect of food: food inhibits absorption
Protein binding: 16% to 42%
Renal impairment: half-life only slightly prolonged (1.6–6 h in patients with creatinine clearance less than 10 mL/min); dosage adjustment only necessary in severe renal impairment
Hepatic impairment: mean half-life 2.6 h in patients with cirrhosis; biliary excretion reduced in patients with common bile duct obstruction

OVERDOSAGE

Excessive doses may cause neuromuscular hyperexcitability or convulsive seizures. Dose-related toxicity can arise with the use of large doses of intravenous penicillin (40–100 MU/d), especially in patients with severe renal impairment. Symptoms include agitation, confusion, asterixis, hallucinations, stupor, coma, multifocal myoclonus, seizures, and encephalopathy. Hypokalemia also has occurred.
In case of overdose, discontinue drug therapy and treat patient symptomatically, using supportive care as required. Hemodialysis may be used if necessary to reduce blood levels of penicillin, although effectiveness is uncertain.

PATIENT INFORMATION

Complete all medication unless otherwise directed by physician. Take medication with a full glass of water on an empty stomach 1 hour before or 2 hours following a meal. Take at regular intervals around the clock. Contact physician if rash, itching, hives, severe diarrhea, shortness of breath or wheezing, black tongue, sore throat, nausea, vomiting, fever, swelling of joints, or unusual bleeding or bruising occurs. Throw away any unused liquid form of penicillin after 7 days when stored at room temperature and after 14 days when stored in refrigerator.

AVAILABILITY

Powder for injection
1-, 2-, 3-, and 4-g vials
2-, 3-, and 4-g infusion bottles
20-g pharmacy bulk package

The information here is provided as guidance only. Prescribers should always consult the manufacturer's current prescribing information.

NAFCILLIN (Nallpen®, Unipen®)

Nafcillin is a semisynthetic penicillinase-resistant penicillin. Although it is 10 times more active than methicillin against staphylococci and streptococci, its high protein binding reduces some of its potency. Nafcillin is available for both oral and parenteral administration. However, the drug is subject to a variable degree of gastric inactivation, and oral administration is seldom used. Because of its lipid solubility and enhanced penetration into the cerebrospinal fluid, nafcillin is the preferred penicillin for staphylococcal central nervous system infections. Because nafcillin is eliminated equally by the kidney and liver, dosage modification is not required in patients with renal insufficiency.

ANTIMICROBIAL ACTIVITY

Gram-positive: *Staphylococcus aureus*, other staphylococci, *Streptococcus pneumoniae*, beta-hemolytic streptococci, *viridans* streptococci.

RESISTANCE

Strains resistant to methicillin are usually resistant to all other penicillinase-resistant penicillins (cross-resistance with cephalosporin derivatives also is frequent). Resistance to any penicillinase-resistant penicillin should be interpreted as clinical evidence of resistance to all, regardless of the fact that minor variations in *in vitro* sensitivity may be encountered when more than one penicillinase-resistant penicillin is tested against the same strain of *Staphylococcus*.

SPECIAL PRECAUTIONS

Use caution using intravenous route of administration due to possibility of thrombophlebitis or extravasation (chemical irritation of perivascular tissues may be severe); make certain tubing is functioning properly and administer nafcillin in recommended concentrations. If patient complains of pain during infusion, stop infusion immediately and evaluate for possible adverse effects.

Estimated incidence of hypersensitivity 1% to 10%; serious and occasionally fatal immediate reactions have occurred. Although anaphylaxis is more frequent after parenteral administration, it can occur with oral forms as well. Accelerated reactions (*eg*, urticaria, laryngeal edema) and delayed reactions (serum sickness–like syndrome) may occur. Reactions are most likely to be immediate and severe in patients with penicillin sensitivity and a history of atopic conditions.

cross-allergenicity with cephalosporins is common in patients with penicillin hypersensitivity.

Desensitization may be considered in patients who have positive skin test results to a penicillin determinant and who have need where no alternative to penicillin exists (*eg*, neurosyphilis, congenital syphilis, or syphilis in pregnancy).

Skin rashes, urticaria, and serum sickness–like reactions may be controlled by antihistamines or corticosteroids if necessary. Unless condition being treated is life-threatening or only amenable to penicillin therapy, discontinuation is recommended.

Bacteriologic studies should be performed to determine causative organisms and their susceptibility.

Use caution in administering broad-spectrum antibiotics to patients with existing or previous gastrointestinal disease. Treatment with broad-spectrum antibiotics alters normal flora of the colon and may permit overgrowth of *Clostridium difficile*, causing antibiotic-associated pseudomembranous colitis. Mild cases usually respond to discontinuation of therapy alone; management of moderate to severe cases should include bacteriologic studies and fluid, electrolyte, and protein supplementation.

(Continued on next page)

INDICATIONS

The primary indication is treatment of infections due to penicillinase-producing staphylococci. Nafcillin may be used to initiate therapy in patients for whom staphylococcal infection is suspected because of the high frequency of penicillinase-producing staphylococci in the community as well as the hospital. If initial therapy is instituted, it should be noted that nafcillin has demonstrated effectiveness only in the treatment of infections due to pneumococci, Group A beta-hemolytic streptococci, and penicillin G–resistant and penicillin G–sensitive staphylococci. If bacteriologic tests determine infection is due to an organism other than those listed, an alternative agent is indicated. For serious or life-threatening infections, oral forms of penicillinase-resistant penicillins should not be relied on for initial therapy.

CONTRAINDICATIONS

Patients with a history of immediate hypersensitivity reactions to any of the penicillins

INTERACTIONS

ORAL: beta-blockers
PARENTERAL: aminoglycosides (parenteral), anticoagulants, heparin
BOTH: chloramphenicol, erythromycin, tetracyclines, oral contraceptives

ADVERSE EFFECTS

See Adverse Effects for amoxicillin-clavulanic acid.

The information here is provided as guidance only. Prescribers should always consult the manufacturer's current prescribing information.

NAFCILLIN (CONTINUED)

SPECIAL PRECAUTIONS *(CONTINUED)*

White blood and differential cell counts should be performed prior to initiation of therapy and every week during therapy with penicillinase-resistant penicillins. Monitor AST and ALT to observe for liver function abnormalities during therapy; this is especially important in newborns and infants receiving higher doses.

Prolonged or repeated antibiotic therapy may result in bacterial or fungal overgrowth of nonsusceptible organisms, leading to secondary infection.

The number of strains of staphylococci resistant to penicillinase-resistant penicillins has been growing. Interpret resistance to any penicillinase-resistant penicillin as evidence of clinical resistance to all. Cross-resistance to cephalosporin derivatives also occurs often.

In streptococcal infections, therapy must be completed to eliminate the organism (*ie*, minimum of 10 days) to prevent sequelae, such as rheumatic fever, from occurring.

In gonococcal infections in which primary or secondary syphilis may be suspected, proper diagnostic procedures, including darkfield examinations and monthly serologic tests for a minimum of 4 months, are indicated. Continuation of clinical and serologic examinations every 6 months for 2 to 3 years is recommended for all cases.

Patients with cystic fibrosis have a higher incidence of adverse effects with extended-spectrum penicillins.

Care should be taken with intravenous administration due to the possibility of thrombophlebitis. Intravenous doses higher than recommended for most penicillins may cause neuromuscular excitability and convulsions.

Avoid subcutaneous and fat layer injections; pain and induration may occur. Inadvertent intravascular administration, including direct arterial injection (or injection immediately adjacent to arteries) has resulted in severe neurovascular damage, including transverse myelitis with permanent paralysis; gangrene, requiring amputation of digits and more proximal portions of extremities; and necrosis and sloughing at the injection site and surrounding area. Other complications include immediate pallor, mottling, or cyanosis of the extremity (both distal and proximal to the injection site), ensuing bleb formation, and severe edema requiring anterior–posterior compartment fasciotomy in the lower extremities. These effects have occurred most frequently in infants and young children. Immediate consultation with a specialist is recommended if any evidence of compromise of blood supply occurs at, proximal to, or distal to the site of injection.

Quadriceps femoris fibrosis and atrophy have occurred after repeated intramuscular injections of penicillin preparations to the anterolateral thigh.

False-positive urine glucose reactions may occur with Clinitest (Ames, Elkhart, IN), Benedicts' solution, or Fehling's solution.

Positive Coombs' test results have occurred.

SPECIAL GROUPS

Children: Safety and efficacy not established in infants or neonates.
Elderly: No modification required.
Renal impairment: No modification required.
Hepatic impairment: No modification required.
Pregnancy: Use only if clearly indicated; controlled human studies not performed.
Breast-feeding: Use caution; excreted in breast milk.

PHARMACOKINETICS AND PHARMACODYNAMICS

Peak serum levels: 1 to 2 h; 7.7 µg/mL with oral dose of 1 g; 40 and 82 µg/mL with intravenous dose 0.5 and 1 g, respectively.
Plasma half-life: 0.5 to 1 h
Bioavailability: 20% to 36% with oral administration
Metabolism: 60% of dose metabolized in liver to inactive metabolites
Elimination: biliary excretion and glomerular filtration
Excretion: approximately 13% of an oral dose and 30% of an intravenous or intramuscular dose is recovered unchanged in the urine in 12 h
Effect of food: cannot be taken with food
Protein binding: 87% to 90%
Renal impairment: half-life 1.8 to 2.8 h in patients with severe renal impairment
Hepatic impairment: half-life 1.2 to 2.3 h in patients with cirrhosis

OVERDOSAGE

Excessive doses may cause neuromuscular hyperexcitability or convulsive seizures. Dose-related toxicity can arise with the use of large doses of intravenous penicillin (40–100 MU/d), especially in patients with severe renal impairment. Symptoms include agitation, confusion, asterixis, hallucinations, stupor, coma, multifocal myoclonus, seizures, and encephalopathy. Hypokalemia also has occurred.

In case of overdose, discontinue drug therapy and treat patient symptomatically, using supportive care as required. Hemodialysis may be used if necessary to reduce blood levels of penicillin, although effectiveness is uncertain.

The information here is provided as guidance only. Prescribers should always consult the manufacturer's current prescribing information.

NAFCILLIN (CONTINUED)

DOSAGE

Parenteral form should be used initially in very serious infections. Severe infections may require very high doses. Oral form may be implemented as soon as clinically indicated.

Adults: For intravenous administration, 3 to 12 g/d. Reduce dose as soon as possible to reduce frequency of phlebitis. For intramuscular administration, 500 mg every 4 to 6 hours; for severe infections, 1 g every 4 to 6 hours.

Elderly: Same as adults.

Children: For intravenous administration, 50 to 200 mg/kg/d in equally divided doses every 4 to 6 hours. For intramuscular administration, 25 mg/kg/d every 12 hours. For oral administration for staph infections, 50 mg/kg/d every 6 hours; for streptococcal pharyngitis, 250 mg every 8 hours for 10 days.*

For intravenous administration in neonates, 10 mg/kg every 12 hours, or one of the following:

For infants over 7 days and over 2000 g, 50 mg/kg/d divided every 6 hours.*

For infants over 7 days and under 2000 g, 50 mg/kg/d divided every 8 hours.*

For infants under 7 days and over 2000 g, 50 mg/kg/d divided every 8 hours.*

For infants under 7 days and under 2000 g, 50 mg/kg/d divided every 12 hours.*

Double dosage for meningitis (eg, normal dose = 50 mg/kg/d; meningitis dose = 200 mg/kg/d).

PATIENT INFORMATION

Complete all medication unless otherwise directed by physician. Take medication with a full glass of water on an empty stomach 1 hour before or 2 hours following a meal. Take at regular intervals around the clock. Contact physician if rash, itching, hives, severe diarrhea, shortness of breath or wheezing, black tongue, sore throat, nausea, vomiting, fever, swelling of joints, or unusual bleeding or bruising occurs. Throw away any unused liquid form of penicillin after 7 days when stored at room temperature and after 14 days when stored in refrigerator.

AVAILABILITY

Capsules—250 mg
Tablets—500 mg
Powder for parenteral administration—1-g and 2-g vials and 10-g bulk vial

OXACILLIN (Bactocill®)

Oxacillin is one of the isoxazolyl class of penicillinase-resistant penicillins. It is available in both oral and parenteral preparations. However, its absorption from the gastrointestinal tract is not as good as cloxacillin and dicloxacillin. The drug is primarily used for the parenteral treatment of serious staphylococcal infections. Most of the drug is excreted in the urine, but some drug is eliminated by biliary excretion. In addition to the usual adverse reactions, oxacillin may produce a transient elevation in liver enzymes.

ANTIMICROBIAL ACTIVITY

Gram-positive: *Staphylococcus aureus*, other staphylococci, *Streptococcus pneumoniae*.

RESISTANCE

See Resistance for dicloxacillin.

SPECIAL PRECAUTIONS

Estimated incidence of hypersensitivity 1% to 10%; serious and occasionally fatal immediate reactions have occurred. Although anaphylaxis is more frequent after parenteral administration, it can occur with oral forms as well. Accelerated reactions (*eg*, urticaria, laryngeal edema) and delayed reactions (serum sickness–like syndrome) may occur. Reactions are most likely to be immediate and severe in patients with penicillin sensitivity and a history of atopic conditions.

Cross-allergenicity with cephalosporins is common in patients with penicillin hypersensitivity.

Desensitization may be considered in patients who have positive skin test results to a penicillin determinant and who have need where no alternative to penicillin exists (*eg*, neurosyphilis, congenital syphilis, or syphilis in pregnancy).

INDICATIONS

Treatment of infections due to penicillinase-producing staphylococci. Oxacillin may be used as initial therapy in patients for whom staphylococcal infection is suspected because of the high frequency of penicillinase-producing strains in the community as well as the hospital.

CONTRAINDICATIONS

Patients with a history of immediate hypersensitivity reactions to any of the penicillins

INTERACTIONS

ORAL: beta-blockers
PARENTERAL: aminoglycosides (parenteral), anticoagulants, heparin
BOTH: chloramphenicol, erythromycin, tetracyclines, oral contraceptives

ADVERSE EFFECTS

See Adverse effects for amoxicillin-clavulanic acid.

(Continued on next page)

The information here is provided as guidance only. Prescribers should always consult the manufacturer's current prescribing information.

OXACILLIN (CONTINUED)

SPECIAL PRECAUTIONS (CONTINUED)

Skin rashes, urticaria, and serum sickness–like reactions may be controlled by anti-histamines or corticosteroids if necessary. Unless condition being treated is life-threatening or only amenable to penicillin therapy, discontinuation is recommended.

Bacteriologic studies should be performed to determine causative organisms and their susceptibility.

Use caution in administering broad-spectrum antibiotics to patients with existing or previous gastrointestinal disease. Treatment with broad-spectrum antibiotics alters normal flora of the colon and may permit overgrowth of *Clostridium difficile*, causing antibiotic-associated pseudomembranous colitis. Mild cases usually respond to discontinuation of therapy alone; management of moderate to severe cases should include bacteriologic studies and fluid, electrolyte, and protein supple-mentation.

White blood and differential cell counts should be performed prior to initiation of therapy and every week during therapy with penicillinase-resistant penicillins. Monitor AST and ALT to observe for liver function abnormalities during therapy; this is especially important in newborns and infants receiving higher doses.

Prolonged or repeated antibiotic therapy may result in bacterial or fungal over-growth of nonsusceptible organisms, leading to secondary infection.

The number of strains of staphylococci resistant to penicillinase-resistant peni-cillins has been growing. Interpret resistance to any penicillinase-resistant peni-cillin as evidence of clinical resistance to all. Cross-resistance to cephalosporin derivatives also occurs often.

In streptococcal infections, therapy must be completed to eliminate the organism (*ie*, minimum of 10 days) to prevent sequelae, such as rheumatic fever, from occurring.

In gonococcal infections in which primary or secondary syphilis may be suspected, proper diagnostic procedures including darkfield examinations and monthly serologic tests for a minimum of 4 months, are indicated. Continuation of clinical and sero-logic examinations every 6 months for 2 to 3 years is recommended for all cases.

Patients with cystic fibrosis have a higher incidence of adverse effects with extended-spectrum penicillins.

Care should be taken with intravenous administration due to the possibility of thrombophlebitis. Intravenous doses higher than recommended for most peni-cillins may cause neuromuscular excitability and convulsions.

Avoid subcutaneous and fat layer injections; pain and induration may occur.

Inadvertent intravascular administration, including direct arterial injection (or injection immediately adjacent to arteries) has resulted in severe neurovascular damage, including transverse myelitis with permanent paralysis; gangrene, requir-ing amputation of digits and more proximal portions of extremities; and necrosis and sloughing at the injection site and surrounding area. Other complications include immediate pallor, mottling, or cyanosis of the extremity (both distal and proximal to the injection site), ensuing bleb formation, and severe edema requiring anterior–posterior compartment fasciotomy in the lower extremities. These effects have occurred most frequently in infants and young children. Immediate consulta-tion with a specialist is recommended if any evidence of compromise of blood supply occurs at, proximal to, or distal to the site of injection.

Quadriceps femoris fibrosis and atrophy have occurred after repeated intramuscular injections of penicillin preparations to the anterolateral thigh.

False-positive urine glucose reactions may occur with Clinitest (Ames, Elkhart, IN), Benedicts' solution, or Fehling's solution.

Positive Coombs' test results have occurred.

PHARMACOKINETICS AND PHARMACODYNAMICS

Peak serum levels: 2.6 to 3.9 μg/mL and 52 to 63 μg/mL after 500 mg oral and intravenous doses, respectively

Plasma half-life: 0.3 to 0.8 h

Bioavailability: 30% to 35% of oral dose

Metabolism: approximately 40% is partially metabo-lized to inactive and active metabolites

Elimination: glomerular filtration and tubular secretion

Excretion: approximately 15% of an oral dose and 45% of an intravenous dose is excreted unchanged in the urine in 12 h

Effect of food: may not be taken with food

Protein binding: 94%

Renal impairment: half-life 0.5 to 2 h in patients with creatinine clearance less than 10 mL/min

Hepatic impairment: no information

OVERDOSAGE

Excessive doses may cause neuromuscular hyperex-citability or convulsive seizures. Dose-related toxic-ity can arise with the use of large doses of intravenous penicillin (40–100 MU/d), especially in patients with severe renal impairment. Symptoms include agitation, confusion, asterixis, hallucinations, stupor, coma, multifocal myoclonus, seizures, and encephalopathy. Hypokalemia also has occurred.

In case of overdose, discontinue drug therapy and treat patient symptomatically, using supportive care as required. Hemodialysis may be used if necessary to reduce blood levels of penicillin, although effec-tiveness is uncertain.

The information here is provided as guidance only. Prescribers should always consult the manufacturer's current prescribing information.

OXACILLIN (CONTINUED)

SPECIAL GROUPS

Children: Safe for use in children.
Elderly: No modification required.
Renal impairment: No modification required.
Hepatic impairment: No modification required.
Pregnancy: Use only when clearly indicated; controlled human studies not performed.
Breast-feeding: Use caution; excreted in breast milk.

DOSAGE

Adults: *PARENTERAL:* For mild to moderate upper respiratory and skin or soft-tissue infections, 250 to 500 mg every 4 to 6 hours. For severe infections (lower respiratory or disseminated), 1 to 2 g every 4 to 6 hours. For very severe infections, very high doses and prolonged therapy may be necessary; do not exceed maximum dose of 12 g/d.
ORAL: For mild to moderate infections of skin or soft tissue or upper respiratory tract, 500 mg every 4 to 6 hours.
Elderly: Same as adults.
Children: *PARENTERAL:* For mild to moderate upper respiratory and skin or soft-tissue infections, 50 mg/kg/d in divided doses every 4 to 6 hours. For severe infections (lower respiratory or disseminated), 100 mg/kg/d in divided doses every 4 to 6 hours. For very severe infections, very high doses and prolonged therapy may be necessary; do not exceed maximum dose of 100 to 300 mg/kg/d.
For infants over 7 days and over 2000 g, 150 mg/kg/d in divided doses every 6 hours.
For infants over 7 days and under 2000 g, 100 mg/kg/d in divided doses every 8 hours.
For infants under 7 days and over 2000 g, 75 mg/kg/d in divided doses every 8 hours.
For infants under 7 days and under 2000 g, 50 mg/kg/d in divided doses every 12 hours.
ORAL: For mild to moderate infections of skin or soft tissue or upper respiratory tract, 50 mg/kg/d in divided doses every 6 hours for at least 5 days.

PATIENT INFORMATION

Complete all medication unless otherwise directed by physician. Take medication with a full glass of water on an empty stomach 1 hour before or 2 hours following a meal. Take at regular intervals around the clock. Contact physician if rash, itching, hives, severe diarrhea, shortness of breath or wheezing, black tongue, sore throat, nausea, vomiting, fever, swelling of joints, or unusual bleeding or bruising occurs. Throw away any unused liquid form of penicillin after 7 days when stored at room temperature and after 14 days when stored in refrigerator.

AVAILABILITY

Capsules—250 mg and 500 mg
Powder for oral solution—250 µg/mL (when reconstituted)

The information here is provided as guidance only. Prescribers should always consult the manufacturer's current prescribing information.

PENICILLIN G

Penicillin G, or *benzylpenicillin*, is a naturally occurring penicillin. Its antimicrobial spectrum consists largely of gram-positive organisms and gram-negative cocci. It is the drug of choice for streptococcal, meningococcal, clostridial, and spirochetal infections. It is also the recommended drug for actinomycosis, anthrax, rat-bite fever, erysipeloid, and periodontal infections. The drug is destroyed rapidly by gastric acid and is available primarily for parenteral administration. The drug is well distributed throughout the body and provides therapeutic concentrations in the cerebrospinal fluid for the treatment of pneumococcal and meningococcal meningitis. The drug has a rapid half-life of 30 minutes. Intramuscular injection of sodium and potassium salts of penicillin is rarely given because of pain and irritation at the injection site.

ANTIMICROBIAL ACTIVITY

Gram-positive: Staphylococci (nonpenicillinase-producing), *Staphylococcus aureus* (nonpenicillinase-producing), streptococci, *Streptococcus pneumoniae*, beta-hemolytic streptococci, *Enterococcus faecalis*, *viridans* streptococci, *Corynebacterium diphtheriae*, *Bacillus anthracis*, *Listeria monocytogenes*.
Gram-negative: *Neisseria gonorrhoeae* (nonpenicillinase-producing), *Neisseria meningitidis*, *Streptobacillus moniliformis*.
Anaerobic: *Clostridium*, *Peptococcus*, *Peptostreptococcus*, *Bacteroides* (*B. fragilis* is resistant), *Fusobacterium*, and *Eubacterium* spp; *Treponema pallidum*, *Actinomyces bovis*.

RESISTANCE

The majority of staphylococci are resistant to penicillin G and penicillin V; *Streptococcus pneumoniae* and *viridans* streptococci have intermediate susceptibility or are resistant to penicillin G; culture and susceptibility tests are high recommended.

SPECIAL PRECAUTIONS

Because alpha-hemolytic streptococci that are resistant to penicillin may be found when patients are receiving oral penicillin for secondary prevention of rheumatic fever, prophylactic drugs other than penicillin can be prescribed in addition to the continuous prophylactic rheumatic fever regimen.
Use caution in administering to neonates; regular and frequent monitoring of organ system function is recommended.
If high doses (> 10 MU) are indicated, administer aqueous penicillin G slowly to prevent electrolyte imbalance from either potassium or sodium content.
In cardiac patients or others requiring sodium restriction, periodic electrolyte determinations and monitoring of cardiac function should be instituted.
Antibiotics used in high doses for short periods to treat gonococcal infection may mask signs of syphilis. Evaluate patients with gonorrhea for syphilis prior to treatment.
See Special Precautions for oxacillin.

SPECIAL GROUPS

Children: Safe for use in children; use caution in neonates.
Elderly: No information.
Renal impairment: Dosage modification required in patients with creatinine clearance < 40 mL/min.
Hepatic impairment: No modification required.
Pregnancy: Probably safe; use with caution.
Breast-feeding: Use caution; excreted in breast milk.

INDICATIONS

For treatment of infections due to susceptible organisms.
Treatment of infection due to penicillinase-producing staphylococci. Methicillin may be used to initiate therapy when staphylococcal infection is suspected because of the high frequency of penicillinase-producing staphylococci in the community as well as the hospital.

CONTRAINDICATIONS

Patients with a history of immediate hypersensitivity reactions to any of the penicillins

INTERACTIONS

ORAL: beta-blockers
PARENTERAL: aminoglycosides (parenteral), anticoagulants, heparin
BOTH: chloramphenicol, erythromycin, tetracyclines, oral contraceptives

ADVERSE EFFECTS

See Adverse Effects for amoxicillin-clavulanic acid.

PHARMACOKINETICS AND PHARMACODYNAMICS

Peak serum levels: 60 µg/mL after intravenous dose of 1 MU; 6 to 8 µg/mL after intramuscular dose of 1 MU.
Plasma half-life: 0.4 to 0.9 h
Bioavailability: widely distributed to extracellular fluids and tissues (except cerebrospinal fluid, eyes, and prostate)
Metabolism: 16% to 30% partially metabolized to penicilloic acids
Elimination: glomerular filtration and tubular secretion
Excretion: 60% in urine after 5 h, primarily unchanged
Effect of food: may not be taken with food
Protein binding: 60% binds to serum proteins, mainly albumin
Renal impairment: half-life 5 h in patients with creatinine clearance < 10 mL/min
Hepatic impairment: minimal change in half-life in severe hepatic impairment

The information here is provided as guidance only. Prescribers should always consult the manufacturer's current prescribing information.

PENICILLIN G (CONTINUED)

DOSAGE

Adults: *See* table below.

Dosage for Specific Infections

Organism or infection	Dosage
Meningococcal meningitis	1–2 MU intramuscularly every 2 h or 20–30 MU/d continuous intravenous drop for 14 d (or until afebrile for 7 d)
Actinomycosis for cervicofacial cases	1–6 MU/d
Thoracic and abdominal disease	12–20 MU/d intravenously for 6 wk; may be followed by oral penicillin V 500 mg every 6 h for 2–3 mo
Clostridial infection	20 MU/d as adjunct to antitoxin
Fusospirochetal infection: severe infections of oropharynx, lower respiratory tract, and genital area	5–10 MU/d
Rat-bite fever (*Spirillum minus*, *S. moniliformis*), Haverhill fever	12–20 MU/d for 3–4 wk
Listeria infection (*L. monocytogenes*) Meningitis (adults) Endocarditis	15–20 MU/d for 2 wk (4 wk for endocartis)
Pasteurella infection (*Pasteurella multocida*) Bacteremia and meningitis	4–6 MU/d for 2 wk
Erysipeloid (*Erysipelothrix rhusiopathiae*) Endocarditis	12–20 MU/d for 4–6 wk
Gram-negative bacillary bacteremia (*Escherichia coli*, *Enterobacter aerogenes*, *Alcaligenes faecalis*, *Salmonella*, *Shigella*, *Proteus mirabilis*	20 MU/d or more
Diphtheria (adjunct to antitoxin to prevent carrier state)	2–3 MU/d in divided doses for 10–12 d
Anthrax (*B. anthracis* is often resistant)	Minimum 5 MU/d; 12–20 MU/d have been used
Streptococcal infection (including *S. pneumoniae*) Bacteremia, pneumonia, emphysema	5–24 MU/d divided doses every 4–6 h
Meningitis	20–24 MU/d for 14 d
Suppurative arthritis, osteomyelitis, mastoiditis, endocarditis, peritonitis, pericarditis	12–20 MU/d for 2–4 wk minimum
Syphilis* Neurosyphilis	12–24 MU/d intravenously (2–4 MU every 4 h) for 10–14 d; benzathine penicillin G 2.4 MU/wk intramuscularly for 3 wk is often recommended on completion of initial therapy
Congenital syphilis (symptomatic or asymptomatic infants	Neonates: 50,000 U/kg/d intravenously every 8–12 h for 10-14 d (if > 1 d of therapy is missed, restart entire course) Infants (after newborn stage): 50,000 U/kg every 4-6 h for 10–14 d
Gonococcal infections (Infants with disseminated gonococcal infection or gonococcal ophthalmia [hospitalization recommended])	(Gonococcal isolate must be proven to be susceptible to penicillin) 100,000 U/kg/d in 2 equal doses (use 4 equal doses in infants < 1 wk); for meningitis, increase dose to 150,000 U/kg/d

*Centers for Disease Control and Prevention: 1989 Sexually transmitted diseases treatment guidelines. MMWR 1989 Sept. 1; 38(no. S-8):1–43.

Elderly: Same as adults.

Children: *PARENTERAL*: 100,000 to 250,000 U/kg/d in divided doses every 4 hours. For infants over 7 days and over 2000 g, 100,000 U/kg/d in divided doses every 6 hours.[†] For infants over 7 days and under 2000 g, 75,000 U/kg/d in divided doses every 8 hours.[†] For infants under 7 days and over 2000 g, 50,000 U/kg/d in divided doses every 8 hours.[†] For infants under 7 days and under 2000 g, 50,000 U/kg/d in divided doses every 12 hours.[†]

†Double dosage for meningitis (eg, normal: 50,000 U/kg/d; meningitis: 100,000 U/kg/d).

Impaired renal function: Reduce dosage by half or double dosing interval in patients receiving high doses with creatinine clearances of 10 to 40 mL/min; reduce dosage by half and double dosing interval in patients with creatinine clearance < 10 mL/min.

OVERDOSAGE

Excessive doses may cause neuromuscular hyperexcitability or convulsive seizures. Dose-related toxicity can arise with the use of large doses of intravenous penicillin (40–100 MU/d), especially in patients with severe renal impairment. Symptoms include agitation, confusion, asterixis, hallucinations, stupor, coma, multifocal myoclonus, seizures, and encephalopathy. Hypokalemia also has occurred. In case of overdose, discontinue drug therapy and treat patient symptomatically, using supportive care as required. Hemodialysis may be used if necessary to reduce blood levels of penicillin, although effectiveness is uncertain.

PATIENT INFORMATION

Complete all medication unless otherwise directed by physician. Take medication with a full glass of water on an empty stomach 1 hour before or 2 hours following a meal. Take at regular intervals around the clock. Contact physician if rash, itching, hives, severe diarrhea, shortness of breath or wheezing, black tongue, sore throat, nausea, vomiting, fever, swelling of joints, or unusual bleeding or bruising occurs. Throw away any unused liquid form of penicillin after 7 days when stored at room temperature and after 14 days when stored in refrigerator.

AVAILABILITY

Penicillin G sodium, powder for injection—5,000,000 U per vial
Penicillin G potassium, injection (premixed, frozen)—1,000,000, 2,000,000, and 3,000,000 U per vial
Penicillin G potassium, powder for injection—5,000,000, 10,000,000, and 20,000,000 U per vial

The information here is provided as guidance only. Prescribers should always consult the manufacturer's current prescribing information.

PENICILLIN G BENZATHINE (Bicillin®)

Penicillin G benzathine is a repository formulation of the drug for intramuscular administration. The benzathine salt of penicillin G is very insoluble and is absorbed very slowly from an intramuscular injection site. This preparation provides very low concentrations of penicillin G that persist for up to 30 days. The low drug levels make this formulation useful only for very susceptible organisms (*eg, Streptococcus pyogenes* and various spirochetes).

ANTIMICROBIAL ACTIVITY

Gram-positive: Streptococci (Groups A, C, G, H, L, and M), beta-hemolytic streptococci, *viridans* streptococci.

RESISTANCE

See Resistance for penicillin G.

SPECIAL PRECAUTIONS

See Special Precautions for oxacillin.

SPECIAL GROUPS

Children: Safe for use in children.
Elderly: No modification required.
Renal impairment: No modification required.
Hepatic impairment: No modification required.
Pregnancy: Use only if clearly indicated; controlled human studies not performed.
Breast-feeding: Use caution; excreted in breast milk.

INDICATIONS

Mild to moderate infections of upper respiratory tract due to susceptible streptococci
Venereal infections (syphilis, yaws, bejel, pinta)
Prophylaxis for rheumatic fever or chorea (also for follow-up prophylactic therapy for rheumatic heart disease and acute glomerulonephritis)

CONTRAINDICATIONS

Do not inject near artery or nerve
Patients with a history of immediate hypersensitivity reactions to any of the penicillins

INTERACTIONS

ORAL: beta-blockers
PARENTERAL: aminoglycosides (parenteral), anti-coagulants, heparin
BOTH: chloramphenicol, erythromycin, tetracyclines, oral contraceptives

PATIENT INFORMATION

Complete all medication unless otherwise directed by physician. Take medication with a full glass of water on an empty stomach 1 hour before or 2 hours following a meal. Take at regular intervals around the clock. Contact physician if rash, itching, hives, severe diarrhea, shortness of breath or wheezing, black tongue, sore throat, nausea, vomiting, fever, swelling of joints, or unusual bleeding or bruising occurs. Throw away any unused liquid forms of penicillin after 7 days when stored at room temperature and after 14 days when stored in refrigerator.

ADVERSE EFFECTS

See Adverse Effects for amoxicillin-clavulanic acid.

PHARMACOKINETICS AND PHARMACODYNAMICS

Peak serum levels: 0.1 to 0.22 U/mL after intramuscular administration of 600,000 U
Plasma half-life: drug very slowly absorbed and detectable for 2 to 4 wks
Bioavailability: wide distribution to body tissues, except to cerebrospinal fluid (unless meninges inflamed) tissue levels are low due to low serum concentrations
Metabolism: no information
Elimination: glomerular filtration and tubular secretion
Excretion: detectable in urine for 12 wks after single injection
Effect of food: for intramuscular use only
Protein binding: 60%
Renal impairment: may considerably delay excretion but serum levels only slightly higher
Hepatic impairment: no information

The information here is provided as guidance only. Prescribers should always consult the manufacturer's current prescribing information.

PENICILLIN G BENZATHINE (CONTINUED)

DOSAGE

Adults: For Group A streptococcal or upper respiratory infections, 1,200,000 U in a single injection. For syphilis (primary, secondary, or latent), 2,400,000 U (one dose); late (tertiary and neurosyphilis), 2,400,000 U at 7-day intervals for three doses. For yaws, bejel, or pinta, 1,200,000 U in a single injection. For prophylaxis for rheumatic fever or glomerulonephritis following as acute attack, 1,200,000 U once a month or 600,000 U every 2 weeks.
Elderly: Same as adults.
Children: Children over 60 lbs, 900,000 U in a single injection. For infants and children below 60 lbs, 300,000–600,000 U. For congenital syphilis in children 2 to 12 years of age, use adult dosage schedule; for children below 2 years of age, 50,000 U/kg body weight.

OVERDOSAGE

Excessive doses may cause neuromuscular hyperexcitability or convulsive seizures. Dose-related toxicity can arise with the use of large doses of intravenous penicillin (40–100 MU/d), especially in patients with severe renal impairment. Symptoms include agitation, confusion, asterixis, hallucinations, stupor, coma, multifocal myoclonus, seizures, and encephalopathy. Hypokalemia also has occurred.

In case of overdose, discontinue drug therapy and treat patient symptomatically, using supportive care as required. Hemodialysis may be used if necessary to reduce blood levels of penicillin, although effectiveness is uncertain.

AVAILABILITY

Needle units:
1 mL containing 600,000 U per cartridge
2 mL containing 1,200,000 U per cartridge
4 mL containing 2,400,000 U per syringe
Single multiple-dose vials, 10 mL size, 300,000 U per mL

PENICILLIN V

Penicillin V is the phenoxymethyl analogue of penicillin G. It is stable in gastric acid and is a suitable formulation for oral dosing. The drug's distribution and elimination are very similar to penicillin G. Its antimicrobial activity is also very similar to penicillin G, except that it is five to 10 times less active than penicillin G against *Haemophilus influenzae* and *Neisseria* species.

ANTIMICROBIAL ACTIVITY

Gram-positive: Staphylococci (nonpenicillinase-producing), *Staphylococcus aureus* (nonpenicillinase-producing), streptococci, *Streptococcus pneumoniae*, beta-hemolytic streptococci, *Enterococcus faecalis*, *viridans* streptococci, *Corynebacterium diphtheriae*, *Bacillus anthracis*, *Listeria monocytogenes*.
Gram-negative: *Neisseria gonorrhoeae*, *Streptococcus moniliformis*.
Anaerobic: *Clostridium*, *Peptococcus*, and *Peptostreptococcus* spp; *Treponema pallidum*, *Actinomyces bovis*.
Streptococci in Groups A, C, G, H, L, and M are very sensitive to penicillin.

RESISTANCE

Group D enterococci, penicillinase-producing bacteria (including most strains of staphylococci). An increasing number of strains of *S. pneumoniae* and *viridans* streptococci have intermediate susceptibility or are resistant to penicillin V; culture and susceptibility tests are highly recommended.

INDICATIONS

(Note: Serious pneumonia, empyema, bacteremia, pericarditis, meningitis, or arthritis should not be treated with oral form of penicillin V during acute stages.)
Treatment of mild to moderately severe infection due to penicillin G–sensitive organisms. Bacteriologic studies, sensitivity tests, and clinical response should guide therapy.
Organism and infection
Streptococcal infection
Infections of upper respiratory tract (including scarlet fever, mild erysipelas); pediatric pharyngitis; otitis media; sinusitis
Prophylaxis for bacterial endocarditis in patients with rheumatic, congenital, or (other) acquired valvular heart disease who are undergoing dental or upper respiratory tract surgery
Pneumococcal infection (mild to moderately severe respiratory tract infections including otitis media)
Staphylococcal infection (mild infections of skin or soft tissue)
Fusospirochetosis (Vincent's infection) of oropharynx, mild to moderately severe

CONTRAINDICATIONS

Patients with a history of immediate hypersensitivity reactions to any of the penicillins

The information here is provided as guidance only. Prescribers should always consult the manufacturer's current prescribing information.

PENICILLIN V (CONTINUED)

SPECIAL PRECAUTIONS
See Special Precautions for oxacillin.

SPECIAL GROUPS
Children: In neonates and infants excretion is considerably delayed.
Elderly: May have age-related renal impairment.
Renal impairment: Modification required if creatinine clearance < 10 mL/min.
Hepatic impairment: No modification required.
Pregnancy: Use only when clearly indicated; controlled human studies not performed.
Breast-feeding: Use caution; excreted in breast milk.

DOSAGE
Adults: General dosage is 125 to 500 mg every 6 hours.

Dosage for Specific Infections

Organism and infection	Dosage
Streptococcal infection	125–250 mg every 6–8 h for 10 d (mild to moderately severe infection)
Infections of upper respiratory tract (including scarlet fever, mild erysipelas); pediatric pharyngitis; otitis media; sinusitis	Amoxicillin is preferred agent; if penicillin V is chosen, use according to amoxicillin monograph
Prophylaxis for bacterial endocarditis* in patients with rheumatic, congenital, or (other) acquired valvular heart disease who are undergoing dental or upper respiratory tract surgery	250–500 mg every 6–8 h until patient is afebrile for at least 2 d
Pneumococcal infection (mild to moderately severe respiratory tract infections including otitis media)	250–500 mg every 6–8 h
Staphylococcal infection (mild infections of skin or soft tissue) Fusospirochetosis (Vincent's infection) of oropharynx, mild to moderately severe	250–500 mg every 6–8 h

American Heart Association Statement. JAMA 1990, 264:2919–2922.

Elderly: Same as adults.
Children: 25 to 50 mg/kg/d in divided doses every 6 to 8 hours.
Impaired renal function: (Creatinine clearance < 10 mL/min) do not exceed 250 mg every 6 hours.

INTERACTIONS
ORAL: beta-blockers
PARENTERAL: aminoglycosides (parenteral), anticoagulants, heparin
BOTH: chloramphenicol, erythromycin, tetracyclines, oral contraceptives

ADVERSE EFFECTS
See Adverse Effects for amoxicillin-clavulanic acid.

PHARMACOKINETICS AND PHARMACODYNAMICS
Peak serum levels: 30 to 60 min; 2.3 to 2.8 µg/mL after 250 mg oral dose
Plasma half-life: 0.5 h
Bioavailability: 60% to 73% of oral dose; wide distribution into body tissues, except to cerebrospinal fluid (unless meninges inflamed)
Metabolism: 35% to 50% is partially metabolized to penicilloic acids
Elimination: glomerular filtration and tubular secretion
Excretion: 30% to 40% excreted unchanged in the urine
Effect of food: food has little or no effect on absorption
Protein binding: 80%
Renal impairment: half-life increased to 4 h in patients with creatinine clearance less than 10 mL/min
Hepatic impairment: no information

OVERDOSAGE
Excessive doses may cause neuromuscular hyperexcitability or convulsive seizures. Dose-related toxicity can arise with the use of large doses of intravenous penicillin (40–100 MU/d), especially in patients with severe renal impairment. Symptoms include agitation, confusion, asterixis, hallucinations, stupor, coma, multifocal myoclonus, seizures, and encephalopathy. Hypokalemia also has occurred.
In case of overdose, discontinue drug therapy and treat patient symptomatically, using supportive care as required. Hemodialysis may be used if necessary to reduce blood levels of penicillin, although effectiveness is uncertain.

PATIENT INFORMATION
Complete all medication unless otherwise directed by physician. Take medication with a full glass of water on an empty stomach 1 hour before or 2 hours following a meal. Take at regular intervals around the clock. Contact physician if rash, itching, hives, severe diarrhea, shortness of breath or wheezing, black tongue, sore throat, nausea, vomiting, fever, swelling of joints, or unusual bleeding or bruising occurs. Throw away any unused liquid forms of penicillin after 7 days when stored at room temperature and after 14 days when stored in refrigerator.

AVAILABILITY
Tablets—125, 250, and 500 mg
Powder for oral solution—125 mg/5 mL and 250 mg/5 mL (when reconstituted)

The information here is provided as guidance only. Prescribers should always consult the manufacturer's current prescribing information.

PENICILLIN G PROCAINE (Wycillin®)

Penicillin G procaine is a repository formulation of the drug for intramuscular administration. The procaine salt of penicillin G is relatively insoluble and is absorbed slowly from an intramuscular injection site. This preparation provides therapeutic serum concentrations for most susceptible organisms for at least 12 hours.

ANTIMICROBIAL ACTIVITY

Gram-positive: Staphylococci (nonpenicillinase-producing), *Staphylococcus aureus* (nonpenicillinase-producing), streptococci (Groups A, C, G, H, L, and M), *Streptococcus pneumoniae*, beta-hemolytic streptococci, *viridans* streptococci, *Corynebacterium diphtheriae, Bacillus anthracis*.
Gram-negative: *Neisseria gonorrhoeae* (nonpenicillinase-producing), *Streptobacillus moniliformis*.
Anaerobic: *Peptococcus, Peptostreptococcus, Fusobacterium,* and *Eubacterium* spp; *Treponema pallidum*.

RESISTANCE

See Resistance for Penicillin G.

SPECIAL PRECAUTIONS

Mental disturbances (anxiety, agitation, combativeness, confusion, depression, hallucinations, seizures, weakness, and expressed "fear of impending death") have been reported in patients after receiving single-dose therapy for gonorrhea; such manifestations may be a reaction to procaine.
Antibiotics used in high doses for short periods to treat gonococcal infection may mask signs of syphilis. Evaluate patients with gonorrhea for syphilis prior to treatment.
See Special Precautions for oxacillin.

SPECIAL GROUPS

Children: Use in neonates should be avoided due to increased risk of sterile abscesses and procaine toxicity.
Elderly: No modification required.
Renal impairment: No modification required.
Hepatic impairment: No modification required.
Pregnancy: Use only if clearly indicated; controlled human studies not performed.
Breast-feeding: Use caution; excreted in breast milk.

INDICATIONS

Treatment of moderately severe infection due to penicillin G–sensitive microorganisms susceptible to low and persistent serum levels that are achieved with this form of penicillin. If continuous high levels are necessary, aqueous penicillin G, intramuscularly or intravenously, is recommended.
(Note: Serious pneumonia, empyema, bacteremia, pericarditis, meningitis, or purulent or septic arthritis due to streptococci or nonpenicillinase-producing staphylococci should be treated with aqueous penicillin G during acute stage.)

CONTRAINDICATIONS

Patients with a history of immediate hypersensitivity reactions to any of the penicillins

INTERACTIONS

ORAL: beta-blockers
PARENTERAL: aminoglycosides (parenteral), anticoagulants, heparin
BOTH: chloramphenicol, erythromycin, tetracyclines, oral contraceptives

PATIENT INFORMATION

Complete all medication unless otherwise directed by physician. Take medication with a full glass of water on an empty stomach 1 hour before or 2 hours following a meal. Take at regular intervals around the clock. Contact physician if rash, itching, hives, severe diarrhea, shortness of breath or wheezing, black tongue, sore throat, nausea, vomiting, fever, swelling of joints, or unusual bleeding or bruising occurs. Throw away any unused liquid forms of penicillin after 7 days when stored at room temperature and after 14 days when stored in refrigerator.

ADVERSE EFFECTS

See Adverse Effects for amoxicillin-clavulanic acid.

PHARMACOKINETICS AND PHARMACODYNAMICS

Peak serum levels: 1 to 4 h, 1.3 to 2.0 and 2.4 to 3.1 µg/mL after intramuscular doses of 600,000 U and 1.2 MU
Plasma half-life: drug slowly absorbed and detectable for 1 to 2 d
Bioavailability: wide distribution to body tissues, except to cerebrospinal fluid (unless meninges inflamed)
Metabolism: no information
Elimination: glomerular filtration and tubular secretion
Excretion: 60% to 90% excreted in urine within 24 to 36 h
Effect of food: for intramuscular use only
Protein binding: 60%
Renal impairment: may considerably delay excretion but serum levels only moderately higher
Hepatic impairment: no information

The information here is provided as guidance only. Prescribers should always consult the manufacturer's current prescribing information.

PENICILLIN G PROCAINE (CONTINUED)

DOSAGE

Adults: 600,000 to 1.2 MU/d intramuscularly in one or two doses to a maximum of 4.8 MU/d for 10 days to 2 weeks.

Dosage for Specific Infections

Organism and infection	Dosage
Pneumococcal infection (moderately severe, uncomplicated pneumonia, otitis media, and paranasal sinus infection)	600,000–1.2 MU/d
Group A streptococcal infection (moderately severe to severe tonsillitis, erysipelas, scarlet fever, upper respiratory tract [otitis media], skin–skin structure infection)	600,000–1.2 MU/d for a minimum of 10 d
Diphtheria: Adjunctive therapy (with antitoxin); also, carrier state	300,000–600,000 U/d
Anthrax (cutaneous)	600,000–1.2 MU/d
Vincent's gingivitis and pharyngitis (fusospirochetosis)	600,000–1.2 MU/d
Erysipeloid	600,000–1.2 MU/d
Rat-bite fever (*Streptobacillus moniliformis* and *Spirillum minus*)	600,000–1.2 MU/d
Gonorrheal infection (uncomplicated with beta-lactamase–negative strains)	4.8 MU divided in two doses per one visit; give 1 g oral probenecid 0.5 h before injection. Take follow-up cultures from original sites of infection 7–14 d after treatment (women should also have test-of-cure cultures taken from both endocervical and anal canals). Gonorrheal endocarditis should be intensively treated with aqueous penicillin G.
Syphilis (primary, secondary, or latent with negative spinal fluid [adults and children over 12 y of age])	600,000 U/d for 8 d; total 4.8 MU
Neurosyphilis* (alternative to penicillin G aqueous regimen)	2–4 MU/d with probenecid 500 mg orally every 6 h for 10–14 d (benzathine penicillin G 2.4 MU/wk for 3 wks is often recommended as follow-up therapy after completion of initial regimen)
Congenital syphilis (symptomatic and asymptomatic infants)	50,000 U/kg/d given once intramuscularly for 10–14 d
Yaws, bejel, and pinta	Same as syphilis in corresponding stage of disease

*Centers for Disease Control and Prevention: 1989 Sexually transmitted diseases treatment guidelines. MMWR 1989 Sept 1, 38 (No. S-8):1–43.

Elderly: Same as adults.

Children: Same as adults. For neonates, 50,000 U/kg intramuscularly once daily. (Note: Use in neonates should be avoided due to increased risk of sterile abscesses and procaine toxicity.)

OVERDOSAGE

Excessive doses may cause neuromuscular hyperexcitability or convulsive seizures. Dose-related toxicity can arise with the use of large doses of intravenous penicillin (40–100 MU/d), especially in patients with severe renal impairment. Symptoms include agitation, confusion, asterixis, hallucinations, stupor, coma, multifocal myoclonus, seizures, and encephalopathy. Hypokalemia also has occurred.

In case of overdose, discontinue drug therapy and treat patient symptomatically, using supportive care as required. Hemodialysis may be used if necessary to reduce blood levels of penicillin, although effectiveness is uncertain.

AVAILABILITY

Injection—300,000 and 500,000 per mL
Injection—600,000 units per 1.2 mL
Injection—1,200,000 units per unit dose
Injection—2,400,000 units per unit dose
Combination package—two 4-mL disposable syringes containing 2,400,000 units penicillin G procaine each and two 500-mg probenecid tablets

The information here is provided as guidance only. Prescribers should always consult the manufacturer's current prescribing information.

PIPERACILLIN (Pipracil®)

Piperacillin sodium is a semisynthetic, broad-spectrum penicillin for parenteral use.

ANTIMICROBIAL ACTIVITY

Gram-positive: Staphylococci (nonpenicillinase-producing), *Staphylococcus aureus* (nonpenicillinase-producing), *Streptococcus pneumoniae*, beta-hemolytic streptococci, *Enterococcus faecalis*, viridans streptococcus.

Gram-negative: *Escherichia coli, Haemophilus influenzae*, (non-beta-lactamase–producing) *Klebsiella* spp, *Neisseria gonorrhoeae, Neisseria meningitidis*, Proteus mirabilis, Salmonella* spp*, *Shigella* spp*, *Moraxella* spp*, *Morganella morganii, Proteus vulgaris, Providencia rettgeri, Yersinia* spp*, *Enterobacter* spp, *Citrobacter* spp, *Pseudomonas aeruginosa, Pseudomonas* spp (including *P. cepacia*, P. maltophilia**, and *P. fluorescens*), *Serratia* spp, *Acinetobacter* spp, *Moraxella (Branhamella) catarrhalis*.

Anaerobic: *Clostridium* (including *C. difficile**), *Peptococcus, Peptostreptococcus, Bacteroides* (non–*B. fragilis* group), *B. asaccharolyticus*, Fusobacterium, Eubacterium*, and *Veillonella* spp, and *Actinomyces bovis**.

**Shown to be active in vitro against these organisms; clinical efficacy has not been established.*

RESISTANCE

Piperacillin is active against beta-lactamase–producing gonococci.
See Resistance for mezlocillin.

SPECIAL PRECAUTIONS

May cause hemorrhagic manifestations associated with abnormalities of coagulation tests; withdrawal of drug should stop bleeding and enable coagulation to return to normal.

Patients with liver disease or those receiving cytotoxic therapy or diuretics have rarely shown a decrease in serum potassium concentrations with high doses of piperacillin.

Positive direct antiglobulin tests have been reported after large doses of piperacillin. Antibiotics used in high doses for short periods to treat gonococcal infection may mask signs of syphilis. Evaluate patients with gonorrhea for syphilis prior to treatment.

In cardiac patients or others requiring sodium restriction, periodic electrolyte determinations and monitoring of cardiac function should be instituted.

See Special Precautions for oxacillin.

SPECIAL GROUPS

Children: Safety not established in children younger than 12 years of age.
Elderly: May have age-related renal impairment.
Renal impairment: Reduced dosage required in patients with creatinine clearance less than 30 mL/min.
Hepatic impairment: Dosage modification not required.
Pregnancy: Use only if clearly indicated; controlled human studies not performed.
Breast-feeding: Use caution; excreted in breast milk.

INDICATIONS

Treatment of infections of the following types due to designated susceptible organisms:
Intra-abdominal (including hepatobiliary and surgical infections):
  E. coli, P. aeruginosa, enterococci, *Clostridium* spp, anaerobic cocci, *Bacteroides* spp (including *B. fragilis*)
Urinary tract:
  E. coli, Klebsiella spp, *P. aeruginosa, Proteus* spp, *P. mirabilis*, enterococci
Gynecologic (including endometritis, pelvic inflammatory disease, and pelvic cellulitis):
  Bacteroides spp (including *B. fragilis*), anaerobic cocci, *N. gonorrhoeae*, and enterococci (*E. faecalis*)
Septicemia:
  E. coli, Klebsiella spp, *Enterobacter* spp, *Serratia* spp, *P. mirabilis, S. pneumoniae*, enterococci, *P. aeruginosa, Bacteroides* spp, anaerobic cocci
Lower respiratory tract:
  E. coli, Klebsiella spp, *Enterobacter* spp, *P. aeruginosa, Serratia* spp, *H. influenzae, Bacteroides* spp, anaerobic cocci
(Note: Improvement may be remarked in cystic fibrosis patients; however, lasting bacterial eradication may not be achieved.)
Skin–skin structure:
  E. coli, Klebsiella spp, *Serratia* spp, *Acinetobacter* spp, *Enterobacter* spp, *P. aeruginosa*, indole-positive *Proteus* spp, *P. mirabilis, Bacteroides* spp (including *B. fragilis*), anaerobic cocci, enterococci
Bone and joint:
  P. aeruginosa, enterococci, *Bacteroides* spp, anaerobic cocci
Gonococcal (uncomplicated gonococcal urethritis)
Perioperative prophylaxis

CONTRAINDICATIONS

Patients with a history of immediate hypersensitivity reactions to any of the penicillins

INTERACTIONS

ORAL: beta-blockers
PARENTERAL: aminoglycosides (parenteral), anticoagulants, heparin
BOTH: chloramphenicol, erythromycin, tetracyclines, oral contraceptives

PATIENT INFORMATION

Complete all medication unless otherwise directed by physician. Take medication with a full glass of water on an empty stomach 1 hour before or 2 hours following a meal. Take at regular intervals around the clock. Contact physician if rash, itching, hives, severe diarrhea, shortness of breath or wheezing, black tongue, sore throat, nausea, vomiting, fever, swelling of joints, or unusual bleeding or bruising occurs. Throw away any unused liquid forms of penicillin after 7 days when stored at room temperature and after 14 days when stored in refrigerator.

The information here is provided as guidance only. Prescribers should always consult the manufacturer's current prescribing information.

PIPERACILLIN (CONTINUED)

DOSAGE

(Note: For serious infection, use intravenous route. When using intramuscular route do not exceed 2 g per injection.)

Adults: 200 to 300 mg/kg/d in four to six divided doses (3–4 g every 4–6 hours as a 20–30 min infusion); maximum daily dose, 24 g (higher doses have been used). Maximum dosage (3–4 g every 4 hours) required for serious *Pseudomonas* infections. For acute, uncomplicated gonococcal urethritis, 2 g administered intravenously or intramuscularly, along with 1 g oral probenecid concurrently or 0.5 hours before. For surgical prophylaxis, 2 g intravenously just before, during surgery, and every 6 hours postoperatively for no more than 24 hours. For cesarean section give first 2-g dose as soon as umbilical cord is clamped; second and third doses should be given intravenously at 4 and 8 hours after first dose, respectively. (Note: When piperacillin is given concurrently with an aminoglycoside it should not be mixed in a syringe or infusion bottle because this may result in inactivation of the aminoglycoside; both drugs should, however, be used in full therapeutic doses.)

Elderly: May have age-related renal impairment; otherwise, same as adults.

Children: Dosage not established, but usually 100 to 300 mg/kg/d in four to six divided doses.

Impaired renal function: 3 to 4 g every 8 hours and 3 to 4 g every 12 hours for creatinine clearances of 10 to 30 and < 10 mL/min, respectively.

ADVERSE EFFECTS

See Adverse Effects for amoxicillin-clavulanic acid.

PHARMACOKINETICS AND PHARMACODYNAMICS

Peak serum levels: 41 to 88 and 98 to 139 µg/mL at 30 min after 2- and 4-g intravenous doses, respectively; 30 to 36 µg/mL at 30 min after 2-g intramuscular dose

Plasma half-life: 0.6 to 1.3 h

Bioavailability: 70% to 80% of intramuscular dose absorbed; widely distributed, including bone, prostate, and heart; low concentrations in cerebrospinal fluid except in presence of meningitis

Metabolism: minimal

Elimination: glomerular filtration, tubular secretion, and biliary excretion

Excretion: 60% to 80% in urine first 24 h, 10% to 20% excreted in bile

Effect of food: for intravenous or intramuscular use only

Protein binding: 16% to 22%

Renal impairment: half-life 2.1 to 6 h in patients with creatinine clearance < 30 mL/min

Hepatic impairment: half-life 1.1 to 2 h in patients with cirrhosis

OVERDOSAGE

Excessive doses may cause neuromuscular hyperexcitability or convulsive seizures. Dose-related toxicity can arise with the use of large doses of intravenous penicillin (40–100 MU/d), especially in patients with severe renal impairment. Symptoms include agitation, confusion, asterixis, hallucinations, stupor, coma, multifocal myoclonus, seizures, and encephalopathy. Hypokalemia also has occurred.

In case of overdose, discontinue drug therapy and treat patient symptomatically, using supportive care as required. Hemodialysis may be used if necessary to reduce blood levels of penicillin, although effectiveness is uncertain.

AVAILABILITY

Vials (freeze-dried piperacillin sodium powder)—2-, 3-, and 4-g and 40-g pharmacy bulk vial

The information here is provided as guidance only. Prescribers should always consult the manufacturer's current prescribing information.

PIPERACILLIN TAZOBACTAM (Zosyn®)

The preparation of *piperacillin* with *tazobactam* is a fixed combination of the broad-spectrum piperacillin with a beta-lactamase inhibitor, tazobactam, which prevents the degradation of piperacillin by certain beta-lactamase enzymes.

ANTIMICROBIAL ACTIVITY

Gram-positive: *Staphylococcus aureus*, other staphylococci, *Staphylococcus pneumoniae*, beta-hemolytic streptococci, *Enterococcus faecalis*, *viridans* streptococci.
Gram-negative: *Escherichia coli*, *Haemophilus influenzae*, *Klebsiella* spp, *Neisseria gonorrhoeae*, *Neisseria meningitidis*, *Proteus mirabilis*, *Morganella morganii*, *Proteus vulgaris*, *Providencia rettgeri*, *Providencia stuartii*, *Enterobacter* spp, *Citrobacter* spp, *Pseudomonas aeruginosa*, *Serratia* spp, *Acinetobacter* spp, *Moraxella (Branhamella) catarrhalis*.
Anaerobic: *Clostridium*, *Peptococcus*, *Peptostreptococcus*, *Bacteroides*, *Fusobacterium*, *Eubacterium*, *Veillonella* spp, *Proteus melanovogenes*.

RESISTANCE

In vitro resistance to piperacillin tazobactam develops slowly (involving multiple step mutation), although some strains of *P. aeruginosa* have developed resistance rather rapidly. Some strains of *E. coli* and *Klebsiella* produce high quantities of beta-lactamase and are resistant to piperacillin tazobactam. Piperacillin tazobactam is not stable in the presence of penicillinase, and strains of *S. aureus* that are resistant to penicillin are likewise resistant to piperacillin tazobactam.
Organisms with new extended-spectrum beta-lactamases that inactivate tazobactam have been reported but are extremely rare.

SPECIAL PRECAUTIONS

May cause hemorrhagic manifestation associated with abnormalities of coagulation tests; withdrawal of drug should stop bleeding and enable coagulation to return to normal.
See Special Precautions for oxacillin.

SPECIAL GROUPS

Children: Dosage not established for children < 12 years of age.
Elderly: May have age-related renal impairment.
Renal impairment: Reduced dosage required in patients with creatinine clearance < 30 mL/min.
Hepatic impairment: Dosage modification not required.
Pregnancy: Use only if clearly indicated; controlled human studies not performed.
Breast-feeding: Use caution; excreted in breast milk.

DOSAGE

Adults: 3.375 (3 g piperacillin and 375 mg tazobactam) every 6 hours.
Elderly: May have age-related renal impairment; otherwise, same as adults.
Children: Dosage not established for children < 12 years of age.
Impaired renal function: Dosage should be reduced to 2.25 g every 6 hours and 2.25 g every 8 hours, respectively, in patients with creatinine clearance of 10 to 30 and < 10 mL/min.

INDICATIONS

Treatment of infections of the following types due to susceptible strains of designated organisms:
Intra-abdominal (appendicitis):
  E. coli, *Bacteroides* spp (including *B. fragilis*)
Gynecologic (including endometritis and pelvic inflammatory disease):
  E. coli
Skin–skin structure:
  S. aureus
Community-acquired pneumonia:
  Haemophilus influenzae

CONTRAINDICATIONS

Patients with a history of immediate hypersensitivity reactions to any of the penicillins

INTERACTIONS

ORAL: beta-blockers
PARENTERAL: aminoglycosides (parenteral), anticoagulants, heparin
BOTH: chloramphenicol, erythromycin, tetracyclines, oral contraceptives

PATIENT INFORMATION

Complete all medication unless otherwise directed by physician. Take medication with a full glass of water on an empty stomach 1 hour before or 2 hours following a meal. Take at regular intervals around the clock. Contact physician if rash, itching, hives, severe diarrhea, shortness of breath or wheezing, black tongue, sore throat, nausea, vomiting, fever, swelling of joints, or unusual bleeding or bruising occurs. Throw away any unused liquid forms of penicillin after 7 days when stored at room temperature and after 14 days when stored in refrigerator.

ADVERSE EFFECTS

See Adverse Effects for amoxicillin-clavulanic acid

PHARMACOKINETICS AND PHARMACODYNAMICS

Peak serum levels: 242 and 24 μg/mL for piperacillin and tazobactam, respectively, at 30 min after 3.375-g dose
Plasma half-life: 0.7 to 1.2 h for both drugs
Bioavailability: widely distributed in body tissues, except cerebrospinal fluid (unless meninges are inflamed)
Metabolism: minimal for piperacillin and approximately 20% for tazobactam
Elimination: glomerular filtration and tubular secretion
Excretion: 60% to 80% in urine as unchanged piperacillin and tazobactam; 10% to 20% of piperacillin excreted in bile
Effect of food: for intravenous and intramuscular use only
Protein binding: 30% for both drugs
Renal impairment: half-life of piperacillin doubles and that of tazobactam increases fourfold in patients with severe renal impairment
Hepatic impairment: 18% to 25% increase in half-life in patients with cirrhosis

OVERDOSAGE

See Overdosage for piperacillin

AVAILABILITY

Vials—2.25, 3.375, and 4.5 g and 40.5-g pharmacy bulk vial

The information here is provided as guidance only. Prescribers should always consult the manufacturer's current prescribing information.

TICARCILLIN (Ticar®)

Ticarcillin disodium is a semisynthetic, extended-spectrum penicillin for parenteral use.

ANTIMICROBIAL ACTIVITY

Gram-positive: Staphylococci (nonpenicillinase-producing), *Staphylococcus aureus* (nonpenicillinase-producing), *Streptococcus pneumoniae*, beta-hemolytic streptococci, *Enterococcus faecalis*.
Gram-negative: *Escherichia coli, Haemophilus influenzae, Klebsiella* spp, *Neisseria gonorrhoeae, Neisseria meningitidis, Proteus mirabilis, Salmonella* spp, *Morganella morganii, Proteus vulgaris, Providencia rettgeri, Enterobacter* spp, *Citrobacter* spp, *Pseudomonas aeruginosa, Serratia* spp, *Acinetobacter* spp
Anaerobic: *Clostridium, Peptococcus, Peptostreptococcus, Bacteroides, Fusobacterium,* and *Eubacterium* spp
In vitro synergism between ticarcillin and gentamicin sulfate, tobramycin sulfate, or amikacin sulfate against particular strains of *P. aeruginosa* has been demonstrated.

RESISTANCE

See Resistance for Mezlocillin.

SPECIAL PRECAUTIONS

May cause hemorrhagic manifestations associated with abnormalities of coagulation tests; withdrawal of drug should stop bleeding and enable coagulation to return to normal.
In cardiac patients or others requiring sodium restriction, periodic electrolyte determinations and monitoring of cardiac function should be instituted.
See Special Precautions for oxacillin.

SPECIAL GROUPS

Children: Safe for use.
Elderly: May have age-related renal impairment.
Renal impairment: Reduced dosage required in patients with creatinine clearance less than 60 mL/min.
Hepatic impairment: No modification required.
Pregnancy: Use only when clearly indicated; controlled human studies not performed.
Breast-feeding: Use caution; excreted in breast milk.

INDICATIONS

Treatment of infections of the following types due to susceptible designated organisms:
Bacterial septicemia, skin and soft tissue, acute and chronic respiratory tract:
  P. aeruginosa, Proteus spp (indole-positive and indole-negative), *E. coli*
Genitourinary tract:
  P. aeruginosa, Proteus spp, *E. coli, Enterobacter, E. faecalis*

CONTRAINDICATIONS

Patients with a history of immediate hypersensitivity reactions to any of the penicillins

INTERACTIONS

ORAL: beta-blockers
PARENTERAL: aminoglycosides (parenteral), anticoagulants, heparin
BOTH: chloramphenicol, erythromycin, tetracyclines, oral contraceptives

PATIENT INFORMATION

Complete all medication unless otherwise directed by physician. Take medication with a full glass of water on an empty stomach 1 hour before or 2 hours following a meal. Take at regular intervals around the clock. Contact physician if rash, itching, hives, severe diarrhea, shortness of breath or wheezing, black tongue, sore throat, nausea, vomiting, fever, swelling of joints, or unusual bleeding or bruising occurs. Throw away any unused liquid forms of penicillin after 7 days when stored at room temperature and after 14 days when stored in refrigerator.

ADVERSE EFFECTS

See Adverse Effects for amoxicillin-clavulanic acid.

The information here is provided as guidance only. Prescribers should always consult the manufacturer's current prescribing information.

TICARCILLIN (CONTINUED)

DOSAGE

(Note: For serious infections, use intravenous route. When using intramuscular route, do not exceed 2 g per injection.)

Adults: For bacterial septicemia, respiratory tract, skin or soft-tissue, intra-abdominal, or female pelvic or genital tract infections: 200 to 300 mg/kg/d in divided doses every 4 to 6 hours by intravenous infusion (3 g every 4 hours or 4 g every 6 hours, depending on weight and severity of infection). Maximum dosage (3–4 g every 4 hours) required for serious *Pseudomonas* infections. For urinary tract infections (complicated), 150 to 200 mg/kg/d in divided doses every 4 to 6 hours by intravenous infusion; (uncomplicated), 1 g every 6 hours intramuscularly or direct intravenous. When ticarcillin is given concurrently with an aminoglycoside, it should not be mixed in a syringe or infusion bottle because this may result in inactivation of the aminoglycoside; both drugs should, however, be used in full therapeutic doses.

Elderly: May have age-related renal impairment; otherwise, same as adults.

Children: (under 40 kg) For bacterial septicemia, respiratory tract, skin and soft-tissue, intra-abdominal, or female pelvic or genital infections: 200 to 300 mg/kg/d in divided doses every 4 to 6 hours by intravenous infusion. For urinary tract infections (complicated), 150 to 200 mg/kg/d in divided doses every 4 to 6 hours by intravenous infusion; (uncomplicated), 50 to 100 mg/kg/d in divided doses every 6 to 8 hours intramuscularly or direct intravenous. Daily dose for children should not exceed adult dosage.

Impaired renal function: Dosage should be reduced to 2 g every 4 hours, 2 g every 8 hours, and 2 g every 12 hours in patients with creatinine clearances of 30 to 60, 10 to 30, and < 10 mL/min, respectively.

PHARMACOKINETICS AND PHARMACODYNAMICS

Peak serum levels: 90 and 29 µg/mL at 30 min after 1- and 3-g intravenous doses; 8.6 to 18 and 22 to 35 µg/mL at 30 to 75 min after 0.5- and 1-g intramuscular dose

Plasma half-life: 0.9 to 1.3 h

Bioavailability: percentage not given; widely distributed in body tissues, except cerebrospinal fluid (unless meninges are inflamed)

Metabolism: approximately 15% is partially metabolized to penicilloic acids

Elimination: glomerular filtration and tubular secretion

Excretion: 80% to 93% excreted unchanged in urine within 24 h

Effect of food: for intravenous or intramuscular use only

Protein binding: 45%

Renal impairment: half-life 3 to 9.4 h in patients with creatinine clearance of 10 to 60 mL/min and 11 to 16 h with creatinine clearance < 10 mL/min

Hepatic impairment: slight prolongation when renal function normal

OVERDOSAGE

Excessive doses may cause neuromuscular hyperexcitability or convulsive seizures. Dose-related toxicity can arise with the use of large doses of intravenous penicillin (40–100 MU/d), especially in patients with severe renal impairment. Symptoms include agitation, confusion, asterixis, hallucinations, stupor, coma, multifocal myoclonus, seizures, and encephalopathy. Hypokalemia also has occurred.

In case of overdose, discontinue drug therapy and treat patient symptomatically, using supportive care as required. Hemodialysis may be used if necessary to reduce blood levels of penicillin, although effectiveness is uncertain.

AVAILABILITY

1-, 3-, and 6-g vials
3-g piggyback bottle
20- and 30-g pharmacy bulk package

The information here is provided as guidance only. Prescribers should always consult the manufacturer's current prescribing information.

TICARCILLIN–CLAVULANIC ACID (Timentin®)

The preparation of *ticarcillin* with *clavulanic acid* is a fixed combination of the broad-spectrum ticarcillin with a beta-lactamase inhibitor, clavulanic acid, that prevents the degradation of ticarcillin by certain beta-lactamase enzymes

ANTIMICROBIAL ACTIVITY

Gram-positive: *Staphylococcus aureus*, other staphylococci, *Streptococcus pneumoniae*, beta-hemolytic streptococci, *Streptococcus faecalis*, *viridans* streptococcus.
Gram-negative: *Escherichia coli, Haemophilus influenzae, Klebsiella* spp, *Neisseria gonorrhoeae, Neisseria meningitidis, Proteus mirabilis, Salmonella* spp, *Morganella morganii, Proteus vulgaris, Providencia rettgeri, Providencia stuartii, Enterobacter* spp, *Citrobacter* spp, *Pseudomonas aeruginosa, Serratia* spp, *Acinetobacter* spp, *Moraxella (Branhamella) catarrhalis*.
Anaerobic: *Clostridium, Peptococcus, Peptostreptococcus, Bacteroides, Fusobacterium, Eubacterium*, and *Veillonella* spp.
In vitro synergism between ticarcillin and gentamicin sulfate, tobramycin sulfate, or amikacin sulfate against particular strains of *P. aeruginosa* has been demonstrated.

RESISTANCE

See Resistance for mezlocillin.
Organisms with new extended-spectrum beta-lactamases that inactivate clavulanic acid have been reported but are extremely rare.

SPECIAL PRECAUTIONS

May cause hemorrhagic manifestations associated with abnormalities of coagulation tests; withdrawal of drug should stop bleeding and enable coagulation to return to normal.
See Special Precautions for oxacillin.

SPECIAL GROUPS

Children: Dosage not established for children younger than 12 years of age.
Elderly: May have age-related renal impairment.
Renal impairment: Reduced dosage required in patients with creatinine clearance < 60 mL/min.
Hepatic impairment: No modification required.
Pregnancy: Use only when clearly indicated; controlled human studies not performed.
Breast-feeding: Use caution; excreted in breast milk.

INDICATIONS

Treatment of infections of the following types due to designated organisms:
Septicemia and bacteremia:
  Klebsiella spp*, *E. coli**, *S. aureus**, *P. aeruginosa**, (and other species)*
Lower respiratory tract:
  *S. aureus, H. influenzae**, and *Klebsiella* spp*
Bone and joint:
  S. aureus
Skin–skin structure:
  S. aureus, Klebsiella spp*, *and* E. coli*
Urinary tract:
  E. coli, Klebsiella spp, *P. aeruginosa*, (and other species)*, *Citrobacter* spp*, *Enterobacter cloacae**, *Serratia marcescens**, and *S. aureus**
Gynecologic (endometritis):
  *Bacteroides melaninogenicus**, *Enterobacter* spp (including *E. cloacae**), *E. coli, Klebsiella pneumoniae**, *S. aureus*, and *Staphylococcus epidermidis*
**Efficacy for this organism for this organ system studied in less than 10 infections.*

CONTRAINDICATIONS

Patients with a history of immediate hypersensitivity reactions to any of the penicillins

INTERACTIONS

ORAL: beta-blockers
PARENTERAL: aminoglycosides (parenteral), anticoagulants, heparin
BOTH: chloramphenicol, erythromycin, tetracyclines, oral contraceptives

PATIENT INFORMATION

Complete all medication unless otherwise directed by physician. Take medication with a full glass of water on an empty stomach 1 hour before or 2 hours following a meal. Take at regular intervals around the clock. Contact physician if rash, itching, hives, severe diarrhea, shortness of breath or wheezing, black tongue, sore throat, nausea, vomiting, fever, swelling of joints, or unusual bleeding or bruising occurs. Throw away any unused liquid forms of penicillin after 7 days when stored at room temperature and after 14 days when stored in refrigerator.

The information here is provided as guidance only. Prescribers should always consult the manufacturer's current prescribing information.

TICARCILLIN–CLAVULANIC ACID (CONTINUED)

DOSAGE

Adults: (Administer intravenous infusion over 30 min) For systemic and urinary tract infections in adults weighing more than 60 kg, 3.1 g (3 g ticarcillin and 100 mg clavulanic acid) every 4 to 6 hours; for adults less than 60 kg, 200 to 300 mg/kg/d (based on ticarcillin content) in divided doses every 6 hours. For gynecologic infections (moderate), 200 mg/kg/d in divided doses every 6 hours; (severe) 300 mg/kg/d in divided doses every 4 hours. Maximum dosage (3.1 g every 4 hours) required for serious *Pseudomonas* infections.

Elderly: May have age-related renal impairment; otherwise, same as adults.

Children: Dosage not established for children younger than 12 years of age.

Impaired renal function: Dosage should be reduced 2 g every 4 hours, 2 g every 8 hours, and 2 g every 12 hours in patients with creatinine clearances of 30 to 60, 10 to 30, and < 10 mL/min, respectively.

ADVERSE EFFECTS

See Adverse Effects for amoxicillin-clavulanic acid.

PHARMACOKINETICS AND PHARMACODYNAMICS

Peak serum levels: 176 and 2.6 μg/mL for ticarcillin and clavulanic acid, respectively, at 30 min after 3.1-g dose

Plasma half-life: 1 to 1.3 h for both drugs

Bioavailability: widely distributed in body tissues, except cerebrospinal fluid (unless meninges are inflamed)

Metabolism: minimal for ticarcillin but extensive for clavulanic acid

Elimination: glomerular filtration and tubular secretion

Excretion: 20% of ticarcillin and 40% of clavulanic acid excreted unchanged in urine in 6 h

Effect of food: for intravenous or intramuscular use only

Protein binding: 45% to 49%

Renal impairment: mean half-life is 4.9 and 2.3 h for ticarcillin and clavulanic acid, respectively, in patients with creatinine clearance of 10 to 30 mL/min; values are 8.5 and 2.9 h with creatinine clearance < 10 mL/min

Hepatic impairment: no information

OVERDOSAGE

Excessive doses may cause neuromuscular hyperexcitability or convulsive seizures. Dose-related toxicity can arise with the use of large doses of intravenous penicillin (40–100 MU/d), especially in patients with severe renal impairment. Symptoms include agitation, confusion, asterixis, hallucinations, stupor, coma, multifocal myoclonus, seizures, and encephalopathy. Hypokalemia also has occurred.

In case of overdose, discontinue drug therapy and treat patient symptomatically, using supportive care as required. Hemodialysis may be used if necessary to reduce blood levels of penicillin, although effectiveness is uncertain.

AVAILABILITY

Powder for injection

3 g ticarcillin and 0.1 g clavulanic acid (in 3.1-g vials, piggyback bottles, and 31-g bulk package)

Solution—3 g ticarcillin and 0.1 g clavulanic acid (in 100-mL premixed frozen vials)

The information here is provided as guidance only. Prescribers should always consult the manufacturer's current prescribing information.

CLASS DESCRIPTION

There are a small number of antibiotics that are not penicillins or cephalosporins but are classified as beta-lactams. These agents fall into only three distinct chemical groups, monobactams, carbapenems, and carbacephems. Currently there is only one drug from each group available for physician use, namely, aztreonam, imipenem, and loracarbef, respectively. A second carbacephem, meropenem, is nearing approval for physician use. Loracarbef differs from a cephalosporin in that the dihydrothiazine ring of the cephalosporin contains a sulfur atom, which in loracarbef has been replaced with a carbon (Fig. 4-1). The molecule is in all other respects similar to cefaclor [1]. The carbapenems are chemically classified as thienamycins (Fig. 4-2) [2]. Aztreonam consists of a four-membered beta-lactam ring joined to a 1-sulfonic acid (ring activator) and is protected by a 4-alpha-methyl group, which provides beta-lactamase resistance (Fig. 4-3) [3].

MECHANISM OF ACTION

The mechanism of action for these beta-lactam antibiotics is similar to that of the penicillins and cephalosporins; they bind to penicillin-binding proteins (PBPs) and thereby interfere with the microorganism's ability to crosslink cell wall components, resulting in a weakened cell wall that eventually ruptures due to internal pressures. The unique characteristics of these agents lie in their affinity for PBPs, resulting in different degrees of microbiologic activity; ability to bind to different PBPs, resulting in activity against certain beta-lactam–resistant bacteria; and resistance to degradation by beta-lactamase. Aztreonam is relatively resistant to degradation by beta-lactamase by virtue of its unique side chains [3]. Loracarbef is also stable against beta-lactamase and has good chemical stability in a variety of media [1]. Both imipenem and meropenem have excellent stability against class I beta-lactamases and bind to a variety of PBPs, which confer a broader spectrum of activity compared with other beta-lactams [2,4,5].

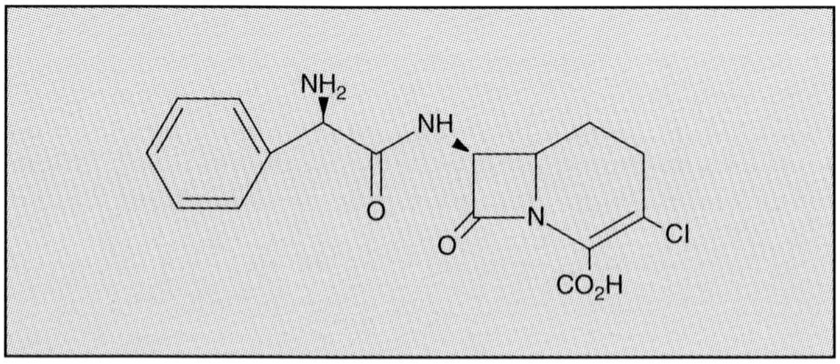

ANTIMICROBIAL ACTIVITY

There are significant differences in antimicrobial activity between these agents. Imipenem and meropenem have strong activity against gram-positive and gram-negative aerobic bacteria, as well as common gram-positive and gram-negative anaerobes. They do not have activity against *Xanthomonas (Pseudomonas) maltophilia* and *Pseudomonas cepacia*. Anaerobic activity is good against the *Bacteroides fragilis* group, other *Bacteroides* species, and *Clostridium* species. Their activity in this regard is generally considered to be roughly equivalent to metronidazole [2,6–8]. In this regard, the microbiologic activity of the carbapenems is very different from the monobactam aztreonam. Aztreonam has a relatively narrow spectrum of activity, being active against most gram-negative aerobic bacteria but not gram-positive aerobes or anaerobes. In regard to its gram-negative activity, it is believed to be roughly equivalent to the aminoglycosides and is frequently employed as an aminoglycoside substitute. In most settings this implies that it is most frequently used in combination with drugs having strong gram-positive activity and, if necessary, anaerobic activity. Typical drug combinations involve nafcillin, oxacillin, methicillin, ampicillin, clindamycin, macrolides, and vancomycin. For anaerobic coverage aztreonam usually is combined with metronidazole or clindamycin—the latter is a particularly good choice because it provides both gram-positive aerobic and anaerobic activity [3,9].

Loracarbef is structurally very similar to cefaclor, and one should not be surprised that their microbiologic spectra are almost identical. Like cefaclor, it is orally absorbed and has activity against most community-acquired respiratory tract, skin and skin structure, and

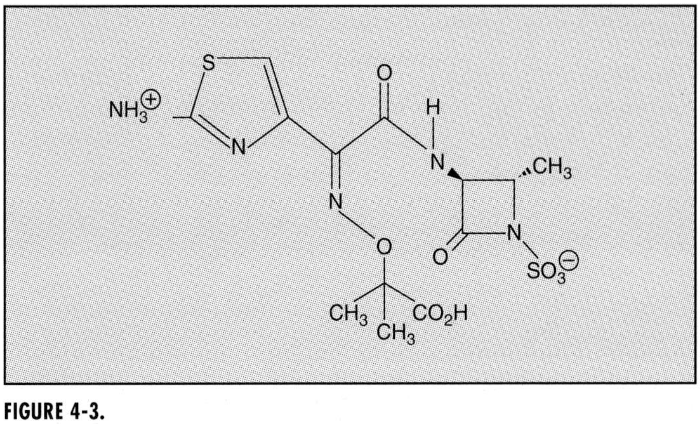

FIGURE 4-1.

The structure of loracarbef.

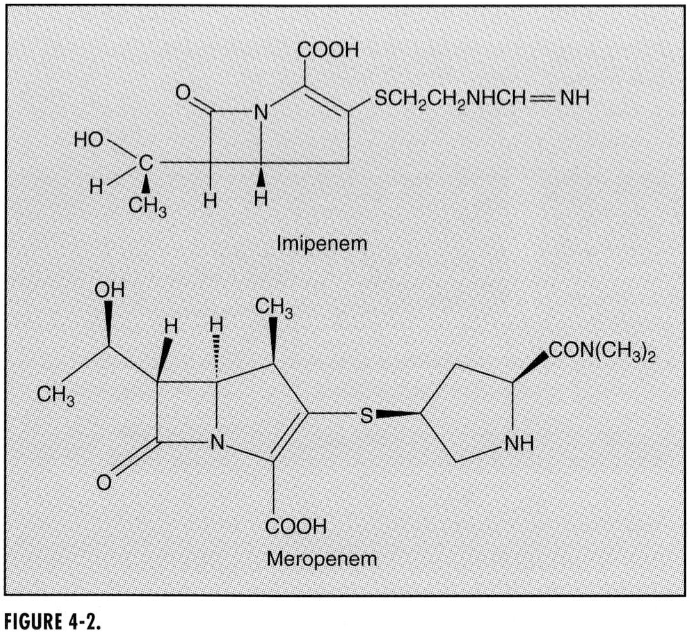

FIGURE 4-2.

Carbapenem structures.

FIGURE 4-3.

The structure of aztreonam.

The information here is provided as guidance only. Prescribers should always consult the manufacturer's current prescribing information.

urinary pathogens. These pathogens include methicillin-sensitive *Staphylococcus aureus*, *Streptococcus pyogenes*, *Haemophilus influenzae*, *Moraxella catarrhalis*, and common Enterobacteriaceae. Loracarbef appears to be somewhat more active against *Escherichia coli* and *Klebsiella pneumoniae* than cefaclor [1,10,11].

PHARMACOKINETICS

The structural similarities of imipenem and meropenem result in similar pharmacokinetic properties. Although structurally dissimilar, aztreonam's pharmacokinetic profile is remarkably similar to the carbapenems. Loracarbef's kinetics are different from all of the other beta-lactams described in this chapter. Imipenem is unique in that it undergoes postexcretory metabolism by dehydropeptidase-I, which is localized in the brush border of the microvillus of the proximal tubule. Cilastatin is coadministered with imipenem to inhibit this metabolism, which also prevents the nephrotoxicity that has been observed in some animal species. A 1:1 combination of cilastatin and imipenem is required to maintain inhibition of renal metabolism for more than 8 hours [2]. Unlike imipenem, meropenem has good stability against human renal dehydropeptidase-I and does not require the coadministration of a dehydropeptidase-I enzyme inhibitor such as cilastatin [12,13].

The half-life of meropenem, imipenem, and cilastatin is approximately 1 hour. These drugs are highly charged at physiologic pH and therefore are not orally absorbed. Like most beta-lactams the charged molecule does not penetrate well into mammalian cells, and its distribution in the body is limited to extracellular water. As such the apparent volume of distribution is low (< 20 L). Both agents are eliminated mainly via the kidneys and therefore are sensitive to alterations in renal function. Cilastatin elimination is more affected by this than that of imipenem [2,12,13].

Aztreonam's half-life is somewhat longer than that of the carbapenems at about 1.7 hours. In all other respects it is similar to other beta-lactams in that it is eliminated mainly via the kidneys and is sensitive to changes in renal function, does not penetrate well into mammalian cells, has a relatively small volume of distribution (< 20 L), and is not highly protein bound (55%–65%) [3,14].

Loracarbef is rapidly and completely absorbed after oral administration, probably because the molecule is more electrically neutral. Its bioavailability is approximately 90%, with peak concentration in serum achieved within 0.5 to 1 hour after administration. After administration of the capsule and suspension (400-mg dose), the peak serum concentrations were 12 and 18 µg/mL. Like most beta-lactams, the protein binding is low (25%), as is the volume of distribution. Like the other agents in this series, loracarbef is eliminated primarily via the kidneys and is therefore sensitive to changes in renal function. In patients with normal renal function, the serum half-life is approximately 1 hour and can increase 32 hours in patients with significant renal impairment [2,15].

DOSAGE ADJUSTMENTS FOR PATIENTS WITH RENAL DYSFUNCTION

Like other beta-lactams, carbapenems, aztreonam, and loracarbef are eliminated almost entirely by renal mechanisms. Tables 4-1 through 4-4 provide dosage adjustment guidelines for these agents in patients with varying degrees of renal dysfunction.

THERAPEUTIC USE

Because of their wide spectrum of activity the carbapenems are particularly useful in infections requiring a broad range of coverage. Imipenem may be used as empiric therapy for nosocomial infections of the respiratory or urinary tract, for intra-abdominal sepsis as a single-agent therapy, or in those situations in which the bacteria are resistant to other agents. Imipenem-cilastatin also is approved for use in complicated skin and skin structure infections (abscesses, ulcers) and gynecologic infections in which polymicrobial infection is highly likely [2,16].

The narrow spectrum of microbiologic activity of aztreonam limits its usefulness as a single agent in empiric therapy. It is useful when the pathogenic organism is known and therefore can play a role in an antibiotic streamlining program. Aztreonam usually is combined with another agent effective against anaerobes and gram-positive aerobes (clindamycin, metronidazole). Aztreonam is approved for use in urinary tract, lower respiratory tract, and intra-abdominal infections. It also has been used to successfully treat osteomyelitis and septic arthritis caused by susceptible gram-negative organisms [3,9,18].

Loracarbef is active gram-positive and gram-negative aerobic organisms, however, it is less active than most of the agents in this

Table 4-1. Dosage Adjustment of Imipenem in Different Degrees of Renal Dysfunction*

Creatinine clearance, L/min/1.73 m^2	Degree of renal function impairment	Fully susceptible organisms	Moderately susceptible organisms (primarily some strains of *Pseudomonas aeruginosa*)
31–70	Mild	500 mg every 8 h	500 mg every 6 h
21–30	Moderate	500 mg every 12 h	500 mg every 8 h
6–20	Severe to marked	250 mg every 12 h	500 mg every 12 h
0–5	None—on hemodialysis	250 mg every 12 h	500 mg every 12 h

*From Merck and Co., Inc [16].

Table 4-2. Dosage Adjustment of Meropenem in Different Degrees of Renal Dysfunction*

Estimated creatinine clearance, *mL/min*	Dosage adjustment (1 dose = 500 mg)
> 80	1 dose every 6 h
51–80	1 dose every 8 h
25–50	1 dose every 12 h
11–24	0.5–1 dose every 12 h
≤ 10	0.5–1 dose every 24 h

*From Leroy et al. [13,17].

The information here is provided as guidance only. Prescribers should always consult the manufacturer's current prescribing information.

chapter. It should be used for less severe infections, such as community-acquired respiratory tract infections, skin and soft tissue infections, and urinary tract infections [1,19]. As an oral agent it is well suited for therapy for ambulatory patients and can be very useful in an antibiotic streamlining program for hospitalized patients.

ADVERSE REACTIONS

Patients treated with imipenem have reported the following side effects: phlebitis at infusion site, nausea, vomiting, diarrhea, and rash. Because imipenem shares the basic beta-lactam nucleus with penicillins and cephalosporins, it can be associated with crossreactivity in those patients with severe beta-lactam allergies and, therefore, should be avoided in these patients [2,16]. Imipenem's most notable adverse reaction involves grand mal seizures and convulsions. The incidence is low (about 1%) and occurs predominantly in elderly patients and those with known predisposing conditions, such as cerebral vascular accident or head trauma. Seizure has been reported in patients with underlying central nervous system pathology or with significant renal dysfunction. The latter is not unexpected because the seizures seem to be dose related (incidence is higher with doses of 4 g/d compared with 2 g/d). Unless dosing adjustments are made, severe renal dysfunction tends to allow the drug to accumulate and therefore can precipitate seizures [2,16]. There is limited clinical evidence suggesting that coadministration of theophylline may also contribute to increased likelihood of seizure activity during imipenem therapy in elderly patients [20]. Although little clinical information is available on meropenem, animal studies suggest that it has less seizure potential than imipenem [21].

Aztreonam and loracarbef are relatively free of adverse events. Loracarbef, the only oral agent presented, is associated with a higher degree of diarrhea compared with the other drugs in this chapter. However, the adverse reaction rate for this complaint (4%) was less than the comparative agents (ie, oral cephalosporins, penicillin–beta-lactamase inhibitor combinations) when investigated in clinical trials. Other frequently reported side effects are headache, vaginal candidiasis, nausea, vomiting, abdominal pain, and rash [1,19]. The most common adverse effect of aztreonam is elevation in liver transaminases (alanine aminotransferase [ALT] and aspartate aminotransferase [AST]), which is reversible with cessation of therapy. Less frequently reported adverse effects include thrombophlebitis at the site of infusion, diarrhea, nausea, vomiting, taste perversion, rash, headache, and dizziness [3,18].

Table 4-3. Dosage Adjustment of Imipenem in Different Degrees of Renal Dysfunction*

Estimated creatinine clearance, mL/min/1.73 m²	Type of infection	Dosage adjustment†
> 30	Urinary tract infection	0.5–1.0 g every 8–12 h
	Moderately severe systemic infections	1–2 g every 8–12 h
	Severe systemic infections	2 g every 6–8 h
10–30		1 or 2 g loading dose; 0.5 dose every 8–12 h
< 10		0.5, 1, or 2 g loading dose; 0.25 loading dose every 6, 8, or 12 h

*From E.R. Squibb and Sons, Inc. [18].
†Dose varies for indication.

Table 4-4. Dosage Adjustment of Loracarbef in Different Degrees of Renal Dysfunction*

Estimated creatinine clearance, mL/min	Dosage adjustment†
> 50	None needed
11–49	0.5 Dose at usual interval
< 10	Dose every 3–5 days; supplemental dose postdialysis

*From Eli Lily and Co. [19].
†Dose varies for indication.

REFERENCES

1. Force RW, Nahata MC: Loracarbef: A new orally administered carbacephem antibiotic. *Ann Pharmacother* 1993, 27:321–328.

2. Buckley MM, Brogden RN, Barradell LB, Goa KL: Imipenem/cilastatin: A reappraisal of its antibacterial activity, pharmacokinetic properties, and therapeutic efficacy. *Drugs* 1992, 44:408–444.

3. Tunkel AR, Scheld WM: Aztreonam. *Infect Control Hosp Epidemiol* 1990, 11:486–494.

4. Yang Y, Livermore DM: Interactions of meropenem with class I chromosomal beta-lactamases. *J Antimicrob Chemother* 1989, 24:S207–S217.

5. Sumita Y, Inoue M, Mitsuhashi S: *In vitro* antibacterial activity and beta-lactamase stability of the new carbapenem SM-7338. *Eur J Clin Microbiol Infect Dis* 1989, 8:908–916.

6. Sheikh W, Pitkin DH, Nadler H: Antibacterial activity of meropenem and selected comparative agents against anaerobic bacteria at seven North American centers. *Clin Infect Dis* 1993, 16:S361–S366.

7. Hoban DJ, Jones RN, Yamane N, *et al.*: *In vitro* activity of three carbapenem antibiotics: Comparative studies with biapenem (L-627), imipenem, and meropenem against aerobic pathogens isolated worldwide. *Diagn Microbiol Infect Dis* 1993, 17:299–305.

8. Lang C, Beuth J, Ko HL, *et al.*: Antibacterial *in vitro* activity of meropenem against 200 clinical isolates in comparison to 11 selected antibiotics. *Int J Med Microbiol Virol Parasitol Infect Dis* 1992, 277:485–492.

9. Westley-Horton E, Koestner JA: Aztreonam: A review of the first monobactam. *Am J Med Sci* 1991, 302:46–49.

The information here is provided as guidance only. Prescribers should always consult the manufacturer's current prescribing information.

10. Knapp CC, Washington JA: *In vitro* activities of LY163892, cefaclor, and cefuroxime. *Antimicrob Agents Chemother* 1988, 32:131–133.

11. Bauernfeind A, Jungwirth R: *In vitro* evaluation of cefpodoxime a new oral cephalosporin of the third generation: Antibacterial activity of cefpodoxime in comparison with cefixime, cefdinir, cefetamet, ceftibuten, loracarbef, cefprozil, BAY 3522, cefuroxime, cefaclor and cefadroxil. *Infection* 1991, 19:353–362.

12. Burman LA, Nilsson-Ehle I, Hutchison M, *et al.*: Pharmacokinetics of meropenem and its metabolite ICI 213,689 in healthy subjects with known renal metabolism of imipenem. *J Antimicrob Chemother* 1991, 27:219–224.

13. Leroy A, Fillastri JP, Borsa-Lebas F, *et al.*: Pharmacokinetics of meropenem (ICI 194,660) and its metabolite (ICI 213,689) in healthy subjects and in patients with renal impairment. *Antimicrob Agents Chemother* 1992, 36:2794–2798.

14. Mattie H: Clinical pharmacokinetics of aztreonam: An update. *Clin Pharmacokinet* 1994, 26:99–106.

15. Lees AS, Andrews JM, Wise R: The pharmacokinetics, tissue penetration and *in vitro* activity of loracarbef, a beta-lactam antibiotic of the carbacephem class. *J Antimicrob Chemother* 1993, 32:853–859.

16. Primaxin® package insert. Merck & Co., Inc. West Point, PA. 1987.

17. Leroy A, Fillastre JP, Etienne I, *et al.*: Pharmacokinetics of meropenem in subjects with renal insufficiency. *Eur J Clin Pharmacol* 1992, 42:535–538.

18. Azactam® package insert. E.R. Squibb & Sons, Inc. Princteon, NJ. 1992.

19. Lorabid® package insert. Eli Lilly & Co. Indianapolis, IN. 1992.

20. Semel JD, Allen N: Seizures in patients simultaneously receiving theophylline and imipenem or ciprofloxacin or metronidazole. *South Med J* 1991, 84:465–468.

21. Patel JB, Giles RE: Meropenem: Evidence of lack of proconvulsive tendency in mice. *J Antimicrob Chemother* 1989, 307–309.

22. Friedrich LV, White RL, Kays MB, *et al.*: Aztreonam pharmacokinetics in burn patients. *Antimicrob Agents Chemother* 1991, 35:57–61.

23. Heikkila A, Renkonen OV, Erkkola R: Pharmacokinetics and transplacental passage of imipenem during pregnancy. *Antimicrob Agents Chemother* 1992, 36:2652–2655.

24. Boucher BA, Hickerson WL, Kuhl DA, *et al.*: Imipenem pharmacokinetics in patients with burns. *Clin Pharmacol Ther* 1990, 48:130–137.

25. Bosso JA, Black PG: The use of aztreonam in pediatric patients: A review. *Pharmacotherapy* 1991, 11:20–25.

26. Stutman HR: Clinical experience with aztreonam for treatment of infections in children. *Rev Infect Dis* 1991, 13:S582–S585.

27. Touny ME, Guinaidy ME, Barry MA, *et al.*: Pharmacokinetics of aztreonam in patients with liver cirrhosis and ascites. *J Antimicrob Chemother* 1992, 30:387–395.

28. Conrad DA, Williams RR, Couchman TL, Lentnek AL: Efficacy of aztreonam in the treatment of skeletal infections due to *Pseudomonas aeruginosa. Rev Infect Dis* 1991, 13:S634–S639.

The information here is provided as guidance only. Prescribers should always consult the manufacturer's current prescribing information.

AZTREONAM (Azactam®)

Asztreonam was originally isolated from *Chromobacterium violaceum*; it is a monobactam antibiotic, which is structurally different from other beta-lactam antibiotics because of a unique monocyclic beta-lactam nucleus. The spectrum of activity is very narrow (gram-negative aerobic organisms), and therefore its empiric clinical use is usually in combination with drugs that have gram-positive aerobic and anaerobic activity.

ANTIMICROBIAL ACTIVITY

Gram-negative aerobes: *Escherichia coli*, *Enterobacter* species, *Klebsiella pneumoniae* and *Klebsiella oxytoca*, *Proteus mirabilis*, *Pseudomonas aeruginosa*, *Serratia marcescens*, *Haemophilus influenzae* (including ampicillin-resistant and other penicillinase-producing strains), *Citrobacter* spp.

Demonstrated *in vitro* activity without clinical documentation of efficacy: *Neisseria gonorrhoeae*, *Proteus vulgaris*, *Morganella morganii*, *Providencia* spp, *Pseudomonas* spp, *Shigella* spp, *Pasteurella multocida*, *Yersinia enterocolitica*, *Aeromonas hydrophila*, *Neisseria meningitidis*. Aztreonam is not active against gram-positive aerobic and anaerobic organisms.

(Note: Aztreonam and aminoglycosides demonstrate synergistic *in vitro* activity against most strains of *P. aeruginosa*, Enterobacteriaceae, and other gram-negative aerobic bacilli.)

RESISTANCE

Aztreonam demonstrates little effect on intestinal flora in *in vitro* studies and is very stable in the presence of beta-lactamases. Aztreonam does not induce chromosomally mediated beta-lactamase production.

SPECIAL PRECAUTIONS

Bacteriologic studies should be performed to determine causative organisms and their susceptibility before initiation of treatment.

Use caution in administering monobactams to patients with sensitivity to penicillin; possible cross-allergenicity and risk of allergic or anaphylactic reaction. If an allergic reaction occurs, discontinue drug. **SERIOUS REACTIONS MAY OCCUR**, requiring epinephrine or other emergency measures (including oxygen, intravenous fluids, intravenous antihistamines, corticosteroids, pressor amines, and airway management).

Bacterial or fungal overgrowth of nonsusceptible organisms, leading to secondary infection, may occur with prolonged or repeated therapy.

Patients with impaired renal or hepatic function should be monitored frequently during therapy.

SPECIAL GROUPS

Children: Safety and efficacy for use in infants and children has not been established.
Elderly: May have age-related renal impairment.
Renal impairment: Reduced dosage necessary.
Hepatic impairment: Reduced dosage may be necessary.
Pregnancy: Use only if clearly indicated; human studies not performed.
Breast-feeding: Excreted in breast milk; decision should be made to discontinue nursing or discontinue agent.
Burn patients: Dosage adjustment needed [22].

INDICATIONS

Treatment of infections of the following types due to susceptible strains of designated organisms or in combination with other agents if broader spectrum coverage is desired empirically:

Urinary tract (complicated and uncomplicated, including pyelonephritis and cystitis, initial and recurrent):
E. coli, *K. pneumoniae*, *P. mirabilis*, *P. aeruginosa*, *Enterobacter cloacae*, *K. oxytoca**, *Citrobacter* spp*, and *S. marcescens**

Lower respiratory tract (including pneumonia and bronchitis):
E. coli, *K. pneumoniae*, *P. aeruginosa*, *H. influenzae*, *P. mirabilis*, *Enterobacter* spp, and *S. marcescens**
(Note: Will not eradicate *P. aeruginosa* consistently from patients with cystic fibrosis [25].)

Septicemia:
E. coli, *P. aeruginosa*, *H. influenzae*, *P. mirabilis*, *Enterobacter* spp, and *S. marcescens*, *K. pneumonia*, and *Citrobacter* spp*

Skin–skin structure:
E. coli, *P. aeruginosa*, *H. influenzae*, *P. mirabilis**, *S. marcescens*, *Enterobacter* spp, *K. pneumoniae*, and *Citrobacter* spp*

Intra-abdominal (including peritonitis):
E. coli, *Klebsiella* spp (including *K. pneumoniae*), *P. aeruginosa*, *H. influenzae*, *P. mirabilis*, *Enterobacter* species (including *E. cloacae**), and *Serratia* spp (including *S. marcescens**), *Citrobacter* spp* (including *C. freundii**)

Gynecologic (including endometritis and pelvic cellulitis):
E. coli, *K. pneumoniae**, *Enterobacter* spp* (including *E. cloacae**), and *P. mirabilis**

Bone infections (including osteomyelitis and septic arthritis) [3,28]:
*P. auruginosa**

**Efficacy for this organism in this type of organ system studied in less than 10 infections.*

CONTRAINDICATIONS

Allergy or hypersensitivity to this antibiotic

INTERACTIONS

Nafcillin sodium, cephradine, metronidazole

The information here is provided as guidance only. Prescribers should always consult the manufacturer's current prescribing information.

AZTREONAM (CONTINUED)

DOSAGE

Adults: For urinary tract infections, 500 mg every 8 to 12 hours. For moderately severe systemic infections, 1 to 2 g every 8 to 12 hours. For severe or life-threatening infections, 2 g every 6 to 8 hours. Maximum recommended dose is 8 g/d. (Note: Intravenous route is recommended for patients who are receiving single doses greater than 1 g or who have bacterial septicemia, parenchymal abscess, peritonitis, or other severe systemic infections. Due to the serious nature of *P. aeruginosa* infection, a dosage of 2 g every 6 to 8 hours is recommended, at least for the onset of therapy.) Duration of therapy depends on severity of infection.

Elderly: May have age-related renal impairment.

Children: Follow dosage guidelines below.

*Dosing Aztreonam in Pediatric Patients**

Age or condition	Dose, *mg/kg*	Interval, *h*
< 1 week	20–30	12–24
1–4 weeks	30	8
4 weeks–24 months	30	8
> 2 years	30	8
Cystic fibrosis	50	6

**Adapted from Bosso and Black [25] and Stutman [26].*

Impaired renal function: Dosage should be halved in patients with estimated creatinine clearance between 10 and 30 mL/min/1.73m² after an initial loading dose of 1 to 2 g is given. In patients with severe renal failure (those on hemodialysis), a dose of 500 mg, 1 g, or 2 g should be given initially, and the maintenance dose should be one fourth of the usual follow-up dose given at 6-, 8-, or 12-hour intervals. For serious or life-threatening infections, an additional one eighth of the initial follow-up dose should be given after each hemodialysis session.

ADVERSE EFFECTS

Local irritation (phlebitis, thrombophlebitis), diarrhea, nausea, vomiting, rash, anaphylaxis, angioedema, bronchospasm, pancytopenia, neutropenia, thrombocytopenia, anemia, leukocytosis, thrombocytosis, abdominal cramps, pseudomembranous colitis, toxic epidermal necrolysis, purpura, erythema multiforme, exfoliative dermatitis, urticaria, petechiae, pruritus, hypotension, transient electrocardiogram changes (ventricular bigeminy and preventricular contractions), hepatitis, jaundice, seizure, confusion, vertigo, paresthesia, insomnia, dizziness, muscular aches, tinnitus, diplopia, mouth ulcer, altered taste, numb tongue, sneezing/nasal congestion, halitosis, vaginal candidiasis, vaginitis, breast tenderness, weakness, headache, fever, malaise, diaphoresis, flushing, chest pain, dyspnea

Laboratory alterations reported during clinical trials include:

Hepatic: increases in AST, ALT, and alkaline phosphatase; signs of hepatobiliary dysfunction occurred in less than 1% of patients

Hematologic: increases in prothrombin, partial thromboplastin times; positive Coombs' test

Renal: increases in serum creatinine

PHARMACOKINETICS AND PHARMACODYNAMICS

Peak serum levels: after intravenous infusions of 500 mg, 1 g, and 2 g levels were 54, 90, and 204 µg/mL respectively, and 1, 3, and 6 µg/mL at 8 h

Serum half-life: 1.7 h

Metabolism: unchanged aztreonam and inactive beta-lactam ring hydrolysis product

Elimination: tubular secretion and glomerular filtration

Excretion: 60% to 70% recovered in urine after 8 h

Effect of food: for parenteral use only

Protein binding: 56%

Renal impairment: prolongs half-life

Hepatic impairment: only slightly prolongs half-life (liver is only a minor pathway of excretion)

Cirrhotic patients with normal renal function may have slightly increased clearance of aztreonam [27] Dose adjustment may be needed

Burn patients: increased volume of distribution; larger doses may be needed [22]

OVERDOSAGE

Aztreonam can be cleared from the blood by hemodialysis or peritoneal dialysis

AVAILABILITY

Single-dose 15-mL capacity vials
500-mg vial
1-g vial
2-g vial
Single-dose 100-mL capacity intravenous infusion bottles with bail bands
500-mg bottle
1-g bottle
2-g bottle

The information here is provided as guidance only. Prescribers should always consult the manufacturer's current prescribing information.

IMIPENEM (Primaxin®)

Imipenem-cilastatin sodium is a combination of imipenem, a thienamycin antibiotic, and cilastatin sodium, the inhibitor of renal dipeptidase and dehydropeptidase-I. It is a broad-spectrum antibiotic for intramuscular and intravenous administration, with activity against gram-positive and gram-negative aerobes as well as anaerobes.

ANTIMICROBIAL ACTIVITY

Gram-positive aerobes: *S. aureus* (including penicillinase-producing strains), Group D *Streptococcus* (including *Enterococcus faecalis* [formerly *S. faecalis*], *Streptococcus pneumoniae*, *Streptococcus pyogenes* (Group A *Streptococcus*), *Streptococcus viridans* group.
Gram-negative aerobes: *Acinetobacter* spp (including *calcoaceticus*), *Citrobacter* spp, *Enterobacter cloacae*, *Escherichia coli*, *Haemophilus influenzae*, *Klebsiella pneumoniae*, *Pseudomonas aeruginosa*.
Gram-positive anaerobes: *Peptostreptococcus* spp.
Gram-negative anaerobes: *Bacteroides* spp (including *fragilis*, *thetaiotaomicron*, *intermedius*), *Fusobacterium* spp (including *necrophorum*).

RESISTANCE

Imipenem is inactive *in vitro* against *Enterococcus faecium* (formerly *S. faecium*), *Xanthomonas (Pseudomonas) maltophilia*, and *Pseudomonas cepacia*.

SPECIAL PRECAUTIONS

Bacteriologic studies should be performed to determine causative organisms and their susceptibility before initiation of treatment.
Use caution in administering carbipenems to patients with sensitivity to penicillin; possible cross-allergenicity and risk of allergic or anaphylactic reaction. If an allergic reaction occurs, discontinue drug. **SERIOUS REACTIONS MAY OCCUR,** requiring epinephrine or other emergency measures (including oxygen, intravenous fluids, intravenous antihistamines, corticosteroids, pressor amines, and airway management).
Use caution in administering broad-spectrum antibiotics to patients with existing or previous gastrointestinal disease. Treatment with broad-spectrum antibiotics alters normal flora of the colon and may permit overgrowth of clostridia, causing antibiotic-associated pseudomembranous colitis. Mild cases usually respond to discontinuation of therapy alone; management of moderate to severe cases should include bacteriologic studies and fluid, electrolyte, and protein supplementation. Bacterial or fungal overgrowth of nonsusceptible organisms, leading to secondary infection, may occur with prolonged or repeated therapy.
Central nervous system (CNS) adverse effects have been reported with use of imipenem and include myoclonic activity, confusion, and seizures. These effects have occurred most often in patients with CNS disorders who also have impaired renal function; however, reports exist in which there has been no underlying or recognized CNS disorder. If adverse CNS effects occur, discontinue drug. Anticonvulsant therapy should be maintained in patients with known seizure disorders.
Patients with known or suspected renal impairment should undergo appropriate evaluation before and during therapy. Total daily dosage should be reduced if renal function is impaired.
Avoid accidental injection into a blood vessel when administering intramuscularly. Some strains of *P. aeruginosa* may develop resistance quickly during single-agent antibiotic therapy (with any of the beta-lactam antibiotics). It is generally recommended that pseudomonal infections be treated using combination therapy with two agents from different antibiotic classes (*ie*, aminoglycosides and fluoroquinolones).

INDICATIONS

(Note: Intramuscular imipenem is not meant for use in therapy for severe or life-threatening infection; this includes bacterial sepsis, endocarditis, or cases of major physical impairment such as shock.)
Imipenem is indicated for the treatment of infections of the following types due to susceptible strains of designated organisms:
Lower respiratory tract (including pneumonia and bronchitis as exacerbation of chronic obstructive pulmonary disease):
S. pneumoniae, H. influenzae
Intra-abdominal (including acute gangrenous or perforated appendicitis or appendicitis with peritonitis):
Group D *Streptococcus* (including *E. faecalis**, *S. viridans* group*, *E. coli*, *K. pneumoniae**, *P. aeruginosa**, *Bacteroides* spp (including *fragilis*, *distasonis**, *intermedius**, *thetaiotaomicron**) *Fusobacterium* spp, and *Peptostreptococcus* spp*
Skin–skin structure (including abscesses, cellulitis, skin ulcers, and wounds):
S. aureus (including penicillinase-producing strains), *S. pyogenes**, group D *Streptococcus* (including *E. faecalis*), *Acinetobacter* spp* (including *A. calcoaceticus**), *Citrobacter* spp*, *E. coli, Enterobacter cloacae, K. pneumoniae**, *P. aeruginosa**, *Bacteroides* spp* (including *B. fragilis**)
Gynecologic (including postpartum endomyometritis):
Group D *Streptococcus* (including *E. faecalis*,* *E. coli*, *K. pneumoniae**, *Bacteroides intermedius**, *Peptostreptococcus* spp*

**Efficacy for this organism in this organ system studied in less than 10 infections.*

CONTRAINDICATIONS

Allergy or hypersensitivity to imipenem or any of the components of the preparation being used (*eg*, lidocaine hydrochloride, amide-type anesthetics)

INTERACTIONS

Probenecid

ADVERSE EFFECTS

Phlebitis or thrombophlebitis, nausea, diarrhea, vomiting, rash, pseudomembranous colitis, hepatitis, gastroenteritis, pruritus, urticaria, fever, seizures, dizziness, somnolence, encephalopathy, tremor, confusion, myoclonus, paresthesia, vertigo, headache, erythema multiforme, toxic epidermal necrolysis, facial edema, flushing, skin texture changes, candidiasis, heartburn, pharyngeal pain, increased salivation, chest discomfort, hyperventilation, dyspnea, transient hearing loss, tinnitus, polyarthralgia, taste perversion, weakness, thoracic spine pain, thrombocytopenia, leukopenia, oliguria or anuria, erythema at injection site, vein induration, psychic disturbances
Laboratory alterations: decreased hemoglobin and hematocrit, increased or decreased leukocytes and platelets, positive Coombs' test, abnormal prothrombin time, decreased serum sodium, increased potassium and chloride, increased blood urea nitrogen and creatinine, presence of protein, erythrocytes, leukocytes, casts bilirubin, or urobilinogen in urine

The information here is provided as guidance only. Prescribers should always consult the manufacturer's current prescribing information.

IMIPENEM (CONTINUED)

SPECIAL GROUPS

Children: Safety and efficacy not established for infants or children under 12 years of age.
Elderly: May have age-related renal impairment.
Renal impairment: Reduced dosage required.
Hepatic impairment: No information.
Pregnancy: Use only when clearly indicated. Dosage adjustment necessary. No fetal accumulation in full-term infants [23].
Breast-feeding: Not known whether excreted in breast milk; caution advised.
Burn patients: Wide interpatient variability; dosage adjustment may be necessary [24].

DOSAGE

(Note: Imipenem should not be mixed or physically added to other antibiotics, although concurrent administration with other antibiotics, such as aminoglycosides, is acceptable.)
Adults: *INTRAMUSCULAR*: For lower respiratory, skin–skin structure, or gynecologic infections of mild to moderate severity, 500 to 750 mg every 12 hours. For intra-abdominal infection, 750 mg every 12 hours. Do not exceed 1500 mg/d.
(Note: Aspiration is necessary to prevent injection into a blood vessel.)

Guidelines for Intravenous Imipenem Dosing in Adults

Type of infection	Fully susceptible organisms	Moderately susceptible organisms (primarily some strains of *P. aeruginosa*)
Mild	250 mg every 6 h	500 mg every 6 h
Moderate	500 mg every 8 h or 500 mg every 6 h	500 mg every 6 h or 1 g every 8 h 1 g every 8 h
Severe, life-threatening	500 mg every 6 h	1 g every 6 h
Urinary tract, uncomplicated	250 mg every 6 h	250 mg every 6 h
Urinary tract, complicated	500 mg every 6 h	500 mg every 6 h

(Note: It is recommended that the total daily dose of imipenem not exceed 50 mg/kg/d or 4 g/d, whichever is lower, due to the high antimicrobial activity of this agent.)
Elderly: May have age-related renal impairment, otherwise, same as adults.
Children: Dosage not established.
Impaired renal function: Patients with creatinine clearance below 70 mL/min/1.73 m^2 need a dosage reduction according to the following equation:

$$\text{Total creatinine clearance (males)} = \frac{(\text{weight in kg}) \times (140 - \text{age})}{(72) \times (\text{creatinine in mg/dL})}$$

$$\text{Total creatinine clearance (females)} = (0.85) \times \text{above value}$$

(Note: Patients with creatinine clearance below 5 mL/min/1.73 m^2 should not receive imipenem unless hemodialysis is performed within 48 hours. There are insufficient data to support the use of imipenem in patients undergoing peritoneal dialysis.)
Patients with creatinine clearance of 6 to 20 mL/min/1.73 m^2 should have 250 mg or 3.5 mg/kg, whichever is lower, every 12 hours for most organisms. There may be an increased risk of seizures in these patients when the 500-mg dose is used.

PHARMACOKINETICS AND PHARMACODYNAMICS

Peak serum levels: 2 h following administration of 500 mg intravenously and intramuscularly, respectively, gave 10 µg/mL and 9.9 µg/mL (1 h after, 45.1 µg/mL and 6.0 µg/mL)
Serum half-life: 2 to 3 h
Metabolism: in kidneys by dehydropeptidase-I
Excretion: in urine, 50% imipenem, 75% cilastatin
Effect of food: for parenteral use only
Protein binding: 20% imipenem, 40% cilastatin
Renal impairment: reduced dosage necessary
Hepatic impairment: no information
Burn patients: adjust dose based on measured 24-h creatinine clearance, if patient has abnormally high or low creatinine [24]

OVERDOSAGE

INTRAMUSCULAR:
Discontinue imipenem and treat patient symptomatically, instituting supportive care as necessary. Imipenem-cilastatin sodium is hemodialyzable, however, its usefulness remains questionable. (In animals studies, signs and symptoms of overdosage included seizures, ataxis, and tremors.)
INTRAVENOUS:
Overdosage information for humans is not available

AVAILABILITY

Imipenem IM, sterile powder
  500 mg imipenem and 500 mg cilastatin
  750 mg imipenem and 750 mg cilastatin
Imipenem IV, sterile powder
  250 mg imipenem and 250 mg cilastatin
  500 mg imipenem and 500 mg cilastatin

The information here is provided as guidance only. Prescribers should always consult the manufacturer's current prescribing information.

LORACARBEF (Lorabid®)

Loracarbef is a synthetic beta-lactam antibiotic of the carbacephem class. Structurally it is very similar to cefaclor. It is an oral agent intended either for less severe community-acquired infections or as streamlining therapy for hospitalized patients after an initial course of parenteral therapy.

ANTIMICROBIAL ACTIVITY

Gram-positive aerobes: *Staphylococcus aureus* (including penicillinase-producing strains), *Staphylococcus saprophyticus, Streptococcus pneumoniae, Streptococcus pyogenes.*
Gram-negative aerobes: *Escherichia coli, Haemophilus influenzae* (including beta-lactamase–producing strains), *Moraxella (Branhamella) catarrhalis* (including beta-lactamase–producing strains).

RESISTANCE

Loracarbef is inactive against methicillin-resistant staphylococci and the enterococcus (as are most beta-lactam antibiotics).

SPECIAL PRECAUTIONS

Bacteriologic studies should be performed to determine causative organisms and their susceptibility before initiation of treatment.
Use caution in administering carbacephems to patients with sensitivity to penicillin; possible cross-allergenicity and risk of allergic or anaphylactic reaction. If an allergic reaction occurs, discontinue drug. **SERIOUS REACTIONS MAY OCCUR,** requiring epinephrine or other emergency measures (including oxygen, intravenous fluids, intravenous antihistamines, corticosteroids, pressor amines, and airway management).
Use caution in administering broad-spectrum antibiotics to patients with existing or previous gastrointestinal disease. Treatment with broad-spectrum antibiotics alters normal flora of the colon and may permit overgrowth of clostridia, causing antibiotic-associated pseudomembranous colitis. Mild cases usually respond to discontinuation of therapy alone; management of moderate to severe cases should include bacteriologic studies and fluid, electrolyte, and protein supplementation. Bacterial or fungal overgrowth of nonsusceptible organisms, leading to secondary infection, may occur with prolonged or repeated therapy.
Patients with known or suspected renal impairment should undergo appropriate evaluation before and during drug therapy. Total daily dosage should be reduced if renal function is impaired.

SPECIAL GROUPS

Children: Safety and efficacy not established for infants under 6 months of age.
Elderly: May have age-related impairment.
Renal impairment: Reduced dosage required.
Hepatic impairment: No information.
Pregnancy: Use only if clearly indicated; human studies not performed.
Breast-feeding: Not known whether excreted in breast milk.

INDICATIONS

Treatment of infections of the following types due to susceptible strains of designated organisms:
Lower respiratory tract (acute bacterial exacerbations of chronic bronchitis):
S. pneumoniae, H. influenzae (including beta-lactamase–producing strains), *M. catarrhalis* including beta-lactamase–producing strains)
Pneumonia:
S. pneumoniae, H. influenzae (non–beta-lactamase–producing strains)*
Upper respiratory tract (otitis media):
S. pneumoniae, H. influenzae (non–beta-lactamase–producing strains), *M. catarrhalis* (including beta-lactamase–producing strains), *S. pyogenes*
Acute maxillary sinusitis*:
S. pneumoniae, H. influenzae (non–beta-lactamase–producing strains), *M. catarrhalis* (including beta-lactamase–producing strains)*
Pharyngitis or tonsillitis:
S. pyogenes (Note: Usual agent of choice is intramuscular penicillin for both treatment and prevention of streptococcal infection, including rheumatic fever. Loracarbef is generally effective; however, data are not yet available to support the efficacy of this agent in the prevention of rheumatic fever)
Skin–skin structure (uncomplicated):
S. aureus (including penicillinase-producing strains), *S. pyogenes*
Urinary tract (cystitis):
*E. coli, S. saprophyticus** (Note: Lower bacterial eradication rates and lower toxicity potential of loracarbef should be weighed against increased eradication rates and increased toxicity potential demonstrated by other approved agents.)
Pyelonephritis (uncomplicated):
E. coli

At this time there are insufficient data to support efficacy in patients with this infection due to beta-lactamase–producing organisms. The bacterial eradication and clinical cure rates were slightly less with loracarbef than with products containing a beta-lactamase inhibitor. The reduced potential for toxicity with loracarbef compared with other agents containing beta-lactamase inhibitors and the susceptibility patterns of common microbes in the given geographic area should be considered when using antimicrobials.

CONTRAINDICATIONS

Allergy or hypersensitivity to loracarbef or cephalosporin-type antibiotics

INTERACTIONS

Probenecid

The information here is provided as guidance only. Prescribers should always consult the manufacturer's current prescribing information.

DOSAGE

Adults: Follow recommended dosage guidelines below.

Adult Loracarbef Dosage Recommendations

Infection	Dosage	Duration, d
Lower respiratory tract Secondary bacterial infection (acute bronchitis)	200–400 mg every 12 h	7
Acute bacterial Exacerbation of chronic bronchitis	400 mg every 12 h	7
Pneumonia	400 mg every 12 h	14
Upper respiratory tract pharyngitis or tonsillitis	200 mg every 12 h*	10
Sinusitis	400 mg every 12 h	10
Skin–skin structure	200 mg every 12 h	7
Uncomplicated urinary tract (uncomplicated cystitis)	200 mg every 24 h	7
Pyelonephritis	200 mg every 24 h	7

*For infections due to S. pyogenes, duration should continue for at least 10 days.

Elderly: Same as adults.

Children: (Infants and children 6 months to 12 years of age) For upper respiratory tract infections (otitis media)*, 30 mg/kg/d in divided doses every 12 hours for 10 days. For pharyngitis or tonsillitis, 15 mg/kg/d in divided doses every 12 hours for 10 days†. For skin–skin structure infections (impetigo), 15 mg/kg/d in divided doses every 12 hours for 7 days.

*Treat otitis media with suspension; suspension is absorbed more rapidly than oral form (clinical studies performed with suspension only). Do not substitute.

†For infections due to S. pyogenes, duration should continue for at least 10 days.

Impaired renal function: Usual dose may be used in patients with creatinine clearance of 50 mL/min or higher. Patients with creatinine clearance in the range of 10 to 49 mL/min should receive half the usual dose at the usual interval or the usual dose at double the usual interval. Patients with creatinine clearance under 10 mL/min should receive the usual dose only every 3 to 5 days, with those on hemodialysis receiving another dose following hemodialysis.

If only serum creatinine is available, the following formula may be used to calculate the value into creatinine clearance (CLCR, mL/min) assuming that renal function is stable:

$$\text{Males} = \frac{(\text{weight in kg}) \times (140 - \text{age})}{(72) \times \text{serum creatinine (mg/100 mL)}}$$

$$\text{Females} = (0.85) \times \text{above value}$$

ADVERSE EFFECTS

Diarrhea, nausea, vomiting, abdominal pain, anorexia, skin rash, urticaria, pruritus, erythema multiforme, headache, somnolence, nervousness, insomnia, nervousness, dizziness, vasodilation, vaginitis, vaginal moniliasis

Laboratory alterations: transient thrombocytopenia, leukopenia, eosinophilia, transient elevations in AST, ALT, and alkaline phosphatase, transient elevations in blood urea nitrogen and creatinine

PHARMACOKINETICS AND PHARMACODYNAMICS

Peak serum levels: 17 µg/mL 0.8 h after a 400-mg dose (increased rate of absorption with suspension in children)

Serum half-life: 1 h, normal renal function

Bioavailability: 90%

Metabolism: no evidence of hepatic metabolism

Elimination: no information

Excretion: < 90% recovered unchanged in urine

Effect of food: (capsules) decreases absorption by 50% to 60%; (suspension) not studied

Protein binding: 25%

Renal impairment: prolongs half-life

Hepatic impairment: not known to affect clearance

OVERDOSAGE

Symptoms may include nausea, vomiting, epigastric distress, and diarrhea. Forced diuresis, peritoneal dialysis, hemodialysis, or hemoperfusion have not been established as useful in cases of overdose; however, hemodialysis has demonstrated effectiveness in speeding the elimination of loracarbef from the plasma of patients with renal failure.

PATIENT INFORMATION

Take medication 1 hour before meals or 2 hours after meals

AVAILABILITY

Pulvules (Eli Lilly and Co., Indianapolis, IN)—200 mg
Oral suspension—100 mg/5 mL and 200 mg/5 mL

The information here is provided as guidance only. Prescribers should always consult the manufacturer's current prescribing information.

MEROPENEM (Merrem®)

Meropenem is a carbapenem antibiotic with a structure and spectrum much like imipenem. This agent offers the advantages of decreased neurotoxicity and increased stability in the presence of renal dehydropeptidase-I.

ANTIMICROBIAL ACTIVITY

NONE: Activities reported here are based on *in vitro* data.

Gram-positive aerobes: *Staphylococcus aureus* (including penicillinase-producing strains), coagulase-negative *Staphylococcus* spp (*saprophyticus, epidermidis*) *Streptococcus pyogenes, Enterococcus faecalis.*

Gram-negative aerobes: *Escherichia coli, Acinetobacter calcoaceticus* (*lwoffi* variant), *Proteus* spp (including *mirabilis* and *vulgaris*), *Klebsiella* spp (including *pneumoniae* and *oxytoca*), *Haemophilus influenzae, Moraxella (Branhamella) catarrhalis, Pseudomonas aeruginosa, Morganella morganii, Enterobacter* spp (including *cloacae* and *aerogenes*), *Citrobacter* spp, *Serratia marcescens, Salmonella* spp.

Gram-positive anaerobes: *Clostridium perfringens, Peptostreptococcus* spp (including *asaccharolyticus*).

Gram-negative anaerobes: *Bacteroides* spp (including *fragilis, thetaiotaomicron, ovatus,* and *vulgatus*), *Fusobacterium* spp (including *necrophorum*).

RESISTANCE

Meropenem has no activity *in vitro* against *Xanthomonas (Pseudomonas) maltophilia, P. cepacia,* and *E. faecium.*

SPECIAL PRECAUTIONS

Bacteriologic studies should be performed to determine causative organisms and their susceptibility before initiation of treatment.

Use caution in administering carbapenems to patients with sensitivity to penicillin; possible cross-allergenicity and risk of allergic or anaphylactic reaction. If an allergic reaction occurs, discontinue drug. **SERIOUS REACTIONS MAY OCCUR** requiring epinephrine or other emergency measures (including oxygen, intravenous fluids, intravenous antihistamines, corticosteroids, pressor amines, and airway management).

Use caution in administering broad-spectrum antibiotics to patients with existing or previous gastrointestinal disease. Treatment with broad-spectrum antibiotics alters normal flora of the colon and may permit overgrowth of clostridia, causing antibiotic-associated pseudomembranous colitis. Mild cases usually respond to discontinuation of therapy alone; management of moderate to severe cases should include bacteriologic studies and fluid, electrolyte, and protein supplementation. Bacterial or fungal overgrowth of nonsusceptible organism, leading to secondary infection, may occur with prolonged or repeated therapy.

Patients with known or suspected renal impairment should undergo appropriate evaluation before and during therapy. Total daily dosage should be reduced if renal function is impaired.

Some strains of *P. aeruginosa* may develop resistance quickly during single-agent antibiotic therapy (with any of the beta-lactam antibiotics). It is generally recommended that *Pseudomonas* infections be treated using combination therapy with two agents from different antibiotic classes (*ie*, aminoglycosides and fluoroquinolones).

INDICATIONS

(Note: The Food and Drug Administration has not approved meropenem at the time of publication.)

CONTRAINDICATIONS

History of allergic reactions to penicillins or cephalosporins

INTERACTIONS

No information

ADVERSE EFFECTS

(Note: These are side effects reported in normal volunteer studies: headache, tiredness, nausea.)

PHARMACOKINETICS AND PHARMACOKINETICS

Peak serum levels: 25 to 30 mg/L following 500-mg dose; 60 mg/L following 1000-mg dose.

Serum half-life: 1 h

Metabolism: moderate amount of metabolism by renal dehydropeptidase-I

Elimination: renal tubular secretion (major); hepatic secretion (minor)

Excretion: 70% to 90% renal; 10% to 30% hepatic

Effect of food: parenteral use only

Protein binding: no information available

Renal impairment: increase in half-time up to 10-fold in anephric patients

Hepatic impairment: minor route of excretion (no specific information available)

The information here is provided as guidance only. Prescribers should always consult the manufacturer's current prescribing information.

MEROPENEM (CONTINUED)

SPECIAL GROUPS

Children: Safety and efficacy for use in infants and children has not been established.
Elderly: Likely age-related decline in renal function.
Renal impairment: Dosage adjustment needed.
Hepatic impairment: No adjustment needed.
Pregnancy: No information available.
Breast feeding: No information available.

DOSAGE

Adults: 500 mg intravenously every 8 hours.
Impaired renal function: *See* table below.

Meropenem Renal Dose Adjustment*

Estimated creatinine clearance, *mL/min*	Dosage/adjustment
> 80	1 dose unit every 6 h
51–80	1 dose unit every 8 h
25–50	1 dose unit every 12 h
11–24	0.5 dose unit every 12 h
≤ 10	0.5 dose unit every 24 h

*Adapted from Leroy et al. [13,17].

OVERDOSAGE

Meropenem is cleared by hemodialysis (extent approximately 20%)

AVAILABILITY

Zeneca Pharmaceuticals Group (Wilmington, DE)

The information here is provided as guidance only. Prescribers should always consult the manufacturer's current prescribing information.

This chapter discusses a variety of organic compounds and antimicrobial agents with diverse chemical structures. These drugs include the glycopeptides—vancomycin and teicoplanin; the polypeptides—bacitracin, gramicidin, and polymyxin; the octose derivatives—lincomycin and clindamycin; the tertiary amine—methenamine; a nitromidazole—metronidazole; a furan—nitrofurantoin; and an acid ester—mupirocin. Some of these compounds are used only topically (*eg*, bacitracin, gramicidin, mupirocin); parenterally (*eg*, vancomycin and teicoplanin); orally (*eg*, methenamine and nitrofurantoin); or by several routes (*eg*, the polymixins, metronidazole, and lincosamines). Some of these drugs are directed mainly toward gram-positive organisms (*eg*, bacitracin, mupirocin, vancomycin, and teicoplanin), others against gram-negative organisms (*eg*, gramicidin, nitrofurantoin, and the polymixins), and others have significant anaerobic activity (*eg*, metronidazole and clindamycin).

BACITRACIN (Cortisporin®, Neosporin®, Polysporin®)

Bacitracin is a water-soluble mixture of polypeptide antibiotics derived from *Bacillus subtilis* (*Bacillus licheniformis*) in 1943. Use is limited to a few gram-positive bacterial infections because of toxicity and a narrow antimicrobial spectrum.

CHEMISTRY AND CLASSIFICATION

Bacitracin possesses a thiazolidine nucleus similar to penicillin but does not have a beta-lactam ring. The nucleus is attached to a peptide containing *D*- and *L*-amino acids.

MECHANISM OF ACTION

Bacitracin inhibits Stage II cell wall peptidoglycan synthesis, the stage of linear polymerization. The drug binds to the lipid pyrophosphate carrier that normally transports cell wall precursors to the membrane of replicating cells, preventing dephosphorylation of the lipid carrier. By blocking dephosphorylation of lipid pyrophosphate to lipid phosphate and inorganic phosphate, the regeneration of lipid carrier is inhibited [1]. Bacitracin also forms a tight complex with magnesium and pyrophosphate [2]. The generation of this complex is responsible for further inhibition of dephosphorylation.

INDICATIONS

Topical preparations containing bacitracin alone or in combination with other antimicrobial agents (neomycin and polymyxin) and corticosteroids are used commonly to treat impetigo and other superficial pyogenic skin infections. Efficacy has not been firmly established. Available formulations include ointments, creams, sprays, powders, and irrigating solutions. Bacitracin is also used for intraoperative irrigations during orthopedic and neurosurgical procedures to prevent postoperative infections. As an alternative to vancomycin and metronidazole, bacitracin also has been used to treat pseudomembranous colitis caused by *Clostridium difficile* [4]. The dose is 25,000 U or 500 mg four times a day for 1 to 3 weeks. The bitter taste of the drug and the nausea it produces limit its use, although placing the powder in a capsule reduces side effects.

ADVERSE EFFECTS

Nephrotoxicity following systemic administration is the major side effect. Local hypersensitivity reactions and anaphylaxis may rarely complicate topical use. Nausea and a bitter taste are common following oral administration.

PHARMACOKINETICS AND PHARMACODYNAMICS

Bacitracin is poorly absorbed from the gastrointestinal tract. When administered parenterally, therapeutic levels are achieved in pleural and ascitic fluid, but transport across the blood–brain barrier into cerebrospinal fluid is limited. The drug is inactivated in tissue and approximately 30% is recovered in urine as the active form. Systemic administration is precluded because of nephrotoxicity [5]. Current use is limited to topical applications to skin and gastrointestinal infections.

DRUG INTERACTIONS

Other nephrotoxic drugs, including aminoglycosides and muscle relaxants

The information here is provided as guidance only. Prescribers should always consult the manufacturer's current prescribing information.

BACITRACIN (CONTINUED)

ANTIMICROBIAL ACTIVITY

Bacitracin is active against gram-positive cocci and bacilli, including *Staphylococcus*, *Clostridium*, *Actinomyces*, and *Fusobacterium* spp [3]. Most *Streptococcus* spp are sensitive, but the drug is less active against group C and G streptococci. Group B strains are resistant. Certain gram-negatives *Neisseria* spp, *Haemophilus influenzae*, and *Treponema pallidum* are sensitive, but most gram-negative bacilli are resistant.

MECHANISM OF BACTERIAL RESISTANCE

The development of resistance is uncommon.

DOSAGE ADJUSTMENT AND RENAL AND HEPATIC FAILURE

Not applicable.

AVAILABILITY

Bacitracin ointment—500 U/g

Cortisporin Ointment (Burroughs Wellcome, Research Triangle Pk, NC) (polymyxin B sulfate–bacitracin zinc–neomycin sulfate–hydrocortisone)—each gram contains polymyxin B sulfate 5,000 U, bacitracin zinc 400 U, neomycin sulfate 3.5 mg, hydrocortisone 10 mg, and special white petrolatum

Cortisporin Ophthalmic Ointment (Burroughs Wellcome)—each gram contains neomycin sulfate 3.5 mg, polymyxin B sulfate 10,000 U, bacitracin zinc 400 U, hydrocortisone 10 mg, and special white petrolatum

Polysporin Ophthalmic Ointment (Burroughs Wellcome)—each gram contains polymyxin B sulfate 10,000 U, bacitracin zinc 500 U, and special white petrolatum

Neosporin original ointment (Burroughs Wellcome)—each gram contains polymyxin B sulfate 5,000 U, bacitracin zinc 400 U, neomycin 3.5 mg

Neosporin Plus (Burroughs Wellcome)—each gram contains bacitracin zinc, neomycin sulfate, and lidocaine

Polysporin Powder (Burroughs Wellcome)—each gram contains polymyxin B sulfate 10,000 U, bacitracin zinc 500 U, and antibiotic powder

Polysporin Ointment (Burroughs Wellcome)—each gram contains polymyxin B sulfate 10,000 U and bacitracin zinc 500 U

The information here is provided as guidance only. Prescribers should always consult the manufacturer's current prescribing information.

GRAMICIDIN (Neosporin Ophthalmic®)

Gramicidin is a polypeptide antibiotic originally produced by *Bacillus brevis*. The drug causes specific permeability changes in lipid bilayers and membranes, allowing the passage of cations. Gramicidin is used only topically because of toxicity.

CHEMICAL COMPOSITION

The drug is an open chain polypeptide with 15 *D*- and *L*-amino acid residues alternating in sequence.

MECHANISM OF ACTION

Typically, lipid constituents of cell membranes are oriented with polar groups aligned along the membrane surface, and nonpolar hydrocarbons directed toward the membrane interior. The nonpolar constituents of the membrane serve as an effective barrier to the passage of small ions, including sodium and potassium. Gramicidin acts as a channel-former. The drug causes the formation of a tube from one surface of the membrane to the other, allowing ions to enter at one side of the membrane and pass through to the other side. Gramicidin produces ion-conducting channels in cell membranes that allow univalent cations but not anions and polyvalent cations to pass [6]. These channels form and disappear in the presence of the drug. Cells are killed because of changes in cellular potassium concentrations.

ANTIMICROBIAL ACTIVITY

Gramicidin is active against gram-positive bacteria, including *Staphylococcus aureus* and *Streptococcus* spp. The drug is used in combination with polymyxin B sulfate and neomycin sulfate. These drugs confer broad-spectrum, aerobic, gram-negative activity to the combination.

MECHANISM OF BACTERIAL RESISTANCE

Serratia marcescens is naturally resistant to gramicidin.

DOSAGE

Adults: One to two drops in affected eye two to four times a day, for 7 to 10 days. In acute infections, more frequent dosing may be necessary.
Children: No special dosage information is available.

INDICATIONS

Gramicidin is available in Neosporin Ophthalmic Solution (Burroughs Wellcome, Research Triangle Pk, NC). Drug-containing eyedrops are used to treat superficial external ocular infections.

ADVERSE EFFECTS

Allergy and hypersensitivity to polymyxin, neomycin, or gramicidin may result from cutaneous and conjunctival sensitization

PHARMACOKINETICS AND PHARMACODYNAMICS

Pharmacokinetics have not been determined because of toxicity produced by systemic administration

DRUG INTERACTIONS

No information

PATIENT INFORMATION

Avoid contamination of applicator tip by contact with eye, finger, or other potentially contaminating sources to preserve sterility of the solution. If redness, irritation, pain, or swelling persists, notify physician.

AVAILABILITY

Ophthalmic solution—10-mL dropper bottle

The information here is provided as guidance only. Prescribers should always consult the manufacturer's current prescribing information.

LINCOMYCIN AND CLINDAMYCIN (Cleocin®, Lincocin®)

Lincomycin was isolated from soil actinomycete *Streptomyces lincolnesis* in 1962. The drug was modified to 7-deoxy, 7-chloro-derivative clindamycin in 1966. The modification increased antimicrobial activity (anaerobes, gram-positive aerobic cocci, and protozoa) and gastrointestinal absorption. *Clindamycin* has replaced lincomycin therapeutically.

CHEMICAL CLASSIFICATION

Lincomycin and clindamycin are weak bases that are water soluble as salts. Lincomycin is available as the hydrochloride salt for oral and parenteral use. Clindamycin is available as the hydrochloride salt for oral use, the palmitate ester is for pediatric suspension, and phosphate ester is for parenteral administration. Clindamycin is a sulfur-containing derivative of octose attached to the amino acid, *trans L-4-n-*propylhygrinic acid.

MECHANISM OF ACTION

The lincosamides are inhibitors of bacterial protein synthesis [7]. Inhibition is accomplished by drug binding to $50S$ subunits of ribosomes. Binding sites may be the same as or closely overlap binding site of macrolides and chloramphenicol. Consequently, each of these drugs may interfere with the activity of the other. Lincosamide antibiotics inhibit the initiation of peptide chain synthesis by interacting with ribosomes that are free of nascent peptides. Inhibition of peptide bond synthesis is produced by interfering with the peptidyl transferase reaction. As protein synthesis inhibitors, the lincosamide are listed as bacteriostatic drugs, although in some instances they may be bacteriocidal. These drugs may potentiate opsonization and phagocytosis of bacteria at subinhibitory concentration [8]. This is thought to be accomplished by altering the bacterial cell surface, resulting in complement fixation, which facilitates phagocytosis and intracellular killing. Clindamycin interferes with the adherence of *Staphylococcus aureus* to fibronectin, preventing colonization [9]. Production of the toxin that causes staphylococcal toxic shock syndrome is inhibited by clindamycin [10]. The drug also inhibits glycocalyx biofilm formation by *S. aureus* [11].

ANTIMICROBIAL ACTIVITY

Clindamycin has a broader spectrum than lincomycin. Sensitive organisms include aerobic gram-positive cocci, gram-negative and gram-positive anaerobes, and certain protozoa [12–15]. Most aerobic gram-negative bacteria are resistant, although *Neisseria meningitidis, Neisseria gonorrhoeae, Haemophilus influenzae,* and *Campylobacter* spp are moderately sensitive. At clinically achievable concentrations, the spectrum of activity of clindamycin includes *Streptococcus pneumoniae, Streptococcus pyogenes, Streptococcus bovis,* and *Streptococcus viridans.* Enterococci are usually resistant. *Staphylococcus epidermidis* and *S. aureus* may be sensitive, but because resistance is possible, sensitivity testing must be performed when treating infections caused by these organisms. Erythromycin-resistant strains of staphylococci may be sensitive to clindamycin or cross-resistant. Occasionally, clindamycin-sensitive, erythromycin-resistant staphylococci treated with clindamycin become rapidly resistant to this drug. This phenomenon is called *disassociated cross-resistance* [16]. Methicillin-resistant strains of *S. aureus* are resistant to clindamycin. Most strains of *Corynebacterium diphtheriae* are sensitive. Although *Nocardia asteroides* is sensitive, clinical data are not available to support the use of clindamycin in treating infections caused by this organism. The drug is bacteriocidal for most gram-positive organisms, including streptococci and staphylococci.

(Continued on next page)

INDICATIONS

Major indications for clindamycin include serious staphylococcal and streptococcal infections in penicillin-allergic patients, especially those with osteomyelitis, septic arthritis, and serious abdominal, pelvic, and respiratory tract infections involving anaerobic flora. Specific indications include intra-abdominal infections that arise from loss of integrity of the bowel (*eg,* perforated ulcers, gangrenous appendicitis, diverticulitis, penetrating abdominal trauma, and abscesses of major organs); pelvic infections (*eg,* chronic salpingitis, endometritis, ovarian abscess, and aseptic abortion); respiratory infections (*eg,* lung abscess, necrotizing pneumonia, aspiration pneumonia, and empyema); polymicrobial infections of the face, floor of the mouth, mediastinum, and retropharyngeal area; diabetic foot infections; and serious polymicrobial soft-tissue infections (*eg,* necrotizing fasciitis and decubitus ulcers) [23–25]. Because of the major role of gram-negative aerobes in these mixed infections, additional chemotherapy, including aminoglycoside, aztreonam, or a third-generation cephalosporin, should be added. Clindamycin may be used in selected cases of malaria, babesiosis, and toxoplasmosis. Topical clindamycin has been used to treat acne vulgaris. Oral clindamycin may be required for severe pustular disease.

ADVERSE EFFECTS

Clindamycin has been associated with hypersensitivity reactions, including rashes, urticaria, Stevens-Johnsons syndrome, and anaphylactoid reactions. Topical clindamycin has been associated with contact dermatitis. Pain at the intramuscular injection site and phlebitis at the site of intravenous infusion may occur. Lincomycin has been associated with hypotension and cardiovascular instability following rapid intravenous administration. Clindamycin has been reported to cause neuromuscular blockade and may potentiate the activity of neuromuscular blocking agents. Bone marrow suppression has been reported but is rare. Elevation of hepatic enzymes may occur in patients receiving lincosamides, but this is often the effect of the drugs on the methodology used to determine enzyme levels and does not indicate liver damage. Antibiotic-associated diarrhea occurs in 2% to 30% of individuals. This is usually self-limited and disappears on discontinuation of the drug. A smaller percentage develop pseudomembranous colitis due to *Clostridium difficile.* This complication may occur following the use of most antimicrobial agents, especially ampicillin and cephalosporins. The spectrum of gastrointestinal toxicity varies from an acute, self-limited, trivial diarrhea to an acute life-threatening colitis with toxic megacolon [26,27]. Diarrhea may occur early during administration or several weeks after discontinuation of the drug. Treatment with antiperistaltic drugs is contraindicated because of the danger of causing toxic megacolon. Oral metronidazole or vancomycin are the drugs of choice. Patients with ileus may require parenteral metronidazole or metronidazole enemas.

The information here is provided as guidance only. Prescribers should always consult the manufacturer's current prescribing information.

LINCOMYCIN AND CLINDAMYCIN (CONTINUED)

ANTIMICROBIAL ACTIVITY *(CONTINUED)*

Clindamycin is active against the *Bacteroides fragilis* group, although some *Bacteroides* subspecies, *Bacteroides vulgatus*, and *Bacteroides thetaiotaomicron* are resistant [17]. The drug is bacteriocidal for some strains of *Bacteroides* and bacteriostatic for others. Clindamycin is active against anaerobic streptococci, *Veillonella* spp, peptococci, *Clostridium perfringens*, *Clostridium tetani*, *Fusobacterium* spp, and *Actinomyces* spp. *Clostridium ramosum* and *C. difficile* are resistant [18]. The resistance of this latter organism accounts for the antibiotic-associated diarrhea and pseudomembranous colitis that occasionally complicate clindamycin treatment. Clindamycin is active against *Toxoplasma gondii*, *Babesia*, and chloroquine-sensitive and -resistant strains of *Plasmodium falciparum*. The drug is also active against *Plasmodium vivax* but not the extraerythrocytic phase. *Mycoplasma pneumoniae* and *Treponema pallidum* are resistant.

MECHANISMS OF BACTERIAL RESISTANCE

Resistance to lincosamides may develop during treatment and has been observed in strains of *S. pyogenes. S. pneumoniae*, *S. aureus*, *S. epidermidis*, *C. diphtheriae*, *H. influenzae*, *Propionibacterium acnes*, and in some anaerobes including *B. fragilis*, *Fusobacterium* spp, *Peptococcus* spp, and *Eubacterium* spp [16,19]. Resistance may result from chromosomal mutations or plasmid transfers [20,21]. Several mechanisms have been implicated, including structural changes in ribosomal binding sites and methylation of the 23*S* ribosomal RNA of the 50*S* ribosome subunit, which prevents attachment of the antibiotic. Resistance of *B. fragilis* has been found to be plasmid mediated [21]. Evidence suggests that resistance in polymicrobial infections may be transferred between species and strains [22]. The plasma-mediated resistance of *Bacteroides* is not caused by metabolism of drug or inhibited uptake but by alterations in target sites. Enzymatic inactivation is not a common mechanism of resistance to lincosamides, although adenylation of lincomycin has been described.

DOSAGE ADJUSTMENTS FOR HEPATIC AND RENAL INSUFFICIENCY

See Pharmacokinetics and Pharmacodynamics.

SPECIAL GROUPS

Children: Monitor organ system functions in children, infants, and neonates. The safety and efficacy of topical solutions in children under 12 years of age have not been established.

Elderly: May tolerate drug-associated diarrhea less well; monitor bowel function.

Renal impairment: Reduced dosage not necessary in mild to moderate impairment.

Hepatic impairment: Reduced dosage not necessary in mild to moderate impairment.

Pregnancy: Safety not established.

Breast-feeding: Decision to discontinue drug or discontinue nursing must be made with respect to the importance of the drug to the mother.

PHARMACOKINETICS AND PHARMACODYNAMICS

Lincomycin and clindamycin are absorbed rapidly from the gastrointestinal tract (90%), and food does not inhibit absorption. Peak serum levels are achieved by 45 minutes. Gastrointestinal absorption is delayed in the elderly, and serum concentrations are higher in patients with renal failure. The hydrochloride salts are bitter and are packaged in capsules. The better-tasting palmitate ester is used in oral suspensions. Clindamycin phosphate is the water-soluble ester used for parenteral administration. The phosphate and palmitate esters are microbiologically inactive, requiring hydrolysis *in vivo* to become active. Clindamycin phosphate ester may be used intramuscularly because it causes little pain and is well absorbed. Following intramuscular injection, a serum peak level is reached in 1 hour in children and in 3 hours in adults. Intravenous administration produces a peak level at the end of infusion. Some drug may be absorbed from the skin following topical use.

Clindamycin diffuses into many tissues but does not cross the blood–brain barrier. Concentrations in sputum approach that of serum. Therapeutic levels are found in dental alveolar bone tissue, pleural, peritoneal, and synovial fluids, the eye, adenoids, tonsils, appendix, fallopian tubes, uterus, wound tissue, and decubitus ulcers [28]. Clindamycin crosses the placenta, and although teratogenic effects have not been found in animals, safety has not been established in pregnant women. Experimentally produced abscesses contain high drug concentrations [29]. The lincosamides are actively transported into neutrophils and macrophages at nine to 50 times the concentration in serum [30,31]. Protein binding varies from 60% to 95% and the half-life from 2 to 2.5 hours. Approximately 10% of the administered drug dose is recovered in the urine. The lincosamides are mainly eliminated in bile, and high concentrations are reached in the gallbladder in the absence of obstruction. The drugs are metabolized in the liver to the biologically active sulfoxide and *N*-demethyl derivatives. The drugs are metabolized in the liver to the biologically active sulfoxide and *N*-demethyl derivatives. The serum half-life is prolonged to 8 to 12 hours in patients with active liver disease, and dosing should be adjusted with moderate to severe liver disease. No dose adjustment is required for kidney dysfunction because most of the drug is eliminated by the liver. In the presence of liver and renal disease, the dose should be reduced significantly. Peritoneal and hemodialysis do not remove clindamycin. High concentrations of clindamycin and metabolites are found in the stool, even after parenteral administration. These compounds persist in stool for long periods of time, and there may be an enterohepatic circulation of clindamycin and metabolites [32]. This leads to suppression of anaerobic flora. The antimicrobial activity in stool may be found for several days after discontinuation of the drug, accounting for the selecting out of resistant organisms, such as *C. difficile* [33].

The information here is provided as guidance only. Prescribers should always consult the manufacturer's current prescribing information.

LINCOMYCIN AND CLINDAMYCIN (CONTINUED)

DOSAGE

Adults: *ORAL:* 150 to 300 mg every 6 hours. For more severe infections, 300 to 450 mg every 6 hours. *PARENTERAL:* For serious infections due to gram-positive cocci and more sensitive anaerobes, 600 to 1200 mg/d in two to four doses. For more severe infections, especially involving anaerobes, 1.2 to 2.7 g/d in two to four divided doses. Dose may be increased for more severe infections. For life-threatening infections due to aerobes or anaerobes 4.8 g/d may be given to adults.
VAGINAL CREAM: For bacterial vaginosis, one applicator-full intravaginally (preferable at bedtime) for 7 consecutive days.
TOPICAL SOLUTION, TOPICAL LOTION, and *TOPICAL GEL:* Apply thin film to affected area twice daily.
Elderly: May have age-related renal impairment; otherwise same as adults.
Children: *ORAL:* (clindamycin hydrochloride). For serious infections 8 to 16 mg/kg/d, divided into three to four doses. For more severe infections, 16 to 20 mg/kg/d, divided into three to four doses (clindamycin palmitate hydrochloride). For serious infections 8 to 12 mg/kg/d, divided into three to four doses. For more serious infections, 13 to 20 mg/kg/d, divided into three to four doses. For children weighing 10 kg or less, 1/2 teaspoon (37.5 mg) three times a day is minimum recommended dosage.
Parenteral: For children less than 1 month of age, 20 to 40 mg/kg/d in three to four doses.

DRUG INTERACTIONS

Clindamycin may potentiate drugs that cause neuromuscular blockade and interfere with the antibacterial activity of erythromycin and chloramphenicol

PATIENT INFORMATION

Take oral clindamycin with food or a full glass of water to reduce esophageal irritation. Vaginal cream and topical solution, lotion, and gel: in case of contact with eyes, rinse thoroughly with cool tap water.

AVAILABILITY

Capsules—75 mg, 150 mg, and 300 mg
Granules for oral solution—75 mg/mL (as palmitate)
Injection—150 mg/mL (as phosphate) in 2-, 4-, 6-mL vials
Vaginal cream—40-g tube with seven disposable applicators
Topical solution—30-mL and 60-mL applicator bottle and 16-oz bottle
Topical lotion—60-mL plastic squeeze bottle
Topical gel—7.5-g and 30-g tubes

The information here is provided as guidance only. Prescribers should always consult the manufacturer's current prescribing information.

METHENAMINE (Hiprex®, Methenamine®, Urex®)

Methenamine, a cyclic hydrocarbon, has been used to treat urinary tract infections since 1894. The drug is not an antibiotic, but a urinary tract antiseptic. Consequently, it has little use in the treatment of urinary tract infections. The niche for this drug is microbial suppression in situations that make infection likely.

CHEMICAL CLASSIFICATION

Methenamine, a condensation of formaldehyde and ammonia, is a tertiary amine with the properties of a monoacidic base. A variety of organic and inorganic compounds may form salts with this base. Methenamine is available as a pure base or a salt of mandelic acid, *ie*, methenamine mandelate, (Mandelamine [Warner-Chilcott, Morris Plains, NJ]), or hippuric acid, *ie*, methenamine hippurate (Hiprex [Marion Merrell Dow, Kansas City, MO] and Urex [3M Pharmaceuticals, St. Paul, MN]). Methenamine is water soluble and makes a weak basic solution at a pH of 8 to 8.5.

MECHANISM OF ACTION

The drug is not intrinsically bacteriocidal, but at an acid pH it hydrolyzes to form formaldehyde and ammonia [34]. Formaldehyde is the active bacteriocidal product, causing bacterial proteins to denature at acid and alkaline pHs. Hydrolysis begins at a pH below 7 and increases as the pH approaches 5. The production of formaldehyde in urine depends on the concentration of methenamine and an acid pH. The longer the drug remains in the urine, the more formaldehyde is produced. The addition of mandelic acid or hippuric acid to form methenamine salts aids in the acidification of the urine [35]. Mandelic and hippuric acids are weak organic acids that are excreted unmetabolized in urine. These organic acids may or may not suffice to acidify the urine. Vitamin C or acid-producing foods, such as cranberry juice, also have been used to potentiate the activity of the drug. Ideally, urinary pH should be maintained at 5.5 or lower. Mandelic acid and hippuric acid are weakly bacteriostatic and add to the total activity of the drug, although large doses of the drug are required to produce bacteriostasis.

ANTIMICROBIAL ACTIVITY

The hydrolysis of methenamine in acid urine to form free formaldehyde provides mild antiseptic effects within the urinary tract directed against gram-positive and gram-negative bacteria and fungi. *Proteus* spp and other urea-splitting organisms are not suppressed by methenamine. These organisms elaborate a urease that produces sufficient quantities of ammonia to render acidification of urine impossible. Under these circumstances, hydrolysis of methenamine does not occur.

MECHANISMS OF BACTERIAL RESISTANCE

None.

SPECIAL GROUPS

Children: Safety and efficacy not established for children under 6 years of age.
Elderly: No information.
Renal impairment: Try to avoid.
Hepatic impairment: Avoid.
Pregnancy: Use with caution.

INDICATIONS

Methenamine and its organic salts are used for chronic suppressive treatment of lower urinary tract infections but not for primary treatment of acute infections [35,36]. Patients with recurrent urinary tract infections, indwelling catheters, and neurogenic bladders are target populations. Because bacterial resistance does not develop, long-term therapy may be safe and effective. Methenamine is used as a prophylactic agent in sexually active women who have a history of recurrent infections and no structural abnormalities of the urinary tract. Trimethoprim–sulfamethoxazole has been shown to be more effective in these patients [37]. Patients with indwelling urinary or suprapubic catheters may not respond to suppressive therapy with methenamine because the urine may be removed from the bladder before sufficient concentrations of formaldehyde are generated. The use of intermittent drainage in such patients allows the drug to stay in urine in the bladder for sufficient periods of time to produce hydrolysis. Methenamine is used commonly as preoperative prophylaxis in patients with bacteriuria who are undergoing urologic procedures, including transurethral prostatic resections, cystoscopy, and gynecologic surgery [38,39].

CONTRAINDICATIONS

Hepatic failure; gastric, pyloric, or duodenal obstruction; allergy; or hypersensitivity

DRUG INTERACTIONS

Sulfonamides, which produce an insoluble complex with methenamine; food or drug products that produce alkaline urine

ADVERSE EFFECTS

Although well tolerated, gastric upset and allergic reactions occur occasionally. Some patients have symptoms of bladder irritation, including dysuria, urgency, frequency, and hematuria.

PHARMACOKINETICS AND PHARMACODYNAMICS

Methenamine and the organic salts methenamine mandelate and methenamine hippurate are quickly absorbed from the gastrointestinal tract, although 10% to 30% may be hydrolyzed in gastric juice. A protective enteric coating reduces gastric hydrolysis. Antimicrobial activity does not develop in blood or other body fluids, except urine, because hydrolysis does not occur at a physiologic pH. Distributed within the total body water, methenamine base diffuses widely into body fluids, including cerebrospinal fluid, ascites, pericardial and pleural fluids, erythrocytes, and vitreous and aqueous humors of the eye. Methenamine is excreted into the urine, with a clearance less than glomerular filtration approximating that of creatinine clearance. The mean half-life is 4.3 hours. Urine bacteriostasis is not achieved for at least 1 to 2 hours after administration of the drug. Because urine in the renal calyx, pelvis, and ureter flows quickly, insufficient formaldehyde is generated in the upper urinary tract.

(Continued on next page)

The information here is provided as guidance only. Prescribers should always consult the manufacturer's current prescribing information.

METHENAMINE (CONTINUED)

DOSAGE

Adults: Two tablets every 6 hours; ensure urinary pH is < 5.5; may increase to two tablets every 4 hours to achieve this pH; methenamine mandelate, 1 g four times a day; methenamine hippurate, 1 g twice a day.
Elderly: Same as adults.
Children: Do not use in children under 6 years of age.

DOSAGE ADJUSTMENTS FOR RENAL AND HEPATIC INSUFFICIENCY

Methenamine and its organic salts should not be given to patients with hepatic insufficiency because of the production of ammonia within gastric juice. Methenamine base is nontoxic in patients with renal insufficiency, but the organic salts may precipitate in the urine, causing crystalluria.

PHARMACOKINETICS AND PHARMACODYNAMICS (CONTINUED)

Antibacterial activity is found only in bladder urine because of the time required to produce sufficient concentrations of formaldehyde. The antibacterial activity in bladder urine remains for a minimum of 6 hours or until urinary voiding. Forced diuresis may diminish the activity of methenamine by rendering the urine alkaline and reducing the concentration of free formaldehyde. About 80% of a 1-g dose is recovered in the urine within 24 hours. Concentrations of formaldehyde of 10 to 20 μg/mL are bacteriostatic; concentrations greater than 30 μg/mL are bacteriocidal. These concentrations may be achieved with a daily dose of 2 or more g/d and a urine volume of 1 to 1.5 L. Increasing the dose will increase the concentration of formaldehyde up to 60 μg/mL.

AVAILABILITY

Urised (Webcon, Ft. Worth, TX)—each tablet contains methenamine 40.8 mg, phenyl salicylate 18.1 mg, methylene blue 5.4 mg, benzoic acid 4.5 mg, atropine sulfate 0.03 mg, and hyoscyamine 0.03 mg
Prosed DS (Star, Pompano Beach, FL)—tablets contain double-strength concentrations as listed above
Uro-Phosphate (Poythress, Richmond, VA)—tablets contain methenamine 300 mg and sodium biphosphate 500 mg
Urex (3M, St. Paul, MN) (methenamine hippurate)
Methenamine mandelate oral suspension (USP)—500 mg/5 mL
Uroqid-acid No. 2 (Beach, Conestee, SC)—tablets contain methenamine mandelate 500 mg and sodium acid phosphate monohydrate 500 mg
Urisedamine (Webcon)—tablets contain methenamine mandelate 500 mg and hyoscyamine 0.15 mg

METRONIDAZOLE (Flagyl®, MetroGel®, Protostat®)

Metronidazole, a 5-nitromidazole synthetic compound, was released in 1959 to treat *Trichomonas vaginalis* infection. In 1970, the drug was found to have activity against anaerobic bacteria and other protozoa. Indeed, this is the most active bacteriocidal drug for anaerobic organisms.

CHEMICAL CLASSIFICATION

Metronidazole (1-[2-hydroxyethyl]-2methyl-5-nitromidazole) is a 5-nitromidazole. It has a molecular weight of 171 D.

INDICATIONS

Metronidazole is used to treat *T. vaginitis* infection, amebic liver abscess and abscesses in other extraintestinal sites, intestinal amebiasis, and giardiasis. The drug may be useful in treating *Blastocystis coli* and *D. medinensis* infections. The major indication for metronidazole, however, is the treatment of anaerobic infections (except *Actinomycosis* and *P. acnes* infections). Abdominal and pelvic infections caused by gut or genitourinary flora are common indications. The pharmacokinetics and bacteriocidal activity of the drug make it extremely useful in treating abscesses in the brain, lung, and solid organs of the abdomen and pelvis; mixed flora osteomyelitis; oral and dental infections; deep soft-tissue infections; and mixed flora infections of the head and neck [49]. Because anaerobic infections are often mixed with aerobes, metronidazole is seldom used alone. In treating mixed aerobic–anaerobic infections, metronidazole is often used in combination with drugs directed at aerobic gram-negative and gram-positive flora. Metronidazole alone is effective in treating *Bacteroides* endocarditis.

(Continued on next page)

The information here is provided as guidance only. Prescribers should always consult the manufacturer's current prescribing information.

METRONIDAZOLE (CONTINUED)

MECHANISM OF ACTION

Metronidazole diffuses into bacteria and certain protozoa, but not into mammalian cells. The nitro group of metronidazole is a preferential electron accepter that has a redox potential lower than that of ferredoxin and flavodoxin, the low redox potential electron transfer proteins normally found only in anaerobic and microaerophilic bacteria. The drug functions as an electron sink when the 5-nitro group is reduced [40,41]. The enzyme nitroreductase, which is found only in anaerobic bacteria, activates metronidazole by reduction. These reduction products are free radicals that are produced only in the absence of oxygen. The nitro ion radical is unstable and along with hydroxylamine derivatives are assumed to be the mediators of toxicity. Reduced metronidazole produces multiple single-strand disruptions of DNA and inhibits replication, transcription, and repair. As metronidazole is activated, the intracellular concentrations of unchanged drug are decreased, producing a gradient that causes further entry of unchanged drug into the organism. This is quickly converted into reduced activated drug, which accounts for the rapid bacteriocidal activity of metronidazole.

ANTIMICROBIAL ACTIVITY

Metronidazole is active against *Entamoeba histolytica*, *Giardia lamblia*, *Trichomonas vaginalis*, *Balantidium coli*, and *Blastocystis hominis* (minimum cidal concentration is 5 µg/mL or less) [42,43]. Amebic cysts and trophozoites are sensitive. The drug is active against a variety of anaerobic and microaerophilic bacteria (minor inhibitory concentration, 16 µg/mL or less). This is the most active drug against strict anaerobes such as *Bacteroides fragilis* and other *Bacteroides* spp [44]. The spectrum of antimicrobial activity includes *Fusobacterium* spp, *Clostridium* spp, anaerobic gram-negative cocci, anaerobic gram-positive cocci, and *Gardnerella vaginalis*. In anaerobic culture, the drug is less active against gram-positive nonsporulating bacilli, such as *Actinomyces*. *Propionibacterium acnes* are often resistant. The drug has poor activity against facultative anaerobes and microanaerophilic streptococci, which are commonly encountered in mixed aerobic–anaerobic infections. Metronidazole is active against oral spirochetes, *Treponema pallidum*, *Campylobacter* spp, and *Helicobacter*. For reasons not clearly understood, the drug has beneficial effects in patients with guinea worm infections (*Dracunculus medinensis*) [45]. Although the drug is not active against this helminth, improvement is thought to result from the immunosuppressant effect of metronidazole.

MECHANISMS OF RESISTANCE

Resistance to the drug develops rarely. Resistant strains of *Bacteriodes fragilis*, *Bacteriodes bivius*, *Bacteriodes distasonis*, and *Bacteriodes melaninogenicus* have been isolated [46]. The mechanism of resistance has not been elucidated, although studies suggest a decrease in bacterial uptake and intracellular reduction of metronidazole [47]. The diminished drug activation may be caused by a decrease in bacterial nitroreductase activity. *T. vaginalis* has been reported to become resistant following long-term therapy [48].

INDICATIONS *(CONTINUED)*

The drug is used to treat nonspecific vaginitis. Currently, metronidazole is considered the drug of choice for the treatment of pseudomembranous colitis due to *C. difficile* [50]. Patients who have ileus or toxic megacolon and are unable to take the drug orally may be treated parenterally [51]. Metronidazole also has been used to treat tetanus. Data are not available for the treatment of syphilis. Patients undergoing elective colon surgery, gynecologic surgery, and emergency appendectomy may be given the drug prophylactically.

ADVERSE EFFECTS

Metronidazole is safe and well tolerated by most patients. Significant reactions are uncommon. The most serious adverse effects involve the central nervous system and include seizures, cerebellar ataxia, encephalopathy, and peripheral neuropathy [52]. Patients with seizure disorders and other neurologic conditions may be sensitive. Reactions are thought to be dose related, especially when the drug is given over an extended period. Peripheral neuropathies have been well described in patients tasking long-term metronidazole for Crohn's disease [53]. Rarely, pseudomembranous colitis follows metronidazole treatment. Gastrointestinal side effects include loss of appetite, nausea, abdominal pain, diarrhea, and vomiting. A metallic taste occurs in about 12% of patients. Uncommon side effects include xerostomia, stomatitis, glossitis, furring of the tongue, syncope, headache, pneumonia, fever, oral and vaginal candidiasis, and reversible neutropenia and thrombocytopenia.

Metronidazole is mutagenic, and the concern that the drug is carcinogenic has been raised. Cancer has been produced in some animal models, but follow-up studies of women treated for long periods of time have not demonstrated an increased rate of cancer [54]. Because metronidazole crosses the placenta, the possibility of teratogenicity has been investigated. Studies in pregnant women have not demonstrated an increased incidence of birth defects or fetal wastage [55]. Nevertheless, the drug should be used only in life-threatening situations during the first trimester of pregnancy.

PHARMACOKINETICS AND PHARMACODYNAMICS

Metronidazole is rapidly and almost completely absorbed following oral administration (90%–95%). Equivalent serum levels are achieved followed oral or intravenous administration. Serum levels of drug are reached within 1 hour of oral dosing, with peaks of 3.7 µg/mL, 9.8 µg/mL, and 11.8 µg/mL after 250-mg, 500-mg, and 1-g doses, respectively. Similar concentrations are achieved with rectal suppositories of 500 mg, 1 g, and 2 g, respectively. Food does not decrease absorption, although there is a delay in reaching peak concentrations. When administered intravenously, metronidazole is infused over a 1-hour period. The usual loading dose is 15 mg/kg, with a maintenance dose of 7.5 mg/kg every 8 hours. Peak and trough levels following this dosing schedule are 26 µg/mL to 18 µg/mL, respectively. Because most anaerobes are sensitive to concentrations of 6 µg/mL or less, these levels are therapeutic. The drug is also absorbed following vaginal application, but peak serum levels are in the low range 1.2 µg/mL). Metronidazole crosses the placenta, producing fetal serum levels equivalent to that of the mother.

(Continued on next page)

The information here is provided as guidance only. Prescribers should always consult the manufacturer's current prescribing information.

METRONIDAZOLE (CONTINUED)

SPECIAL GROUPS

Children: Safety and efficacy not established except for use of oral form for the treatment of amebiasis.

Elderly: Pharmacokinetics may be altered.

Renal impairment: No information.

Hepatic impairment: Prolonged metabolism resulting in accumulation of drug in plasma; reduce dosage with caution.

Pregnancy: Intravenous, oral, and vaginal gel preparations; use only when clearly indicated.

Breast-feeding: Decision to stop therapy or stop nursing must be made with respect to the importance of the drug to the mother.

DOSAGE

Intravenous administration must be by slow intravenous drip infusion only. Intravenous ad mixtures containing metronidazole and other drugs should be avoided. Do not use equipment containing aluminum (*eg*, needles, cannulae) that may come in contact with the drug solution. Intravenous preparations should not be given by direct intravenous injection due to the low pH of the reconstituted product. Intravenous preparations must be diluted and neutralized for intravenous infusion.

Adults: (parenteral [*INTRAVENOUS*] for anaerobic infection): give loading dose 15 mg/kg intravenous infused over 1 hour, followed by a maintenance dose of 7.5 mg/kg intravenous infused over 1 hour every 6 hours. Do not exceed maximum of 4 g/24 h. For colorectal surgical prophylaxis: 15 mg/kg infused over 30 to 60 minutes and completed approximately 1 hour before surgery and 7.5 mg/kg infused over 30 to 60 minutes at 6 and 12 hours after initial dose period. *ORAL* (for trichomoniasis in female patients, dosage should be individualized for each patient by the physician): 1-day regimen: 2 g as a single dose or in divided doses (1 g each) on same day; 7-day regimen: 250 mg every 8 hours for 7 consecutive days. Do not administer in first trimester of pregnancy; do not use 1-day regimen for patients who are pregnant. If repeated courses are required, an interval of 4 to 6 weeks is recommended between treatments. For male patients, individualize dosage as for female patients.

For amebiasis: 750 mg every 8 hours for 7 to 10 days.

For amebic liver abscess: 500 or 750 mg every 8 hours for 5 to 10 days.

For anaerobic bacterial infections (use intravenous preparations initially for serious infections): 7.5 mg/kg every 6 hours for 7 to 10 days or longer in cases of bone or joint infection, lower respiratory tract infections, or endocardium. Do not exceed 4 g/d.

VAGINAL GEL: One applicator-full intravaginally twice a day (morning and evening) for 5 days.

Children: Safety and efficacy not established except for tablet form to treat amebiasis. For amebiasis, 35 to 50 mg/kg/d (24 h) in divided doses every 8 hours for 10 days.

Impaired renal function: Doses need not be reduced in anuric patients because accumulated metabolites may be removed rapidly by hemodialysis.

Severe hepatic function impairment: Reduce dosage according to degree of impairment; use caution and monitor plasma metronidazole levels closely.

PHARMACOKINETICS AND PHARMACODYNAMICS *(CONTINUED)*

There is very little protein binding (10% or less). Metronidazole penetrates almost all tissues at a volume distribution of almost 80% of body weight. Therapeutic levels are found in fluids and tissues, including amniotic fluid, cerebrospinal fluid, pleural fluid, middle ear fluid, breast milk, saliva, seminal fluid, vaginal secretions, dental alveolar bone, the unobstructed biliary tree, and abscess fluid in liver, spleen, and brain [56]. The drug reaches one third to one half of serum levels in the aqueous humor. Metronidazole is metabolized by the liver, forming an acid metabolite, a hydroxy derivative, acetyl metronidazole, metronidazole glucuronide, and the glucuronide conjugate of hydroxy metronidazole [57]. The hydroxy metabolite, which has approximately 30% of the activity of the unchanged drug, is one of the major biologic products. Sixty to eighty percent of metronidazole and its metabolites are excreted in the urine, and 6% to 15% in the feces.

The hydroxy metabolite accumulates in patients with renal disease, although this is usually not problematic because the drug and metabolites are excreted by hepatic mechanisms. Dosage adjustment is not necessary unless there is also liver failure. The drug is eliminated during peritoneal dialysis, and dose reduction is not required in patients undergoing chronic ambulatory peritoneal dialysis. Metronidazole is eliminated during hemodialysis, and a replacement dose is required following dialysis. Normal drug half-life is 8 hours, but it is reduced to approximately 2.5 hours in patients undergoing hemodialysis. A 50% reduction in dosage is recommended for people with severe liver disease.

Metronidazole has little impact on fecal flora because the drug is rapidly reduced by bowel flora. A significant decrease in fecal flora occurs in patients who are receiving large doses of drug or drug plus an oral aminoglycoside or who have diarrhea while on the drug. Because of this capacity, metronidazole may be used for the treatment of short loop syndrome, Crohn's disease, and as a preoperative bowel preparation.

DRUG INTERACTIONS

The drug increases the half-life and hypoprothrombinemic effect of warfarin. Drug interactions occur with phenobarbital, phenytoin, and cimetidine. A disulfiram-like reaction may occur in patients consuming alcohol and metronidazole.

PATIENT INFORMATION

Prolonged use and large doses in patients with blind loop syndrome, Crohn's disease, recurrent *Trichomonas* infection, and so forth may lead to peripheral neuropathy and other neurotoxicity. Avoid alcohol consumption when taking metronidazole. Topical gel only: avoid contact with eyes. Vaginal gel only: do not engage in vaginal intercourse during treatment with metronidazole.

AVAILABILITY

For intravenous infusion—single-dose vials containing 500 mg metronidazole equivalent

Tablets—250 mg and 500 mg

Vaginal gel—7-g tube with 5-g vaginal applicator

The information here is provided as guidance only. Prescribers should always consult the manufacturer's current prescribing information.

MUPIROCIN (Bactroban®)

Mupirocin is a topical antimicrobial produced by *Pseudomonas fluorescens*. The drug is available only as a topical preparation, and its activity is directed only against gram-positive cocci.

CHEMICAL CLASSIFICATION
The drug is a crotonic acid ester of 9 hydroxynonanoic acid.

MECHANISM OF ACTION
Mupirocin inhibits bacterial protein synthesis by binding reversibly and specifically to bacterial isoleucyl transfer-RNA synthetase [58]. The drug inhibits isoleucine incorporation into protein sequences.

ANTIMICROBIAL ACTIVITY
Mupirocin is active against *Staphylococcus aureus* (methicillin-resistant and beta-lactamase–producing strains), *Staphylococcus epidermidis*, *Staphylococcus saprophyticus*, and *Streptococcus pyogenes*.

MECHANISMS OF BACTERIAL RESISTANCE
Recently, resistant strains of *S. aureus* have emerged during mupirocin therapy [59]. The exact mechanism has not been determined.

DRUG ADMINISTRATION FOR RENAL AND HEPATIC INSUFFICIENCY
Not applicable.

DOSAGE
Apply a small amount of ointment to affected areas three times a day. The same dose is recommended for nasal staphylococcal carriers. Dosing recommendations for the elderly and children are similar. Caution is advised when treating patients with renal failure and infections involving large surface areas because of the potential of polyethylene glycol absorption.

INDICATIONS
Mupirocin ointment is indicated for the treatment of impetigo due to *S. aureus* and group A streptococcus [60]. The ointment has been used to eradicate the nasal carriage of *S. aureus* for prolonged periods of time [61]. This strategy may be attempted in treating patients with recurrent furunculosis. The assumption is that such patients inoculate their skin with bacteria from the nose.

ADVERSE REACTIONS
Allergy or hypersensitivity to mupirocin

DRUG INTERACTIONS
No information

ADVERSE EFFECTS
Burning, stinging, pruritus, and pain of the skin may follow dermal application. Stinging and drying of the nasal mucosa have been reported with intranasal use [61]. Mupirocin ointment contains polyethylene glycol, which may be absorbed from open wounds and damaged skin. Absorption of large quantities of polyethylene glycol may cause renal impairment.

PHARMACOKINETICS AND PHARMACODYNAMICS
Mupirocin is formulated in a topical, water-miscible ointment base containing polyethylene glycol. There is no measurable systemic absorption after topical application to the skin covered with occlusive dressings.

AVAILABILITY
Ointment—1-g, 15-g and 30-g tubes

The information here is provided as guidance only. Prescribers should always consult the manufacturer's current prescribing information.

NITROFURANTOIN (Macrobid®, Macrodantin®, Nitrofurantoin®)

Nitrofurantoin is a member of the family of synthetically manufactured nitrofuran compounds. The drug was first used clinically in 1953 as a microcrystal and marketed as Furadantin (Norwich Eaton, Norwich, NY). In 1967 a macrocrystalline form of drug was prepared—Macrodantin (Norwich Eaton). Nitrofurantoins are indicated exclusively in the treatment of urinary tract infections caused by susceptible organisms.

CHEMICAL AND CLASSIFICATION

The nitrofurans are 5-nitro-2-furaldehyde derivatives. Nitrofurantoin is *O*-(5-nitrofurfurylideneamino)-hydantoin. This class of compounds has a heterocyclic ring, composed of 4 carbon and 1 oxygen atoms.

MECHANISM OF ACTION

The mechanism of action of the 5-nitrofurans is still not clearly understood, although evidence suggests that the reduction of the 5-nitro group in the nitro anion results in bacterial toxicity. The nitro anion causes the production of superoxide, oxygen-free radicals, and other toxic oxygen products that are selectively toxic to microbial cells but not to mammalian cells [62]. Nitrofurantoin is also capable of inhibiting a variety of microbial enzymatic systems. The drug's ability to produce damage to DNA in bacteria is the cause of cell death. The reductive activation of nitrofurantoin is critical in producing DNA damage and the bacteriocidal effect [63].
The selective microbial toxicity is a function of its pharmacokinetics as well as bacterial activation. Nitrofurantoin is excreted rapidly by the kidney. Drug levels are low in serum and tissue and high in urine. Although tissues such as lung and liver may activate nitrofurantoin, bacteria reduce the drug much more rapidly.

ANTIMICROBIAL ACTIVITY

Nitrofurantoin has a wide spectrum of activity that includes common gram-positive and gram-negative urinary tract pathogens [64]. Organisms found to have a minimum inhibitory concentration ≤ 32 µg/mL are considered to be susceptible. Such a concentration is readily achieved in urine. *Escherichia coli* is the most sensitive gram-negative aerobe, and *Enterobacter* and *Klebsiella* are less susceptible. *Pseudomonas aeruginosa* is almost always resistant, and most *Proteus* spp are moderately resistant. Nitrofurantoin is active against enterococci and some staphylococcal species, including *S. aureus*, *S. epidermidis*, and *S. saprophyticus*. Although streptococci (including *Streptococcus pneumoniae*), *Neisseria*, and *Bacteroides* are usually sensitive, standard oral doses do not produce sufficient serum or tissue concentrations to be active against these organisms. *Salmonella* and *Shigella* spp are sensitive *in vitro*.

MECHANISM OF BACTERIAL RESISTANCE

Sensitive bacteria do not usually become resistant to nitrofurantoin.

DOSAGE ADJUSTMENT FOR RENAL AND HEPATIC INSUFFICIENCY

Nitrofurantoin should not be used in patients with renal or liver disease.

INDICATIONS

Nitrofurantoin is used in the treatment of acute lower urinary tract infections caused by sensitive bacteria. The drug is considered a second-line drug for patients who are allergic to sulfonamides, penicillins, and tetracyclines. The advent of fluroquinolones has left few, if any, indications for this drug. Nitrofurantoin is not indicated for renal cortical infections or perinephric abscesses because of poor concentration of drug. The drug is occasionally used as a single daily dose to prevent urinary tract infections in women with a history of recurrent urinary tract infection. Organisms recovered from the urine of such patients usually remain sensitive despite recurrence because nitrofurantoin-resistant organisms do not appear in the stool and the sensitivity of intestinal flora remains unaltered [65]. Because the organisms that cause urinary tract infections usually come from the gut flora, these organisms remain sensitive to nitrofurantoin.

ADVERSE EFFECTS

Adverse reactions range from mild to severe, and life-threatening severe events are rare. Most are reversible. The most common effect is dose-related gastrointestinal irritation, manifested as nausea and vomiting. The macrocrystalline drug has fewer gastrointestinal side effects, and diarrhea is uncommon.

Hypersensitivity reactions may involve skin, liver, and lungs. Drug fever, a lupuslike syndrome, and anaphylaxis have been described. Dermatologic allergic syndromes vary and include maculopapular erythematous rashes, urticaria, and angioneurotic edema [66]. These usually subside when the drug is discontinued.

Hepatic toxicity, which is rare, includes acute hepatocellular disease, chronic active hepatitis associated with hypergammaglobulinemia and antinuclear antibodies, and cholestatic jaundice [67,68]. The latter may be associated with rash and eosinophilia. Discontinuation of the drug often results in reversibility. Parotitis, pancreatitis, and thyroiditis have been described.

Nitrofurantoin is associated with a variety of pulmonary reactions, including acute bronchitis, asthma, and pneumonia [69]. Pulmonary symptoms may occur 5 to 10 days after therapy has begun and are manifested by shortness of breath, cough, and fever, with or without pulmonary infiltrates on chest radiograph. The latter typically occur at the bases and may be associated with pleural effusions. Eosinophilia is common (60%–80%); allergy and cell-mediated immunity are suspected. The disease usually abates with discontinuation of drug or in response to steroids in 1 to 3 weeks. Unfortunately the process recurs on rechallenge [70]. Subacute pneumonia and chronic lung involvement may be manifested by interstitial fibrosis with chronic cough and shortness of breath [69]. Chronic pulmonary disease is more common in women and, as with liver disease, hypergammaglobulinemia and antinuclear antibodies may be noted. The onset is insidious and fever uncommon. The mechanism may be related to the generation of toxic oxygen radicals producing lung injury [71]. An immunologic element is also suspected because some patients respond to steroids. Many will improve on discontinuation of the drug, but two thirds have radiologic evidence of fibrosis, which is usually irreversible [72].

(Continued on next page)

The information here is provided as guidance only. Prescribers should always consult the manufacturer's current prescribing information.

NITROFURANTOIN (CONTINUED)

SPECIAL GROUPS

Children: Contraindicated in children under 1 month of age.
Elderly: May have age-related renal impairment.
Renal impairment: Contraindicated in patients with significant renal function impairment (creatinine clearance less than 60 mL/min or clinically significant elevated serum creatinine); otherwise, no dosage reduction required. Monitor renal function in prolonged therapy.
Pregnancy: Use only when clearly indicated. Human studies not performed.
Breast-feeding: Decision should be made to discontinue nitrofurantoin or discontinue nursing with respect to the importance of the drug to the mother.

DOSAGE

Adults: 100 mg capsule every 12 hours.
Elderly: Same as adults.
Children: Drug is contraindicated in children under 1 month of age. For older children, 5 to 7 mg/kg/24 h given in four divided doses.

ADVERSE EFFECTS *(CONTINUED)*

The drug's effect on hematologic enzyme systems results in its being contraindicated in pregnant women and in infants under 1 month of age. Acute hemolytic anemia may be provoked in patients who are glucose-6-phosphate dehydrogenase–deficient. Megaloblastic anemia, thought to be due to folic acid deficiency, may also occur.

Several neurologic syndromes are well known. An ascending sensorimotor polyneuropathy in a glove stocking distribution is one of the major side effects and is encountered in patients with renal insufficiency [73]. The sensory loss is usually more profound than motor weakness. Pain is also common. Demyelination and degeneration of nerve fibers are noted. Because the peripheral neuropathy may be irreversible, the drug should be discontinued at first appearance of paresthesias. Additional neurologic toxicities include cranioneuropathy, retrobulbar neuritis, and pseudotumor cerebri. Direct toxic activity of the drug is suspected.

INTERACTIONS

Magnesium trisilicate antacids and uricosuric agents (*eg,* probenecid and sulfinpyrazone)

PATIENT INFORMATION

Take with food to enhance tolerance and improve drug absorption. Patients who are unable to tolerate microcrystalline nitrofurantoin may be able to tolerate Macrodantin without nausea. Avoid antacids and uricosuric agents.

AVAILABILITY

Macrodantin capsules— 25 mg, 50 mg, and 100 mg
Macrobid (Procter & Gamble, Cincinnati, OH)— (nitrofurantoin monohydrate–macrocrystals) 100 mg
Nitrofurantoin capsules—50 and 100 mg

PHARMACOKINETICS AND PHARMACODYNAMICS

Oral nitrofurantoin is rapidly and completely (94%) absorbed from the gut. The drug is available as a suspension for oral administration. Nitrofurantoin has limited solubility in water. The macrocrystalline form is absorbed more slowly from the gastrointestinal tract and has a reduced gastrointestinal toxicity profile (nausea, vomiting) compared with the microcrystal. Although the macrocrystal is absorbed slowly, the same percentage of drug as the microcrystal is recovered in the urine in 24 hours because the kinetics are the same. Therapeutic levels are not achieved in most tissues, including the renal cortex. The drug's serum half-life is about 20 minutes in people with normal renal function. Approximately two thirds of the drug is rapidly metabolized in tissue. Inactivation occurs in most body tissues, although the liver and lung play major metabolic roles. The remaining one third of the drug is rapidly excreted into urine by glomerular filtration and active tubular secretion and reabsorption [74]. Nitrofurantoin is a weak acid, and in an acid urine more of the drug is undissociated (nonionized). The undissociated drug is more easily reabsorbed, with less appearing in the urine. In alkaline urine, more of the drug is dissociated (ionized), and little is reabsorbed. Consequently, more appears in the urine. Unfortunately, antibacterial efficacy is diminished in alkaline urine. As a caveat, urine should not be alkalinized when using nitrofurantoin. The average dose of drug produces a urine concentration of approximately 200 µg/mL in patients with normal renal function. Because the concentration in the urine is related to creatinine clearance, the concentration of drug in the urine of azotemic patients may be insufficient to be active against urinary tract pathogens. This occurs when the glomerular filtration rate is less than 30 mL/min [75]. Nitrofurantoin may accumulate in the serum of patients with a creatinine clearance of less than 60 mL/min. Blood levels in such instances may range between 5 to 7 µg/mL and produce systemic toxicity. Nitrofurantoin is removed by hemodialysis but should not be used in uremic patients. The drug is contraindicated in newborns and premature infants. The parenteral formulation is no longer available.

The information here is provided as guidance only. Prescribers should always consult the manufacturer's current prescribing information.

POLYMYXINS
(Colistimethate sodium®, Colistin sulfate®, Polymyxin B sulfate®)

Polymyxins A–E, a family of cyclic basic polypeptides, are produced by *Bacillus polymyxa*. Only polymyxins B and E are available for use because the other compounds are too toxic. The polymyxins are active against gram-negative aerobes. Polymyxin B became available in 1947 and polymyxin E in 1961.

CHEMICAL CLASSIFICATION

Polymyxin B and E are cyclic basic polypeptides with molecular weights of approximately 1100 D that differ in only one of 10 amino acids. One unit of polymyxin B sulfate is equivalent to 0.1 µg of polymyxin base. Colistin (polymyxin E) is available as the methanesulfonate (colistimethate) and the sulfate.

MECHANISM OF ACTION

Polymyxins contain hydrophilic and hydrophobic portions, acting as cationic surface-active compounds or detergents. Polymyxin B and E accumulate in bacterial cell membranes, interacting with membrane anionic phospholipids. The fatty acid portion of the drugs extends into the hydrophobic portion of phospholipid, and the polypeptide rings bind to exposed anionic phosphate groups in the membrane. This surfactant effect results in distortion or disruption of the cell membrane, with loss of permeability, leakage of protein and nucleic acids, and inhibition of metabolic processes [76]. This effect also occurs in mammalian cells and accounts for the nephrotoxicity and neuro-toxicity of these compounds [77]. Cell walls rich in phospholipids are damaged by the polymyxins, resulting in breaks to the osmotic barrier and leakage of intracellular materials. The binding of the polymyxins to phos-pholipids may result in inhibition of endotoxin (lipopolysaccharide) activity [78–80]. These drugs may interfere with the physiologic effects of bacteria lipopolysaccharides that produce the syndrome of endotoxemia. Antibacterial activity is lost in the presence of the divalent cations calcium and magnesium, which stabilize membranes by competitively preventing the polymyxins from binding to negatively charged phosphate groups [81]. This occurs at physiologic concentrations of calcium and may account for the discrepancy between *in vitro* and *in vivo* activity. Calcium also interferes with the effect of polymyxins on bacterial endotoxins [82].

ANTIMICROBIAL ACTIVITY

Polymyxins are bacteriocidal for most gram-negative aerobes, except *Proteus* spp [83]. Gram-positive organisms are resistant because the thick cell walls prevent the drugs from reacting with the outer cell membrane [84]. The natural resistance of *Proteus* and other species may be the result of the drugs' inability to gain access to the outer cell membrane [85]. The antibacterial spectra of polymyxins B and E are identical, and there is complete cross-resistance. On a weight basis, polymyxin B sulfate is more active than colistin methanesulfonate. These drugs were used primarily to treat *Pseudomonas* infections and other resistant gram-negative bacilli, including members of the *Klebsiella-Enterobacter* group. Gram-positive organisms, obligate anaerobes, *Proteus*, *Providencia*, *Neisseria*, and *Serratia* spp are natu-rally resistant. The combination of trimethoprim–sulfamethoxizole and polymyxins is synergistic and has been used to treat *Xanthomonas cepacia* and *Xanthomonas maltophilia* infections [86].

INDICATIONS

Currently, polymyxins are rarely used because they have been replaced by aminoglycosides, third-generation cephalosporins, quinolones, monobactams, penems, and so forth. Their niche had been the treatment of serious *Pseudomonas aeruginosa* infections, especially complicated burns, severe urinary tract infections, pneumonia, and meningitis. Patients with meningitis requiring polymyxin should be treated intrathecally and intravenously. The intrathecal dose of polymyxin B is 5 to 10 mg/d in adults and 2 mg/d in children under 2 years of age. Intrathecal injections may be given for as long as 5 days. Urinary tract infections may be treated with intramuscular colis-timethate. The use of polymyxin–neomycin in bladder irri-gations in patients with an indwelling catheter has its advocates. The dose if 40 mg/L of neomycin and 20 mg/L of polymyxin B; 1 L/d of irrigation is recommended. Oral decontamination of the gut with polymyxin E or B has been used in patients with granulocytopenia. Polymyxin is usually combined with neomycin and amphotericin in treating such patients. Creams, solutions, and sprays of polymyxins have been used in the treatment of certain skin infections, including external otitis, as well as ulcerations of the cornea. Topical formulations are often combined with neomycin and bacitracin. Oral polymyxin E sulfate has been used to treat children with enteropathogenic *Escherichia coli* infections [87]. Polymyxins have been combined with sulfamethoxazole–trimethoprim to treat *X. maltophilia* and *X. cepacia* infections [11].

ADVERSE EFFECTS

The polymyxins are associated with nephrotoxicity and neurotoxicity. At a serum concentration greater than 2 µg/mL, many patients develop paresthesias in glove stock-ing or circumoral distribution [88]. This may be associated with vertigo, light-headedness, ataxia, flushing, difficulty with speech, somnolence, and confusion. Neurotoxicity subsides with discontinuation of the drug. Polymyxins cause neuromuscular blockade, a curarelike action, and with high serum concentrations, apnea may occur [89]. This results from rapid absorption from serous surfaces during surgery or rapid parenteral administration in patients with renal failure. Aminoglycosides potentiate neuromuscular blockade [90]. Intravenous calcium chloride partially reverses the curarelike effect due to polymyxin. Neuromuscular blockade due to aminoglycosides is more completely reversed by calcium. Polymyxin B is more nephrotoxic than colistin. Nephrotoxicity is potentiated by aminoglycosides and other nephrotoxic drugs. Kidney disease is characterized by proteinuria, cylindruria, and cells in the sediment. Acute tubular necrosis has been reported [91]. Nephrotoxicity reverses with discontinuation of treat-ment. Renal damage may occur in the first few days of treatment or after the drug is discontinued. Allergic reac-tions are rare. Polymyxins release histamine, and urticaria and shock have been described after rapid intravenous infu-sion [92]. Pain at the site of intramuscular injection is common. Topical sensitivity reactions produced by polymyxin–neomycin formulations are usually due to the neomycin component. Intrathecal drug administration may produce signs of meningeal irritation, including headache and neck stiffness.

The information here is provided as guidance only. Prescribers should always consult the manufacturer's current prescribing information.

POLYMYXINS (CONTINUED)

MECHANISM OF BACTERIAL RESISTANCE

Resistance in gram-positive organisms is caused by the inability of the drug to penetrate the cell wall to gain access to the membrane. Resistance in gram-negative organisms may be caused by a similar mechanism or because of diminished binding to the cell membrane.

DOSAGE ADJUSTMENT FOR RENAL AND HEPATIC INSUFFICIENCY

Hepatic insufficiency: No data.
Significant reduction in dosage is required with renal failure.

SPECIAL GROUPS

Children: Accepted for use in children.
Elderly: May have age-related renal impairment.
Renal involvement: Use with extreme caution; monitor function and serum drug levels.
Hepatic impairment: No information.
Pregnancy: Safety not established for use in pregnancy.
Breast-feeding: No information.

DOSAGE

Adults: *INTRAVENOUS*: 15,000 to 25,000 kg/d in normal renal function. *INTRAMUSCULAR*: not recommended for routine use due to severe pain at injection site. Colistimethate sodium may be given intramuscularly. Doses of 2.5 to 5.0 mg/kg/24 h in two to four divided doses in patients with normal renal function. *INTRATHECAL*: especially for *Pseudomonas* meningitis, 50,000 kg/d in a single dose for 3 to 4 days followed by 50,000 U once every other day for a minimum of 2 weeks after cerebrospinal fluid cultures are negative and glucose content is normal.
Elderly: May have age-related renal impairment; otherwise same as adults.
Children: *INTRAVENOUS*: same as adults. Infants with normal renal function may receive up to 40,000 U/kg/d. *INTRAMUSCULAR*: not recommended for children. *INTRATHECAL*: for children greater than 2 years of age, 20,000 once a day for 3 to 4 days or 25,000 U every other day. A dose of 25,000 U once every other day should be continued for a minimum of 2 weeks after cerebrospinal fluid cultures are negative.
Impaired renal function: *INTRAVENOUS* only: use 15,000 U/kg/d or less; intramuscular should not be used. *INTRATHECAL*: usual dosing.
Significant reduction in dosage is required with renal failure.

PHARMACOKINETICS AND PHARMACODYNAMICS

Polymyxin B and colistin are not well-absorbed from the gastrointestinal tract. This attribute has led to the use of these drugs in the treatment of bacterial diarrhea in infants. Gastrointestinal absorption may occur in neonates, and care must be taken when using the drugs in this patient population. Following intramuscular injections of the polymyxins, high concentrations appear in the liver and kidneys. These drugs do not cross the blood–brain barrier, even in the presence of inflammation, and diffusion into synovial and pleural fluid and the biliary tree is poor. Colistimethate is less painful than polymyxin B sulfate when administered intramuscularly. The methanesulfontion of polymyxin E, however, inactivates the amino acids, eliminating the antibacterial effect until the drug is hydrolyzed to colistin base. Colistimethate is hydrolyzed gradually in muscle to polymyxin E. The polymyxins are excreted slowly by glomerular filtration; there is no tubular secretion or reabsorption. Delayed elimination is due to binding of the drug to tissues. This binding also accounts for the large volume of distribution. Polymyxins accumulate in patients with renal disease, which may potentiate toxicity. Sodium colistimethate is excreted more quickly than the free base because there is less tissue binding. Colistin sulfate is available for oral, intramuscular, and intravenous use. Polymyxin B sulfate may be given intravenously, intramuscularly, intrathecally, orally, topically, by aerosol, and endobronchially. Colistimethate is given intramuscularly. Colistimethate may be given intravenously, but it requires a slow infusion that may result in inadequate tissue and serum levels because the drug may be excreted by the kidneys before hydrolysis so active base can occur. The serum half-life of polymyxin B is 6 to 7 hours, and colistin 2 to 4.5 hours. The serum half-life of the polymyxins in anuric patients is 48 to 72 hours. Therefore, dosing must be reduced in patients with renal failure. The appearance of active drug in the urine may be delayed following intramuscular administration, but colistimethate is excreted more rapidly than polymyxin B and E sulfate. All drugs are found in the urine 2 to 3 days after cessation of therapy. Peritoneal dialysis removes small amounts (1 mg/h), but hemodialysis has no effect on serum concentrations. The polymyxins are used topically in concentrations of 0.1%, often in combination with other antibiotics (neomycin or bacitracin). Polymyxin B is also used for bladder irrigations and irrigations of serous surfaces, such as the pleura and peritoneum, during surgery. This practice may be dangerous because polymyxins are absorbed and toxic levels may be reached.

DRUG INTERACTIONS

Neuromuscular blocking agents; muscle relaxants used in anesthesia; aminoglycosides

PATIENT INFORMATION

Drugs should be avoided in patients with renal disease and myasthenia gravis

AVAILABILITY

Polymyxin B sulfate (Aerosporin [Burroughs Wellcome, Research Triangle Pk, NC]) for intramuscular, intravenous, intrathecal, topical, oral, and inhalation use
Colistin sulfate (Coly-Mycin [Parke-Davis, Morris Plains, NJ]) for intramuscular or intravenous administration. The powder is also available for oral administration.
Colistimethate sodium (Coly-Mycin M [Parke-Davis, Morris Plains, NJ]), a colistin derivative, is used for the intramuscular treatment of urinary tract infections

The information here is provided as guidance only. Prescribers should always consult the manufacturer's current prescribing information.

VANCOMYCIN AND TEICOPLANIN
(Vancocin HCL®, Vancoled®)

Vancomycin is a soluble glycopolypeptide antibiotic with a narrow spectrum directed against gram-positive bacteria. This compound was discovered in 1956 as a derivative of *Streptomyces orientalis*. First used in the era of penicillin-resistant staphylococci, vancomycin played a secondary role because of relative toxicity when compared with methicillin. The first commercial preparations contained as much as 30% foreign substances, which contributed to the major side effects. Purification led to current, less toxic preparations. With the appearance of methicillin-resistant staphylococci, vancomycin has reemerged as an important drug for the treatment of serious gram-positive infections caused by methicillin-resistant *Staphylococcus aureus*, *Staphylococcus epidermidis*, *Enterococcus*, *Propionibacterium*, and *Corynebacterium* spp. Vancomycin is also useful in treating antibiotic-associated colitis due to *Clostridium difficile*, systemic staphylococcal infections in patients with chronic renal failure undergoing dialysis, and gram-positive prosthetic infections. Nomograms have been developed to calculate dosing schedules for patients with chronic renal disease. The ability to determine serum vancomycin concentrations is widely available. These two factors have allowed clinicians to dose vancomycin safely.

Teicoplanin, a new glycopeptide derived from *Actinoplanus teichomyceticus*, has antimicrobial activity similar to vancomycin but has different pharmacologic properties. Although not yet available in the United States, the drug has been widely used in Europe for treating gram-positive coccal infections including *S. aureus* and enterococcal species. Teicoplanin is more active than vancomycin.

CHEMICAL CLASSIFICATION

Vancomycin is a complex tricyclic glycopeptide with a molecular weight of approximately 1450 D. The drug consists of a disaccharide (glucose and vancosamine), two beta-hydroxychlorotyrosines, three substituted phenylglycines, *N*-methylleucine, and an aspartic acid residue. These subunits are connected in a seven-member peptide chain, constructed into three large rings by two ether bonds and a carbon–carbon bond. Vancomycin chloride has a peak solubility at pH 3–5, which decreases with increasing pH. In physiologic saline or distilled water, vancomycin has a pH of 4.

Teicoplanin is a mixture of six glycopeptides, each having a similar heptapeptide base, and an aglycone containing aromatic amino acids with *D*-mannose and *N*-acetyl-*D*-glycosamine as sugars. Unlike other glycopeptides, it has an acyl substituent that is a fatty acid. This makes teicoplanin more lipophilic than vancomycin.

MECHANISM OF ACTION

By inhibiting cell wall synthesis, vancomycin is bacteriocidal for multiplying organisms. Inhibition occurs during the second stage of cell wall assembly of linear peptidoglycan polymers [93,94]. The drug complexes with *D*-alanyl-*D*-alanine precursors. Tight binding of vancomycin and *D*-alanyl-*D*-alanine causes steric hindrance of the attachment of the precursors to the enzyme peptidoglycan synthetase. By binding to the terminal carboxyl group of *D*-alanyl-*D*-alanine of the *N*-acetyl glucosamine *N*-acetyl-muramic acid peptide, vancomycin inhibits polymerization of linear peptidoglycan by the enzyme. Penicillins and cephalosporins act during the third stage of cell wall synthesis by inhibiting cross-linkages of pentapeptide side chains with peptidoglycan. As a consequence, crossresistance between vancomycin and beta-lactams does not occur. Vancomycin has been found to injure protoplasts by altering the permeability of cytoplasmic membranes of bacteria and to inhibit RNA synthesis [95–97]. Because vancomycin acts by several mechanisms, the development of resistance has been uncommon. Teicoplanin affects cell wall synthesis by forming complexes with terminal *D*-alanyl-*D*-alanine cell wall precursors, thus inhibiting polymerization of peptidoglycan [98].

INDICATIONS

Vancomycin has excellent activity against most gram-positive organisms, although it remains a second-line drug for many infections. For patients with significant allergies to beta-lactam drugs and serious infections due to *S. aureus* (eg, bacteremia, pneumonia, meningitis, septic joint infections, and endocarditis) vancomycin is the drug of choice. The drug may be used to treat osteomyelitis, although clindamycin has superior kinetics. Vancomycin is indicated in the treatment of serous infections due to methicillin-resistant *S. aureus* and non-*aureus* staphylococci [112]. Bacteremia and infections of prostheses, indwelling cannulas, A-V shunts, grafts, an so forth are common examples. Foreign bodies may have to be removed to achieve cure. Combination therapy with rifampin or an aminoglycoside is often required in prostheses-associated infections. Vancomycin is indicated in the treatment of serious streptococcal and enterococcal infections in the penicillin-allergic patient. The latter organisms may require the addition of an aminoglycoside (gentamicin). The drug is effective in the treatment of highly resistant *S. pneumoniae* [113]. Vancomycin is the drug of choice for serious *Corynebacterium* infections in patients with prostheses, underlying cancer, or neutropenia [114]. Oral vancomycin (125 mg four times a day) is useful in treating pseudomembraneous colitis caused by *C. difficile* [115]. Oral drug is much more effective than intravenous therapy because of the low fecal concentration of vancomycin following intravenous administration. Currently metronidazole is preferred because of the recent emergence of vancomycin-resistant enterococcal strains thought to arise from the selective pressure of the drug on gut flora. For infants and children with *C. difficile* colitis, the oral dose is 500 mg/1.73 m^2 every 6 hours. When treating patients with pseudomembranous colitis and ileus, the drug may be given orally or by nasogastric tube in a dose of 500 mg every 5 or 6 hours in addition to full therapeutic parenteral doses of vancomycin and metronidazole. Oral vancomycin is also used to treat staphylococcal pseudomembranous enterocolitis. The drug is used in the empiric treatment of neutropenic patients with fever when there is a high likelihood of gram-positive infection. Vancomycin is indicated to prevent bacterial endocarditis in penicillin-allergic patients with valvular heart lesions who are undergoing dental and lower respiratory tract invasive procedures. The recommended dose is 1 g of drug given intravenously over 60 minutes before the procedure; no repeat dose is required. For prophylaxis in patients undergoing invasive gastrointestinal or genitourinary procedures, vancomycin in the above dose schedule plus gentamicin 1.5 mg/kg is given. The drugs may be repeated in 8 to 12 hours. Vancomycin is used as prophylaxis for the insertion of prosthetic heart valves at a dose of 15 mg/kg 1 hour prior to surgery and 10 mg/kg immediately following surgery.

(Continued on next page)

The information here is provided as guidance only. Prescribers should always consult the manufacturer's current prescribing information.

VANCOMYCIN AND TEICOPLANIN (CONTINUED)

ANTIMICROBIAL ACTIVITY

At concentrations ranging from 1 to 5 µg/mL, vancomycin inhibits strains of *S. aureus* and *S. epidermidis* (methicillin-sensitive and -resistant strains) [99,100]. A small percentage of strains may require higher concentrations (10–20 µg/mL). Most non-*aureus* staphylococci, including *S. epidermidis*, *S. hominis*, *S. sprophyticus*, and *S. warneri* are susceptible, although *S. hemolyticus* is relatively resistant. The production of biofilms by staphylococci on foreign bodies may account for the persistence of organisms in the presence of bacteriocidal concentrations of drug. Vancomycin is bacteriocidal for groups A, C, and G streptococci, *Streptococcus pneumoniae*, including multiple resistant stains, *Streptococcus viridans*, and *Streptococcus bovis*. The drug is often not bacteriocidal for *Enterococcus* spp, but aminoglycosides act synergistically with vancomycin and the combination is usually bacteriocidal at clinically achievable concentrations [101]. Recently, isolates of resistant *Enterococcus faecium*, *Enterococcus fecalis*, and *Leuconostoc* have been reported [102]. *Corynebacterium jeikeium*; *Clostridium* spp, including *C. perfringens*, *C. difficile*, and *C. tetani*; *Bacillus anthracis*; *Corynebacterium diphtheria*; and microaerophilic and anaerobic streptococci are sensitive. The susceptibility of *Actinomyces*, *Listeria*, and lactobacilli is variable. Vancomycin is not active against most aerobic and anaerobic gram-negative bacilli, mycobacteria, chlamydiae, and rickettsiae. The drug is active against *Flavobacterium meningosepticum*, and cases of meningitis due to this organism have been successfully treated with vancomycin [103]. Organisms sensitive to teicoplanin include staphylococcal species (methicillin-sensitive and -resistant); streptococci, including the *viridans* group, *S. pneumoniae*, and groups A, B, C, G, and F; and anaerobic gram-positive bacilli, including *C. difficile*, *C. perfringens*, *Listeria monocytogenes*, and *C. jeikeium*. Inhibitory concentrations range from 0.025 to 3.1 µg/mL [98,99,104]. Some strains of *S. epidermidis* and *S. hemolyticus* are more resistant to teicoplanin than vancomycin. For susceptible organisms, teicoplanin is two to four times more active than vancomycin. Teicoplanin is bacteriocidal for growing cells. Although it is the most active antimicrobial agent available for *Enterococcus faecalis*, it is usually not bacteriocidal for this species. Teicoplanin is not active against mycobacteria, fungi, and gram-negative aerobes and anaerobes. The drug may interact synergistically with rifampin and aminoglycosides against staphylococci, streptococci, enterococci, and *Listeria*.

MECHANISMS OF RESISTANCE

Certain sensitive strains of organisms lack autolysin and are tolerant in the presence of vancomycin [100,105]. Biofilm development on prosthetic devices may lead to treatment failure. The appearance of vancomycin resistance in *Enterococcus* species is well documented, and some cross-resistance between vancomycin and teicoplanin has been noted [102,106,107]. This resistance appears to be the result of mutations that change the building blocks of cell wall synthesis. In some resistant strains, *D*-alanyl-*D*-alanine is replaced by *D*-alanine-*D*-lactose. Vancomycin does not attack to this cell wall precursor, and this novel substituted monomer allows the organism to synthesize new cell walls. Resistance among *E. faceium* has been reported to be plasmid mediated [106].
The mechanism of teicoplanin resistance, although not clear, is assumed to be based on the cells' incorporation of precursors other than *D*-alanyl-*D*-alanine into peptidoglycan production.

INDICATIONS *(CONTINUED)*

Oral antibiotic prophylactic regimens to prevent indigenous infections in patients with neutropenia often combine vancomycin with antifungal agents and drugs active against gram-negative aerobes.
Teicoplanin is used in many of the situations that are considered indications for vancomycin [116]. The drug may be used less frequently (one to two times daily) and appears to be less nephrotoxic and ototoxic. Teicoplanin may be given to patients who develop allergic reactions or neutropenia when given vancomycin. Staphylococcal infections (methicillin-resistant and -sensitive strains) (*eg*, pneumonia, bacteremia, septic arthritis, and endocarditis) have been treated successfully. The presence of foreign bodies and prostheses reduces efficacy rates. The drug may be used to treat serious enterococcal infections due to vancomycin-resistant organisms, but cross-resistance has emerged as a problem. Teicoplanin has been used to treat peritonitis complicating peritoneal dialysis.

ADVERSE EFFECTS

The current formulation of vancomycin is relatively safe, and the most common side effects include fever, chills, phlebitis at the intravenous infusion site, and the "red man" syndrome (as many as 35% of patients) [117]. Hypersensitivity maculopapular rashes, reversible eosinophilia, thrombocytopenia, and leukopenia are also well described. Rashes may respond to steroid or antihistamine treatment. Auditory and, rarely, vesticular toxicity may occur, but with careful dosing in patients with renal insufficiency, ototoxicity is now uncommon [118]. Aminoglycosides may potentiate ototoxicity, especially in the elderly. Nephrotoxicity is dose related and may resolve following discontinuation of the drug [119]. Antibiotic-associated *C. difficile* colitis has been reported following intravenous vancomycin.
Teicoplanin is less toxic than vancomycin. Intramuscular injections may be associated with mild pain, but absorption is excellent. Phlebitis following intravenous administration is uncommon, as is the "red man" syndrome. Ototoxicity and nephrotoxicity are also uncommon. Reversible neutropenia has been described in about 2% of patients. Rashes and transient liver function abnormalities have been reported.

PHARMACOKINETICS AND PHARMACODYNAMICS

Vancomycin is poorly absorbed from the gastrointestinal tract, except in rare instances of patients with pseudomembranous colitis and renal failure. Oral administration produces high concentration in stool, accounting for efficacy in the treatment of *C. difficile* infections. Intramuscular injections of vancomycin have been associated with sterile abscesses and severe pain at the injection site. Consequently, parenteral administration is almost exclusively intravenous. Phlebitis may follow intravenous infusions.

(Continued on next page)

The information here is provided as guidance only. Prescribers should always consult the manufacturer's current prescribing information.

VANCOMYCIN AND TEICOPLANIN (CONTINUED)

DOSAGE

The vancomycin dose for patients with normal renal function is 30 mg/kg/d or 2 g/d in two to four divided doses. This produces peak and trough levels in the therapeutic range. Trough levels should be measured within 1 hour of the next dose. The therapeutic trough concentration should be in the 5 to 10 µg/mL range for twice-a-day dosing and 10 to 15 µg/mL for four-times-a-day dosing. Peak levels should be measured within 1 to 2 hours of an intravenous infusion. The optimal range is 25 to 40 µg/mL. Pediatric dosing in newborns is 15 mg/kg given intravenously slowly every 12 hours during the first week of life; in infants 8 to 30 days old it is 15 mg/kg every 8 hours; in older infants and children it is 10 mg/kg every 6 hours. For infants and children with staphylococcal central nervous system infections the dose is 15 mg/kg every 6 hours. Serum levels must be monitored, especially in premature infants. Special consideration is given when administering vancomycin to patients with renal failure because of the potential of accumulating toxic levels of drug. A loading dose of 15/kg can be given to all adults, including patients with abnormal renal function; however, subsequent dosing must be reduced. Creatinine clearance can be used to determine vancomycin dosing using the patient's age, sex, and creatinine clearance values [108].

$$\text{Creatinine clearance (mL/min/kg)} = \frac{(140\text{-age}) \times (1.0 \text{ for males; } 0.85 \text{ for females})}{72 \times \text{serum creatinine} \times \text{wt(kg)}}$$

Several techniques for dosing are available: 1) Dose (mg/kg/24 h) = 15.4 × creatinine clearance (measured in mL/min/kg) [109]; 2) Give loading dose, then one daily dose (mg/kg/24 h) = (15 × creatinine clearance + 150) [110]; 3) Give 1 g every 36 hours for serum creatinines 1.5 to 5 mg/100 mL and 1 g every 10 to 14 days when the creatinine is greater than 5 mg/100 mL [111]. Serum vancomycin concentrations in such patients should be monitored at least weekly to prevent toxicity.

Significant amounts of vancomycin can be removed by peritoneal dialysis but not hemodialysis. No dose modification is required in patients undergoing hemodialysis. In patients undergoing peritoneal dialysis, the peritoneal penetration of serum vancomycin is variable. To treat peritonitis caused by gram-positive organisms in patients receiving chronic intermittent peritoneal dialysis, the drug should be administered peritoneally. Vancomycin kinetics are more predictable in chronic ambulatory peritoneal dialysis (CAPD) patients. Intravenous vancomycin given to CAPD patients produces peritoneal levels about 25% of serum levels. With intraperitoneal administration of 30 mg/kg of vancomycin to CAPD patients, there is sufficient absorption (approximately 60%) to result in therapeutic serum levels. Peritoneal clearance of drug is greater with CAPD than with intermittent peritoneal dialysis. In order to maintain therapeutic serum levels in CAPD patients, additional drug must be added to dialysis fluid. Concentrations given by dialysate approximate targeted serum levels (25 µg/mL). Monitoring serum levels is essential in such patients and will help determine dosing for supplemental intraperitoneal or intravenous drug. Hemofiltration effectively removes vancomycin and is used in treating patients with overdose.

Other patient factors affect vancomycin kinetics. The half-life in patients with third-degree burns is reduced, and higher doses are needed. Obesity results in a larger volume of distribution, requiring that dosing be calculated on total body weight. Vancomycin clearance is delayed in patients with liver disease, and such patients should have serum concentrations closely monitored.

DOSAGE ADJUSTMENTS FOR RENAL AND HEPATIC INSUFFICIENCY

See Pharmacokinetics and Pharmacodynamics.

PHARMACOKINETICS AND PHARMACODYNAMICS *(CONTINUED)*

To prevent this complication, the drug should be reconstituted in 100 to 250 mL of 0.9% NaCl or 5% dextrose in water and administered over 30 to 60 minutes, not exceeding a rate of 15 mg/min. Rapid administration has been associated with histamine release from mast cells and basophils, causing the "red man" syndrome. Manifestations are characterized by flushing, pruritus, erythema, maculopapular rash, painful muscle spasms, anaphylactic-like reactions, and cardiac arrest. Although antihistamines and steroids are often added to the infusion to prevent this complication, steroids may precipitate vancomycin. The mixture of these drugs is to be discouraged. Slowing the rate of vancomycin infusions prevents this complication.

Following intravenous administration, vancomycin is distributed in a biphasic way. The drug is 55% bound to protein and has a half-life that ranges from 3 to 13 hours (average of 6 hours) in patients with normal renal function. The half-life is prolonged to 7 to 9 days in patients with anuria. With normal renal function, 80% to 90% of the administered dose is recovered in urine in 24 hours. The drug is eliminated almost exclusively by glomerular filtration, not by tubular secretion or reabsorption. There is a linear relationship between vancomycin clearance and creatinine clearance, with a ratio of about 70%. The difference between these rates is caused by the protein binding of vancomycin. Following intravenous infusion, serum levels at 2 hours are 2 to 10 µg/mL for a dose of 500 mg; 25 µg/mL for a dose of 1 g; and 45 µg/mL for a 2-g dose. Following a 500-mg dose an average level of 8 µg/mL is found, but after repeated dosing plasma levels may reach 50 µg/mL. Following a 1-g dose, peak and trough levels are 20 to 50 µg/mL and 5 to 10 µg/mL, respectively, and concentrations in the urine range from 100 to 300 µg/mL. After oral dosing of 500 mg every 6 hours, levels of 1000 to 9000 µg/mL are found in the stool; with oral dosing of 125 mg, stool concentrations range from 100 to 800 µg/mL. Although some drug may be found in the stool of some patients given intravenous drug, must have undetectable drug levels. Vancomycin does not cross the blood–brain barrier in patients without meningeal inflammation, although bacteriocidal levels (1%-30% of serum levels) may be reached in patients with meningitis. Supplemental doses of drug (3–5 mg) may be given intrathecally to patients with meningitis who do not respond to intravenous drug. The drug diffuses into synovial, ascitic, pericardial, and pleural fluid (50%-75% of serum levels). The penetration of vancomycin into peritoneal dialysis fluid is variable and undependable. Vancomycin is not concentrated in bile, although 30% to 50% of serum levels may be reached. The drug does not penetrate ocular tissue adequately. Vancomycin diffuses into abscess fluid at therapeutic concentrations, but penetration into bone is variable.

(Continued on next page)

The information here is provided as guidance only. Prescribers should always consult the manufacturer's current prescribing information.

VANCOMYCIN AND TEICOPLANIN (CONTINUED)

SPECIAL GROUPS

Children: Confirm desired serum drug concentrations in premature infants and full-term neonates. Administration with anesthetic agents has been associated with the "red man" syndrome. No specific dosage information for teicoplanin, although an increase in the loading dose may be required.

Elderly: Age-related renal impairment may require reduced dosing for both drugs.

Renal impairment: As above.

Hepatic involvement: No information.

Pregnancy: Use only when clearly indicated; limited studies performed for vancomycin; no information on teicoplanin.

Breast-feeding: Decision to discontinue drug or discontinue nursing must be made with respect to the importance of the drug to the mother for vancomycin. No information on teicoplanin.

DOSAGE

Vancomycin:

Adults: *ORAL:* 500 mg to 2 g/d in divided doses every 6 to 8 hours for 7 to 10 days; for *C. difficile*–associated colitis, 125 mg may be as effective as the 500-mg regimen. *PARENTERAL:* Infusion preferred over a period of at least 60 minutes, 500 mg intravenously every 6 hours or 1 g intravenously every 12 hours. For prevention of bacterial endocarditis in dental or upper respiratory procedures as an alternative regimen (*eg*, penicillin-allergic patients) 1 g intravenously over 1 hour, starting 1 hour prior to procedure. For prophylaxis in genitourinary or gastrointestinal procedures (*eg*, penicillin-allergic patients) 1 g intravenously over 1 hour plus 1.5 mg/kg gentamicin, starting 1 hour prior to procedure. Dose may be repeated once, 8 hours after first dose.

Elderly: Renal function may be reduced; *see* Pharmacokinetics and Pharmacodynamics.

Children: *ORAL: See* Indications. *PARENTERAL:* Infusion is preferred over a period of at least 60 minutes 10 mg/kg every 6 hours. For infants and neonates, give initial dose of 15 mg/kg followed by 10 mg/kg every 12 hours for neonates in the 1st week of life and every 8 hours thereafter up to age of 1 month. For dental or upper respiratory prophylaxis in penicillin-allergic children, 20 mg/kg starting 1 hour prior to procedure. For prophylaxis in genitourinary or gastrointestinal procedures in penicillin-allergic children, 20 mg/kg plus 2 mg/kg gentamicin intravenously 1 hour prior to procedure; dose may be repeated once, 8 hours after first dose.

Impaired renal function: *See* Pharmacokinetics and Pharmacodynamics.

Teicloplanin:

Adults: Loading and maintenance dose is 6 mg/kg followed by 3 mg/kg/d, which may need to increase in *S. aureus* endocarditis or septicemia.

Elderly: Half-life usually increased; otherwise, dose same as adults.

Children: No information.

Impaired renal function: Usual dose for first 3 days; vary dose based on serum creatinine and creatinine clearance.

PHARMACOKINETICS AND PHARMACODYNAMICS *(CONTINUED)*

There is no significant absorption of teicoplanin from the gastrointestinal tract. The drug may be given intramuscularly or intravenously. Teicoplanin is soluble as a sodium salt at physiologic pH and is well tolerated and absorbed following intramuscular injections. The half-life in serum is from 40 to 70 hours, and the drug may be given once daily. The drug has excellent tissue and cellular penetration and is slowly released from tissues because it is lipophilic. Teicoplanin has superior water solubility at physiologic pHs compared with vancomycin. The drug is highly bound to protein (90%), which probably accounts for delayed elimination and thus a longer half-life. The standard recommendation is a loading dose of 6 mg/kg followed by a daily dose of 2 to 3 mg/kg, which should yield adequate serum levels (10–3 µg/mL peak–trough concentrations). Recent studies indicate that seriously ill patients require twice daily dosing during the first few days of therapy. Such patients may require serum levels at a trough concentration of 5 to 10 mg/mL and peak of 25 to 30 mg/mL. To reach this level, intravenous loading doses of 6 to 7 mg/kg given every 12 hours for three doses, followed by single daily doses of the same amount, may be necessary. For pediatric dosing doses of 10 mg/kg/d for children and 6 mg/kg for neonates are recommended. Dosage adjustment for renal failure is required because serum concentrations are related to creatinine clearance. Supplemental doses following hemodialysis are not required, suggesting that the drug is not removed by hemodialysis. There is no information on dosage adjustment for hepatic insufficiency.

DRUG INTERACTIONS

Because of incompatibility with many drugs, intravenous vancomycin should be administered alone. Drug interactions include steroids, heparin at high concentrations, methicillin, and chloramphenicol. Other nephrotoxic drugs, including aminoglycosides, may potentiate nephrotoxicity.

PATIENT INFORMATION

Teicoplanin is currently not available. Marion Merrill Dow is the manufacturer.

AVAILABILITY

Vancomycin pulvules—125 mg, 250 mg
Powder for oral solution—1-g and 10-g bottles
Powder for injection—500-mg, 1-g, and 5-g viles and in 10-g pharmacy bulk packages. Teicoplanin, as supplied by manufacturer, Marion Merrill Dow (Kansas City, MO)

The information here is provided as guidance only. Prescribers should always consult the manufacturer's current prescribing information.

REFERENCES

1. Siewart G, Strominger JL: Bacitracin: An inhibitor of the dephosphorylation of lipid pyrophosphate, an intermediate biosynthesis of peptidoglycan of bacterial cell walls. *Proc Natl Acad Sci U S A* 1967, 57:767.

2. Storm DR, Strominger JL: Binding of bacitracin to cells and protoplasts of micrococcus lysodeikticus. *J Biol Chem* 1974, 249:1823–1827.

3. Kucers A: Bacitracin and Gramicidin. In *The Use of Antibiotics*, edn 4. Edited by Kucers A, Bennet N McK. London: William Heinemann Medical Books; 1987:751–753.

4. Tedesco FJ: Bacitracin therapy in antibiotic-associated pseudomembranous colitis. *Dig Dis Sci* 1980, 25:783–784.

5. Meleny FL, Johnson BA: Bacitracin. *Am J Med* 1949, 7:794–806.

6. Harold FM, Baarda JR: Gramicidin, valinomycin, and cation permeability of *Streptococcus faecalis*. *J Bacteriol* 1967, 94:53–60.

7. Contreras A, Vasquez D: Cooperative and antagonistic interactions of peptidyl-tRNA and antibiotics with bacterial ribosomes. *Eur J Biochem* 1977, 74:539–547.

8. Milatovic D, Breveny I, Verhoef J: Clindamycin enhances opsonization of *Staphylococcus aureus*. *Antimicrob Agents Chemother* 1983, 24:413–417.

9. Proctor RA, Olbrantz PJ, Mosher DF: Subinhibitory concentrations of antibiotics alter fibronectin binding to *Staphylococcus aureus*. *Antimicrob Agents Chemother* 1983, 24:823–826.

10. Schlievert PM, Kelly JA: Clindamycin-induced suppression of toxic shock syndrome-associated exotoxin production. *J Infect Dis* 1984, 149:471.

11. Mayberry-Carson KJ, Mayberry WR, Tober-Meyer BK, *et al.*: An electron microscope study of the effect of clindamycin on adherence of *Staphylococcus aureus* to bone surfaces. *Microbios* 1986, 45:21–32.

12. Philips I, Fernandes R, Warren C: *In vitro* of erythromycin, lincomycin, and clindamycin. *BMJ* 1970, 2:89–90.

13. Tally FP, Cuchural GJ, Jacobus NV, *et al.*: Susceptibility of the *Bacteroides fragilis* group in the United States in 1981. *Antimicrob Agents Chemother* 1983, 23:536–540.

14. Tate GW Jr, Martin RG: Clindamycin in the treatment of human ocular toxoplasmosis. *Can J Ophthalmol* 1977, 12:188–195.

15. Miller LH, Glew RH, Wyler DJ, *et al.*: Evaluation of clindamycin in combination with quininine against multidrug-resistant strains of *Plasmodium falciparum*. *Am J Trop Med Hyg* 1974, 23:565–569.

16. Watanakunakorn C: Clindamycin therapy of *Staphylococcus aureus* endocarditis: Clinical relapse and development of resistance to clindamycin, lincomycin, and erythromycin. *Am J Med* 1976, 60:419–425.

17. Cuchural GJ Jr, Tally FP, Jacobus NV, *et al.*: Susceptibility of the *Bacteroides fragilis* group in the United States: Analysis by site of isolation. *Antimicrob Agents Chemother* 1988, 32:717–722.

18. Wilkins TD, Thiel T: Resistance of some species of *Clostridium* to clindamycin. *Antimicrob Agents Chemother* 1973, 3:136–137.

19. Salaki JS, Black R, Tally FP, *et al.*: *Bacteroides fragilis* resistant to the administration of clindamycin. *Am J Med* 1976, 60:426–428.

20. Semel JD, Trenhome GM, Levin S: Gentamicin and clindamycin resistant *Staphylococcus aureus*. *Am J Med Sci* 1980, 280:4–9.

21. Tally FP, Snydman DR, Gorbach SL, *et al.*: Plasmid mediated transferable resistance to clindamycin and erythromycin in *Bacteroides fragilis*. *J Infect Dis* 1979, 139:83–88.

22. Tally FP, Cuchural GJ Jr, Malamy MH: Mechanisms of resistance and resistance transfer in anaerobic bacteria: Factors influencing antimicrobial therapy. *Rev Infect Dis* 1984, 6(suppl 1):260–269.

23. Chow AW, Montgomerie JZ, Guze LB: Parenteral clindamycin therapy for severe anaerobic infections. *Arch Intern Med* 1974, 134:78–82.

24. Fass RJ, Ruiz DE, Garner WG, *et al.*: Clindamycin and gentamicin for aerobic and anaerobic sepsis. *Arch Intern Med* 1977, 137:28–38.

25. Gorbach SL, Thadepalli H: Clindamycin in pure and mixed anaerobic infections. *Arch Intern Med* 1974, 134:87–92.

26. Tedesco FJ, Barton RW, Albers DH: Clindamycin-associated colitis: A prospective study. *Ann Intern Med* 1974, 81:429–433.

27. Condon RE, Anderson MJ: Diarrhea and colitis in clindamycin treated surgical patients. *Arch Surg* 1978, 113:794–797.

28. Panzer JD, Brown DC, Epstein WL, *et al.*: Clindamycin levels in various body tissues and fluids. *J Clin Pharmacol* 1972, 12:259–262.

29. Joiner KA, Lowe BR, Dzink JL, *et al.*: Antibiotic levels in infected and sterile abscesses in mice. *J Infect Dis* 1981, 143:487–494.

30. Johnson JD, Hand WL, Francis JB, *et al.*: Antibiotic uptake by alveolar macrophages. *J Lab Clin Med* 1980, 95:429–439.

31. Prokesch RC, Wand WL: Antibiotic entry into human polymorphonuclear leukocytes. *Antimicrob Agents Chemother* 1982, 23:373–380.

32. Keusch GT, Present DH: Summary of the workshop on clindamycin colitis. *J Infect Dis* 1976, 133:578–587.

33. Silva J Jr, Fekety R: Clostridia and antimicrobial enterocolitis. *Ann Rev Med* 1981, 32:327–333.

34. Musher DM, Griffith DP: Generation of formaldehyde from methenamine: Effect of pH and concentration and antibacterial effect. *Antimicrob Agents Chemother* 1974, 6:708–711.

35. Gleckman R, Alvarez S, Joubert DW, *et al.*: Drug therapy reviews: Methenamine mandelate and methenamine hippurate. *Am J Hosp Pharm* 1979, 36:1509–1512.

36. Brumfitt W, Cooper J, Hamilton-Miller JMT: Prevention of recurrent urinary tract infections in women: A comparative trial between nitrofurantoin and methenamine hippurate. *J Urol* 1981, 126:71–74.

37. Harding GKM, Ronald AR: A controlled study of antimicrobial prophylaxis of recurrent urinary infection in women. *N Engl J Med* 1974, 291:597–601.

38. Olsen JM, Friss-Moller A, Jensen SK, *et al.*: Cefotaxime for prevention of infectious complications in bactiruric men undergoing transurethral prostatic resection: A controlled comparison with methenamine. *Scand J Urol Nephrol* 1983, 17:299–301.

39. Tyreman NO, Andersson PO, Kroon L, *et al.*: Urinary tract infection after vaginal surgery: Effect of prophylactic treatment with methenamine hippurate. *Acta Obstet Gynecol Scand* 1986, 65:731–733.

40. Edwards DI, Mathison GE: The mode of action of metronidazole against *Trichomonas vaginalis*. *J Gen Microbiol* 1970, 63:297–302.

41. Edwards DI, Dye M, Carne H: The selective toxicity of antimicrobial nitroheterocyclic drugs. *J Gen Microbiol* 1973, 76:135–145.

42. Gillin FD, Diamond LS: Inhibition of clonal growth of *Giardia lamblia* and *Entamoeba histolytica* by metronidazole, quinacrine and other antimicrobial agents. *J Antimicrob Chemother* 1981, 8:305–316.

43. Sutter VL, Finegold SM: Susceptibility of anaerobic bacteria to 23 antimicrobial agents. *Antimicrob Agents Chemother* 1976, 10:736–752.

44. Bartlett JG, Dezfulian M, Joiner K: Relative efficacy and critical interval of antimicrobial agents in experimental infections involving *Bacteroides fragilis*. *Arch Surg* 1983, 118:181–184.

45. Padonu KO: A controlled trial of metronidazole in the treatment of dracunculiasis in Nigeria. *Am J Trop Med Hyg* 1973, 22:42–44.

46. Philips I, Warren C, Taylor E, *et al.*: The antimicrobial susceptibility of anaerobic bacteria in a London teaching hospital. *J Antimicrob Chemother* 1981, 8:17–26.

47. Tally FP, Snydman DR, Schimell MJ, *et al.*: Mechanisms of antimicrobial resistance of *Bacteroides fragilis*. In *Metronidazole: Proceedings of the 2nd International Symposium on Anaerobic Infections. Geneva, April 1979*. Edited by Philips I, Collier J. London: The Royal Society of Medicine and Academic Press; New York: Grune and Stratton; 1979: 19–24.

The information here is provided as guidance only. Prescribers should always consult the manufacturer's current prescribing information.

48. Muller M, Meingassner JG, Miller WA, *et al.*: Three metronidazole-resistant strains of *Trichomonas vaginalis* from the United States. *Am J Obstet Gynecol* 1980, 138:808–812.

49. Molavi A, LeFrock JL, Prince RA: Metronidazole. *Med Clin North Am* 1982, 66:121–133.

50. Bolton RP, Culshaw MA: Faecal metronidazole concentrations during oral and intravenous therapy for antibiotic associated colitis due to *Clostridium difficile*. *Gut* 1986, 27:1169–1172.

51. Kleinfeld DI, Sharpe RJ, Donta ST: Parenteral therapy for antibiotic-associated pseudomembranous colitis. *J Infect Dis* 1988, 157:389.

52. Kusumi RK, Plouffe JF, Wyatt RH, *et al.*: Central nervous system toxicity associated with metronidazole therapy. *Ann Intern Med* 1980, 93:59–60.

53. Duffy LF, Daum F, Fisher SE, *et al.*: Peripheral neuropathy in Crohn's disease patients treated with metronidazole. *Gastroenterology* 1985, 88:681–684.

54. Beard CM, Noller KL, O'Fallon WM, *et al.*: Cancer after exposure to metronidazole. *Mayo Clin Proc* 1988, 63:147–153.

55. Robbie MO, Sweet RL: Metronidazole use in obstetrics and gynecology: A review. *Am J Obstet Gynecol* 1983, 145:865–881.

56. Templeton R: Metabolism and pharmacokinetics of metronidazole: A review. In *Metronidazole: Proceedings of the International Metronidazole Conference, Montreal*. Edited by Feingold SM. Amsterdam: Exerpta Medica; 1977:28–37.

57. Stambaugh JE, Feo LG, Manthei RW: The isolation and identification of the urinary oxidative metabolites of metronidazole in man. *J Pharmacol Exp Ther* 1968, 161:373–381.

58. Chren M-M, Bickers DR: Drugs used in dermatological disorders. In *Modern Pharmacology*, edn 4. Edited by Craig CR, Stitzel RE. Boston: Little, Brown & Co; 1994:530–534.

59. Hirschmann JV: Topical antibiotics in dermatology. *Arch Dermatol* 1988, 124:1691–1700.

60. Leyden JJ: Review of mupirocin ointment in the treatment of impetigo. *Clin Pediatr* 1992, 31:549–553.

61. Doebbling BN, Breneman DL, Neu HC, *et al.*: Elimination of *Staphylococcus aureus* nasal carriage in health care workers: Analysis of six clinical trials with calcium mupirocin ointment: The Mupirocin Collaborative Study Group. *Clin Inf Dis* 1993, 17:466–474.

62. McCalla DR, Reuvers A, Kaiser C: Mode of action of nitrofurazone. *J Bacteriol* 1970, 104:1126–1134.

63. McCalla DR: Biological effects of nitrofurans. *J Antimicrob Chemother* 1977, 3:517–520.

64. Chamberlain RE: Chemotherapeutic properties of prominent nitrofurans. *J Antimicrob Chemother* 1976, 2:325–336.

65. Winberg J, Bergstrom T, Lincoln K, *et al.*: Treatment trials in urinary tract infection with special reference to the effect of antimicrobials on the fecal and periurethral flora. *Clin Nephrol* 1973, 1:142–148.

66. Koch-Weser J, Sidel VW, Dexter M, *et al.*: Adverse reactions to sulfisoxazole, sulfamethoxazole, and nitrofurantoin. *Arch Intern Med* 1971, 128:399–404.

67. Goldstein LI, Ishak KG, Burns W: Hepatic injury associated with nitrofurantoin therapy. *Am J Digest Dis* 1974, 19:987–998.

68. Sharp JR, Ishak KG, Zimmerman HJ: Chronic active hepatitis and severe hepatic necrosis associated with nitrofurantoin. *Ann Intern Med* 1980, 92:14–19.

69. Holmberg L, Boman G, Bottinger LE, *et al.*: Adverse reactions to nitrofurantoin: Analysis of 921 reports. *Am J Med* 1980, 69:733–738.

70. Nicklaus TM, Snyder AB: Nitrofurantoin pulmonary reaction: A unique syndrome. *Arch Intern Med* 1968, 121:151–155.

71. Sasame HA, Boyd MR: Superoxide and hydrogen peroxide production and NADPH oxidation stimulated by nitrofurantoin in lung microsomes: Possible implications for toxicity. *Life Sci* 1979, 24:1091–1096.

72. Sovijarvi ARA, Lemola M, Stenius B, *et al.*: Nitrofurantoin-induced acute, subacute, and chronic pulmonary reactions. *Scand J Resp Dis* 1977, 58:41–50.

73. Felts JH, Hayes DM, Gergen JA, *et al.*: Neural, hematologic, and bacteriologic effects of nitrofurantoin in renal insufficiency. *Am J Med* 1971, 51:331–339.

74. Schirmeister J, Stephani F, Willmann H, *et al.*: Renal handling of nitrofurantoin in man. *Antimicrob Agents Chemother* 1966, 1965:223–226.

75. Sachs J, Geer T, Noell P, *et al.*: Effect of renal function on urinary recovery of orally administered nitrofurantoin. *N Engl J Med* 1968, 278:1032–1035.

76. Storm DR, Rosenthal KS, Swanson PE: Polymyxin and related peptide antibiotics. *Ann Rev Biochem* 1977, 46:723–763.

77. Kunin CM, Bugg A: Binding of polymyxin antibratus to tissue: The major determinant of distribution and persistence in the body. *J Infect Dis* 1971, 124:394–400.

78. Warner SJ, Mitchell D, Savage N, *et al.*: Dose-dependent reduction of lipopolysaccharide pyrogenicity by polymyxin B. *Biochem Pharmacol* 1985, 34:3995–3998.

79. Cavaillon JM, Haeffner-Cavaillon N: Polymyxin B inhibition LPS-induced interleukin-1 secretion by human monocytes is dependent upon the LPS origin. *Mol Immunol* 1986, 23:965–969.

80. Rifkind D: Prevention of polymyxin B of endotoxin lethality in mice. *J Bacteriol* 1966, 93:1463–1464.

81. Nicas TI, Hancock RE: Alteration of susceptibility to EDTA, polymyxin B and gentamicin in *Pseudomonas aeruginosa* by divalent cation regulation of outer membrane protein H1. *J Gen Microbiol* 1983, 129:509–517.

82. Davis SD, Ianetta A, Wedghood RJ: Activity of colistin against *Pseudomonas aeruginosa*: Inhibition by calcium. *J Infect Dis* 1971, 124:610–612.

83. Hoeprich PD: The polymyxins. *Med Clin North Am* 1970, 54:1257-1265.

84. LaPorte DC, Rosenthal KS, Storm DR: Inhibition of *Escherichia coli* growth and respiration by polymyxin B covalently attached to agarose beads. *Biochemistry* 1977, 16:1642–1648.

85. Peterson AA, Fesik SW, McGroarty EJ: Decreased binding of antibiotics to lipopolysaccharides from polymyxin-resistant strains of *E. coli* and *Salmonella typhimurium*. *Antimicrob Agents Chemother* 1987, 31:230–237.

86. Nord C-E, Wadstrom T, Wretlind B: Synergistic effect of combinations of sulfamethoxazole, trimethoprim, and colistin against *Pseudomonas maltophilia* and *Pseudomonas cepacia*. *Antimicrob Agents Chemother* 1974, 6:521–523.

87. Marsden HB, Hyde WA: Colistin methane sulphonate in childhood infections. *Lancet* 1962, ii:740–742.

88. Fekety FR, Norman PS, Cluff LE: The treatment of gram-negative bacillary infections with colistin: The toxicity and efficacy of large doses in 48 patients. *Ann Intern Med* 1962, 57:214–229.

89. Lindesmith LA, Baines RD, Bigelow DB, *et al.*: Reversible respiratory paralysis associated with polymyxin therapy. *Ann Intern Med* 1968, 68:318–327.

90. Singh YN, Marshall IG, Harvey AL: Depression of transmitter release and post junctional sensitivity during neuromuscular block produced by antibiotics. *Br J Anaesth* 1979, 51:1027–1033.

91. Koch-Weser J, Sidel VW, Federman EB, *et al.*: Adverse effects of sodium colistamethate manifestations and specific reaction rates during 317 course of therapy. *Ann Intern Med* 1970, 72:857–868.

92. Sanders WE, Sanders CC: Toxicity of antibacterial agents: Mechanism of action in mammalian cells. *Ann Rev Pharmacol Toxicol* 1979, 19:53–83.

The information here is provided as guidance only. Prescribers should always consult the manufacturer's current prescribing information.

93. Perkins HR, Nieto M: The chemical basis for the action of the vancomycin group of antibiotics. *Ann N Y Acad Sci* 1974, 235:348–363.

94. Cheung RPF, DiPiro JT: Vancomycin: An update. *Pharmacotherapy* 1986, 6:153–169.

95. Jordan DC, Innis WE: Selective inhibition of ribonucleic acid synthesis in *Staphylococcus aureus* by vancomycin. *Nature* 1959, 184:1894–1895.

96. McHenry MC, Gavan TL: Vancomycin. *Pediatr Clin North Am* 1983, 30:31–47.

97. Barna JC, Williams DH: The structure and mode of action of glycopeptide antibiotics of the vancomycin group. *Annu Rev Microbiol* 1984, 38:339–357.

98. Williams AH, Gruneberg RN: Teicoplanin. *J Antimicrob Chemother* 1984, 14:441–445.

99. LaGast H, Dodion P, Klastersky J: Comparison of pharmacokinetics and bacteriocidal activity of teicoplanin and vancomycin. *J Antimicrob Chemother* 1986, 18:513–520.

100. Watanakunakorn C: Mode of action and *in vitro* activity of vancomycin. *J Antimicrob Chemother* 1984, 14(Suppl):7–18.

101. Harwick HJ, Kalmanson GM, Guze LB: *In vitro* activity of ampicillin or vancomycin combined with gentamicin or streptomycin against enterococci. *Antimicrob Agents Chemother* 1973, 4:383–387.

102. Uttley AC, Collins CH, Naidoo J, *et al.*: Vancomycin-resistant enterococci. *Lancet* 1988, i:57–58.

103. Aber RC, Wennersten C, Moellering RC Jr: Antimicrobial susceptibility of flavobacteria. *Antimicrob Agents Chemother* 1978, 14:483–487.

104. Pallanza R, Berti M, Goldstein BP, *et al.*: Teicoplanin: *In vitro* and *in vivo* evaluation and comparison to other antibiotics. *J Antimicrob Chemother* 1983, 11:419–425.

105. Geraci JE, Wilson WR: Vancomycin therapy for infective endocarditis. *Rev Infect Dis* 1981, 3:S250–5258.

106. LeClercq R, Derlot E, Duval J, *et al.*: Plasmid-mediated resistance to vancomycin and teicoplanin in *Enterococcus faecium. N Engl J Med* 1988, 319:157–161.

107. Johnson AP: Resistance to vancomycin and teicoplanin: An emerging clinical problem. *Clin Microbiol Rev* 1990, 3:280–291.

108. Cockcroft DW, Gault MH: Prediction of creatinine clearance from serum creatinine. *Nephron* 1976, 16:31–41.

109. Moellering RC Jr, Krogstad DJ, Greenblatt DJ: Vancomycin therapy in patients with impaired renal function: A nomogram for dosage. *Ann Intern Med* 1981, 96:343–346.

110. Nielsen HE, Hansen HE, Korsager B, *et al.*: Renal excretion of vancomycin in kidney disease. *Acta Med Scand* 1975, 197:261–264.

111. Eykyn S, Philip I, Evans J: Vancomycin for staphylococcal shunt infections in patients on regular hemodialysis. *BMJ* 1970, 3:80–82.

112. Cafferkey MT, Hone R, Keane CT: Antimicrobial chemotherapy of septicemia due to methicillin-resistant *Staphylococcus aureus. Antimicrob Agents Chemother* 1985, 28:819–823.

113. Dajani AS: Antibiotic-resistant pneumococci. *Pediatr Infect Dis* 1982, 1:143–144.

114. Riebel W, Frantz N, Adelstein D, *et al.*: *Corynebacterium* JK: A cause of nosocomial device-related infection. *Rev Infect Dis* 1986, 8:42–49.

115. Fekety R, Silva J, Armstrong AJ, *et al.*: Treatment of antibiotic-associated enterocolitis with vancomycin. *Rev Infect Dis* 1981, 3(Suppl):S273–S281.

116. Williams AH, Grunberg RN: Teicoplanin revisited. *J Antimicrob Chemother* 1988, 22:397–401.

117. Polk RE, Healy DP, Schwartz LB, *et al.*: Vancomycin and the red-man syndrome: Pharmacodynamics of histamine release. *J Infect Dis* 1988, 157:502–507.

118. Bailie GR, Neal D: Vancomycin ototoxicity and nephrotoxicity: A review. *Med Toxicol Adverse Drug Experience* 1988, 3:376–386.

119. Glew RH, Pavuk RA, Shuster A, *et al.*: Vancomycin pharmacokinetics in patients undergoing chronic intermittent peritoneal dialysis. *Int J Clin Pharmacol Ther Toxicol* 1982, 20:559–563.

The information here is provided as guidance only. Prescribers should always consult the manufacturer's current prescribing information.

CLASS DESCRIPTION

Erythromycin is the prototype of the macrolide class of antibiotics, and it was first introduced to treat pneumococcal, streptococcal, and other gram-positive infections in 1952 [1]. Erythromycin, derived from a metabolite of *Streptomyces erythreus*, is a naturally occurring substance with a 14–carbon ring structure. Other naturally occurring macrolides include oleandomycin, josamycin, spiramycin, and mide-camycin. Recently introduced agents, such as clarithromycin, roxithromycin, dirithromycin, and flurithromycin, are semisynthetic compounds with modifications of the 14-membered macrolide ring, as is troleandomycin [2]. Azithromycin is a 15-membered azalide with a methyl-substituted nitrogen at position 9. Sixteen-membered macrolides include the semisynthetic rokitamycin and miokamycin and the naturally occurring josamycin, midecamycin, and spiramycin. Only erythromycin, troleandomycin, azithromycin, and clar-ithromycin currently are marketed in the United States (Table 6-1). Roxithromycin has been in use in Europe and elsewhere for almost a decade. Spiramycin is available from Rhône-Poulenc-Rorer (Fort Washington, PA) for the treatment of cryptosporidiosis in patients with AIDS. The major advances of the new "macrolides" azithromycin and clarithromycin include their intracellular activity, pharmacokinetics, longer half-life, and better gastrointestinal toler-ance. As a class, the macrolides are well absorbed from the gastroin-testinal tract, and only erythromycin is currently available in an intravenous preparation. Dirithromycin is currently in the final stages of development.

The streptogramins are a class of compounds similar to the macrolides and lincosamides. The naturally occurring pristinamycin consists of two macrolactone components, pristinamycin I_A and pristinamycin II_A. These two components are synergistic and bacteri-cidal when combined as the investigational streptogramin RP-59500, or Synercid (Rhône-Poulenc-Rorer, Fort Washington, PA) [3]. This drug is being developed as a parenteral agent and has bactericidal activity against *Staphylococcus aureus* (including methicillin-resistant strains) and *Enterococcus* spp, among other gram-positive bacteria.

CHEMISTRY AND CLASSIFICATION

All of the macrolides are modifications of the macrolide ring struc-ture associated with erythromycin. They are lipophilic agents with a central lactone ring and amino- or natural sugars attached. The macrolides have been classified chemically according to the number of members (usually carbon atoms) in the ring. Most of the available agents have 14-membered rings. Azithromycin is an azalide with a 15-membered ring, and its C-9 has been replaced with a nitrogen atom. The new modified macrolide structures (such as methylation of the C-OH group at position 6 in clarithromycin and the methy-lated addition of the inserted nitrogen at position 9 of azithromycin) are protected against inactivation by metabolism or decomposition to inactive ketal derivatives, as is the case with erythromycin. Dirithromycin is formed by condensation of erythromycylamine with 2-(2-methoxyethoxy) acetaldehyde diethylacetal [2].

MECHANISM OF ACTION

Macrolides and azalides share a common mechanism of action in inhibiting bacterial protein synthesis by binding to the 50S compo-nent of the 70S ribosomal subunit. The macrolides also stimulate the dissociation of peptidyl transfer RNA (tRNA) from the ribosomes. The end result blocks translocation of amino acids during the synthesis of the elongating peptide chain [2]. Erythromycin results in bacteriostatic inhibition of *S. aureus* but is bactericidal for *Streptococcus pyogenes* and *Streptococcus pneumoniae* [4]. The strep-togramins are postulated to inhibit bacterial protein synthesis by diminishing the size of the exit channel for the growing polypeptide, resulting in accumulation on ribosomes that in turn might decrease the concentration of tRNA within the bacterial cell by decreasing the activity of peptidyl tRNA [5].

ANTIMICROBIAL ACTIVITY

Erythromycin has demonstrable *in vitro* activity against *viridans* streptococci, *S. pyogenes*, *S. pneumoniae*, *S. aureus* (except methicillin-resistant strains), *Corynebacterium* spp, *Neisseria gonorrhoeae*, *Listeria monocytogenes*, *Moraxella (Branhamella) catarrhalis*, *Mycoplasma pneu-moniae*, *Legionella pneumophila*, and *Chlamydia trachomatis*. Variable activity has been demonstrated for *Haemophilus influenzae* and anaer-obic organisms [4]. Erythromycin usually is not considered active against Enterobacteriaceae, but significant clinical activity has been demonstrated in the presence of an alkaline pH [6].

The new macrolides (clarithromycin and azithromycin) are active against the same organisms but can inhibit *M. pneumoniae*, *Legionella* spp, and *Chlamydia pneumoniae* at lower concentrations. They also are more active against *H. influenzae*, *Mycobacterium avium* complex, and other atypical mycobacteria, as well as the agent of Lyme disease, *Borrelia burgdorferi* [7]. Because of its high intracellular concentration,

Table 6-1. Macrolides Available in the United States

Drug Name	Trade Name	Manufacturer	Dosage Forms
Erythromycin	E.E.S., Ery-Tab, EryPed	Abbott	Oral*
	E-mycin	Boots	
	ERYC	Parke-Davis	
	Ilosone, Ilotycin	Dista	
Troleandomycin	Tao	Roerig	Oral
Azithromycin	Zithromax	Pfizer/Roerig	Oral
Clarithromycin	Biaxin	Abbott	Oral

*Available as an intravenous preparation as erythromycin lactobionate from several manufacturers.

The information here is provided as guidance only. Prescribers should always consult the manufacturer's current prescribing information.

azithromycin is more active against *C. trachomatis* and *Toxoplasma gondii*, and clarithromycin is very active against *Helicobacter pylori*.

The developmental streptogramin antibiotic Synercid is particularly active against streptococci and staphylococci, and it retains activity against methicillin-resistant *S. aureus*. This drug also may be active against enterococcal species and against erythromycin-resistant strains of *S. pneumoniae* as well as *Clostridium* species and *Listeria monocytogenes* [8,9].

Because of their intracellular concentration, macrolides can enhance phagocytic killing of bacteria, and some of these drugs may affect chemotaxis and the intracellular respiratory burst. In these capacities the macrolides may be considered as immunomodulatory [10,11].

MECHANISMS OF RESISTANCE

Resistance to macrolides is mediated by methylation of adenine residues in the ribosome that interfere with binding of the macrolide [4]. This resistance, known as *MLS resistance* (for macrolide, lincosamide, and streptogramin), may be chromosomal or transferable and may be constitutive or inducible. The prevalence of MLS resistance is highly variable geographically. Macrolide resistance in *S. pneumoniae* and *S. pyogenes* has been less than 5% in the United States, but recent increases have occurred. *S. aureus* resistance is more common.

PHARMACOKINETICS

Erythromycin must be protected with enteric coating or esterification to prevent its degradation to an inactive ketal. When administered orally, erythromycin achieves peak serum concentrations 2 to 4 hours after a 500-mg dose, is usually less than 4 µg/mL, and is widely distributed, with levels in bronchial secretions, middle ear and sinus fluids, and lung tissue above the minimal inhibitory concentration (MIC) for most respiratory pathogens. Lower levels are found in spinal fluid and brain. Only 4% to 5% of administered drug appears in the urine, and most of the dose is excreted by the liver in bile [4].

Clarithromycin and azithromycin have some pharmacologic advantages over erythromycin, with excellent bioavailability (55% and 37%, respectively), longer half-lives (3.5–4.7 hours and as high as 48 hours, respectively), and good to excellent intracellular concentration [12]. Azithromycin can be given once daily for 5 days or less, and clarithromycin is administered twice daily, usually for 10 days. Although very low serum concentrations of azithromycin (0.4 µg/mL) are found, high concentrations in respiratory tract tissue and prostate (1–9 mg/kg) are maintained for 4 to 8 days after a single 500-mg dose [13].

DOSAGE ADJUSTMENTS IN RENAL AND HEPATIC INSUFFICIENCY

For erythromycin, no adjustment is necessary if hepatic function is normal. This is probably true also for azithromycin, but data are limited. Clarithromycin should be reduced or administered at longer intervals for patients with creatinine clearances below 30 mL/min. If renal function is normal, clarithromycin can be administered normally to patients with liver impairment, but reduced doses of erythromycin and clarithromycin should be used in the presence of renal failure.

INDICATIONS

The macrolides are useful in the treatment of upper respiratory tract infections, including pharyngitis, sinusitis, and otitis due to susceptible organisms. Erythromycin is still quite useful in these infections and in Legionnaire's disease, *M. pneumoniae* infection, and in some cutaneous infections. The new macrolides are indicated for streptococcal pharyngitis and tonsillitis; pneumococcal sinusitis; acute exacerbations of chronic bronchitis due to *H. influenzae*, *S. pneumoniae*, and *M. catarrhalis*; pneumonia due to *M. pneumoniae* or *S. pneumoniae*; and staphylococcal and streptococcal skin and soft-tissue infections. In addition, azithromycin in a single 1-gm dose is effective for chlamydial urethritis and cervicitis [7]. Both drugs are effective in the treatment of *M. avium* complex infections in patients with AIDS.

ADVERSE REACTIONS

The macrolides generally are considered to be very safe drugs. Gastrointestinal reactions, especially nausea and vomiting, occur in up to 20% of erythromycin-treated patients. Lower rates are found with the new macrolide agents. Hepatotoxicity does occur with some erythromycin preparations, and these are less frequent with the new derivatives. Transient deafness also may occur with erythromycin, and intravenous administration may be associated with phlebitis.

INTERACTIONS

Because erythromycin and troleandomycin stimulate hepatic microsomal activity with cytochrome P-450 complexes, impaired clearance of theophylline, methylprednisolone, cyclosporine, phenytoin, carbamazepine, warfarin, midazolam, triazolam, digoxin, ergotamine compounds, barbiturates, and bromocriptine may occur [14]. Less interaction is expected with clarithromycin and azithromycin, although monitoring is recommended. Recently erythromycin has been found to interact with the antihistamines astemizole and terfenadine and cause cardiac arrhythmias, including torsades de pointes and ventricular tachycardia. Although these effects have not been reported with the new macrolides, caution should be exercised.

PATIENT INFORMATION

The macrolides are best taken on an empty stomach, but food may be taken simultaneously to minimize nausea. Azithromycin should not be used with aluminum- or magnesium-containing antacids. Clarithromycin should not be used in pregnant women unless no alternative agents are available. As with other antibiotics, patients should discontinue medication in the presence of rash, difficulty breathing, wheezing, swelling of the lips, jaundice, severe diarrhea, or abdominal cramps.

The information here is provided as guidance only. Prescribers should always consult the manufacturer's current prescribing information.

REFERENCES

1. Haight TM, Finland M: The antibacterial action of erythromycin. *Proc Soc Exp Biol Med* 1952, 81:175–183.

2. Mazzei T, Mini E, Novelli A, *et al.*: Chemistry and mode of action of macrolides. *J Antimicrob Chemother* 1993, 31(suppl C):1–9.

3. Barriere JC, Bouanchaud DH, Paris JM, *et al.*: Antimicrobial activity against *Staphylococcus aureus* of semisynthetic injectable streptogramins: RP 59500 and related compounds. *J Antimicrob Chemother* 1992, 30(suppl A):1–8.

4. Neu HC: The development of macrolides: Clarithromycin in perspective. *J Antimicrob Chemother* 1991, 27(suppl A):1–9.

5. Aumercier M, Bouhallab S, Capmau M-L, *et al.*: RP 59500: A proposed mechanism for its bactericidal activity. *J Antimicrob Chemother* 1992, 30(suppl A):9–14.

6. Zinner SH, Sabath LD, Casey JI, *et al.*: Erythromycin and alkalinization of the urine in the treatment of urinary tract infections due to gram-negative bacilli. *Lancet* 1971, i:1267–1268.

7. Neu HC: New macrolide antibiotics: Azithromycin and clarithromycin. *Ann Intern Med* 1992, 6:517–519.

8. Fremaux A, Sissia G, Cohen R, *et al.*: *In vitro* antibacterial activity of RP 59500, a semisynthetic streptogramin, against *Streptococcus pneumoniae*. *J Antimicrob Chemother* 1992, 30(suppl A):19–23.

9. Brumfitt W, Hamilton-Miller JMT, Shah S: *In vitro* activity of RP 59500, a new semisynthetic streptogramin antibiotic, against gram-positive bateria. *J Antimicrob Chemother* 1992, 30(suppl A):29–37.

10. McDonald PJ, Pruul H: Macrolides and the immune system. *Scand J Infect Dis* 1992, 83(suppl):34–40.

11. Gemmell CG: Macrolides and host defences to respiratory tract pathogens. *J Hosp Infect* 1991, 19(suppl A):11–19.

12. Williams JD, Sefton AM: Comparison of macrolide antibiotics. *J Antimicrob Chemother* 1993, 31(suppl C):11–16.

13. Foulds G, Shepard RM, Johnson RB: The pharmacokinetics of azithromycin in human serum and tissues. *J Antimicrob Chemother* 1990, 25(suppl A):73–82.

14. Periti P, Mazzei T, Mini E, *et al.*: Pharmacokinetic drug interactions of macrolides. *Clin Pharmacokinet* 1992, 23:106–131.

The information here is provided as guidance only. Prescribers should always consult the manufacturer's current prescribing information.

AZITHROMYCIN (Zithromax®)

Azithromycin is a new azalide derivative of erythromycin and differs chemically by the insertion of a methylated nitrogen as the 15th member of the macrolide ring.

It is well absorbed (37%) from the gastrointestinal tract after oral absorption and accumulates in tissue of the respiratory tract and prostate at levels several times higher than its low serum concentrations. Because the half-life is very long (up to 48 hours), the drug only has to be administered once daily, and a total of 5 days of treatment is recommended. (Shorter courses may prove useful.) Azithromycin can be used to treat upper and lower respiratory tract infections and skin and soft-tissue infections due to susceptible pathogens. A special use for this drug is in the single dose (1 g) treatment of chlamydial urethritis and cervicitis. Studies indicate its utility in *M. avium* complex infections in patients with AIDS. Side effects are less frequent than with erythromycin.

ANTIMICROBIAL ACTIVITY

Gram-positive aerobes: *Staphylococcus aureus, Streptococcus pyogenes, Streptococcus pneumoniae, Streptococcus agalactiae, Streptococcus* spp, *viridans* streptococcus.
Gram-negative aerobes: *Haemophilus influenzae, Haemophilus ducreyi, Moraxella catarrhalis, Bordetella pertussis, Legionella pneumophila, Campylobacter jejuni, Neisseria gonorrhoeae.*
Anaerobes: *Bacteroides bivius, Clostridium perfringens, Peptostreptococcus* spp.
Other: *Borrelia burgdorferi, Chlamydia trachomatis, Mycoplasma pneumoniae, Chlamydia pneumoniae, Treponema pallidum, Ureaplasma urealyticum.*

RESISTANCE

Less active than erythromycin against most *Staphylococcus* and *Streptococcus* spp (but more active against other species, including many gram-negative bacteria considered resistant to erythromycin).

SPECIAL PRECAUTIONS

Azithromycin is safe and effective in the treatment of community-acquired pneumonia of mild severity due to *S. pneumoniae* and *H. influenzae* in patients who are able to undergo outpatient oral therapy. Azithromycin should not be used in patients who cannot undergo outpatient therapy or in those who demonstrate any of the following: nosocomially acquired infection, known or suspected bacteremia, conditions requiring hospitalization (including moderate to severe pneumonia), significant underlying health problems inhibitory of good response (including immunodeficiency or functional asplenia), or patients who are elderly or debilitated. Do not use to treat gonorrhea or syphilis at normal or higher doses. High-dose, short-period treatment of nongonococcal urethritis may mask or delay symptoms of incubating gonorrhea or syphilis. All patients with sexually transmitted urethritis or cervicitis should undergo seriologic testing for syphilis and cultures for gonorrhea at time of diagnosis. (Although not recommended because of gastrointestinal intolerance, azithromycin 2 g orally [single dose] is effective in the treatment of uncomplicated gonorrhea.)
Use with caution in patients with hepatic function impairment. Azithromycin is eliminated primarily by the liver.
Ventricular arrhythmias, including ventricular tachycardia and torsades de pointes, have been reported in patients with prolonged QT intervals in trials with macrolide agents, especially in combination with terfenadine (however, no reports with azithromycin in particular).

INDICATIONS

Treatment of mild-to-moderate infections of the following types due to susceptible strains of designated organisms:
Lower respiratory tract (acute exacerbations of chronic obstructive pulmonary disease):
 H. influenzae, M. catarrhalis, S. pneumoniae (community-acquired pneumonia of mild severity for oral, outpatient therapy only) *S. pneumoniae* or *H. influenzae*
Upper respiratory tract (streptococcapharyngitis or tonsillitis as an alternative to first-line therapy):
 S. pyogenes
(Note: Penicillin is the usual drug of choice in *S. pyogenes* infection and in prophylaxis of rheumatic fever; some strains may be resistant to azithromycin. Susceptibility tests are recommended.)
Skin–skin structure (uncomplicated):
 S. aureus, S. pyogenes, S. agalactiae
Sexually transmitted disease (nongonococcal urethritis or cervicitis):
 C. trachomatis (1 g orally [single dose])

CONTRAINDICATIONS

Allergy or hypersensitivity to azithromycin or any of the macrolide antibiotics

INTERACTIONS

Although erythromycin is known to interact with several drugs including methylprednisolone, theophylline, carbamazepine, cyclosporin, phenytoin, and warfarin, these interactions have not been reported for azithromycin. Single-dose azithromycin does not affect warfarin clearance. Also, interactions with terfenidine have not been reported with azithromycin. Nonetheless, physicians should follow patients closely when these drugs are used with the macrolide/azalide drugs. Aluminum and magnesium-containing antacids reduce the maximum serum concentration of azithromycin, and they should not be administered concurrently.

ADVERSE EFFECTS

Vomiting, nausea, diarrhea, angioedema (rare), cholestatic jaundice (rare)
Multiple-dose regimen: Palpitations, chest pain, flatulence, melena, monilia, vaginitis, nephritis, dizziness, vertigo, somnolence, fatigue, photosensitivity
Single-dose regimen: Vomiting, vaginitis
Lab test abnormalities: Increased serum creatinine, phosphokinase, potassium, alanine aminotransferase, gamma-glutamyl transferase, and aspartate aminotransferase; leukopenia; neutropenia; decreased platelet count; elevated serum alkaline phosphatase, bilirubin, blood urea nitrogen, serum creatinine, blood glucose, lactic dehydrogenase, and serum phosphate
(Note: In multiple-dose clinical trials in more than 3000 patients, three patients discontinued therapy due to treatment-related liver enzyme abnormalities and one due to renal abnormalities.)

The information here is provided as guidance only. Prescribers should always consult the manufacturer's current prescribing information.

AZITHROMYCIN (CONTINUED)

SPECIAL GROUPS

Children: Safety and efficacy not established for children under 16 years of age.
Elderly: No dosage adjustment necessary in absence of hepatic or renal impairment.
Renal impairment: No data are available; use with caution.
Hepatic impairment: Use with caution; reduced dosage recommended.
Pregnancy: Use only when clearly indicated; no studies performed.
Breast-feeding: Use with caution; not known whether excreted.

DOSAGE

Adults: For mild-to-moderate acute bacterial exacerbations of chronic obstructive pulmonary disease, pneumonia, pharyngitis, or tonsillitis (as second-line therapy), and uncomplicated skin–skin structure infection: 500 mg as a single dose on first day followed by 250 mg/d in single doses on days 2 to 5 (for a total of 1.5 g). For nongonococcal urethritis or cervicitis due to *C. trachomatis*, one single 1-g dose. (3-d regimens of 500 mg/d are under investigation.)
Elderly: No dosage adjustment necessary in absence of hepatic or renal impairment. Same as adults.
Children: Safety and efficacy not established for children under 16 years of age.
Renal impairment: No information.

PHARMACOKINETICS AND PHARMACODYNAMICS

Peak serum levels: 0.4 µg/mL in 2 to 3 h
Plasma half-life: (average terminal half-life) 68 h
Bioavailability: 40%
Metabolism: no information
Excretion: primarily excreted unchanged in bile; 4.5% excreted unchanged in urine
Effect of food: food decreases absorption and serum concentration levels
Protein binding: 50%
Renal impairment: no data; use with caution
Hepatic impairment: use with caution

OVERDOSAGE

No information

PATIENT INFORMATION

Take on an empty stomach (1 hour before or 2 hours after meals). Do not use aluminum- or magnesium-containing antacids simultaneously with azithromycin.

AVAILABLILTY

Capsules—250 mg

The information here is provided as guidance only. Prescribers should always consult the manufacturer's current prescribing information.

CLARITHROMYCIN (Biaxin®)

Clarithromycin is a 14-membered semisynthetic macrolide that produces higher serum and tissue levels than erythromycin and is usually administered twice daily for 10 days. Clarithromycin is useful in the treatment of upper and lower respiratory infections and in skin and soft-tissue infections caused by susceptible pathogens, including *Chlamydia pneumoniae*. Studies also indicate its potential usefulness in the treatment of *Helicobacter pylori* infections and for the control of *Mycobacterium avium* complex infections in patients with AIDS. This drug produces adverse effects similar to those of erythromycin but at considerably lower frequencies.

ANTIMICROBIAL ACTIVITY

Gram-positive aerobes: *Staphylococcus aureus, Streptococcus pyogenes, Streptococcus pneumoniae, Streptococcus agalactiae, Streptococcus* sp, *viridans* streptococcus, *Listeria monocytogenes.*
Gram-negative aerobes: *Haemophilus influenzae, Moraxella catarrhalis, Bordetella pertussis, Legionella pneumophila, Campylobacter jejuni, Neisseria gonorrhoeae, Pasteurella multocida.*
Anaerobes: *Bacteroides melaninogenicus, Clostridium perfringens, Propionibacterium acnes, Peptococcus niger.*
Other: *Borrelia burgdorferi, Chlamydia trachomatis, Mycoplasma pneumoniae, C. pneumoniae, H. pylori.*

RESISTANCE

Erythromycin-resistant pneumococci and streptococci are likely to be resistant. Variable resistance is reported for penicillin-resistant pneumococci. Staphylococci may be more susceptible to clarithromycin than erythromycin, but most strains of methicillin-resistant *S. aureus* are resistant to clarithromycin. Although strains of *H. influenzae* might be reported by the microbiology laboratory as resistant, there is additional activity of the 14-hydroxy-metabolite of the drug against this organism. The combined activity of the parent drug with the metabolite may be effective clinically against *H. influenzae* strains reported as intermediately susceptible.

SPECIAL PRECAUTIONS

As with other antibiotics, pseudomembranous colitis and antibiotic associated colitis may occur. Clarithromycin is excreted primarily by the liver and kidney. In the presence of severe renal impairment (with or without hepatic insufficiency), the dose or frequency of administration should be altered accordingly. In elderly patients with severe renal impairment, similar adjustments should be made. Clarithromycin should not be given to pregnant women, except where no alternate therapy is appropriate or available. Caution is advised in the administration of this drug to lactating women and children younger than age 12 because its safety and efficacy have not been completely established.

INDICATIONS

Treatment of infections of the following types due to susceptible strains of designated organisms
Adults:
Upper respiratory:
  (Pharyngitis or tonsillitis): *S. pyogenes*
  (Acute maxillary sinusitis): *S. pneumoniae, H. influenzae, M. catarrhalis*
Lower respiratory tract (acute exacerbation of chronic bronchitis):
  H. influenzae, M. catarrhalis, S. pneumoniae (pneumonia), *M. pneumoniae, S. pneumoniae*
Skin–skin structure (uncomplicated):
  S. aureus, S. pyogenes
Children:
Acute otitis media:
  H. influenzae, M. catarrhalis, S. pneumoniae
Acute maxillary sinusitis:
  S. pneumoniae, H. influenzae, M. catarrhalis
Pharyngitis or tonsillitis:
  S. pyogenes
Skin–skin structure (uncomplicated):
  S. aureus, S. pyogenes

CONTRAINDICATIONS

Allergy or hypersensitivity to clarithromycin or macrolide antibiotics

INTERACTIONS

Serum concentrations and area under the concentration curve for theophylline compounds might be slightly increased in the presence of clarithromycin due to a slight decrease in clearance. Similarly, carbamazepine pharmacokinetics may be altered slightly by clarithromycin. Only limited data are available regarding the interaction of clarithromycin with terfenidine and astemazole. Physicians should monitor patients receiving clarithromycin with these drugs. Also, although not reported, physicians should consider the possibility of drug interactions with drugs known to interact with erythromycin (*see* erythromycin).

ADVERSE EFFECTS

(Note: Studies of pneumonia comparing erythromycin base or erythromycin stearate with clarithromycin showed fewer gastrointestinal adverse effects with clarithromycin-treated patients.)

The information here is provided as guidance only. Prescribers should always consult the manufacturer's current prescribing information.

CLARITHROMYCIN (CONTINUED)

SPECIAL GROUPS

Children: Safety and efficacy not established for children under 12 years of age.
Elderly: Maximum concentrations of clarithromycin and its metabolite and the area under the curve may be increased. Effects are parallel with known age-related renal impairment. No increase in adverse effects has been observed. Reduce dosage in severe renal impairment.
Renal impairment: Reduced dosage or prolonged dosage intervals necessary in severe impairment with or without coexisting hepatic impairment.
Hepatic impairment: No dosage adjustment necessary when renal function is normal.
Pregnancy: Use with caution only when no alternative exists. Studies indicate the potential for harm to fetus. If pregnancy occurs during use, advise patient of hazards.
Breast-feeding: Excreted in breast milk, use with caution.

DOSAGE

Adults: For pharyngitis or tonsillitis, 250 mg every 12 hours for 10 days. For acute maxillary sinusitis, 500 mg every 12 hours for 14 days. For uncomplicated skin–skin structure infection, 250 mg every 12 hours for 7 to 14 days. Dosage guidelines for lower respiratory tract infections are listed in the table below.

Dosage Recommendations for Drug Indication

Infection	Dosage, *every 12 h*	Duration, *d*
Acute exacerbation of chronic bronchitis due to:		
S. pneumoniae	250 mg	7–14
M. catarrhalis	250 mg	7–14
H. influenzae	500 mg	7–14
Pneumonia due to:		
S. pneumoniae	250 mg	7–14

Elderly: In absence of renal or hepatic impairment, same as adults.
Children: Dosage not established for children under 12 years of age.
Renal or hepatic impairment: No dosage adjustment is necessary in hepatic impairment if renal function is normal; however, in severe renal functional impairment with or without coexisting hepatic impairment, reduced doses or prolonged dosage intervals are recommended.

PHARMACOKINETICS AND PHARMACODYNAMICS

Peak serum levels: 1 to 3 µg/mL in 1.7 h
Plasma half-life: 3 to 7 h
Bioavailability: 50%
Metabolism: metabolized to active metabolite (14-OH clarithromycin)
Excretion: primarily renal; rate approximately that of glomerular filtration
Effect of food: delays onset of absorption and metabolism; no effect on bioavailability (may take without regard to meals)
Protein binding: no information
Renal impairment: reduced dosages or increased intervals required in severe impairment
Hepatic impairment: no dosage adjustment required when renal function is normal

OVERDOSAGE

No information

PATIENT INFORMATION

Clarithromycin may be taken without regard to meals

AVAILABILITY

Tablets—250 mg and 500 mg

The information here is provided as guidance only. Prescribers should always consult the manufacturer's current prescribing information.

ERYTHROMYCIN
(EES®, E-mycin®, EYRC®, EryPed®, Ery-Tab®, Ilosone®, Ilotycin®)

Erythromycin is the prototypic macrolide and contains a 14–carbon ring with sugar side chains. This drug was introduced in clinical medicine in 1952 and has been used to treat streptococcal and pneumococcal infections. Serum concentrations are relatively low, but some tissue and intracellular accumulation occurs. Current indications include streptococcal pharyngitis and other upper and lower respiratory tract infections and skin and skin structure infections due to susceptible organisms as well as the treatment of pertussis, diphtheria, erythrasma, intestinal amebiasis, neonatal conjunctivitis, and so forth. The intravenous preparation remains first-line therapy for Legionnaire's disease. Erythromycin produces nausea and vomiting in up to 20% of treated patients, and several important drug interactions exist. Most preparations require administration four times daily for 10 to 14 days.

ANTIMICROBIAL ACTIVITY

Gram-positive aerobes: *Staphylococcus aureus, Streptococcus pyogenes, Streptococcus pneumoniae, Streptococcus agalactiae, viridans* streptococcus, *Listeria monocytogenes, Corynebacterium diphtheriae, Corynebacterium minutissimum.*
Gram-negative aerobes: *Haemophilus influenzae**, *Moraxella catarrhalis, Bordetella pertussis, Legionella pneumophila, Neisseria gonorrhoeae.*
Other: *Chlamydia trachomatis, Mycoplasma pneumoniae, Treponema pallidum, Ureaplasma urealyticum, Entamoeba histolytica.*
**See* Resistance, below.

RESISTANCE

Many strains of *H. influenzae* are resistant to erythromycin alone but are susceptible to erythromycin and sulfonamides in combination.

SPECIAL PRECAUTIONS

Use caution in hepatic impairment; erythromycin is excreted primarily by the liver. Erythromycin has been associated with hepatotoxicity (cholestatic hepatitis). Reports have been most common for erythromycin estolate but also have occurred with other erythromycin salts. Symptoms may include malaise, nausea, vomiting, abdominal cramps, and fever. Jaundice may or may not manifest. Severe abdominal pain may mimic the pain of biliary colic, pancreatitis, perforated ulcer, or an acute abdominal surgical problem. In addition, symptoms and liver function tests have resembled findings associated with extrahepatic obstructive jaundice. Generally, symptoms have followed 1 to 2 weeks of continuous therapy; but they may develop after a few days of treatment. Effects subside when the drug is discontinued. Serious allergic reactions (including anaphylaxis) have occurred with erythromycin.

INDICATIONS

Treatment of mild-to-moderate infections of the following types due to susceptible strains of designated organisms:
Upper respiratory tract:
 S. pyogenes (group A beta-hemolytic streptococci), *S. pneumoniae, H. influenzae* (with concomitant sulfonamides)
Lower respiratory tract:
 S. pyogenes (group A beta-hemolytic streptococci), *S. pneumoniae*
Respiratory tract:
 M. pneumoniae
Skin–skin structure:
 S. pyogenes, S. aureus (resistant staphylococci may emerge)
Pertussis (whooping cough):
 B. pertussis
Diphtheria:
 As an adjunct to antitoxin in infection due to *C. diphtheriae*, to prevent establishment of carriage and to eradicate the organisms in carriers
Erythrasma:
 C. minutissimum
Intestinal amebiasis:
 E. histolytica (oral only)
(Note: Extraenteric amebiasis necessitates treatment with other agents.)
Pelvic inflammatory disease (acute):
 N. gonorrhoeae (as an alternative to penicillin)
Conjunctivitis of neonates, pneumonia of infants, and urogenital infection in pregnant patients:
 C. trachomatis
Urethral, endocervical, or rectal (uncomplicated):
 C. trachomatis (when tetracyclines are contraindicated or intolerated)
Nongonococcal urethritis:
 U. urealyticum (when tetracyclines are contraindicated or intolerated)
Primary syphilis:
 T. pallidum (oral erythromycin; as an alternative to penicillin)
Legionnaire's disease:
 L. pneumophila (initial intravenous therapy preferred, 1 g every 6 h) (Note: No controlled studies performed; *in vitro* data suggest effectiveness.)
Rheumatic fever (prophylaxis):
 As an alternative to penicillin
Bacterial endocarditis (prophylaxis):
 As an alternative to penicillin

CONTRAINDICATIONS

Allergy or hypersensitivity to erythromycin or other macrolide antibotics. Preexisting liver disease (erythromycin estolate only).

The information here is provided as guidance only. Prescribers should always consult the manufacturer's current prescribing information.

ERYTHROMYCIN (CONTINUED)

SPECIAL GROUPS

Children: Safe for use in children.
Elderly: No dosage reduction necessary in normal hepatic function.
Renal impairment: No dosage reduction necessary in normal hepatic function.
Hepatic impairment: Reduced dosage necessary; use with caution.
Pregnancy: Safety not established.
Breast-feeding: Excreted in breast milk. Erythromycin is considered compatible with nursing by the American Academy of Pediatrics. Possible adverse effects in infant include modified bowel flora, pharmacologic effects, and interference with fever work-up.

DOSAGE

Adults: *PARENTERAL*: (Use only when oral use is impossible or when severity of infection necessitates immediate high serum levels. Oral therapy should replace intravenous [IV] therapy as soon as clinically possible. Continuous infusion is preferable, but intermittent infusion in periods of 20 to 60 min at intervals of 6 hours or less also may be effective. Because ertythromycin is irritating, IV push is not acceptable.) For severe infection, 15 to 20 mg/kg/d, up to 4 g/d in very severe infections. *ORAL*: 250 mg (or 400 mg ethylsuccinate) every 6 hours, or 500 mg every 12 hours, or 333 mg every 8 hours. Dosage may be increased up to 4 g/d or more based on the severity of the infection. For twice-a-day dosage, give 500 mg every 12 hours (not recommended with doses > 1 g/d).
Elderly: In absence of hepatic impairment, same as adults.
Children: (Note: No specific parenteral dosage was given.) Oral: 30 to 50 mg/kg/d in divided doses; base dosage on age, weight, and severity of infection. Dosage may be doubled in severe infection.
Hepatic impairment: Reduced dosage required. Use with caution.

AVAILABILITY

Erythromycin lactobionate: Powder for injection—
  500 mg (as lactobionate) per vial or piggyback vial
Erythromycin base:
Tablets (enteric coated)—250 mg; 333 mg; and 500 mg
Tablets (polymer coated particles)—333 mg and 500 mg
Tablets (delayed release)—333 mg
Tablets (film coated)—250 mg and 500 mg
Capsules (delayed release, enteric coated pellets)—
  250 mg
Capsules (delayed release)—250 mg
Erythromycin estolate:
Tablets—500 mg (as estolate)
Capsules—250 mg (as estolate)
Suspension—125 mg (as estolate)/5 mL and 250 mg
  (as estolate)/5 mL
Erythromycin stearate:
Tablets (film coated)—250 mg and 500 mg
Erythromycin ethylsuccinate:
Tablets (chewable)—200 mg (as ethylsuccinate)
Tablets—400 mg (as ethylsuccinate)
Suspension—200 mg (as ethylsuccinate)/5 mL
Suspension—400 mg (as ethylsuccinate)/5 mL
Suspension—100 mg (as ethylsuccinate)/2.5 mL
Powder for oral suspension—200 mg
  (as ethylsuccinate)/5 mL reconstituted
Granules for oral suspension—400 mg
  (as ethylsuccinate)/5 mL reconstituted

INTERACTIONS

Erythromycin is an inhibitor of microsomal liver enzymes and may result in the decreased clearance or metabolism of several drugs such as theophylline, carbamazepine, methylprednisolone, cyclosporine, warfarin, triazolam, and bromocriptime. Also, digoxin bioavailability is increased by erythromycin in some patients. Recently, the concurrent administration of erythromycin with antihistamines, terfenidine and astemazole, resulted in cardiac arrythmias and torsades de pointes in some patients. These drugs should not be used with erythromycin.

ADVERSE EFFECTS

Serious allergic reactions (including anaphylaxis) have occurred. Symptoms of mild allergic reactions include rash, pruritis, urticaria, bullous fixed eruptions, and eczema (*see* Special Precautions). Other adverse effects include venous irritation (IV only), phlebitis (IV only), anorexia, vomiting, ototoxicity, hepatotoxicity (most frequent with erythromycin estolate), and ventricular arrhythmias.

PHARMACOKINETICS AND PHARMACODYNAMICS

Peak serum levels: no information
Plasma half-life: 1.4 h
Bioavailability: 0.3 to 1.9 µg/mL (higher with estolate)
Metabolism: hepatic (demethylation)
Excretion: significant quantities excreted in bile, and < 5% (oral) and 12% to 15% (IV) excreted unchanged in urine
Effect of food: base or stearate should be taken on an empty stomach; estolate, ethylsuccinate, and delayed-release base may be taken without regard to meals
Protein binding: 70% to 74%
Renal impairment: no dosage reduction necessary
Hepatic impairment: reduce dosage; use with caution

OVERDOSAGE

Symptoms include nausea, vomiting, epigastric distress, and diarrhea. Reversible mild acute pancreatitis has occurred, and hearing loss (with or without tinnitus and vertigo) may occur, particularly in patients with renal or hepatic impairment.
If overdose occurs, induce evacuation of unabsorbed drug. Unless five times the normal dose has been ingested, gastrointestinal decontamination is usually not necessary. Prediction of minimal toxicity should not be predicted unless amount ingested is known and only a single agent is involved. Allergic reactions should be treated with conventional therapy. Neither hemodialysis nor peritoneal dialysis is especially effective.

PATIENT INFORMATION

Take medication on an empty stomach (1 hour before or 2 hours after meals); medication may be taken with food if stomach upset occurs. Some types of erythromycin base enteric coated tablets may be taken without regard to meals; package literature should be consulted. Finish all medicine. Take each dose with a sufficient amount of water. Contact physicians if nausea, vomiting, diarrhea, stomach cramps, yellow discoloration of the skin or eyes, darkened urine, pale stools, or unusual fatigue occurs.

The information here is provided as guidance only. Prescribers should always consult the manufacturer's current prescribing information.

CLASS DESCRIPTION

Quinolones are a class of antimicrobial agents that are all structurally similar, completely synthetic, and highly effective in the treatment of many different types of infectious diseases, primarily those caused by bacteria. The quinolone antimicrobial agents are analogues of nalidixic acid, which was developed and introduced in 1962 [1]. The older analogues, pipemidic acid, oxolinic acid, and cinoxacin, were developed later. Shortly thereafter the development of the newer quinolones progressed rapidly and was spearheaded by the insertion of a fluorine at the 6-position in the basic nucleus. This chemical modification enhances and broadens the antibacterial activity of these agents, thus leading to the discovery of newer 4-quinolones with antibacterial activities 1000 times that of nalidixic acid [1,2]. The clinical importance of the newer quinolones is based on their broad antibacterial spectrum, unique mechanism of action, good absorption from the gastrointestinal tract after oral administration, excellent tissue distribution, availability for intravenous administration, and low incidence of adverse reactions [2,3].

CHEMISTRY AND CLASSIFICATION

Although the quinolones are structurally similar compounds, they can be divided into four general groups, *ie*, naphthyridines, cinnolines, pyridopyrimidines, and quinolones (Fig. 7-1). The addition of an oxygen at the 4-position in the basic nucleus provides a common skeleton, 4-*oxo*-1,4-dihydro-quinolone, more commonly called *4-quinolone*. The naphthyridines (nalidixic acid and enoxacin) are 8-*aza*-4-quinolones because they have an additional nitrogen in the 8-position. The cinnoline cinoxacin is a 2-*aza*-4-quinolone because it has an additional nitrogen in the 2-position. The pyridopyrimidines have additional nitrogens in the 6- and 8-positions and are called 6,8-diaza-4-quinolones. All of the other highly active agents (ciprofloxacin, lomefloxacin, norfloxacin, and ofloxacin) are classified as 4-quinolones [2,3]. Additional compounds have been synthesized and are undergoing development.

MECHANISM OF ACTION

The identification of the enzyme DNA gyrase, or topoisomerase II, by Gellert *et al*. [4] in 1976 led to our current understanding of the mechanism of action of the quinolones. These drugs inhibit DNA topoisomerase (gyrases), of which four subunits (two A monomers and two B monomers) have been defined. The topoisomerases, which have been found in every organism examined, supercoil strands of bacterial DNA in the bacterial cell. Each chromosomal domain is transiently nicked during supercoiling, which results in single-stranded DNA. When supercoiling is completed, the single-stranded DNA state is abolished by an enzyme that seals the nicked DNA. Thus, the enzyme DNA gyrase, or topoisomerase II, (nicking-closing enzyme), nicks double-stranded DNA, introduces supercoils, and seals the nicked DNA [4,5]. It is thought that the A subunits introduce the nicks, the B subunits supercoil, and then the A subunits seal the nick they produced initially. The newer 4-quinolones may affect both the A and B subunits of DNA gyrase because mutations that affect the B subunit change the bacterial sensitivity to the 4-quinolones. Also, the bactericidal activity of the quinolones is reduced substantially if RNA or protein synthesis is inhibited. The newer 4-quinolones are bactericidal.

The next major advance was the ability to manipulate the nucleus of the 4-quinolones, which led to the development of newer compounds with improved antimicrobial activity and pharmacokinetic profiles [2,3,6]. Key modifications to the basic molecule have been made at the N-1, C-5, C-6, C-7, and C-8 positions (Fig. 7-1). These modifications have resulted in enhanced DNA gyrase inhibitory activity, increased absorption, longer half-life, and broader antibacterial activity. Table 7-1 shows some of the improvements brought about by some of the modifications at key positions in the basic molecule.

ANTIMICROBIAL ACTIVITY

The newer 4-quinolones are very active against enteric gram-negative aerobic bacteria and are generally active against other aerobic gram-negative organisms [7]. These drugs are moderately active against *Pseudomonas auerginosa* and have activity against staphylococci. With the potential for the development of resistance by these organisms, they have variable activity against streptococci. Currently available quinolones are not active against anaerobic bacteria. Table 7-2 provides the *in vitro* antimicrobial activity of selected 4-quinolones.

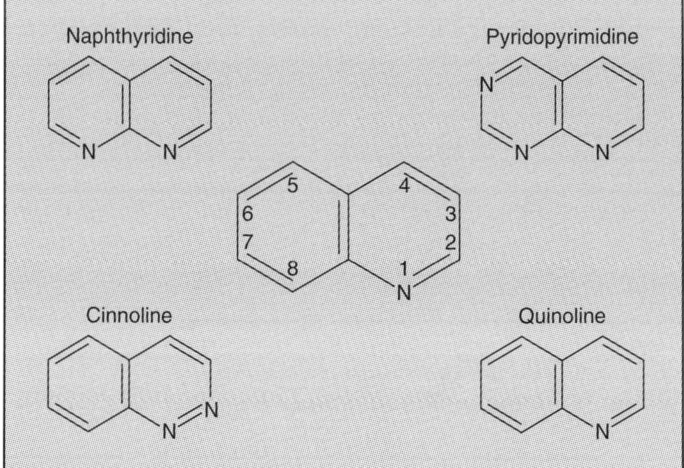

FIGURE 7-1.

Chemical structure of the four general groups of the 4-quinolones and its system of ring numbering. (*From* Andriole [14]; with permission.)

Table 7-1. Modifications in the Quinolone Nucleus

Change	Effect
Addition of a fluorine atom to position 6	Enhances DNA gyrase inhibitory activity and provides activity against staphylococci
Addition of a second fluoro group at position 8	Results in increased absorption and a longer half-life
Addition of a piperazine group at position 7	Results in increased activity against staphylococci and adds activity against *Pseudomonas*
Substitution of the piperazine group with a methyl group	Provides increased oral absorption and a longer half-life
Addition of a cyclopropyl group at position 1, an amino group at position 5, and a fluorine group at position 8	Results in increased activity against *Mycoplasma* and *Chlamydia*

The information here is provided as guidance only. Prescribers should always consult the manufacturer's current prescribing information.

QUINOLONES

MECHANISMS OF BACTERIAL RESISTANCE

Serial exposure of both gram-positive and gram-negative aerobic bacteria to subinhibitory concentrations of the quinolones *in vitro* leads to the selection of bacterial variants with reduced susceptibility to the drug. The affected strains may exhibit crossresistance to other quinolones. The mechanism of resistance usually involves either 1) mutations in the gene coding for DNA gyrase, so that there is reduced quinolone affinity for the A or B subunit or 2) mutations that change the outer membrane porins, particularly OmpF, and thus alter quinolone permeation [8,9].

PHARMACOKINETICS

All of the currently available quinolones are well absorbed from the gastrointestinal tract after oral administration, and most are excreted by the kidney into the urine. Some are metabolized in the liver. The pharmacokinetic properties of selected newer quinolones are shown in Table 7-3 [10]. Quinolones provide good tissue distribution, with excellent interstitial fluid levels, entry into phagocytic cells, and urinary concentrations after oral administration (Tables 7-3 and 7-4). Also, both oral and intravenous preparations are available for some of the newer quinolones. Table 7-5 lists the currently available quinolones by generic name, trade name, manufacturer, and mode of administration.

Table 7-2. *In Vitro* Activity of Selected 4-Quinolones

Organism	Nalidixic Acid	Ciprofloxacin	Enoxacin	Norfloxacin	Ofloxacin	Lomefloxacin
Gram-negative aerobes						
Escherichia coli	8 (4–128)	0.03 (0.015–0.06)	0.5 (0.25–1)	0.125 (0.06–0.5)	0.125 (0.06–0.25)	1 (0.03–128)
Klebsiella pneumoniae	8 (1–128)	0.125 (0.06–0.25)	0.5	0.25 (0.125–1)	0.25	0.5
Enterobacter spp	32 (4–128)	0.125 (0.03–0.5)	0.5 (0.25–4)	0.5 (0.125–2)	0.5 (0.125–1)	0.5 (0.064–16)
Citrobacter spp	8 (4– >100)	0.03 (0.03–0.06)	0.5	0.25 (0.125–0.5)	0.5	1 (0.25–32)
Serratia marcescens	> 128 (16– > 256)	1 (0.25–2)	2 (0.5–4)	1 (0.5–8)	1 (0.25–2)	4 (0.064–128)
Shigella spp	4	0.03 (0.015–0.06)	0.125	0.06 (0.03–0.125)	0.125 (0.06–0.125)	0.25 (0.01–1)
Salmonella spp	8 (4–8)	0.015 (≤ 0.015–0.03)	0.25 (0.125–0.25)	0.125 (0.06–0.125)	0.125 (0.06–0.125)	0.5 (0.01–2)
Proteus mirabilis	16 (4–32)	0.06 (0.03–0.125)	0.5 (0.25–1)	0.25 (0.125–0.5)	0.25 (0.25–0.5)	1 (0.06–64)
Proteus spp (indole-positive)	8 (4–16)	0.06	0.25 (0.25–0.5)	0.125 (0.06–0.125)	0.25	0.5 (0.06–8)
Morganella morganii	8 (2–8)	0.015 (0.015–0.03)	0.25 (0.25–0.5)	0.125 (0.3–0.25)	0.125 (0.125–0.25)	0.25 (0.25–2)
Pseudomonas aeruginosa	≥ 128	0.5 (0.25–1)	4 (2–8)	2 (0.06–8)	4 (2–4)	8 (0.06–> 256)
Haemophilus influenzae	1 (1–2)	0.015 (0.015–0.03)	0.125 (0.06–0.25)	0.06 (0.03–0.125)	0.03 (0.03–0.06)	0.25 (< 0.25–0.5)
Legionella pneumophila	NA	(0.03–0.125)	NA	(0.125–0.5)	NA	0.25
Neisseria gonorrhoeae	1 (1–2)	≤ 0.015	0.03 (0.015–0.06)	0.06 (0.015–0.125)	0.3 (0.015–0.06)	< 0.25
Neisseria meningitidis	2	0.004	0.06	0.03	0.015	0.25 (< 0.25–< 0.25)
Gram-negative anaerobes						
Bacteroides fragilis	128 (64–256)	8 (4–32)	32 (16–128)	64 (16–> 128)	4 (4–8)	16 (4–32)
Bacteroides spp	256	16 (16–32)	32 (32–64)	128 (128–256)	NA	8 (2–32)
Gram-positive aerobes						
Staphylococcus aureus (MS)	≥ 128 (32–>128)	0.5 (0.25–1)	2 (1–4)	2 (1–4)	0.5 (0.25–1)	2 (< 0.25–16)
Staphylococcus aureus (MR)	> 64 (32–128)	0.5 (0.5–1)	2	2	0.5 (0.25–0.5)	2 (< 0.25–32)
Staphylococcus epidermidis	> 64 (64–128)	0.25 (0.125–0.5)	1	2 (1–4)	0.5 (0.25–1)	2
Streptococcus pneumoniae	≥ 128 (64– ≥ 256)	1 (0.5–2)	16	16 (4–16)	2 (1–2)	16 (< 0.25–32)
Streptococcus pyogenes	≥ 128	1 (0.5–2)	8 (8–16)	16 (8–32)	4	8 (2–32)
Streptococcus agalactiae	> 128 (>128–512)	1 (0.5–2)	16 (16–32)	16 (8–32)	2 (1–4)	8 (4–16)
Enterococcus	> 128 (64–> 128)	2 (0.5–2)	8 (8–16)	8 (4–32)	2 (2–4)	8 (2–8)
Gram-positive anaerobes						
Peptococcus	256	2	8	8	4	8 (0.5–16)
Peptostreptococcus	≥ 64	1 (0.5–8)	8	4 (2–4)	2	8 (0.5–16)
Clostridium spp	≥ 256	16 (8–32)	32 (32–64)	64 (32–128)	16 (8–16)	32 (< 0.25–128)

*Mean value and range.
MIC—minimum inhibitory concentration; MR—methicillin-resistant; MS—methicillin-sensitive; NA—not available.

The information here is provided as guidance only. Prescribers should always consult the manufacturer's current prescribing information.

Table 7-3. Pharmacokinetic Properties of Selected Newer Quinolones

Drug	Dose, *mg*	C_{max}, *mg/L*	Half-life, *h*	Protein binding, %	Bioavailability, %	VD, *L*	Urinary Excretion, % Unchanged	Urinary Excretion, % Metabolites
Ciprofloxacin	500	2–3	3–4.5	35	85	250	30–60	10
Norfloxacin	400	1.5	3–4.5	15	80	225	20–40	20
Ofloxacin	400	3.5–5	5–6	8–30	85–95	100	70–90	5–10
Enoxacin	400	2–3	4–6	43	90	190	50–55	15
Lomefloxacin	400	3	8	10	95	190	65	10

C_{max}—peak serum concentration; VD—volume of distribution.

Table 7-4. Penetration of Selected Quinolones Into Body Fluids and Tissues

	Ciprofloxacin	Norfloxacin	Ofloxacin	Enoxacin	Lomefloxacin
Blister fluid	++++	++++	++++	++++	—
Saliva	++	++	+++	+++	—
Bronchial secretions	++	—	+++	++++	++++
Pleural fluid	+++	—	—	—	—
Nasal secretions	+++	+++	++++	++++	—
Tears	++	++	+++	++	—
Sweat	+	+	++	++	—
Cerebrospinal fluid	+	—	++	—	—
Prostatic fluid	+++	++	++++	++	++++
Ejaculate	+++++	—	++++	++++	—
Lung	++++	—	++++	+++++	—
Kidney	+++++	+++++	+++++	++++	—
Bone	++++	—	++	++	—
Skin	++++	—	—	++++	—
Muscle	++++	—	—	++++	—
Fat	++++	—	—	+++	—

+—area under the curve (AUC) ratios or concentration ratios < 0.1; ++—AUC ratios or concentration ratios 0.1–0.5; +++—AUC ratios or concentration ratios 0.5–1; ++++—AUC ratios or concentration ratios 1–4; +++++—AUC ratios or concentration ratios > 4.

Table 7-5. Quinolone Antimicrobial Agents

Agent	Trade Name	Manufacturer	Dosage Forms
Cinoxacin	Cinobac	Oclassen (San Rafael, CA)	Oral
Ciprofloxacin	Cipro	Miles (West Haven, CT)	Oral, intravenous, ophthalmic
Enoxacin	Penetrex	Rhone-Poulenc Rorer (Fort Washington, PA)	Oral
Lomefloxacin	Maxaquin	Searle and Co. (Chicago, IL)	Oral
Naladixic acid	NegGram	Sanofi Winthrop (New York, NY)	Oral
Norfloxacin	Chibroxin	Merck Sharp and Dohme (West Point, PA)	Oral, ophthalmic
	Noroxin	Merck Sharp and Dohme	
Ofloxacin	Floxin	McNeil (Springhouse, PA)	Oral, intravenous

The information here is provided as guidance only. Prescribers should always consult the manufacturer's current prescribing information.

DOSAGE ADJUSTMENTS FOR RENAL AND HEPATIC INSUFFICIENCY

For patients whose creatinine clearance rate is below 50 mL/min, dosage adjustments of ofloxacin and lomefloxacin are suggested because these drugs are excreted largely unchanged in the urine and undergo minimal hepatic metabolism [2,10,11]. The suggested adjustment for ofloxacin and lomefloxacin is a standard dose given at intervals of 24 hours in patients with creatinine clearances of 10 to 50 mL/min and one half the standard dose every 24 hours in patients with creatinine clearances of less than 10 mL/min. Dosage adjustments for ciprofloxacin, norfloxacin, and enoxacin may be necessary for patients with moderate renal insufficiency, but only when the creatinine clearance rate is substantially depressed (*eg*, < 30 mL/min), when maintenance doses can be given at 18- to 24-hour intervals. Also, studies indicate that in patients undergoing hemo- or peritoneal dialysis, a maintenance dose of ciprofloxacin should be given after dialysis and then at 24-hour intervals.

For patients with hepatic disease without concomitant renal insufficiency, no dosage adjustment is needed for the quinolones, except possibly for enoxacin. However, norfloxacin and ciprofloxacin may accumulate in patients with severe hepatic failure [2].

INDICATIONS

Certain infectious diseases are amenable to oral therapy: these include infections of the respiratory tract, especially those that are chronic; urinary tract infections, except urosepsis; bone and joint infections; skin and soft-tissue infections; certain gastrointestinal infections; some sexually transmitted diseases; and some pelvic infections. Adequate evidence of efficacy with the newer quinolones, particularly ciprofloxacin and ofloxacin, has been demonstrated by clinical investigation in most of these infectious diseases [12,13]. Enoxacin and lomefloxacin have been efficacious in some of these infections; norfloxacin in urinary tract infections and some sexually transmitted diseases; and cinoxacin and nalidixic acid in urinary tract infections only. Indications for the quinolones that have been approved by the Food and Drug Administration are given in Table 7-6.

ADVERSE REACTIONS

Toxicities with the early newer quinolones were low. Compared with other commonly used antimicrobial agents, the fluoroquinolones can be considered relatively safe [3,11,12]. Gastrointestinal disturbances (nausea, diarrhea, vomiting, and dyspepsia) are the adverse reactions reported most frequently (2%–5%). Central nervous system (CNS) reactions (1%–2%) may occur in the form of headache, dizziness, tiredness, or insomnia. Severe neurotoxic reactions are rare (< 0.5%) and include psychotic reactions, hallucinations, depression, and grand mal seizures, which are reversible with cessation of therapy. Thus, the quinolones should be used with caution in patients with known or suspected CNS disorders (*eg*, epilepsy) or other conditions predisposing to seizures. Hypersensitivity reactions also are rare (0.4%–1%) and include erythema, pruritus, urticaria, and rash. Equally rare are episodes of hypotension, tachycardia, nephrotoxic reactions (crystalluria) with elevated serum creatinine levels, thrombocytopenia, leukopenia, and anemia. Transient elevations in liver enzymes have been observed rarely [3,10,12].

Moderate to severe phototoxicity, manifested by an exaggerated sunburn reaction, has been observed in patients who are exposed to direct sunlight while receiving some members of the quinolone class of drugs, especially lomefloxacin. Patients should be instructed to avoid excessive sunlight, and therapy should be discontinued if phototoxicity occurs.

DRUG INTERACTIONS

Nalidixic acid–glucuronide conjugates may produce a false-positive reaction for urine glucose when tested with Benedicts' solution but not with glucose oxidase strips. Nitrofurantoin interferes with the therapeutic action of nalidixic acid.

Some of the newer quinolones increase theophylline plasma concentrations, *eg*, enoxacin (111%), ciprofloxacin (23%), and ofloxacin (12%). The 4-*oxo* metabolite of the piperazine ring is thought to compete with theophylline for hepatic enzymes and interfere with theophylline clearance [2,3]. Theophylline doses probably should be halved in patients receiving enoxacin. No routine reduction in theophylline dose is recommended for patients receiving ciprofloxacin, ofloxacin, or lomefloxacin, but theophylline levels should be monitored.

Caffeine clearance is interfered with by the newer quinolones. Enoxacin increases the plasma concentration of caffeine by 41% and reduces the clearance by 78%. Ciprofloxacin increases the half-life of caffeine only modestly (15%), and ofloxacin and lomefloxacin only minimally [2,3].

Some fluoroquinolones form chelates with alkaline earth and transition metal cations. Administration of quinolones with antacids containing calcium, aluminum, or magnesium; with sucralfate; with divalent or trivalent cations, such as iron; or with multivitamins containing zinc may substantially interfere with the absorption of the quinolones, resulting in low systemic levels so that simultaneous oral administration should be avoided. These agents should not be taken within the 2-hour period before or after quinolone administration. Also, the absorption of some quinolones may be affected minimally by food.

The quinolones may interact to varying degrees with other drugs, including warfarin, H_2 receptor antagonists, cyclosporine, rifampin, and nonsteroidal anti-inflammatory drugs (NSAIDs). The concomitant administration of an NSAID with a quinolone may increase the risk of CNS stimulation and convulsive seizures. Disturbances of blood glucose, including symptomatic hyper- and hypoglycemia have been

Table 7-6. Approved Indications for Quinolones

Agent	FDA–Approved Indications
Cinoxacin	Urinary tract
Ciprofloxacin	Lower respiratory tract; skin and skin structure, bone and joint; urinary tract; gastrointestinal (infectious diarrhea); uncomplicated (urethral or cervical) gonorrhea; conjunctivitis
Enoxacin	Urinary tract; uncomplicated (urethral or cervical) gonorrhea
Lomefloxacin	Acute bacterial exacerbations of chronic bronchitis; urinary tract (treatment and perioperative prophylaxis)
Nalidixic acid	Urinary tract
Norfloxacin	Urinary tract; uncomplicated (urethral or cervical) gonorrhea; conjunctivitis
Ofloxacin	Lower respiratory tract; uncomplicated (urethral or cervical) gonorrhea; *Chlamydia trachomatis* urethritis or cervicitis skin and skin structure (uncomplicated); urinary tract; prostatitis (less than 10 patients)

The information here is provided as guidance only. Prescribers should always consult the manufacturer's current prescribing information.

reported, usually in diabetic patients receiving concomitant treatment with an oral hypoglycemic agent or insulin. In these patients, careful monitoring of blood glucose is recommended, and the quinolone should be discontinued if a hypoglycemic reaction occurs.

PATIENT INFORMATION

Patients should be advised to 1) drink fluids liberally; 2) avoid taking antacids, sucralfate, vitamins, or food except 2 hours before or after taking their quinolone, even though the influence of food on quinolone absorption may be minimal; 3) exercise caution while performing activities requiring alertness and coordination (*eg*, operating an automobile or machinery) because dizziness or lightheadedness may occur; 4) avoid excessive sunlight or artificial ultraviolet light; and 5) discontinue the quinolone and contact their physician if tremors, restlessness, or confusion occurs or a rash or other allergic reaction develops.

NOTE: Quinolones have not been approved for use in pediatric patients. Their use in pregnancy and in nursing mothers is not encouraged.

REFERENCES

1. Lesher GY, Froelich EJ, Gruett MD, *et al.*: 1,8-napthyridine derivatives: A new class of chemotherapeutic agents. *J Med Pharm Chem* 1962, 5:1063.

2. Andriole VT: Quinolones. In *Infectious Diseases*. Edited by Gorbach SL, Bartlett JG, and Blacklow NR. Philadelphia: W.B. Saunders; 1992: 244–253.

3. Andriole VT: Quinolones. Encyclopedia of Human Biology. London: Academic Press. 1991, 6:399–410.

4. Gellert M, Mizuuchi K, O'Dea MH, *et al.*: Nalidixic acid resistance: A second genetic character involved in DNA gyrase activity. *Proc Natl Acad Sci U S A* 1977, 74:4772.

5. Smith JT, Lewin CS: Chemistry and mechanisms of action of the quinolone antibacterials. In *The Quinolones*. Edited by Andriole VT. London: Academic Press; 1988: 23–81.

6. Neu HC: Quinolone antimicrobial agents. *Ann Rev Med* 1992, 43:465–486.

7. Phillips I, King A, Shannon K: *In vitro* properties of the quinolones. In *The Quinolones*. Edited by Andriole VT. London: Academic Press; 1988: 83–117.

8. Hooper DC, Wolfson JS: Mode of action of the new quinolones: New data. *Eur J Clin Microbiol Infect Dis* 1991, 10:223–231.

9. Aoyama H, Fujimaki K, Sato K, *et al.*: Clinical isolate of *Citrobacter freundii* highly resistant to new quinolones. *Antimicrob Agents Chemother* 1988, 32:922–924.

10. Bergan T: Pharmacokinetics of fluorinated quinolones. In *The Quinolones*. Edited by Andriole VT. London: Academic Press; 1988: 119–154.

11. Stahlmann R, Lode H: Safety overview: Toxicity, adverse effects and drug interactions. In *The Quinolones*. Edited by Andriole VT. London: Academic Press; 1988: 201–233.

12. Andriole VT: The future of the quinolones. *Drugs* 1993, 45(Suppl 3):1–7.

13. Andriole VT: Clinical overview of newer 4-quinolone antibacterial agents. In *The Quinolones*. Edited by Andriole VT. London: Academic Press; 1988: 155–200.

14. Andriole VT: Quinolones. In *Principles and Practice of Infectious Diseases*, edn 3. Edited by Mandell GL, Douglas RG, and Bennett JE. New York: Churchill Livingstone:1989.

The information here is provided as guidance only. Prescribers should always consult the manufacturer's current prescribing information.

CINOXACIN (Cinobac®)

Cinoxacin is one of the earlier compounds of the quinolone class of antimicrobial agents. It is derived from the cinnoline nucleus, is identified by and additional nitrogen in the 2-position of the nucleus, and also is referred to as *2-aza-4-quinolones*. Cinoxacin is a yellow-white crystalline solid with a pK_8 of 4.7. It is insoluble in water, poorly soluble in lipids, and soluble in alkaline solution. Cinoxacin is rapidly and almost completely absorbed from the gastrointestinal tract after oral administration and produces excellent peak serum levels and high urinary concentrations, which are bactericidal for susceptible microorganisms. Concentrations in human prostatic tissue range from 0.6 to 6.3 µg/g and in renal tissue exceed those in serum. Urine concentrations are decreased in patients with impaired renal function.

Cinoxacin is approved for use in adult patients with urinary tract infections. It is supplied in 250- and 500-mg capsules, given either four times or two times daily, respectively, to achieve a total daily dose of 1 g. Cinoxacin can be taken without regard to meals.

ANTIMICROBIAL ACTIVITY

Gram-negative: *Enterobacter* spp, *Escherichia coli*, *Klebsiella* spp, *Proteus mirabilis*, *Proteus vulgaris*.

RESISTANCE

Enterococcus spp, *Pseudomonas* spp, *Staphylococcus* spp, and *Streptococcus* spp are resistant.

SPECIAL PRECAUTIONS

Gastrointestinal disturbances, *ie*, nausea, diarrhea, vomiting, and dyspepsia, are the most frequent adverse reactions (2%–5%) during therapy with the quinolones. *Warning*: Central nervous system (CNS) stimulation resulting in convulsions, tremor, restlessness, lightheadedness, confusion, or hallucinations may occur, although the incidence of CNS reactions is low (0.5%–2%). Use with caution in patients with known or suspected CNS disorders (*eg*, epilepsy, severe cerebral arteriosclerosis) or other conditions predisposing to seizures. If CNS effects occur, discontinue administration. Serious and occasionally fatal hypersensitivity reactions have occurred with quinolone use (in some cases, after first dose). Reactions may include hypotension, tachycardia, loss of consciousness, tingling, pharyngeal, or facial edema, dyspnea, erythema, urticaria, rash, and pruritus. If reaction occurs, discontinue administration. Treatment with broad-spectrum antibiotics alters normal flora of the colon and may permit overgrowth of clostridia, causing antibiotic-associated pseudomembranous colitis. Mild cases usually respond to discontinuation of therapy alone; management of moderate to severe cases should include bacteriologic studies; fluid, electrolyte, and protein supplementation; and administration of an agent active against *Clostridium difficile*. Prolonged or repeated use of antibiotic agents may cause bacterial or fungal overgrowth of nonsusceptible organisms, lead to secondary infection.
Ophthalmologic abnormalities (*eg*, cataracts, multiple punctate lenticular opacities) have occurred with quinolone use. In multiple-dose therapy, ophthalmic tissue levels were significantly higher than plasma levels. No casual relationship is yet established. Crystalluria has occurred in volunteers using 800 to 1600 mg norfloxacin, and crystalluria related to ciprofloxacin has occurred rarely. Although this effect is not expected with normal doses of 400 mg twice daily, the patient should have sufficient fluid intake to ensure hydration and normal urinary output. Do not exceed recommended daily dose. Avoid substances that alkaline urine.
Reduced dosage is necessary in patients with renal function impairment.
Photosensitivity reactions have occurred with quinolone use. Excessive sunlight and artificial ultraviolet light should be avoided, and the agent should discontinue in cases of an photosensitivity. Regular monitoring of organ functions (*eg*, renal, hepatic, and hematopoietic) is advised during prolonged therapy.

INDICATIONS

Treatment of infections of the following types due to susceptible strains of designated organisms:
Urinary tract infection (initial and recurrent):
E. coli, P. mirabilis, P. vulgaris, Klebsiella spp (including *K. pneumoniae*, and *Enterobacter* spp)

CONTRAINDICATIONS

Allergy or hypersensitivity to fluoroquinolones or the quinolone group of antibacterial agents (cinoxacin and nalidixic acid)

INTERACTIONS

Theophylline, caffeine, probenecid

ADVERSE EFFECTS

Incidence < 3%: nausea, rash, urticaria, pruritus, and edema.
Incidence < 1%: anorexia, vomiting, abdominal cramps, diarrhea, insomnia, tingling sensation, perineal burning, photophobia, tinnitus, and elevations in blood urea nitrogen, alanine aminotranferase, aspartate aminotransferase, serum creatinine, and alkaline phosphatase.

PHARMACOKINETICS AND PHARMACODYNAMICS

Peak serum levels: 15 µg/mL 6 h after 500-mg dose
Plasma half-life: 1.5 h
Bioavailability: not affected by meals
Metabolism: approximately 30%, to inactive metabolites
Excretion: 97% recovered in urine in 24 h, 60% unchanged
Effect of food: reduced peak serum concentrations by 30%; total absorption unaffected
Protein binding: 60% to 70%
Renal impairment: reduced dosage necessary; not recommended if patient is anuric
Hepatic impairment: use with caution in patients with liver disease
Area under the curve: 50 µgh/mL

The information here is provided as guidance only. Prescribers should always consult the manufacturer's current prescribing information.

CINOXACIN (CONTINUED)

SPECIAL GROUPS

Children: Do not use; safety and efficacy not established.
Elderly: May have age-related renal impairment requiring reduced dosage.
Renal impairment: Reduced dosage necessary.
Hepatic impairment: No information.
Pregnancy: Not approved for use in pregnancy.
Breast-feeding: Not known whether excreted in breast milk. Not recommended for use in nursing mothers.

DOSAGE

Adults: For urinary tract infection, 1 g/d in 2 to 4 divided doses (500 mg twice a day or 250 mg four times a day) for 7 to 14 days. For preventive therapy against urinary tract infections, 250-mg single dose at bedtime for up to 5 months.
Elderly: May have age-related renal impairment; otherwise, same as adults.
Children: Safety and efficacy not established.
Impaired renal function: Dosage must be individualized based on serum drug concentrations or creatinine clearance, monitored during treatment by appropriate assay procedures.
The following maintenance dosage guide for patients with renal impairment is suggested:

Maintenance Dosage Guide for Patients With Renal Impairment

Creatinine clearance, mL/min/1.73 m^2	Dosage
> 80	500 mg twice a day
80–50	250 mg three times a day
< 50–20	250 mg twice a day
< 20	250 mg every day

OVERDOSAGE

Empty stomach by inducing vomiting or by gastric lavage. Maintain adequate hydration.

PATIENT INFORMATION

May be taken without regard to meals.
Drink plenty of fluids.
Discontinue drug and contact physician if rash or other allergic reaction occurs.

AVAILABILITY

Capsules—250 mg and 500 mg

The information here is provided as guidance only. Prescribers should always consult the manufacturer's current prescribing information.

CIPROFLOXACIN (Cipro®)

Ciprofloxacin, approved for use in 1987, is one of the newer compounds of the fluoroquinolone class of antimicrobial agents. Derived from the quinolone nucleus, it is a light yellow crystalline substance that is slightly soluble in water. Ciprofloxacin is rapidly absorbed from the gastrointestinal tract after oral administration, produces very adequate peak serum levels, and has excellent penetration into extravascular tissues and other body compartments. It diffuses into lung, skin, fat, muscle, cartilage, and bone and in bronchial secretions, sputum, skin blister fluid, lymph, peritoneal fluid, bile, aqueous and vitreous humors of the eye, and in low amounts into the cerebrospinal fluid. Ciprofloxacin produces high concentrations in urine and prostatic tissue. Urine concentrations are decreased in patients with severely impaired renal function. An intravenous preparation and an ophthalmic solution of ciprofloxacin are also available.

Ciprofloxacin is approved for use in adult patients with infections of the lower respiratory tract, skin–skin structure, bone and joint, urinary tract, and gastrointestinal tract (infectious diarrhea), uncomplicated (urethral/cervical) gonorrhea, and conjunctivitis. It can be taken orally without regard to meals, although the preferred time is 2 hours after meals.

ANTIMICROBIAL ACTIVITY

Gram-negative: *Acinetobacter* spp, *Aeromonas* spp*, *Brucella melitensis*, *Campylobacter* spp, *Citrobacter* spp*, *Edwardsiella tarda*, *Enterobacter* spp*, *Escherichia coli*, *Haemophilus ducreyi*, *Haemophilus influenzae*, *Haemophilus parainfluenzae*, *Klebsiella pneumoniae*, *Klebsiella* spp, *Legionella* spp, *Listeria monocytogenes*, *Moraxella (Branhamella) catarrhalis*, *Morganella morganii*, *Neisseria gonorrhoeae*, *Neisseria meningitidis*, *Pasteurella multocida*, *Proteus mirabilis*, *Proteus vulgaris*, *Providencia rettgeri*, *Providencia stuartii*, *Pseudomonas aeruginosa*, *Salmonella* spp, *Serratia* spp*, *Shigella* spp, *Vibrio* spp, *Yersinia enterocolitica*.
Gram-positive: *Staphylococcus aureus*† coagulase-negative spp, *epidermidis*, *hemolyticus*, and *saprophyticus*, *Streptococcus* (*faecalis, pneumoniae, pyogenes*).
*May be species dependent.
†Includes methicillin-susceptible and -resistant strains.

RESISTANCE

Most strains of streptococci are only moderately susceptible, as are *Mycobacterium tuberculosis*, *Mycobacterium fortuitum*, and *Chlamydia trachomatis*. Additionally, some strains of *P. aeruginosa* and methicillin-resistant staphylococci may develop resistance rapidly.

SPECIAL PRECAUTIONS

See Special Precautions for cinoxacin.

SPECIAL GROUPS

Children: Do not use; safety and efficacy not established.
Elderly: May have age-related renal impairment affecting pharmacokinetics.
Renal impairment: Reduced dosage necessary.
Hepatic impairment: No information.
Pregnancy: No adequate studies. Only use if potential benefit justifies potential risk to fetus. Studies indicate potential for harm to fetus.
Breast-feeding: Excreted in breast milk; ingestion levels appear to be low. Avoid use unless absolutely necessary.

INDICATIONS

Treatment of infections of the following types due to susceptible strains of designated organisms:
Oral intravenous: Lower respiratory tract: *E. coli, K. pneumoniae, Enterobacter cloacae, P. mirabilis, P. aeruginosa, Haemophilus influenzae, H. parainfluenzae, H. pneumoniae*
Skin or skin structure: *E. coli, K. pneumoniae, E. cloacae, P. mirabilis, P. vulgaris, P. stuartii, M. morganii, Citrobacter freundii, S. pyogenes, P. aeruginosa, S. aureus* (penicillinase- and nonpenicillinase-producing), and *S. epidermidis*
Bone and joint: *E. cloacae, Serratia marcescens, P. aeruginosa*
Urinary tract: *E. coli, K. pneumoniae, E. cloacae, S. marcescens, P. mirabilis, P. rettgeri, M. morganii, Citrobacter diversus, Citrobacter freundii, P. aeruginosa, S. epidermidis, S. faecalis*
Infectious diarrhea: *E. coli* (enterotoxigenic strains), *Campylobacter jejuni, Shigella flexneri**, and *Shigella sonnei**
Uncomplicated (urethral or cervical) gonorrhea
OPHTHALMIC: Corneal ulcers: *P. aeruginosa, S. marcescens*, *S. aureus, S. epidermidis, S. pneumoniae, Streptococcus* (*viridans* group)*
Conjunctivitis: *S. aureus, S. epidermidis, S. pneumoniae**
*Efficacy of this drug in this organ system studied in fewer than 10 infections.

CONTRAINDICATIONS

Allergy or hypersensitivity to fluoroquinolones or the quinolone group of antibacterial agents (cinoxacin and nalidixic acid)

INTERACTIONS

Antacids containing aluminum, magnesium or calcium; sucralfate; or divalent and trivalent cations, such as iron or zinc salts; caffeine; anticoagulants; probenecid; cyclosporine; theophylline

ADVERSE EFFECTS

The following have occurred with an incidence of < 1%: acidosis, interstitial nephritis, renal failure, polyuria, urinary retention, urethral bleeding, vaginal candidiasis, renal calculi, angina pectoris, atrial flutter, cardiopulmonary arrest, cerebral thrombosis, myocardial infarction, ventricular ectopy, postural hypotension, bronchospasm, dyspnea, epistaxis, hemoptysis, hiccups, laryngeal or pulmonary edema, pulmonary embolism, bad taste in mouth, eye pain, tinnitus, nystagmus, restlessness, oral or cutaneous candidiasis, interstitial perforation, gastrointestinal bleeding, nightmares, irritability, tremor, ataxia, anorexia, urticaria, flushing, hyperpigmentation, erythema nodosum, hepatic necrosis, exacerbation of myasthenia gravis, dysphasia, agranulocytosis, cholestatic jaundice. Nausea, abdominal pain, diarrhea*, vomiting, headache, dizziness, fatigue, lethargy, malaise, somnolence, drowsiness, dry mouth, constipation, flatulence, rash, pruritus, visual disturbances, vaginitis, hypertension, hypotension*, paresthesia, palpitations, syncope, chills, edema, insomnia (rare with all except ofloxacin), pseudomembranous colitis*, confusion*, hypersensitivity*, toxic epidermal necrosis, Stevens-Johnson syndrome, hallucinations*, seizures or convulsions*, psychotic reactions*, exfoliative dermatitis
*See also Special Precautions for cinoxacin.

(Continued on next page)

The information here is provided as guidance only. Prescribers should always consult the manufacturer's current prescribing information.

CIPROFLOXACIN (CONTINUED)

DOSAGE

Adults: Duration of treatment is based on severity of infection; usual duration is 7 to 14 days, with discontinuation at 2 days after signs and symptoms of infection have resolved. Bone or joint infection may require treatment for 4 to 6 weeks or longer.

Dosage Guidelines

Infection	Severity	Dose and route	Frequency	Daily dose
Urinary tract	Mild or moderate	250 mg orally	Every 12 h	500 mg orally
		200 mg intravenously		400 mg intravenously
	Severe	500 mg orally	Every 12 h	1000 mg orally
		400 mg intravenously		800 mg intravenously
Respiratory tract	Mild or moderate	500 mg orally	Every 12 h	1000 mg orally
Bone or joint		400 mg intravenously		800 mg intravenously
Skin or skin structure	Severe	750 mg orally	Every 12 h	1500 mg
Diarrhea, infectious	Mild, moderate, or severe	500 mg orally	Every 12 h	1000 mg

OPHTHALMIC SOLUTION: [Note: Not for injection into the eye.] For corneal ulcers, two drops in affected eye every 15 minutes for first 6 hours, then two drops in affected eye every 30 minutes for remainder of first day; on second day, two drops in eye every 1 hour. For days 3 to 14, two drops in eye every 4 hours. Treatment may be continued beyond 14 days if corneal reepithelialization has not occurred.

For bacterial conjunctivitis, one to two drops into conjunctival sacs every 2 hours while awake for 2 days, then one to two drops every 4 hours while awake for ensuing 5 days.

Elderly: May have age-related renal impairment (*see* Special Groups); otherwise, same as adults.

Children: Dosage not established.

Impaired renal function: Dosage must be individualized based on serum drug concentrations or creatinine clearance, monitored during treatment by appropriate assay procedures, and adjusted accordingly.

Recommended Doses in Varying Degrees of Renal Function

Creatinine clearance, mL/min	Usual dose
> 50	250–500 mg every 12 h
30–50	250–500 mg every 18 h
5–29	250–500 mg every 24 h
Hemodialysis or peritoneal dialysis	(after dialysis)

ADVERSE EFFECTS *(CONTINUED)*

Abnormal laboratory values may include:

Increased: alanine aminotranferase, aspartate amino-transferase, alkaline phosphatase, lactic-dehydrogenase, bilirubin, platelet count, erythrocyte sedimentation rate, serum creatinine, blood urea nitrogen, γ-glutamyltransferase, serum amylase, uric acid, blood glucose, potassium, bleeding/prothrombin time, monocytes, triglycerides and cholesterol

Decreased: platelets, blood glucose, potassium, hemo-globin and hematocrit

Other: eosinophilia, leukopenia, pancytopenia, neutropenia, crystalluria or cylindruria or candiduria, hematuria, glycosuria or pyuria, proteinuria or albu-minuria, anemia, leukocytosis

OPHTHALMIC: Burning, discomfort, lid margin crusting, crystals or scales, foreign body sensation, itching, conjunctival hyperemia, bad taste, corneal staining, keratopathy or keratitis, allergic reactions, lid edema, tearing, photophobia, corneal infiltrates, nausea, decreased vision

OVERDOSAGE

Empty stomach by inducing vomiting or by gastric lavage. Maintain adequate hydration. (Note: One patient developed oliguric acute renal failure after ingestion of 21 g of ciprofloxacin [serum concentration 12 µg/mL]. The patient responded to pred-nisone therapy.)

Hemodialysis or peritoneal dialysis may be useful in removal of drug from circulation, especially in patients with renal function impairment.

PATIENT INFORMATION

May be taken without regard to meals; however, ideal dosing time is 2 hours following a meal. Drink plenty of fluids. Discontinue drug and contact physician if rash or other allergic reaction occurs. Avoid excessive sunlight and artificial ultraviolet light.

AVAILABILITY

Tables—250 mg, 500 mg, and 750 mg

Injection—200 mg in 20-mL vials and 400 mg in 40-mL vials

Ophthalmic solution—2.5-mL and 5-mL dispensers

PHARMACOKINETICS AND PHARMACODYNAMICS

Peak Serum Levels

Plasma concentration, µg/mL	Dose, mg
Oral	
1.2	250
2.4	500
4.3	750
5.4	1000
Intravenous	
4.3	400

Area Under the Curve

µg, h/mL	Dose, mg
Oral	
4.8	250
11.6	500
20.2	750
30.8	1000
Intravenous	
4.8	200
11.6	400

Plasma half-life: *ORAL:* 4 h; 5 to 6 h

Bioavailability: *ORAL:* 70% to 80%; *INTRAVENOUS:* no information

Metabolism: *ORAL:* four metabolites identified in urine, accounting for 15% of dose; *INTRAVENOUS:* three metabolites identified in urine, accounting for approximately 10% of dose

Excretion: (urinary excretion usually complete within 24 h) *ORAL:* 40% to 50% recovered unchanged in urine; *INTRAVENOUS:* 50% to 70% recovered

Effect of food: *ORAL:* absorption delayed (2 h); overall absorption unaffected

Protein binding: *ORAL:* 20% to 40%; INTRAVENOUS: same

Renal impairment: *ORAL/INTRAVENOUS:* half-life slightly prolonged; may require reduced dosage

Hepatic impairment: *ORAL/INTRAVENOUS:* only small amounts recovered from bile

The information here is provided as guidance only. Prescribers should always consult the manufacturer's current prescribing information.

ENOXACIN (Penetrex®)

Enoxacin, approved for use in 1992, is one of the newer compounds of the fluoroquinolone class of antimicrobial agents. It is derived from the napthyridine nucleus, as is nalidixic acid, and is an ivory to slightly yellow powder, which in dilute aqueous solutions is unstable in strong sunlight. Enoxacin is rapidly absorbed (approximately 90%) from the gastrointestinal tract after oral administration and produces adequate peak serum levels, particularly with the 400-mg dose. Enoxacin is excreted primarily by the kidney and provides high concentrations in the urine, which are decreased in the elderly and in other patients with impaired renal function. Enoxacin diffuses into the cervix, fallopian tubes, and myometrium, and into kidney tissue and prostate in concentrations higher than plasma.

Enoxacin is approved for use in adult patients with urinary tract infections and in patients with uncomplicated urethral or cervical gonorrhea. The effect of food on the absorption of enoxacin has not been studied. Enoxacin has a significant drug/drug interaction with theophylline (decreases clearance of theophylline) and caffeine.

ANTIMICROBIAL ACTIVITY

Gram-negative: *Aeromonas* spp*, *Citrobacter* spp*, *Escherichia coli, Klebsiella pneumoniae, Klebsiella* spp*, *Morganella morganii, Neisseria gonorrhoeae, Proteus mirabilis, Proteus vulgaris, Providencia alcalifaciens, Providencia stuartii, Pseudomonas aeruginosa, Serratia* spp*.
Gram-positive: *Staphylococcus (epidermidis, saprophyticus)*†.
May be species dependent.
†*Includes methicillin-susceptible and -resistant strains.*

RESISTANCE

Cross-resistance with other quinolones has been demonstrated.

SPECIAL PRECAUTIONS

Not effective in treatment of syphilis. High doses of antibiotics given for short periods of time to treat gonorrhea may delay or mask symptoms of incubating syphilis. When diagnosed with gonorrhea, all patients should undergo serologic testing for syphilis. If enoxacin is used as treatment, perform follow-up serologic test in 3 months.
Animal tests demonstrate decreased spermatogenesis and subsequent decreased fertility after doses producing plasma levels three times greater than those of the recommended therapeutic human dosage.
(*See also* Special Precautions for cinoxacin.)

SPECIAL GROUPS

Children: Do not use; safety and efficacy not established.
Elderly: Plasma concentrations are 50% higher.
Renal impairment: Reduced dosage necessary.
Hepatic impairment: No information.
Pregnancy: No adequate studies. Only use if potential benefit justifies potential risk to fetus. Studies indicate potential for harm to fetus.
Breast-feeding: Not known whether excreted. Not recommended for use in nursing mothers.

INDICATIONS

Treatment of infections of the following types due to susceptible strains of designated organisms:
Sexually transmitted diseases (uncomplicated urethral or cervical gonorrhea): *N. gonorrhoeae*
Urinary tract: (uncomplicated) *E. coli, S. epidermidis*, *S. saprophyticus*; (complicated) *E. coli, K. pneumoniae, P. mirabilis, P. aeruginosa, S. epidermidis, Enterobacter cloacae*
Efficacy of this drug in this organ system studied in less than 10 infections.

CONTRAINDICATIONS

Allergy or hypersensitivity to fluoroquinolones or the quinolone group of antibacterial agents (cinoxacin and nalidixic acid)

INTERACTIONS

Antacids containing aluminum, magnesium or calcium, products containing iron or zinc; sucralfate; bismuth subsalicylate; caffeine; digoxin; anticoagulants; cyclosporine; theophylline (major interaction); nonsteroidal anti-inflammatory agents

ADVERSE EFFECTS

The following have occurred with an incidence of <1%: Anorexia, bloody stools, gastritis, stomatitis, nervousness, anxiety, tremor, agitation, myoclonus, depersonalization, hypertonia, urticaria, hyperhidrosis, mycotic infection, erythema multiforme, vertigo, unusual taste, tinnitus, conjunctivitis, dyspnea, cough, epistaxis, vaginal moniliasis, urinary incontinence, renal failure, asthenia, back or chest pain, myalgia, arthralgia, tachycardia, vasodilatation, purpura
(*See also* Adverse Effects for ciprofloxacin.)

PHARMACOKINETICS AND PHARMACODYNAMICS

Peak serum levels: 0.83 µg/mL with 200-mg dose, 2 µg/mL with 400-mg dose (50% higher in elderly patients)
Plasma half-life: 3 to 6 h
Bioavailability: 90%
Metabolism: five metabolites identified in urine, accounting for 15% to 20% of dose
Excretion: > 40% excreted unchanged in urine
Effect of food: not studied
Protein binding: 40%
Renal impairment: clearance reduced; dosage adjustment necessary
Hepatic impairment: some isozymes of the cytochrome P-450 hepatic microsomal enzyme system are inhibited by enoxacin, resulting in significant drug interactions with certain agents (*see* Interactions)
Area under the curve: 16 µg h/mL per 400-mg dose

OVERDOSAGE

Empty stomach by inducing vomiting or by gastric lavage. Maintain adequate hydration. Hemodialysis or peritoneal dialysis may be useful in removal of drug from circulation, especially in patients with renal function impairment.

The information here is provided as guidance only. Prescribers should always consult the manufacturer's current prescribing information.

ENOXACIN (CONTINUED)

DOSAGE

Adults: (1 hour before or 2 hours following meals) For urinary tract infection (uncomplicated), 200 mg every 12 hours (400 mg/d) for 7 days; (complicated) 400 mg every 12 hours (800 mg/d) for 14 days. For uncomplicated gonorrhea, 400 mg in a single dose.

Elderly: May have age-related renal impairment (*see* Special Groups and Pharmacokinetics); otherwise, same as adults.

Children: Safety and efficacy not established.

Impaired renal function: Dosage must be individualized based on serum drug concentrations or creatinine clearance, monitored during treatment by appropriate assay procedures, and adjusted accordingly.

PATIENT INFORMATION

Take medication 1 hour before or 2 hours after meals. Drink plenty of fluids.

Discontinue drug and contact physician if rash or other allergic reaction occurs.

Avoid excessive sunlight and artificial ultraviolet light.

AVAILABILITY

Tablets—200 mg and 400 mg

LOMEFLOXACIN (Maxaquin®)

Lomefloxacin, approved for use in 1992, is one of the newer compounds of the fluoroquinolone class of antimicrobial agents. It is derived from the quinoline nucleus and is a pale yellow powder that is slightly soluble in water. Lomefloxacin is rapidly absorbed from the gastrointestinal tract after oral administration and produces adequate peak serum concentrations. It is excreted primarily by the kidney and provides high concentrations in the urine, which are decreased in the elderly and in other patients with impaired renal function. Lomefloxacin diffuses into bronchial mucosa and prostatic tissue in concentrations higher than in plasma. Lomefloxacin has a long half-life that permits once-daily dosing.

Lomefloxacin is approved for use in adult patients with acute bacterial exacerbations of chronic bronchitis (except when *Streptococcus pneumoniae* is suspected) and in patients with urinary tract infections. It is associated with moderate to severe phototoxicity. Patients must be instructed to avoid sunlight and artificial ultraviolet light while receiving lomefloxacin.

ANTIMICROBIAL ACTIVITY

Gram-negative: *Aeromonas* spp*, *Citrobacter* spp*, *Enterobacter* spp, *Escherichia coli*, *Hafnia alvei*, *Haemophilus influenzae*, *Haemophilus parainfluenzae*, *Klebsiella pneumoniae*, *Klebsiella* spp, *Legionella* spp, *Moraxella (Branhamella) catarrhalis*, *Morganella morganii*, *Proteus mirabilis*, *Proteus vulgaris*, *Providencia alcalifaciens*, *Providencia rettgeri*, *Pseudomonas aeruginosa*, *Salmonella* spp, *Serratia* spp
Gram-positive: *Staphylococcus aureus*[†], *epidermidis*[†], *saprophyticus*.
*May be species dependent.
[†]Includes methicillin-susceptible and -resistant strains.

RESISTANCE

The following are generally resistant: group A, B, D, and G streptococci, *S. pneumoniae*, *Pseudomonas cepacia*, *U. urealyticum*, *Mycoplasma hominis*, and anaerobic bacteria. Cross-resistance has occurred with other quinolones.

INDICATIONS

Treatment of infections of the following types due to susceptible strains of designated organisms:
Lower respiratory tract (acute exacerbation of chronic bronchitis): *H. influenzae*, *M. (Branhamella) catarrhalis* (Note: Lomefloxacin is not indicated for the empiric treatment of the above condition if the known or suspected organism is *S. pneumoniae* [*see* Special Precautions].)
Urinary tract: (uncomplicated) *E. coli*, *K. pneumoniae*, *P. mirabilis*, *S. saprophyticus*; (complicated) *E. coli*, *K. pneumoniae*, *P. mirabilis*, *P. aeruginosa*, *C. diversus*, *Enterobacter cloacae*
Perioperative prophylaxis: To reduce incidence of urinary tract infection in postoperative period following transurethral surgery

CONTRAINDICATIONS

Allergy or hypersensitivity to fluoroquinolones or the quinolone group of antibacterial agents (cinoxacin and nalidixic acid)

INTERACTIONS

Antacids containing aluminum, magnesium, or calcium; sucralfate; nonsteroidal anti-inflammatory agents; probenecid; anticoagulants; theophylline

ADVERSE EFFECTS

The following have occurred with an incidence of <1%: Dysuria, hematuria, strangury, micturition disorder, anuria, leukorrhea, intermenstrual bleeding, perineal pain, vaginal moniliasis, orchitis, epididymitis, hypotension, tachycardia, bradycardia, arrhythmia, extrasystoles, cyanosis, cardiac failure, angina pectoris, myocardial infarction, pulmonary embolism, cerebrovascular disorder, cardiomyopathy, phlebitis, dyspnea, respiratory infection, epistaxis, respiratory disorder, bronchospasm, cough, increased sputum, stridor, coma, hyperkinesia, tremor, vertigo, nervousness, anorexia, anxiety, agitation, increased appetite, depersonalization, paroniria, gastrointestinal inflammation or bleeding, *(Continued on next page)*

The information here is provided as guidance only. Prescribers should always consult the manufacturer's current prescribing information.

LOMEFLOXACIN (CONTINUED)

SPECIAL PRECAUTIONS

Not indicated for empiric treatment of acute bacterial exacerbation of chronic bronchitis when suspected or known pathogen is *S. pneumoniae*. (Use only if sputum gram stain shows adequate quality of specimen, and a predominance of gram-negative and not gram-positive organisms exists.)
Moderate to severe phototoxicity reactions.
Avoid excessive sunlight or artificial ultraviolet light.
(*See also* Special Precautions for cinoxacin.)

SPECIAL GROUPS

Children: Do not use; safety and efficacy not established.
Elderly: Plasma clearance reduced by 25%, area under the curve increased by 33%; possibly due to age-related renal impairment.
Renal impairment: Reduced dosage necessary.
Hepatic impairment: Cirrhosis does not decrease the nonrenal clearance of lomefloxacin; dosage adjustment should be based on degree of renal function and plasma concentrations.
Pregnancy: No adequate studies. Only use if potential benefit justifies potential risk to fetus. Studies indicate potential for harm to fetus.
Breast-feeding: Not known whether excreted in breast milk. Not recommended for use in nursing mothers.

DOSAGE

Adults: (May be taken without regard to meals.) For lower respiratory tract infection (acute exacerbation of chronic bronchitis), 400 mg/d in a single dose for 10 days. For urinary tract infection (cystitis), 400 mg/d in a single dose for 10 days; for complicated urinary tract infections, 400 mg in a single dose for 14 days. For prophylaxis in transurethral procedures, give a single dose of 400 mg 2 to 6 hours before surgery when oral therapy for prophylaxis is appropriate.
Elderly: May have age-related renal impairment (*see* Special Groups); otherwise, same as adults.
Children: Safety and efficacy not established.
Impaired renal function: In patients with creatinine clearances greater than 10 but less than 40 mL/min and in dialysis patients, an initial loading dose of 400 mg followed by maintenance doses of 200 mg/d for remainder of treatment is recommended. Lomefloxacin is not removed significantly by hemodialysis (3% in 4 hours). Dosage must be individualized based on serum drug concentrations or creatinine clearance, monitored during treatment by appropriate assay procedures, and adjusted accordingly.

ADVERSE EFFECTS *(CONTINUED)*

dysphagia, tongue discoloration, bad taste in mouth, earache, tinnitus, conjunctivitis, eye pain, urticaria, eczema, skin exfoliation, skin disorder, flushing, increased sweating, back or chest pain, asthenia, facial edema, flulike symptoms, decreased heat tolerance, purpura, lymphadenopathy, increased fibrinolysis, thirst, gout, hypoglycemia, leg cramps, arthralgia, myalgia, abnormalities of urine specific gravity or serum electrolytes
The following have occurred with an incidence of $\geq 1\%$: Nausea, headache, photosensitivity, dizziness, and diarrhea
(*See also* Adverse Effects for ciprofloxacin.)

PHARMACOKINETICS AND PHARMACODYNAMICS

Peak serum levels: 4.2 µ/mL with 400-mg dose
Plasma half-life: 8 h
Bioavailability: 95% to 98%
Metabolism: approximately 9% recovered in urine as glucuronide metabolite
Excretion: renal; 65% recovered unchanged in urine (plasma clearance reduced by 25% in elderly patients, and area under the curve increased by 33%—possibly due to age-related renal impairment)
Effect of food: delays absorption (time to maximum plasma concentration prolonged by 41%; maximum plasma concentration decreased by 18%; area under the curve decreased by 12%)
Protein binding: 10%
Renal impairment: dosage adjustment necessary
Hepatic impairment: no information

Area Under the Curve

µg, h/mL	Dose, mg
5.6	100
10.9	200
26.1	400

OVERDOSAGE

Empty stomach by inducing vomiting or by gastric lavage. Maintain adequate hydration.
Hemodialysis or peritoneal dialysis may be useful in removal of drug from circulation, especially in patients with renal function impairment.

PATIENT INFORMATION

May be taken without regard to meals. Drink plenty of fluids.
Discontinue drug and contact physician if rash or other allergic reaction occurs.
Avoid excessive sunlight and artificial ultraviolet light.

AVAILABILITY

Tablets—400 mg

The information here is provided as guidance only. Prescribers should always consult the manufacturer's current prescribing information.

NALIDIXIC ACID (NegGram®)

Nalidixic acid is the first in the series of the quinolone class of antimicrobial agents. It is derived from the napthyridine nucleus, as in enoxacin, and is a pale yellow crystalline substance and a very weak organic acid. It is only slightly soluble in water but is soluble in dilute alkali and stable in urine. Nalidixic acid is rapidly absorbed from the gastrointestinal tract after oral administration, produces very high peak serum concentrations, is partially metabolized in the liver, and is rapidly excreted through the kidneys into the urine.

Nalidixic acid is approved for use in patients with urinary tract infections.

ANTIMICROBIAL ACTIVITY

Gram-negative: *Enterobacter* spp, *Escherichia coli*, *Klebsiella* spp, *Proteus mirabilis*, *Proteus vulgaris*, *Morganella morganii*, *Providencia rettgeri*.

RESISTANCE

Pseudomonas strains are generally resistant.

SPECIAL PRECAUTIONS

Perform blood counts and renal and liver function tests periodically for therapy continuing longer than 2 weeks.

Use with caution in patients with liver disease.

If no clinical response is seen within 48 hours, culture and sensitivity tests should be repeated. Underdosage may predispose to emergence of bacterial resistance. (*See also* Special Precautions for cinoxacin.)

SPECIAL GROUPS

Children: Safety and efficacy not established.

Elderly: May have age-related renal impairment.

Renal impairment: Reduced dosage may be necessary.

Hepatic impairment: Use with caution in patients with liver disease.

Pregnancy: No adequate studies. Only use if potential benefit justifies potential risk to fetus. Studies indicate potential for harm to fetus. Not recommended for use in pregnancy.

Breast-feeding: Appears in mother's milk and may be harmful to the newborn. As with other quinolones, nalidixic acid is not recommended for use in nursing mothers.

DOSAGE

Adults: 1 g every 6 hours (4 g/d) for 1 to 2 weeks. For prolonged therapy, total daily dose may be reduced to 2 g after initial treatment period. Underdosage during initial treatment may lead to bacterial resistance.

Elderly: May have age-related renal impairment; otherwise, same as adults.

Children: For children 12 years of age and younger, base dosage on body weight. Recommended total daily dose is 25 mg/kg/d in four divided doses every 6 hours. For prolonged therapy, total daily dose may be reduced to 15 mg/kg/d. Not recommended for use in prepubescent children.

Impaired renal function: Although caution should be used when administering nalidixic acid to patients with severe renal failure, therapeutic concentrations of the drug in the urine, without increased toxicity due to drug accumulation in the blood, have been observed in patients with creatinine clearances as low as 2 mL/min to 8 mL/min for patients who received full dosage.

INDICATIONS

Treatment of infections of the following types due to susceptible strains of designated organisms:

Urinary tract: Gram-negative organisms, including most *Proteus* spp, *Klebsiella*, *Enterobacter*, and *E. coli*

CONTRAINDICATIONS

Allergy of hypersensitivity to fluoroquinolones or the quinolone group of antibacterial agents (cinoxacin and nalidixic acid)

INTERACTIONS

Nalidixic acid–glucuronide conjugates may produce false–positive reaction for urine, glucose when tested with Benedicts', Fehling's solutions or clinitest reagent tablets (Ames, Elkhart, IN) but not with glucose oxidase, clinistix reagent strips (Ames, Elkhart, IN), or tes-tape (Eli Lilly, Indianapolis, IN)

ADVERSE EFFECTS

Drowsiness, weakness, cholestasis (rare), metabolic acidosis (rare), a few cases of sixth cranial nerve palsy have been observed
(*See also* Adverse Effects for ciprofloxacin.)

PHARMACOKINETICS AND PHARMACODYNAMICS

Peak serum levels: 20 to 40 μ/mL 1 to 2 h after a 1-g dose

Plasma half-life: 1.5 h

Bioavailability: no information

Metabolism: partially, in liver, to active metabolite hydroxynalidixic acid; hydroxy metabolite represents 30% of active drug in blood and 85% in urine

Excretion: renal

Effect of food: no information

Protein binding: no information

Renal impairment: dosage adjustment usually not necessary

Hepatic impairment: no information

Area under the curve: no information

OVERDOSAGE

Symptoms include toxic psychosis, convulsions, increased intracranial pressure, or metabolic acidosis. Vomiting, nausea, and lethargy also may occur. Reactions are short lived due to the rapid excretion of the drug. Gastric lavage is indicated if overdosage is realized early. After absorption has occurred, increased fluid intake is recommended as well as supportive care (*eg*, oxygen or artificial respiration). Anticonvulsant therapy may be indicated in severe cases.

PATIENT INFORMATION

Drink plenty of fluids.

Discontinue drug and contact physician if rash or other allergic reaction occurs.

AVAILABILITY

Suspension—250 mg/5 mL in 1-pint bottles
Caplets—250 mg, 500 mg, and 1 g

The information here is provided as guidance only. Prescribers should always consult the manufacturer's current prescribing information.

NORFLOXACIN (Chibroxin®, Noroxin®)

Norfloxacin, approved for use in 1986, is the first of the newer compounds of the fluoro-quinolone class of antimicrobial agents. This yellow-white crystalline solid is derived from the quinoline nucleus and is only slightly soluble in water. Norfloxacin is rapidly absorbed from the gastrointestinal tract after oral administration and produces adequate peak serum levels. It is eliminated through metabolism and biliary and renal excretion. Concentrations of norfloxacin in urine are decreased in the elderly and in other patients with impaired renal function. Norfloxacin diffuses into the uterus/cervix, vagina, fallopian tube, testicle, seminal fluid, and kidney and prostate tissues. An ophthalmic solution is also available.

Norfloxacin is approved for use in adult patients with urinary tract infections, uncomplicated urethral or cervical gonorrhea, and conjunctivitis. Food may decrease absorption of oral norfloxacin.

ANTIMICROBIAL ACTIVITY

Gram-negative: *Acinetobacter* spp*, *Aeromonas* spp, *Alcaligenes* spp, *Campylobacter* spp, *Citrobacter* spp*, *Edwardsiella tarda*, *Enterobacter* spp*, *Escherichia coli*, *Flavobacterium* spp, *Hafnia alvei*, *Klebsiella pneumoniae*, *Klebsiella* spp*, *Morganella morganii*, *Neisseria gonorrhoeae*, *Neisseria meningitidis*, *Proteus mirabilis*, *Proteus vulgaris*, *Providencia alcalifaciens*, *Providencia rettgeri*, *Providencia stuartii*, *Pseudomonas aeruginosa*, *Salmonella* spp, *Serratia* spp*, *Shigella* spp, *Vibrio* spp*, *Yersinia enterocolitica*.
Gram-positive: *Staphylococcus aureus*†, and *epidermidis*, *hemolyticus*, and *saprophyticus*; *Streptococcus* spp, *Enterococcus* spp; and *Bacillus cereus*.
*May be species dependent.
†Includes methicillin-susceptible and -resistant strains.

RESISTANCE

Resistance development is most common in the following: *P. aeruginosa*, *K. pneumoniae*, *Acinetobacter* spp, and enterococci. Not active against obligate anaerobes.

SPECIAL PRECAUTIONS

See Special Precautions for cinoxacin.

SPECIAL GROUPS

Children: Do not use; safety and efficacy not established.
Elderly: Elimination prolonged; absorption unaffected.
Renal impairment: Reduced dosage necessary.
Hepatic impairment: No information.
Pregnancy: No adequate studies. Only use if potential benefit justifies potential risk to fetus. Studies indicate potential for harm to fetus. Not recommended for use in pregnancy.
Breast-feeding: Not detected in breast milk after administration of low doses. Not recommended for use in nursing mothers.

DOSAGE

Adults: (1 hour before or 2 hours after meals) for uncomplicated urinary tract infections due to *E. coli*, *K. pneumoniae*, or *P. mirabilis*, 400 mg every 12 hours (800 mg/d) for 3 days; for uncomplicated urinary tract infections due to other organisms, 400 mg every 12 hours (800 mg/d) for 7 to 10 days. For complicated urinary tract infections, 400 mg every 12 hours (800 mg/d) for 10 to 21 days. For uncomplicated gonorrhea, 800 mg in a single dose.
Elderly: May have age-related renal impairment (*see* Special Groups); otherwise, same as adults.
Children: Safety and efficacy not established.
Impaired renal function: Dosage must be individualized based on serum drug concentrations or creatinine clearance, monitored during treatment by appropriate assay procedures, and adjusted accordingly. In patients with creatinine clearances of 30 mL/min or less the recommended dosage is one 400-mg tablet once daily for the duration of therapy.

INDICATIONS

Treatment of infections of the following types due to susceptible strains of designated organisms:
Urinary tract: (uncomplicated) *Enterococcus faecalis*, *E. coli*, *K. pneumoniae*, *P. mirabilis*, *P. aeruginosa*, *S. epidermidis*, *S. saprophyticus*, *C. freundii**, *Enterobacter aerogenes**, *Enterobacter cloacae**, *P. vulgaris**, *S. aureus**, *S. agalactiae**; (complicated) *E. faecalis*, *E. coli*, *K. pneumoniae*, *P. mirabilis*, *P. aeruginosa*, *Serratia marcescens**, *N. gonorrheae*
*Efficacy of this drug against this organism studied in less than 10 infections.

CONTRAINDICATIONS

Allergy of hypersensitivity to fluoroquinolones or the quinolone group of antibacterial agents (cinoxacin and nalidixic acid)

INTERACTIONS

Antacids containing aluminum magnesium, or calcium; sucralfate; or products containing iron or zinc salts
Nitrofurantoin, theophylline, anticoagulants, cyclosporine, probenecid

ADVERSE EFFECTS

Erythema, erythema multiforme, hepatitis, pancreatitis, stomatitis, arthralgia, myoclonus (rare) (*See also* Adverse Effects for ciprofloxacin)

PHARMACOKINETICS AND PHARMACODYNAMICS

Peak serum levels: 0.8 µg/mL with 200 mg; 1.5 µg/mL with 40 mg
Plasma half-life: 3 to 4.5 h
Bioavailability: 30% to 40%
Metabolism: 5% to 8% recovered as metabolites
Excretion: renal, biliary, and metabolism; 26% to 32% recovered unchanged in urine
Effect of food: may decrease absorption
Protein binding: 10% to 15%
Renal impairment: serum half-life 6.5 h; dosage adjustment not usually necessary (Note: In patients with creatinine clearances of ≤ 30 mL/min, the recommended dosage is one 400-mg tablet daily for the duration of therapy.)
Hepatic impairment: no information
Area under the curve: 5.4 µg h/mL per 400 mg

OVERDOSAGE

Empty stomach by inducing vomiting or by gastric lavage. Maintain adequate hydration. Hemodialysis or peritoneal dialysis may be useful in removal of drug from circulation, especially in patients with renal function impairment.

PATIENT INFORMATION

Take medication 1 hour before or 2 hours after meals
Drink plenty of fluids
Discontinue drug and contact physician if rash or other allergic reaction occurs
Avoid excessive sunlight and artificial ultraviolet light
May increase the effects of caffeine

AVAILABILITY

Tablets—400 mg

The information here is provided as guidance only. Prescribers should always consult the manufacturer's current prescribing information.

OFLOXACIN (Floxin®)

ANTIMICROBIAL ACTIVITY

Ofloxacin, approved for use in 1991, is one of the newer members of the fluoroquinolone class of antimicrobial agents. Derived from the quinoline nucleus, it is an off-white to pale-yellow crystalline substance with varying solubility (pH dependent) in aqueous solutions. Ofloxacin is rapidly absorbed from the gastrointestinal tract after oral administration, produces adequate peak serum concentrations, and diffuses into the lung, cervix, ovary, and prostatic tissues. It is excreted primarily by the kidney and provides high concentrations in the urine, which are decreased in the elderly and in other patients with impaired renal function. An intravenous preparation is also available.

Ofloxacin is approved for use in adult patients with infections of the lower respiratory tract, uncomplicated skin or skin structure infections, uncomplicated urethral or cervical gonorrhea, chlamydia urethral or cervicitis, prostatitis, and urinary tract infections. The effect of food on the absorption of ofloxacin has not been studied.

ANTIMICROBIAL ACTIVITY

Gram-negative: *Acinetobacter* spp, *Aeromonas* spp*, *Campylobacter* spp*, *Citrobacter* spp*, *Enterobacter* spp*, *Escherichia coli*, *Haemophilus influenzae*, *Haemophilus parainfluenzae*, *Klebsiella pneumoniae*, *Klebsiella* spp*, *Legionella* spp, *Moraxella (Branhamella) catarrhalis*, *Morganella morganii*, *Neisseria gonorrhoeae*, *Neisseria meningitidis*, *Plesiomonas shigelloids*, *Proteus mirabilis*, *Proteus vulgaris*, *Providencia rettgeri*, *Providencia stuartii*, *Pseudomonas aeruginosa*, *Pseudomonas fluorescens*, *Salmonella* spp, *Serratia* spp*, *Shigella* spp, *Vibrio* spp*, *Xanthomonas (Pseudomonas) maltophilia*, *Yersinia enterocolitica*, and *Staphylococcus*.

Gram-positive: *Staphylococcus aureus*[†], and *Staphylococcus* (*epidermidis*[†] and *saprophyticus*), *Streptococci** (*agalactiae, pneumoniae, pyogenes*).

*May be species dependent.
[†]Includes methicillin-susceptible and -resistant strains.

RESISTANCE

Strains of streptococci not listed, *Enterococcus* spp, and anaerobes are resistant. Not active against *Treponema pallidum*.

SPECIAL PRECAUTIONS

Not effective in treatment of syphilis. High doses of antibiotics given for short periods of time to treat gonorrhea may delay or mask symptoms of incubating syphilis. When diagnosed with gonorrhea, all patients should undergo serologic testing for syphilis. If ofloxacin is used as treatment, perform follow-up serologic test in 3 months.
(*See also* Special Precautions for cinoxacin.)

SPECIAL GROUPS

Children: Do not use; safety and efficacy not established.
Elderly: Half-life increased slightly (6–8 hours compared with normal 5 hours); absorption unaffected.
Renal impairment: Reduced dosage necessary.
Hepatic impairment: No information.
Pregnancy: No adequate studies. Only use if potential benefit justifies potential risk to fetus. Studies indicate potential for harm to fetus. Not recommended for use in pregnancy.
Breast-feeding: Concentrations in breast milk after a 200-mg dose were similar to those found in plasma of mother. Not recommended for use in nursing mothers.

INDICATIONS

Treatment of infections of the following types due to susceptible strains of designated organisms:
Lower respiratory tract (acute bacterial exacerbations of chronic bronchitis or community-acquired pneumonia): *H. influenzae*, *S. pneumoniae*
Sexually transmitted diseases: Acute, uncomplicated urethral or cervical gonorrhea due to *N. gonorrhoeae*; nongonococcal urethritis or cervicitis due to *Chlamydia trachomatis*; (mixed infections of urethra and cervix due to both *N. gonorrhoeae* and *C. trachomatis*)
Skin or skin structure (uncomplicated): *S. aureus, S. pyogenes, P. mirabilis**
Urinary tract: Uncomplicated cystitis due to *Citrobacter diversus, Enterobacter aerogenes, E. coli, K. pneumoniae, P. mirabilis, C. diversus*, P. aeruginosa**; complicated due to *E. coli, K. pneumoniae, P. mirabilis, C. diversus*, P. aeruginosa**
Prostatis: *E. coli*
*Efficacy of this drug for this organism studied in less than 10 infections.

CONTRAINDICATIONS

Allergy or hypersensitivity to fluoroquinolones or the quinolone group of antibacterial agents (cinoxacin and nalidixic acid)

INTERACTIONS

Antacids containing aluminum, magnesium or calcium; sucralfate; or divalent or trivalent cations such as iron or zinc salts; anticoagulants; theophylline

ADVERSE EFFECTS

Vaginal discharge, genital pruritus, chest pain, dysgeusia, sleep disorders, nervousness, anorexia
The following occurred with an incidence of < 1%: burning, pain, irritation of female genitalia; dysmenorrhea; menorrhagia; metrorrhagia, urinary frequency or pain, vasodilatation, cough, rhinorrhea, photophobia, anxiety, cognitive change, dream abnormalities, euphoria, vertigo, arthralgia, asthenia, diaphoresis, myalgia, thirst, vasculitis, weight loss.
(*See also* Adverse Effects for ciprofloxacin.)

PHARMACOKINETICS AND PHARMACODYNAMICS

Peak Serum Levels 1 to 2 Hours After Dosing

µg, h/mL	Dose, mg
Oral	
1.5	200
2.4	300
2.9	400
Intravenous	
2.7	200
4	400

(Continued on next page)

The information here is provided as guidance only. Prescribers should always consult the manufacturer's current prescribing information.

OFLOXACIN (CONTINUED)

DOSAGE

Adults: (Note: Patients receive the same systemic antimicrobial therapy with equivalent doses of oral and intravenous ofloxacin. No safety data are available to support use of intravenous form for more than 10 days; therefore, a switch to the oral form or other appropriate therapy should be made after 10 days.) Usual dose is 200 to 400 mg every 12 hours; see the following guidelines for both oral and intravenous therapy:

Dosage Recommendations

Infection	Description	Dose, mg	Frequency	Duration	Daily dose, mg
Lower respiratory tract	Exacerbation of chronic bronchitis	400	Every 12 h	10 d	800
Sexually transmitted diseases	Pneumonia	400	Every 12 h	10 d	800
	Acute, uncomplicated gonorrhea; cervicitis or urethritis due to *C. trachomatis*	400	Single dose	1 d	400
	Cervicitis or urethritis due to *C. trachomatis* and *N. gonorrhoeae*	300	Every 12 h	7 d	600
Skin or skin structure	Mild or moderate	300	Every 12 h	7 d	600
		400	Every 12 h	10 d	800
Urinary tract	Cystitis due to *E. coli* or *K. pneumoniae*	200	Every 12 h	3 d	400
	Cystitis due to other organisms	200	Every 12 h	7 d	400
	Complicated urinary tract infections	200	Every 12 h	10 d	400
Prostatitis	*E. coli*	300	Every 12 h	6 wk	600

Note: Intravenous infusion only. Do not administer intramuscularly, intrathecally, intraperitoneally, or subcutaneously. Avoid rapid or bolus intravenous infusion. Administer slowly over a period of at least 60 minutes. All preparations must be diluted before use (see manufacturer's information).

Elderly: May have age-related renal impairment (*see* Special Groups); otherwise, same as adults.

Children: Safety and efficacy not established.

Impaired renal function: Dosage must be based on serum drug concentrations or creatinine clearance, monitored during treatment by appropriate assay procedures and adjust accordingly.

Recommended Doses in Varying Degrees of Renal Function

Creatinine clearance, mL/min	Dosage adjustment	Dosage interval
> 50	None	Every 12 h
10–50	None	Every 24 h
< 10	One half recommended dose	Every 24 h

ADVERSE EFFECTS *(CONTINUED)*

Plasma half-life: *ORAL:* 5 to 7 h; *INTRAVENOUS:* 5 to 10 h (Elimination is biphasic; half-lives are approximately 4 to 5 h and 20 to 25 h, although accumulation at steady state can be estimated using a half-life of 9 h. Steady-state concentrations are achieved after four doses and are 50% higher than concentrations after a single dose.)

Bioavailability: *ORAL:* approximately 98%; *INTRAVENOUS:* no information

Metabolism: < 5% recovered in urine as desmethyl or *N*-oxide metabolites

Excretion: renal (and 4%–8% in feces) *ORAL:* 70% to 80% recovered unchanged in urine

Effect of food: not studied

Protein binding: *ORAL/INTRAVENOUS:* 32%

Renal impairment: clearance reduced; dosage adjustment necessary

Hepatic impairment: no information

Area Under the Curve

µg, h/mL	Dose, mg
Oral	
14.1	200
21.2	300
31.4	400
Intravenous	
43.5	400

OVERDOSAGE

Empty stomach by inducing vomiting or by gastric lavage. Maintain adequate hydration.

Hemodialysis or peritoneal dialysis may be useful in removal of drug from circulation, especially in patients with renal function impairment.

PATIENT INFORMATION

Do not take medication with food

Drink plenty of fluids

Discontinue drug and contact physician if rash or other allergic reaction occurs

Avoid excessive sunlight and artificial ultraviolet light

AVAILABILITY

Tablets—200 mg, 300 mg, and 400 mg

Injection—200 mg in 50-mL single-use containers and 400 mg in 10- and 20-mL single-use vials and 100-mL single-use bottles (both preservative free)

The information here is provided as guidance only. Prescribers should always consult the manufacturer's current prescribing information.

CLASS DESCRIPTION

The reports in 1932 by Gerhard Domagk documenting the protective activity of Prontosil against murine streptococcal infections ushered in the modern era of antibiotic therapy. This prototypical sulfa drug was an outgrowth of the German aniline dye industry and had been commercially available for several decades. Prontosil, which is chemically known as sulfachrysoidine, inhibits bacterial growth through the release of para-aminobenzenesulfonamide (Fig. 8-1). The drug was first used in the 1930s, and subsequent modifications of the sulfanilamide compound produced unpleasant side effects while expanding the antibacterial spectrum of activity. Subsequent modifications further altered pharmacokinetic properties so that some compounds are more soluble and are particularly useful in the treatment of urinary tract infections, whereas other nonabsorbable sulfonamides are used only for gastrointestinal disorders.

Trimethoprim is a 2,4-diaminopyrimidine inhibitor of folic acid metabolism through its action on dihydrofolate reductase (Fig. 8-2). Because its interference in bacterial pyrimidine synthesis is due to its inhibition of a different enzyme than the sulfonamides, the combination of trimethoprim and sulfonamides has been shown to result in synergistic potentiation of antibacterial efficacy. Since 1968, when Bushby and Hitchings first demonstrated the antibacterial synergism of sulfonamides plus trimethoprim, this combination has gained clinical acceptance globally. The combination has wide antimicrobial activity and is currently used to treat infections as disparate as bacterial urinary tract infections acquired in the community to the most common opportunistic infection in patients with AIDS, *Pneumocystis carinii* pneumonia.

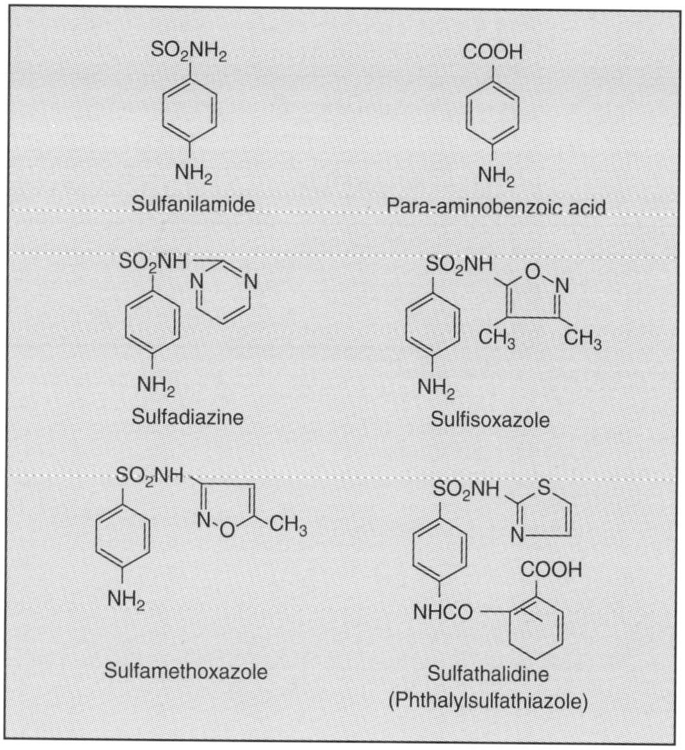

CHEMISTRY AND CLASSIFICATION

A wide array of sulfonamides that are currently used clinically are all sulfanilamide derivatives and thus are structurally similar to para-aminobenzoic acid (PABA), a factor required by bacteria for folic acid synthesis (Fig. 8-1). A free amino group at the 4 position is associated with enhanced activity. Increased activity due to increased PABA inhibition is associated with substitutions at the sulfonyl radical attached to the one carbon (as seen with sulfadiazine, sulfisoxazole, and sulfamethoxazole, all of which are more active than the parent compound, sulfanilamide). These substitutions determine other pharmacologic properties, including absorption, solubility, and gastrointestinal tolerance. The sulfonamides can be divided into four clinically useful groups: 1) short- or medium-acting sulfonamides; 2) long-acting sulfonamides; 3) sulfonamides limited to the gastrointestinal tract; and 4) topical sulfonamides.

Trimethoprim is a 2,4-diaminopyrimidine, synthesized as a dihydrofolate reductase inhibitor, and is structurally unique (Fig. 8-2). Although it has been used clinically as monotherapy in some locations such as Finland, the widespread dissemination of trimethoprim-resistant genes to plasmids and transposons has tended to limit most of its usage to combination antibacterial therapy with sulfonamides [1].

MECHANISMS OF ACTION

Sulfonamides are bacteriostatic and inhibit bacterial cell growth by competitively inhibiting the incorporation of PABA into a tetrahydropteroic acid (Fig. 8-3). Sulfonamides may have a higher affinity for the microbial tetrahydropteroic acid synthetase than the natural substrate PABA. The ultimate result of decreased folic acid synthesis is decreased bacterial nucleosides, with subsequent inhibition of bacterial growth. Trimethoprim potentiates the activity of sulfonamides by inhibiting dihydrofolate reductase and thus synergistically inhibiting the ability of bacteria to use environmental PABA in the formation of folic acid and nucleotide precursors.

ANTIMICROBIAL ACTIVITY

Sulfonamides exhibit *in vitro* inhibitory activity against a broad spectrum of gram-positive and gram-negative bacteria as well as *Actinomyces*, *Chlamydia*, *Plasmodia*, and *Toxoplasma* (Table 8-1). However, the global spread of antibiotic-resistant genes via plasmids and transposons has resulted in severe limitations in the *in vivo* spectrum of activity for this class of drugs [2]. *In vitro* antimicrobial

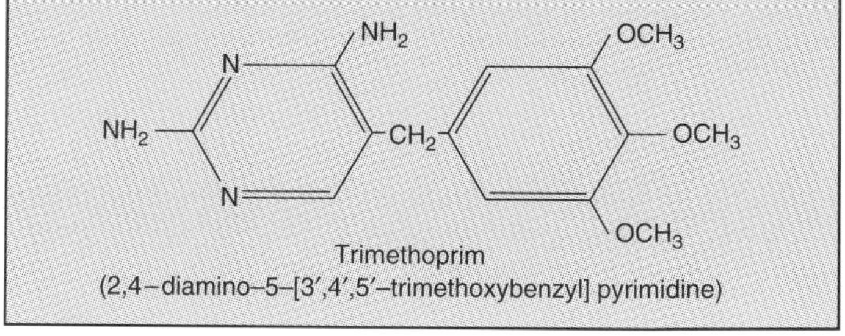

FIGURE 8-1.

Chemical structure of sulfonamides.

FIGURE 8-2.

Chemical structure of trimethoprim.

The information here is provided as guidance only. Prescribers should always consult the manufacturer's current prescribing information.

susceptibility testing of sulfonamides may be influenced by a variety of parameters, including inoculum size and the composition of the test media, particularly the concentrations of PABA and thymidine, which can be inhibitory in test media. Trimethoprim generally has a similar spectrum of action as the sulfonamides but is rarely used as monotherapy. Trimethoprim is quite active *in vitro* against many gram-positive and most gram-negative rods, except for *Pseudomonas aeruginosa* and *Bacteroides* species, *Treponema pallidum*, *Mycobacterium tuberculosis*, and *Mycoplasma* species. Most anaerobes and enterococcij6 are resistant to both trimethoprim and sulfa [3].

The combination of trimethoprim-sulfamethoxazole is active *in vitro* against many isolates of *Staphylococcus aureus*, *Streptococcus pyogenes*, *Streptococcus pneumoniae*, *Escherichia coli*, and other aerobic gram-negative rods, including *Pseudomonas pseudomallei* and *Xanthomonas* species (Table 8-1). Trimethoprim combined with sulfamethoxazole or dapsone has been highly effective in the treatment of *P. carinii* pneumonia [4], *Listeria monocytogenes* [5], *Branhamella catarrhalis* [6], and atypical mycobacteria [7].

The optimal ratio for *in vitro* synergism of trimethoprim-sulfa in combination is 1:20 [8]. Variation in resistance to one or the other drug of the combination of organisms *in vivo*, as well as pharmacologic variations in different hosts, explains some of the variations that my be seen *in vivo* and in clinical efficacy.

MECHANISMS OF RESISTANCE

Resistance to sulfonamides and trimethoprim is widespread and found increasingly in both community and nosocomial bacterial strains, including many streptococci, staphylococci, enterobacteriaceae, as well as *Pseudomonas* species [9]. Resistance to one sulfonamide generally predicts resistance to the whole class. Resistance may develop via mutation or via the acquisition of extrachromosomal elements, *ie*, plasmids or transposons [10]. Through either means, resistance may result from either overproduction of PABA or a structural change in the dihydroptoate synthetase or dihydrofolate reductase enzymes that result in enzymes with lower affinity for the antibiotic substrate. Changes in cellular permeability and metabolic requirements also have been noted as causes of increased resistance to sulfonamides and trimethoprim.

PHARMACOKINETICS

Sulfonamides may be administered orally for community-acquired infections, but several drugs of this class may be used intravenously. In the treatment of severely ill patients with trimethoprim plus sulfonamides, the intravenous preparation is used frequently. As noted below, other sulfonamide preparations are available, including ophthalmologic preparations as topical agents in the form of silver sulfadiazine and mafenide acetate for burn patients. Oral nonabsorbable sulfonamides are described below.

The short- and medium-acting sulfonamides are generally rapidly absorbed from the small intestine and stomach. Compounds with N-1 substitutions are poorly absorbed. Topical sulfonamides may be absorbed and detectable in the blood (Table 8-2) [11]. Drugs are generally well distributed throughout the body, entering the cerebral spinal fluid and the synovial, pleural, and peritoneal fluids, with concentrations approaching 80% of serum levels. Blood and tissue levels are related to the degree of protein binding and lipid solubility. Sulfonamides administered in pregnancy readily cross the placenta and are present in fetal blood and amniotic fluid.

Sulfonamides are acetylated and glucuronidated in the liver, and both free and metabolized drug may appear in the urine. Urinary excretion is more rapid for those sulfonamides with low pKa values (*eg*, sulfisoxazole), and alkalinization of the urine increases excretion by this route. Plasma half-lives vary widely, are inversely related to lipid solubility, but are not clearly related to the degree of protein binding. Small amounts of sulfonamides are found in bile, human milk, prosthetic secretions, saliva, and tears.

Trimethoprim is absorbed readily from the gastrointestinal tract, with peak serum levels occurring 1 to 4 hours after ingestion, which approach 1 µg/mL. Coadministration of sulfonamides does not effect the rate of absorption or serum levels of trimethoprim. Trimethoprim is distributed widely in tissues, and 60% to 80% of the dose will be excreted in the urine via a tubular secretion within 24 hours after administration. Trimethoprim also is excreted in the bile. Unlike sulfamethoxazole, the excretion rate of trimethoprim is increased with acidification of the urine, and urinary concentrations in healthy subjects are usually in excess of the minimum inhibitory concentration of most urinary pathogens.

The combination of trimethoprim-sulfamethoxazole can be given in the usual doses to patients with creatinine clearances of 30

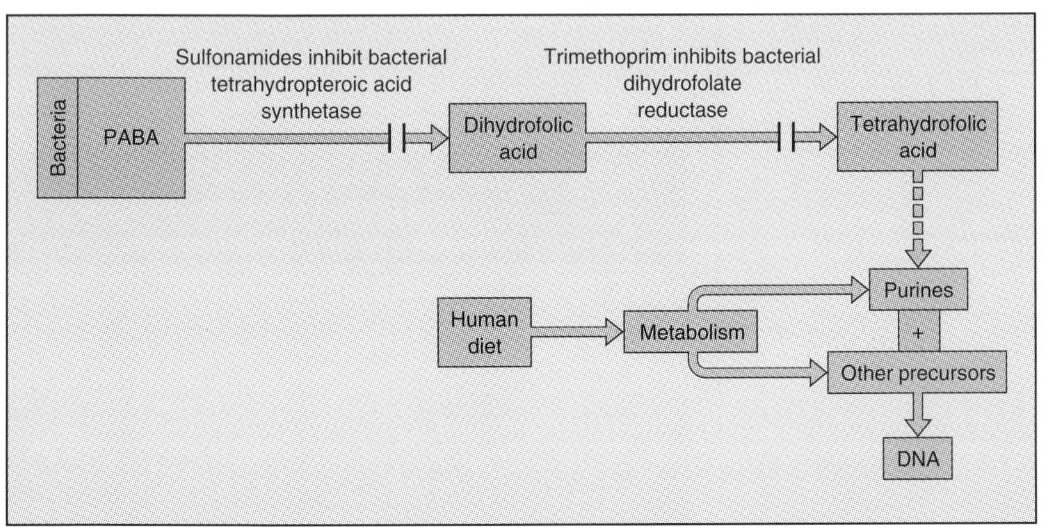

FIGURE 8-3.

Sulfonamides and trimethoprim inhibit two necessary sequential steps involved in bacterial DNA synthesis that are not essential for humans, who have other dietary sources of substrate that can be metabolized into purines and other DNA precursors. PABA—para-aminobenzoic acid.

The information here is provided as guidance only. Prescribers should always consult the manufacturer's current prescribing information.

mL/min or greater. One half the usual daily dose can be given to patients with creatinine clearances of 15 to 30 mL/min, but trimethoprim-sulfamethoxazole is not recommended for use in those patients with clearances less than 15 mL/min. Both trimethoprim and nonacetylated sulfamethoxazole are removed by hemodialysis. Patients needing chronic peritoneal dialysis can receive the equivalent of one double-strength trimethoprim-sulfamethoxazole tablet every 48 hours.

INDICATIONS

Sulfonamides were previously used as monotherapy in the management of acute urinary tract infections, but increasing resistance has diminished their effectiveness. However, sulfonamides alone may be quite effective in the treatment of infections due to *Nocardia aster-oides* [12] and in the management of infections due to rifampin-resistant atypical mycobacteria (Table 8-3) [13]. Sulfonamides have been used to treat toxoplasmosis and malaria in combination with pyrimethamine and are often used in combination with erythromycin for the treatment of acute and chronic otitis media [14]. Melioidosis, dermatitis herpetiformis, lymphogranuloma venereum, and chancroid have responded to sulfonamides [12]. Sulfasalazine (Azulfidine) has been used in the treatment of Crohn's disease [15] and other inflammatory disorders [16].

However, because of the increasing resistance to sulfamides, the combination of trimethoprim and sulfa has been used increasingly in situations in which sulfonamides alone were previously used, such as in the management of acute urinary tract infections including cystitis. Many upper respiratory pathogens are susceptible to trimethoprim-sulfa, and thus this regimen may be useful for the treatment of acute bronchitis and pneumonia due to sensitive organisms [18,19]. In many parts of the world, the combination is useful in the management of bacillary dysentery [20,21], but the increasing prevalence of resistance has reduced the efficacy of this regimen [22]. Increasing resistance also has limited the usefulness of trimethoprim-sulfa for the management of sexually transmitted diseases [23], although it may be useful in treating chancroid and lymphogranuloma venereum [24]. The combination also has been used in the management of brucellosis [25], mycetoma, *Nocardia* infection [26], Melioidosis, and Whipple's disease [27]. In addition to *P. carinii* [30,31] and *Toxoplasma gondii* [32], the combination has been clinically useful in the management of *Isospora belli* infection in immunocompromised hosts.

Sulfonamides alone have been used in the prophylaxis of patients against recurrent attacks of rheumatic fever, but the drugs are not

Table 8-1. *In vitro* Activity of Sulfonamides and Trimethoprim Alone and in Combination Against Representative Organisms*

Organism	Range of MIC, µg/mL[†]		
Gram-positive	Sulfonamide	Trimethoprim	Combination[‡]
Staphylococcus aureus	8–64	0.15–2	0.04–16
Staphylococcus epidermidis	—	0.02	—
Streptococcus pneumoniae	4–128	0.004–5	0.05–15
Streptococcus pyogenes	0.5–16	0.02–1	0.015–0.4
Enterococcus faecalis	25–250	0.15–4.0	0.05–4.0
Corynebacterium diphtheriae	25–75	0.15–0.5	0.05–0.15
Listeria monocytogenes	3–75	0.05–1.5	0.015–0.15
Bacillus anthracis	12–100	—	—
Propionebacterium acnes	—	0.07	—
Clostridium perfringens	—	2–50	—
Gram-negative			
Escherichia coli	4–64	0.01– >5	0.005– > 5
Klebsiella pneumoniae	8–128	0.15–5	0.05–3.1
Proteus mirabilis	8–128	0.15–1.5	0.05–0.15
Serratia marcescens	25– > 1000	0.8–50	0.4–50
Salmonella spp	16–128	0.01–0.4	0.05–0.15
Shigella spp	2–32	0.04–0.8	0.02–0.5
Vibrio cholerae	—	0.2	0.2
Haemophilus influenzae	1–16	0.1–12.5	0.04–12.5
Neisseria gonorrhoeae	4–32	0.2–128	0.15– > 5
Neisseria meningitidis	0.25– > 10	3.1–50	0.01–1.6
Pseudomonas aeruginosa	> 100	50– >100	3.1–100
Xanthomonas maltophilia	–	> 32	> 32
Bacteroides fragilis	–	> 4.0	> 4.0
Other			
Nocardia spp	0.1	3–100	1.5
Chlamydia trachomatis	2–16	20	2–16

*From Wharton et al. [30] and EORTC International Antimicrobial Therapy Project Group [34]; with permission.
[†]Minimum inhibitory concentration (MIC) varies with method, inoculum size, and media used. Acquisition of resistance plasmids and transposons may increase MICs. MBCs may be higher.
[‡]Trimethoprim: sulfa ratio 1:20.

Table 8-2. Pharmacokinetics of Commonly Used Sulfonamides*

Drug	Peak blood level, µg/mL[†]	Serum, % in cerebrospinal fluid	Plasma half-life, h	Protein binding, %
Sulfadiazine	30–60	40–80	17	45
Sulfisoxazole	40–50	30–50	5–6	92
Sulfamethoxazole	80–100	25–30	11	70
Sulfadoxine	50–75	20–30	100–230	80–98

*From Wallace et al. [7]; with permission.
[†]Approximate free sulfonamide level after a 2-g oral dose.

Table 8-3. Clinical Indications for the Use of Sulfonamides and Trimethoprim for the Prevention of Infectious Diseases

Prevention of

Recurrent urinary tract infections

Traveler's diarrhea

Pneumocystis carinii pneumonia

Gram-negative septicemia in neutropenic patients

Rheumatic fever

The information here is provided as guidance only. Prescribers should always consult the manufacturer's current prescribing information.

effective for the management of established streptococcal pharyngitis (Table 8-4). Trimethoprim-sulfa is frequently used for the prophylaxis of recurrent urinary tract infection and has been used to prevent traveler's diarrhea. However, the increasing prevalence of resistance to trimethoprim-sulfa has limited its usefulness for both these indications. In addition to the use of trimethoprim sulfa for the treatment of severe protozoal infections in immunocompromised hosts, the prophylactic use of trimethoprim-sulfa has been shown to reduce the incidence of gram-negative bacteremia in neutropenic patients [33,34].

Table 8-4. Clinical Indications for the Use of Sulfonamides With Trimethoprim or Other Drugs for the Treatment of Infectious Diseases

		Indicated uses of sulfonamide	
Clinical condition*	Usual causative species	Trimethoprim	Plus other drugs
Urinary tract infection	Enterobacteriaceae	+	
Prostatitis	Enterobacteriaceae	+	
Dysentery	*Shigella* spp	+	
Enteric fever	*Salmonella* spp	+	
Otitis media	*Streptococcus pneumoniae, Haemophilus flu*	+/-	Erythromycin
Bronchitis	*Streptococcus pneumoniae, Haemophilus flu*	+	
Chancroid	*Haemophilus ducreyi*	+/-	
Lymphogranuloma venereum	*Chlamydia trachomatis*	+/-	
Granuloma inguinale	*Calymmatobacterium granulomatis*	+/-	
Brucellosis	*Brucella* spp	+	
Listeriosis	*Listeria monocytogenes*	+	
Melioidosis	*Pseudomonas pseudomallei*	+	
Nocardiosis	*Nocardia asteroides*	+/-	
Atypical mycobacteriosis	*Mycobacterium fortuitum* and *ulcerans*	+/-	Other antimycobacterial drugs
Leprosy	*Mycobacterium leprae*	+/-	Other antimycobacterial drugs
Whipple's disease	*Tropherema whipplelii*	+	
Pneumocystosis	*Pneumocystis carinii*	+	
Isosporiasis	*Isospora belli*	+	
Malaria	*Plasmodium* spp	+/-	Pyrimethamine
Toxoplasmosis		+/-	Pyrimethamine

*Susceptibility testing is generally desirable when feasible given the increasing prevalence of resistant organisms.
+ —use only with trimethoprim; +/- —can be used with or without trimethoprim.

REFERENCES

1. Mennish ML, Salam MA, Hossain MA, *et al.*: Antimicrobial resistance of *Shigella* isolates in Bangladesh: 1983–1990: Increasing frequency of strains multiply resistant to ampicillin, trimethoprim-sulfamethoxazole, and nalidixic acid. *J Clin Infect Dis* 1992, 14:1055–1060.

2. Then RL: Mechanisms of resistance to trimethoprim, the sulfonamides and trimethoprim-sulfamethoxazole. *Rev Infect Dis* 1982, 4:261–269.

3. Najjar A, Murray BE: Failure to demonstrate a consistent *in vitro* bactericidal effect of trimethoprim sulfamethoxazole against enterococci. *Antimicrob Agents Chemother* 1987, 31:808–810.

4. Wofsy CB: Use of trimethoprim-sulfamethoxazole in the treatment of *Pneumocystis carinii* pneumonitis in patients with acquired immunodeficiency syndrome. *Rev Infect Dis* 1987, 9:S184–S191.

5. Armstrong RW, Slater B: *Listeria monocytogenes* meningitis treated with trimethoprim-sulfamethoxazole. *J Pediatr Infect Dis* 1986, 5:712–713.

6. Riley TV, Degiovanni C, Hoyne GF: Susceptibility of *Branhamella catarrhalis* to sulphamethoxazole and trimethoprim. *J Antimicrob Chemother* 1987, 19:39–43.

7. Wallace RJ Jr, Swanson JM, Silcox VA, Bullen MG: Treatment of nonpulmonary infections due to *Mycobacterium fortuitum* and *Mycobacterium chelonei* based on *in vitro* susceptibility. *J Infect Dis* 1985, 152:500–514.

8. O'Brien TF, Acar JF, Altmann G, *et al.*: Laboratory surveillance of synergy between and resistance to trimethoprim and sulfonamides. *Rev Infect Dis* 1982, 4:351–357.

9. Goldstein FW, Papadopoulou B, Acar JF: The changing of trimethoprim resistance in Paris, with a review of worldwide experience. *Rev Infect Dis* 1986, 8:725–737.

10. Burchall JJ, Pelwell L, Fling ME: Molecular mechanisms of resistance to trimethoprim. *Rev Infect Dis* 1982, 4:246–254.

11. Pater RB, Welling PG: Clinical pharmacokinetics of co-trimoxazole (trimethoprim/sulfamethoxazole). *Clin Pharmacokinet* 1980, 5:405–423.

The information here is provided as guidance only. Prescribers should always consult the manufacturer's current prescribing information.

12. Salter AJ: Trimethoprim sulfamethoxazole: an assessment of more than 12 years of use. *Rev Infect Dis* 1982, 4:196–236.

13. Ahn CH, Wallace RJ Jr, Steel LC, Murphy DT: Sulfonamide-containing regimens for disease caused by rifampin-resistant *Mycobacterium kansasii. Am Rev Respir Dis* 1987, 135:10–16.

14. Bernard PA, Stenstrom RJ, Feldman W, *et al.*: Randomized controlled trial comparing long-term sulfonamide therapy to ventilation tubes for otitis media with effusion. *Pediatrics* 1991, 88:215–222.

15. Peppercorn MA: Sulfasalazine: Pharmacology, clinical use, toxicity, and related new drug development. *Ann Intern Med* 1984, 3:377–384.

16. Pullar T, Hunter JA, Capell HA: Sulphasalazine in rheumatoid arthritis: A double-blind comparison of sulphasalazine with placebo and sodium aurothiomalate. *BMJ* 1983, 287:1102–1106.

17. Meares EM Jr: Prostatitis: Review of pharmacokinetics and therapy. *Rev Infect Dis* 1982, 4:475–483.

18. Stamey TA: Recurrent urinary tract infections in female patients: an overview of management and treatment. *Rev Infect Dis* 1987, 9:S195–S208.

19. Schmidt U, Sen P, Kapila R, *et al.*: Clinical evaluation of intravenous trimethoprim sulfamethoxazole for serious infections. *Rev Infect Dis* 1982, 4:332–337.

20. DuPont HL, Reves RR, Galindo E, *et al.*: Treatment of travelers' diarrhea with trimethoprim-sulfamethoxazole and with trimethoprim alone. *N Engl J Med* 1982, 307:841–844.

21. DuPont HL, Evans DG, Rios N, *et al.*: Prevention of traveler's diarrhea with trimethoprim-sulfamethoxazole. *Rev Infect Dis* 1982, 4:533–539.

22. Threlfall EJ, Rowe B, Huq I: Plasmid-encoded multiple antibiotic resistance in *Vibrio cholerae* El Tor from Bangladesh [Letter]. *Lancet* 1980, i:1247–1248.

23. Centers for Disease Control: 1985 STD treatment guidelines. *MMWR* 1985, 34(suppl):4S.

24. Plourde PJ, D'Costa LJ, Agoki E, *et al.*: A randomized, double-blind study of the efficacy of fleroxacin versus trimethoprim-sulfamethoxazole in men with culture-proven chancroid. *J Infect Dis* 1992, 165:949–952.

25. Shehabi A, Shakir K, el-Khateeb M, *et al.*: Diagnosis and treatment of 106 cases of human brucellosis. *J Infect Dis* 1990, 20:5–10.

26. Wallace RJ, Septimus EJ, Williams JH, *et al.*: Use of trimethoprim-sulfamethoxazole for the treatment of infections due to *Noccardia. Rev Infect Dis* 1982, 4:315–325.

27. Viteri AL, Greene JF Jr, Chandler JB Jr: Whipple's disease, successful response to sulfamethoxazole-trimethoprim. *Am J Gastroenterol* 1981, 75:309–314.

28. Freerksen E, Alvarenga AE, Legguizamo O, *et al.*: A new short-term combination therapy of leprosy. *Chemotherapy* 1991, 37:353–363.

29. Wallace RJ, Wissk, Bushby MB, *et al.*: *In vitro* activity of trimethoprim and sulfamethoxazole against nontuberculosis mycobacteria. *Rev Infect Dis* 1982, 4:326–331.

30. Wharton JM, Coleman DL, Wofsy CB, *et al.*: Trimethoprim-sulfamethoxazole or pentamidine for *Pneumocystis carinii* pneumonia in the acquired immunodeficiency syndrome. *Ann Intern Med* 1985, 105:37–44.

31. Klein NC, Duncanson FP, Lenox TH, *et al.*: Trimethoprim-sulfamethoxazole versus pentamidine for *Pneumocystis carinii* pneumonia in AIDS patients: results of a large prospective randomized treatment trial. *AIDS* 1992, 6:301–305.

32. Canessa A, DelBono V, De Leo P, *et al.*: Cotrimoxazole therapy for *Toxoplamsa gondii* encephalitis in AIDS patients. *Eur J Clin Microbiol Infect Dis* 1992, 11:125–130.

33. Wade JC, Schimpff SC, Hargadon MT, *et al.*: A comparison of trimethoprim-sulfamethoxazole plus nystatin with gentamicin plus nystatin in the prevention of infections in acute leukemia. *N Engl J Med* 1981, 304:1057–1062.

34. EORTC International Antimicrobial Therapy Project Group: Trimethoprim-sulfamethoxazole in the prevention of infection in neutropenic patients. *J Infect Dis* 1984, 150:372–379.

The information here is provided as guidance only. Prescribers should always consult the manufacturer's current prescribing information.

MAFENIDE (Sulfamylon®)

Mafenide (para-aminomethybenzine sulfonamide) is formulated as a cream for use in the topical treatment of burns. However, its use is limited by metabolic acidosis caused by carbonic and hydrase inhibition due to the absorption of the nonsulfa moiety of the compound. The drug has bacteriostatic activity against gram-negative and gram-positive bacteria. However, because of increasing resistance among Enterobacteriaceae and *S. aureus* and intrinsic resistance due to *P. aeruginosa*, its efficacy in recent years has been limited. Clinical decisions to use mafenide should be made in conjunction with knowledge of prevailing epidemiologic trends. In addition, obtaining burn specimens for susceptibility testing is advisable before embarking on a long-term therapeutic course. The compound is used topically to reduce the bacterial population in avascular tissue of second- and third-degree burns.

SPECIAL PRECAUTIONS

Studies of effect on reproduction capabilities and in pregnancy have not been performed. Not recommended for treatment of women of childbearing potential unless benefit outweighs risk (*eg*, more than 20% of total body surface has burn injury).

Use of mafenide may inhibit carbonic anhydrase and may result in metabolic acidosis, often compensated by hyperventilation. Close monitoring of acid–base balance is required, especially in patients with extensive second-degree or partial thickness burns or those with pulmonary or renal function impairment. (Some patients treated for burns have experienced unexplained syndrome of marked hyperventilation with subsequent respiratory alkalosis; etiology and significance of this are unknown.) If acidosis occurs and is difficult to control, discontinue therapy for 24 to 48 hours while maintaining fluid therapy to help restore acid–base balance. Use with caution in patients with acute renal impairment.

SPECIAL GROUPS

Children: Use with caution in children with extensive burns because of the possibility of significant systemic absorption.
Elderly: May have age-related renal impairment; acute impairment requires caution.
Renal Impairment: Use with caution in acute impairment.
Hepatic impairment: Use with caution in patients with severe hepatic disease.
Pregnancy: No studies performed; use only when benefits outweigh risk (*see* Special Precautions).
Breast-feeding: Not known whether excreted. Because potential for harm is not known, decision to discontinue nursing or discontinue drug is necessary.

INDICATIONS

Adjunctive treatment of second- and third-degree burns

CONTRAINDICATIONS

Allergy or hypersensitivity to mafenide. Incidence of cross-sensitivity to other sulfonamides is unknown.

INTERACTIONS

Because mafenide is only used topically because it is applied to burn surfaces, appreciable blood levels may be achieved. There are no unique interactions associated with mafenide, but attention should be paid to the potential for some of the generic interactions of sulfonamides with other medications that very sick burn patients may be receiving.

ADVERSE EFFECTS

Allergic: rash, itching, facial edema, swelling, hives, blisters, erythema, eosinophilia
Dermatologic: pain or burning on application, excoriation of new skin (rare), bleeding of skin (rare)
Metabolic: acidosis, increase in serum chloride
Respiratory: tachypnea or hyperventilation, decrease in arterial P_{CO_2}
Other: one case of bone marrow depression and one case of acute attack of porphyria have been reported; fatal hemolytic anemia with disseminated intravascular coagulation (presumably related to a glucose-6-phosphate dehydrogenase [G-6-PD] deficiency) has been reported; diarrhea has been reported with accidental ingestion.

PHARMACOKINETICS AND PHARMACODYNAMICS

Peak serum levels: no information
Serum half-life: no information
Bioavailability: no percentage given; diffuses through devascularized areas and is absorbed
Protein binding: no information
Metabolism: rapidly converted to a metabolite (*p*-carboxybenzenesulfonamide)
Excretion: metabolite is cleared through the kidneys
Renal impairment: no information
Hepatic impairment: no information

The information here is provided as guidance only. Prescribers should always consult the manufacturer's current prescribing information.

MAFENIDE (CONTINUED)

DOSAGE

Adults: Apply a thickness of 1/16 inch to clean debrided wound with sterile gloved hand once or twice daily. Thicker application not recommended. Burned areas should be covered with cream at all times; reapply to areas from which it has been removed (*eg*, by activity of patient). If necessary, use a thin layer of dressing; however, dressings are usually not required. Bathe patient daily in whirlpool, shower, or bed to aid debridement. Continue treatment until healing is well progressed or until area is graft-ready. Do not withdraw if infection is still possible. Discontinue only if allergic reaction occurs.

Elderly: May have age-related renal impairment; acute impairment requires caution.

Children: No dosage given; safety not established.

Renal impairment: Use with caution in acute impairment.

OVERDOSAGE

Because mafenide is used topically, overdosage would be very difficult to achieve through its normal means of administration. There have been no reports of the oral ingestion of the cream resulting in clinical problems. The major clinical management problem with high concentrations of mafenide systemically is that its metabolites *p*-carboxybenzene-sulfonamide and *c*-carboxybenzene-sulfonamide inhibit carbonic anhydrase, which may result in systemic metabolic acidosis. If acidosis occurs and becomes different to control, attempts can be made to compensate with respiratory alkalosis if the patient is intubated, or metabolic parameters may be shifted through the use of buffered bicarbonate solutions, which can be administered intravenously. However, if the patient has pulmonary dysfunction or difficulty in metabolic regulation because of renal insufficiency the sulfamylon cream should be removed from surfaces where it has been applied.

PATIENT INFORMATION

Contact physician immediately if hyperventilation occurs, if condition worsens, or if irritation occurs

AVAILABILITY

Cream (*Sulfamylon*, Dow B. Hickam, Inc., Sugar Land, TX), 85 mg/g (as acetate) (contains EDTA, parabens, and metabisulfite)

SULFACETAMIDE (Sultrin®)

Although *sulfacetamide* preparations were initially used in the management of urinary tract infections because of their preferential renal excretion, the resulting blood levels were too low for satisfactory systemic effects. Thus, sulfacetamide preparations are presently only in clinical use as ophthalmologic suspensions and ointments. Sulfacetamide sodium USP is available for treating conjunctivitis due to susceptible bacteria and as adjunctive therapy of trachoma, either alone or in combination with corticosteroids. Some of the preparation names include: Bleph, Cetamide, Isoph, and Sulamyd.

Sulfacetamide is a highly soluble sulfonamide available for treating conjunctivitis due to susceptible bacteria and as adjunctive therapy for trachoma. It may be used in combination with sulfathiazole and sulfabenzamide as a triple sulfa cream and topical agent for treatment of bacterial vaginosis due to *Haemophilus (Gardnerella) vaginalis*. The drugs are not given systemically because other sulfa drugs are more bioavailable, but small amounts may be absorbed when applied to the eye or intravaginally. In one case, a patient who had previously developed a bullous reaction to an oral sulfonamide developed Stevens-Johnson syndrome after exposure to the combination drug applied intravaginally. Cases of myelosuppression also have been described in conjunction with topical sulfonamides. Because of the increasing prevalence of resistance of many potential ophthalmologic pathogens (*eg*, staphylococci, *Haemophilus influenzae*, and so forth), this preparation is often not first-line therapy. Susceptibility testing of conjunctival drainage may assist in evaluating the appropriate regimen in the treatment of bacterial conjunctivitis.

INDICATIONS

Conjunctivitis, corneal ulcer, adjunctive treatment in systemic sulfonamide therapy of trachoma, other superficial ocular infections due to susceptible organisms

CONTRAINDICATIONS

Allergy or hypersensitivity to sulfonamides or any ingredients in the preparations

INTERACTIONS

Sulfacetamide preparations are incompatible with silver preparations. Sulfacetamide currently is not given systemically so therefore the interactions with albumen binding drugs such as Warfarin is theoretical. For ophthalmologic treatment, sufficient systemic levels of sulfonamides most likely will not be sustained to result in potentiating methotrexate toxicity or the hypoglycemic effect of chlorpropamide and tolbutamide.

The information here is provided as guidance only. Prescribers should always consult the manufacturer's current prescribing information.

SULFACETAMIDE (CONTINUED)

ANTIMICROBIAL ACTIVITY

Sulfacetamide is active against a wide range of gram-positive and gram-negative bacteria due to its restriction of the synthesis of folic acid (by competition with para-aminobenzoic acid), which is necessary for the growth of such organisms.

RESISTANCE

A significant number of staphylococcal isolates are completely resistant to sulfa agents. Sulfonamides are inactivated by aminobenzoic acid present in purulent exudates.

SPECIAL PRECAUTIONS

For topical ophthalmic use only; do not inject.
Sulfonamides have caused serious hypersensitivity reactions (Stevens-Johnson syndrome, fever, skin rash, gastrointestinal effects, bone marrow depression) in patients with no prior history of sulfonamide sensitivity.
Sulfacetamide preparations are incompatible with silver preparations.
Nonsusceptible organisms (including fungi) may proliferate with the use of ophthalmic ointment or ophthalmic solution.
Sensitization is possible when agent is readministered irrespective of the route of administration; cross-sensitivity between different sulfonamides may occur.
Discontinue use if signs of sensitivity manifest.
Ophthalmic ointments may retard corneal healing.
Use care to avoid contaminating dropper tip of ophthalmic solution.

SPECIAL GROUPS

Children: Do not use in infants under 2 months of age.
Elderly: May have age-related renal impairment (*see* Special Precautions).
Renal Impairment: Use with caution (*see* Special Precautions).
Hepatic impairment: Use with caution (*see* Special Precautions).
Pregnancy: Contraindicated at term; in earlier stages, use only when benefits outweigh risk.
Breast-feeding: Safe for use, except in nursing premature infants or those with hyperbilirubinemia or G-6-PD dehydrogenase deficiency.

DOSAGE

Adults: *SOLUTION*: one to two drops into lower conjunctival sac every 2 to 3 hours during daytime. *OINTMENT*: apply small amount on conjunctival sac four times daily and at bedtime.
Elderly: Same as adults.
Children: No special dosage given.

ADVERSE EFFECTS

Local irritation (stinging, burning), secondary infection
(Note: An isolated incident of Stevens-Johnson syndrome was reported in a patient who experienced a previous bullous reaction to an oral sulfonamide, and a single case of local hypersensitivity was reported that progressed to a fatal systemic lupus erythematosus–like syndrome)

PHARMACOKINETICS AND PHARMACODYNAMICS

Data are not available regarding the pharmacokenetic and pharmacodynamic properties of topical sulfonamide. The drug is felt to have very low toxicity in the amounts to which individuals are exposed when treated topically for ophthalmologic problems.

OVERDOSAGE

No information

PATIENT INFORMATION

Avoid contamination of applicator tip by contact with fingers or surfaces

AVAILABILITY

Ophthalmic solution—2.5-mL, 5-mL, and 15-mL dropper bottles
Ophthalmic ointment—3.5-g tubes

The information here is provided as guidance only. Prescribers should always consult the manufacturer's current prescribing information.

SULFACYTINE

Sulfacytine is an orally bioavailable sulfonamide that has generally been used to treat uncomplicated urinary tract infections due to susceptible organisms, particularly Enterobacteriaceae. This drug can be given every 6 hours and has a spectrum of activity comparable with other more commonly used orally bioavailable sulfonamides. Because of the increasing emergence of resistance to sulfonamides, susceptibility testing should be performed prior to the initiation of therapy with this agent.

ANTIMICROBIAL ACTIVITY
Active against a broad spectrum of both gram-negative and gram-positive bacteria as well as protozoa. Bacteriostatic ability is due to competitive antagonism of para-aminobenzoic acid (PABA), which is essential to folic acid synthesis.

RESISTANCE
Organisms may develop resistance to sulfacytine by mutation, resulting in either microbial overproduction of PABA or a structural change in a folic acid synthesizing enzyme that has a lowered affinity for the sulfonamide. Resistance may also be mediated by plasmids that may encode for the production of drug-resistant enzymes or may result in decreased bacterial cell permeability to sulfonamides.

SPECIAL PRECAUTIONS
No specific precautions have been noted with sulfacytine, independent of those precautions associated with other sulfa drugs that are systemically absorbed (*eg*, sulfamethoxazole).

SPECIAL GROUPS
Children: Not recommended for use in children under 14 years of age (except for treatment of infants with congenital toxoplasmosis, as adjunctive therapy with pyrimethamine).
Elderly: May have age-related renal impairment (*see* Special Precautions).
Renal Impairment: Use with caution (*see* Special Precautions).
Hepatic impairment: Use with caution (*see* Special Precautions).
Pregnancy: Contraindicated at term; in earlier stages, use only when benefits outweigh risk.
Breast-feeding: Safe for use, except in nursing premature infants or those with hyperbilirubinemia or G-6-PD deficiency.

DOSAGE
Adults: Give loading dose of 500 mg, followed by maintenance dose of 250 mg every 6 hours for 10 days.
Elderly: May have age-related renal impairment (*see* Special Precautions); otherwise, same as adults.
Children: Not recommended for use in children under 14 years of age.
Impaired renal or hepatic function: Usual doses can be given until creatinine clearance exceeds 30 mL/min; one-half daily dose for creatinine clearance 15 to 30 mL/min; do not use if creatinine clearance is less than 15 mL/min; sulfonamides are removed by dialysis. No dosage change is necessary with hepatic insufficiency.

INDICATIONS
Infections of the following types due to susceptible strains of designated organisms:
Urinary tract (pyelonephritis/cystitis; in absence of uropathy or foreign bodies): *E. coli, Klebsiella-Enterobacter, S. aureus, P. mirabilis, P. vulgaris*

CONTRAINDICATIONS
No contraindications have been noted that are different from other sulfa drugs

INTERACTIONS
No interactions have been noted with sulfacytine, independent of other sulfa drugs

ADVERSE EFFECTS
No adverse effects have been noted with sulfacytine, independent of other sulfa drugs

PHARMACOKINETICS AND PHARMACODYNAMICS
Peak serum levels: "free" serum levels of 5 to 15 mg/dL may be therapeutic for most infections; avoid levels greater than 20 mg/dL
Plasma half-life: no information
Bioavailability: approximately 70% to 100% of an oral dose is absorbed
Metabolism: in the liver by conjugation, acetylation, and other pathways to inactive metabolites
Excretion: renal, by glomerular filtration; tubular reabsorption occurs in varying degrees
Effect of food: no information
Protein binding: no information
Renal impairment: use with caution
Hepatic impairment: use with caution

OVERDOSAGE
No overdose information is available beyond that known for other sulfa drugs

PATIENT INFORMATION
No additional patient information is necessary beyond that used when prescribing other topical sulfa drugs

AVAILABILITY
Tablets—250 mg

The information here is provided as guidance only. Prescribers should always consult the manufacturer's current prescribing information.

SULFADIAZINE

Sulfadiazine is a highly active sulfonamide that can be given orally every 4 to 6 hours. The drug attains high blood and cerebrospinal fluid levels and is associated with low protein binding and lower solubility than most other short- or medium-acting sulfonamides. Because of its favorable pharmacokinetic properties, it is often given in combination with pyrimethamine (*see* below), particularly to treat infection with *Toxoplasma gondii*. By itself, the drug has been used as an adjunct in the treatment of chloroquine-resistant strains of *Plasmodium falciparum* and in the management of meningitis and acute otitis media due to susceptible *Haemophilus influenzae*. The drug also has been used in the management of chancroid, trachoma, conjunctivitis, nocardiosis, and urinary tract infections. However, because the increases in global resistance of bacteria in parasites against sulfonamides are equally relevant in regard to sulfadiazine, ongoing epidemiologic surveillance and susceptibility testing of clinical isolates are warranted when this drug is used.

ANTIMICROBIAL ACTIVITY

Sulfadiazine has a similar spectrum of activity as that of the other sulfonamides against a wide array of gram-positive and gram-negative aerobic bacteria, but the increasing prevalence of bacterial resistance genes has limited its usefulness as an antibacterial agent. However, sulfadiazine USP (2-sulfanil-amidopyridine) is highly active against *T. gondii* and maintains high blood and cerebrospinal levels in association with its low protein binding compared with other sulfonamides.

RESISTANCE

Bacteria may develop resistance by mutation, resulting in either microbial overproduction of PABA or a structural change in a folic acid synthesizing enzyme that has lower affinity sulfadiazine. Resistance has also been mediated by plasmids that may code for the production of drug-resistant enzymes or may result in decreased bacterial cell permeability to sulfonamides. Concerns regarding the possibility of the development of *in-vivo* resistance to sulfadiazine by *T. gondii* trophozoites has resulted in the standard usage of sulfadiazine only in combination with another antiparasitic agent, such as pyrimethamine.

SPECIAL PRECAUTIONS

Like other sulfonamides, sulfadiazine may result in nausea, vomiting, diarrhea, rash, fever, headache, depression, jaundice, hepatic necrosis, and serum sickness. Nephrotoxicity is uncommon. Acute hemolytic anemia (sometimes related to G-6-PD deficiency) is also uncommon, and other hematologic toxicities such as aplastic anemia, agranulocytosis, and clinically significant thrombocytopenia are rare. Hypersensitivity reactions that have been reported include erythema nodosum, erythema multiforme (including Stevens-Johnson syndrome), drug eruption, vasculitis, and anaphylaxis.

SPECIAL GROUPS

Children: Do not use in infants under 2 months of age (except for treatment of congenital toxoplasmosis as adjunctive therapy with pyrimethamine).
Elderly: May have age-related renal impairment (*see* Special Precautions).
Renal Impairment: Use with caution (*see* Special Precautions).
Hepatic impairment: Use with caution (*see* Special Precautions).
Pregnancy: Contraindicated at term; in earlier stages, use only when benefits outweigh risk.
Breast-feeding: Safe for use, except in nursing premature infants or those with hyperbilirubinemia or G-6-PD deficiency.

INDICATIONS

Infections of the following types due to susceptible strains of designated organisms:
Malaria: As adjunctive therapy due to chloroquine-resistant strains of *Plasmodium falciparum*, with pyrimethamine
Meningitis: Meningococcal (when organism is susceptible and for prophylaxis when sulfonamide-sensitive Group A strains are prevalent)
Otitis media (acute): *H. influenzae* (with erythromycin)
Toxoplasmosis: As adjunctive therapy with pyrimethamine
Chancroid, inclusion conjunctivitis, nocardiosis, trachoma, urinary tract infection (pyelonephritis or cystitis in absence of uropathy or foreign bodies)

CONTRAINDICATIONS

The contraindications are the same for sulfadiazine as for any of the other sulfonamides

INTERACTIONS

Sulfadiazine may displace warfarin from albumen binding sites, thus increasing the anticoagulant activity. Anticoagulant dosage should therefore be reduced during sulfadiazine therapy. Sulfadiazine may displace methotrexate from its bound protein, thereby increasing methotrexate toxicity. It may increase the hypoglycemic effect of chlorpropamide and tolbutamide. Sulfadiazine may potentiate the action of thiazide diuretics, phenytoin, and uricosuric agents. Sulfonamide activity may be increased because of displacement from binding sites by indomethacin, phenylbutazone, salicylates, and probenecid. Activity of sulfadiazine may be decreased by procaine and other local anesthetics derived from PABA.

ADVERSE EFFECTS

No specific adverse effects have been noted with sulfadiazine, beyond those noted with other systemically absorbed sulfa drugs (*eg*, sulfamethoxazole)

PHARMACOKINETICS AND PHARMACODYNAMICS

Peak serum levels: "free" serum levels of 5 to 15 mg/dL may be therapeutic for most infections; avoid levels over 20 mg/dL
Plasma half-life: no information
Bioavailability: approximately 70% to 100% of an oral dose is absorbed
Metabolism: in the liver by conjugation, acetylation, and other pathways to inactive metabolites
Excretion: renal, by glomerular filtration; tubular reabsorption occurs in varying degrees
Effect of food: no information
Protein binding: no information
Renal impairment: use with caution
Hepatic impairment: use with caution

The information here is provided as guidance only. Prescribers should always consult the manufacturer's current prescribing information.

SULFADIAZINE (CONTINUED)

DOSAGE

Adults: Give loading dose of 2 to 4 mg, followed by maintenance dose of 4 to 8 g/d in divided doses every 4 to 6 hours. For prevention of recurrent attacks of rheumatic fever in patients over 30 kg, give 1 g/d; in patients under 30 kg, give 0.5 g/d. (Note: Not recommended for initial therapy of streptococcal infection.)

Elderly: May have age-related renal impairment (*see* Special Precautions); otherwise, same as adults.

Children: Infants and children over 2 months of age, give loading dose of 75 mg/kg (or 2 g/m^2) and maintenance dose of 120 to 150 mg/kg/d (4 g/m^2/d) in divided doses every 4 to 6 hours. For infants under 2 months of age as adjunctive therapy with pyrimethamine in treatment of congenital toxoplasmosis, give loading dose of 75 to 100 mg/kg and maintenance dose of 100 to 150 mg/kg/d in divided doses every 6 hours. (Note: Contraindicated in infants under 2 months of age for any use other than that specified above.)

Impaired renal or hepatic function: Usual doses can be given until creatinine clearance exceeds 30 mL/min; one-half daily dose for creatinine clearance 15 to 30 mL/min; do not use if creatinine clearance is less than 15 mL/min; sulfonamides are removed by dialysis. No dosage change is necessary with hepatic insufficiency.

OVERDOSAGE

No overdose information is available beyond that known for other sulfa drugs

PATIENT INFORMATION

No additional patient information is necessary beyond that used when prescribing other topical sulfa drugs

AVAILABILITY

Tablets—500 mg

SULFADOXINE-PYRIMETHAMINE (Fansidar®)

Sulfadoxine is a very long-acting sulfonamide that has been sold in combination with *pyrimethamine*. Sulfadoxine has a half-life of 100 to 230 hours and reaches a peak serum level of 51 to 76 µg/mL 2.5 to 6 hours after an oral dose of 500 mg. The combination is known as Fansidar® (Roche, Nutley, NJ) and is active in the treatment and prophylaxis of malaria due to chloroquine-resistant *Plasmodium falciparum*. It also has been used for the secondary prophylaxis for *Pneumocystis carinii* pneumonia and toxoplasmosis in patients with AIDS.

Fatalities have occurred as a result of Stevens-Johnson syndrome and toxic epidermal necrolysis. Because of its long half-life, the potential for any rash to evolve and pose serious clinical problems has led to a decrease in the frequency of using this combination. In addition, some strains of *P. falciparum* from Southeast Asia and South America have been found to be resistant. Thus, careful knowledge of the susceptibility patterns of malaria in specific locales is critical in allowing appropriate clinical decisions regarding use of this combination. Because of the very long half-life and potential for significant toxicity, the use of sulfadoxine by pregnant women is discouraged.

ANTIMICROBIAL ACTIVITY

Sulfadoxine-pyrimethamine is an antimalarial agent, effective because of reciprocal potentiation of its components, which is achieved by sequential blockade of two enzymes involved in the biosynthesis of acid within parasites. Pyrimethamine inhibits enzyme dihydrofolate reductase, which catalyzes reduction of dihydrofolate to tetrahydrofolate and is important to cellular biosynthesis of purines, pyrimidines, and some amino acids.

Sulfadoxine inhibits bacteria and protozoa by interference with microbial folic acid synthesis by competitively inhibiting the incorporation of PABA into tetrahydropteroic acid, thereby preventing the incorporation into dihydropteroate, which is necessary to the generation of microbial DNA.

Sulfadoxine has a higher affinity for the microbial enzyme tetrahydropteroic acid synthetase than the natural substrate PABA.

INDICATIONS

Treatment of malaria due to *P. falciparum* in patients for whom chloroquine resistance is suspected or known.

Prophylaxis of malaria for travelers to areas where chloroquine-resistant *P. falciparum* malaria is endemic. It should be noted that resistant strains may be encountered; it is therefore still possible to contract malaria regardless of prophylaxis.

Sulfadoxine-pyrimethamine has been used as a prophylaxis for *P. carinii* pneumonia in patients with AIDS, most commonly as a second-line agent.

CONTRAINDICATIONS

Allergy or hypersensitivity to sulfonamides or pyrimethamine

Documented megaloblastic anemia due to folate deficiency

Severe renal impairment, liver parenchymal damage, or blood dyscrasias

Because of the unknown teratogenic potential of pyrimethamine and the extremely long half-life of sulfadoxine, the combination is not recommended for the prophylaxis and treatment of malaria in pregnant women

INTERACTIONS

Antifolic agents (methotrexate, sulfonamides, trimethoprim-sulfamethoxazole).

Sulfadoxine may displace warfarin from albumen binding sites thereby increasing its anticoagulant activity. Sulfonamides may also displace methotrexate from bound protein thereby increasing methotrexate toxicity. *(continued on next page)*

The information here is provided as guidance only. Prescribers should always consult the manufacturer's current prescribing information.

SULFADOXINE-PYRIMETHAMINE (CONTINUED)

RESISTANCE

Organisms may develop resistance by mutation resulting in either microbial over-production of PABA or a structural change in a folic acid synthesizing enzyme that has a lowered affinity for sulfadoxine and/or pyrimethamine. Resistance may also be mediated by plasmids that may code for the production of drug resistant enzymes such as hydropteroate synthetase, or it may result in decreased microbial cell permeability to sulfonamides.

SPECIAL PRECAUTIONS

Fatalities associated with sulfadoxine-pyrimethamine have occurred as a result of severe reactions (including Stevens-Johnson syndrome and toxic epidermal necrolysis). Discontinue use if skin rash occurs, if any blood count is reduced significantly, or if active secondary bacterial or fungal infection occurs.
Contraindicated as prophylactic agent in patients with severe renal impairment or marked liver parenchymal damage.
Pyrimethamine is mutagenic in laboratory animals and human bone marrow following 3 to 4 consecutive daily doses totaling 200 to 300 mg. Testicular changes have been seen in rats treated with 105 mg/kg/d of the combination and with 15 mg/kg/d of pyrimethamine alone.
Use with caution in patients with possible folate deficiency, severe allergy, or bronchial asthma. Microscopic urinalysis and renal function tests should be performed during therapy for patients with impaired renal function.
Hemolysis may occur in patients with G-6-PD deficiency.
Discontinue drug if signs of folic acid deficiency develop. Administer folinic acid (leucovorin) 5 to 15 mg intramuscularly daily for at least 3 days if recovery from depressed platelet or white cell counts is too slow.

SPECIAL GROUPS

Children: Do not use in infants under 2 months of age.
Elderly: May have age-related renal impairment (*see* Special Precautions).
Renal impairment: Use with caution (*see* Special Precautions).
Hepatic impairment: Use with caution (*see* Special Precautions).
Pregnancy: Contraindicated at term; in earlier stages, use only when benefits outweigh risk.
Breast-feeding: Discontinue nursing during treatment.

DOSAGE

Adults: For acute malarial attack, two to three tablets. For malarial prophylaxis, one table per week or two tablets every 2 weeks.
Elderly: May have age-related renal impairment (*see* Special Precautions); otherwise, same as adults.
Children: *See* table below.

Dosage of Sulfadoxine-Pyrimethamine (Fansidar®) for Malaria Treatment and Prophylaxis in Children and Adolescents

Age, y	Acute malarial attack, tablets*	Malarial prophylaxis†	
		Once weekly, tablets	Once every 2 weeks, tablets
9–14	2	0.75	1.5
4–8	1	0.5	1
<4	0.5	0.25	0.5

*Single dose used in sequence with quinine or alone.
†Take first dose 1 to 2 days before departure to an endemic area; continue administration throughout stay and for 4 to 6 weeks after return.

Impaired renal or hepatic function: Use with caution. Contraindicated in severe renal impairment or marked liver parenchymal damage (*see* Special Precautions).

INTERACTIONS *(CONTINUED)*

Sulfadoxine may potentiate the hypoglycemic effect of chlorpropamide and talbutamide. Sulfadoxine may potentiate the action of thiazide diuretics, phenytoin, and uricosuric agents. Sulfadoxine activity may be potentiated by indomethacin, phenolbutizone, salicylates, and probenecid. Activity of sulfadoxine may be decreased by procaine and other local anesthetics derived from PABA.

ADVERSE EFFECTS

Sulfadoxine may cause nausea, vomiting, diarrhea, rash, fever, headache, depression, jaundice, hepatic necrosis, and a serum sickness–type illness. Toxicity is uncommon. Hematologic abnormalities include acute hemolytic anemia, sometimes related to G-6-PD deficiency, as well as less commonly aplastic anemia, agranulocytosis, and clinically significant thrombocytopenia. Because of the extremely long half-life of sulfadoxine, the hypersensitivity reactions have occasionally been extremely serious and rarely fatal, including Stevens-Johnson syndrome. More frequently, and less clinically serious, are erythema nodosum, erythema multiforme, drug eruption, vasculitis, and anaphylaxis.

PHARMACOKINETICS AND PHARMACODYNAMICS

Peak serum levels: 51 to 76 µg/mL in 2.5 to 6 h (sulfadoxine) and 0.13 to 0.4 µg/mL in 1.5 to 8 h (pyrimethamine) after a one-tablet dose
Plasma half-life: 100 to 231 h (sulfadoxine) and 54 to 148 h (pyrimethamine)
Bioavailability: sulfadoxine is readily absorbed from the gastrointestinal tract; it is highly protein bound and therefore has a long half-life of 100 to 230 h
Metabolism: sulfadoxine undergoes minimal hepatic metabolism
Excretion: renal
Effect of food: food has not been shown to affect gastrointestinal absorption
Protein binding: 80% to 98% protein bound
Renal impairment: use with caution because of long half-life and renal excretion, which is the primary mode of elimination
Hepatic impairment: no contraindication for use with patients with mild hepatic insufficiency; use with caution in patients with severe disease

OVERDOSAGE

Monitor renal and hematopoietic systems for a minimum of 1 month after overdose. Administer leucovorin 5 to 15 mg intramuscularly daily for 3 days or longer to correct depressed platelet or white cell counts.

PATIENT INFORMATION

If undergoing prophylaxis therapy, it should be noted that it is still possible to contract malaria regardless of agent used. Medical attention should be sought immediately in the event of febrile illness.
Contraceptive measures should be taken to prevent pregnancy during therapy.

AVAILABILITY

Tablets—500 mg sulfadoxine with 25 mg pyrimethamine

The information here is provided as guidance only. Prescribers should always consult the manufacturer's current prescribing information.

SULFAMETHIZOLE (Thiosulfil®)

Sulfamethizole is most commonly used for the treatment of urinary tract infections, particularly those due to Enterobacteriaceae and, less frequently, *Staphylococcus aureus*. Because of the increasing development of resistance to sulfonamides, it is recommended that urinary cultures and susceptibilities be obtained prior to initiation of therapy. The drug has been combined previously with tetracycline, but this preparation is available only in Europe. The drug has been combined with a urinary analgesic, phenazopyridine.

ANTIMICROBIAL ACTIVITY

Sulfamethizole exhibits an inhibitory activity against a broad spectrum of gram-positive and gram-negative bacteria, as well as actinomyces, chlamydia, plasmodia, and toxoplasma. However, resistance to sulfamethizole is widespread and increasing and is found between one third and more than one half of community and nosocomial strains of bacteria, including Staphylococci, Enterobacteriaceae, *Neisseria meningitidis*, and *Pseudomonas* species. Susceptibility testing should be performed when using sulfamethoxazole as monotherapy, even for uncomplicated community-acquired infections.

RESISTANCE

Resistance may develop by mutation, either resulting in microbial overproduction of PABA, or a structural change in a folic acid–synthesizing enzyme that has a lowered affinity for sulfonamide. A former mechanism has been implicated in resistant strains of *Neisseria gonorrhea* and *S. aureus*, and the latter has been found in strains of *Escherichia coli*. Resistance may also be mediated by plasmids that may code for the production of drug-resistant enzymes such as dihydropteroate synthetase, or it may result in decreased bacterial cell permeability to sulfonamides. More than one mechanism of resistance to sulfonamides may be present in a single bacterial isolate.

SPECIAL PRECAUTIONS

Elderly patients receiving certain diuretics (especially thiazide) concurrently have increased incidence of thrombocytopenia and purpura.
May prolong prothrombin time in patients receiving the anticoagulant warfarin.
May inhibit hepatic metabolism of phenytoin; be alert for possible excessive phenytoin effect.
May interfere with Jaffé alkaline picrate reaction assay for creatinine, resulting in an overestimation of approximately 10% in the range of normal values.

SPECIAL GROUPS

Children: Do not use in infants under 2 months of age.
Elderly: May have age-related renal impairment (*see* Special Precautions).
Renal Impairment: Use with caution (*see* Special Precautions).
Hepatic impairment: Use with caution (*see* Special Precautions).
Pregnancy: Contraindicated at term; in earlier stages, use only when benefits outweigh risk.
Breast-feeding: Safe for use, except in nursing premature infants or those with hyperbilirubinemia or G-6-PD deficiency.

INDICATIONS

Infections of the following types due to susceptible strains of designated organisms:
Urinary tract (pyelonephritis or cystitis in absence of uropathy or foreign bodies): *E. coli*, *Klebsiella-Enterobacter*, *P. mirabilis*, and *P. vulgaris*

CONTRAINDICATIONS

Allergy or hypersensitivity to sulfonamides. Patients with documented megaloblastic anemia due to folate deficiency. Patients with severe renal impairment and/or liver parenchymal damage or blood dyscrasias.

INTERACTIONS

No interactions have been noted with sulfamethizole, independent of other sulfa drugs

ADVERSE EFFECTS

No adverse effects have been noted with sulfamethizole, independent of other sulfa drugs

PHARMACOKINETICS AND PHARMACODYNAMICS

Peak serum levels: no information
Plasma half-life: no information
Bioavailability: 95%
Metabolism: less than 5% of a given dose is acetylated
Excretion: renal
Effect of food: no information
Protein binding: no information
Renal impairment: use with caution
Hepatic impairment: use with caution

OVERDOSAGE

The amount of a single dose that is associated with symptoms of overdosage or is likely to be life threatening has not been reported. Signs and symptoms of overdosage with sulfamethizole include anorexia, colic, nausea, vomiting, headache, dizziness, drowsiness, and unconsciousness. Fever, hematuria, and crystalluria may be noted. Blood dyscrasias and jaundice are potential late manifestations of overdosage. General principles of treatment include the immediate discontinuation of the drug, instituting gastric lavage or emesis, forcing oral fluids, and administering intravenous fluids if urine output is low and renal function is normal. The patient should be monitored with blood counts and appropriate blood chemistries, including electrolytes. If the patient becomes cyanotic, the possibility of methemoglobinemia should be considered, and if present, the condition should be treated appropriately with intravenous 1% methaline blue. If significant blood dyscrasia or jaundice occurs, specific therapy should be instituted for these complications. Peritoneal dialysis is not effective, and hemodialysis is only moderately effective in removing sulfonamides.

The information here is provided as guidance only. Prescribers should always consult the manufacturer's current prescribing information.

SULFAMETHIZOLE (CONTINUED)

DOSAGE

Adults: 0.5 to 1 g every 6 to 8 hours.

Elderly: May have age-related renal impairment (*see* Special Precautions); otherwise same as adults.

Children: Infants and children over 2 months of age, 30 to 45 mg/kg/d in divided doses every 6 hours.

Impaired renal or hepatic function: Usual doses can be given until creatinine clearance exceeds 30 mL/min; one-half daily dose for creatinine clearance 15 to 30 mL/min; do not use if creatinine clearance is less than 15 mL/min; sulfonamides are removed by dialysis. No dosage change is necessary with hepatic insufficiency.

PATIENT INFORMATION

Sulfamethizole is used for the treatment of urinary tract infections caused by sensitive organisms. If this drug is prescribed, it is important that a urine culture be obtained prior to initiating therapy. It is advisable to drink lots of fluids (at least eight glasses of fluids a day) while taking this drug.

AVAILABILITY

Tablets—500 mg

SULFAMETHOXAZOLE (Gantanol®)

Sulfamethoxazole is a medium-duration, orally bioavailable sulfonamide that is generally used for the management of urinary tract infections. It is the sulfonamide that has been combined successfully with trimethoprim for synergism. As a single agent, its primary use has been in the treatment of uncomplicated urinary tract infections caused by susceptible strains of Enterobacteriaceae and, less frequently, *Staphylococcus aureus*. Because of the increasing resistance of community-derived isolates, routine testing of urinary tract isolates is recommended if patients are placed on this medication. The most commonly sold preparation containing sulfamethoxazole is a combination with phenazopyridine, a urinary analgesic.

ANTIMICROBIAL ACTIVITY

Sulfamethoxazole exhibits an inhibitory activity against a broad spectrum of gram-positive and gram-negative bacteria, as well as actinomyces, chlamydia, plasmodia, and toxoplasma. However, resistance to sulfamethoxazole is widespread and increasing and is found between one third and more than one half of community and nosocomial strains of bacteria, including Staphylococci, Enterobacteriaceae, *Neisseria meningitidis*, and *Pseudomonas* species. Susceptibility testing should be performed when using sulfamethoxazole as monotherapy, even for uncomplicated community-acquired infections.

RESISTANCE

Resistance may develop by mutation, either resulting in microbial overproduction of PABA, or a structural change in a folic acid–synthesizing enzyme that has a lowered affinity for sulfonamide. The former mechanism has been implicated in resistant strains of *Neisseria gonorrhea* and *S. aureus*, and the latter has been found in strains of *Escherichia coli*. Resistance may also be mediated by plasmids that may code for the production of drug-resistant enzymes such as dihydropteroate synthetase, or it may result in decreased bacterial cell permeability to sulfonamides. More than one mechanism of resistance to sulfonamides may be present in a single bacterial isolate.

INDICATIONS

Infections of the following types due to susceptible strains of designated organisms:

Meningitis: Meningococcal (when organism is susceptible and when sulfonamide-sensitive Group A strains are prevalent)

Otitis media (acute): *H. influenzae* (with erythromycin)

Toxoplasmosis: As adjunctive therapy with pyrimethamine

Urinary tract (pyelonephritis/cystitis; in absence of uropathy or foreign bodies): *E. coli*, *Klebsiella-Enterobacter*, *Proteus mirabilis*, and *Proteus vulgaris*

Chancroid, inclusion conjunctivitis, nocardiosis, trachoma

CONTRAINDICATIONS

Allergy or hypersensitivity to sulfonamides. Patients with documented megaloblastic anemia due to folate deficiency. Patients with severe renal impairment and/or liver parenchymal damage or blood dyscrasias.

INTERACTIONS

No interactions have been noted with sulfamethoxazole, independent of other sulfa drugs

ADVERSE EFFECTS

No adverse effects have been noted with sulfamethoxazole, independent of other sulfa drugs

The information here is provided as guidance only. Prescribers should always consult the manufacturer's current prescribing information.

SULFAMETHOXAZOLE (CONTINUED)

SPECIAL PRECAUTIONS

Elderly patients receiving certain diuretics (especially thiazide) concurrently have increased incidence of thrombocytopenia and purpura.

May prolong prothrombin time in patients receiving the anticoagulant warfarin.

May inhibit hepatic metabolism of phenytoin; be alert for possible excessive phenytoin effect.

May interfere with Jaffé alkaline picrate reaction assay for creatinine, resulting in an overestimation of approximately 10% in the range of normal values.

SPECIAL GROUPS

Children: Do not use in infants under 2 months of age. Insufficient data exist on prolonged or repeated therapy in chronic renal disease of children under 6 years of age.

Elderly: May have age-related renal impairment (*see* Special Precautions).

Renal Impairment: Use with caution (*see* Special Precautions).

Hepatic impairment: Use with caution (*see* Special Precautions).

Pregnancy: Contraindicated at term; in earlier stages, use only when benefits outweigh risk.

Breast-feeding: Discontinue nursing during therapy.

DOSAGE

Adults: For mild to moderate infection, give initial dose of 2 g, followed by maintenance dose of 1 g in the morning and 1 g in the evening thereafter. For severe infection, give initial dose of 2 g, followed by maintenance dose of 1 g every 8 hours.

Elderly: May have age-related renal impairment (*see* Special Precautions); otherwise, same as adults.

Children: For infants and children over 2 months of age, give initial dose of 50 to 60 mg/kg and maintenance dose of 25 to 30 mg/kg in the morning and evening. Do not exceed 75 mg/kg/d. An alternative regimen is 50 mg/kg/d in divided doses every 12 hours, not exceeding 3 g/24 h.

Impaired renal or hepatic function: Usual doses can be given until creatinine clearance exceeds 30 mL/min; one-half daily dose for creatinine clearance 15 to 30 mL/min; do not use if creatinine clearance is less than 15 mL/min; sulfonamides are removed by dialysis. No dosage change is necessary with hepatic insufficiency.

PHARMACOKINETICS AND PHARMACODYNAMICS

Peak serum levels: 38 µg/mL in 2 hours after single 1-g oral dose

Plasma half-life: 10 h

Bioavailability: widely distributed; no percentages given

Metabolism: in liver, predominantly by N_4-acetylation, although the glucuronide conjugate has been identified

Excretion: renal; by glomerular filtration and tubular secretion

Effect of food: no information

Protein binding: 70%

Renal impairment: increased half-life requires dosage adjustment (creatinine clearance < 30 mL/min)

Hepatic impairment: use with caution (*see* Special Precautions)

OVERDOSAGE

The amount of a single dose that is associated with symptoms of overdosage or is likely to be life threatening has not been reported. Signs and symptoms of overdosage with sulfamethoxazole include anorexia, colic, nausea, vomiting, headache, dizziness, drowsiness, and unconsciousness. Fever, hematuria, and crystalluria may be noted. Blood dyscrasias and jaundice are potential late manifestations of overdosage. General principles of treatment include the immediate discontinuation of the drug, instituting gastric lavage or emesis, forcing oral fluids, and administering intravenous fluids if urine output is low and renal function is normal. The patient should be monitored with blood counts and appropriate blood chemistries, including electrolytes. If the patient becomes cyanotic, the possibility of methemoglobinemia should be considered, and if present, the condition should be treated appropriately with intravenous 1% methaline blue. If significant blood dyscrasia or jaundice occurs, specific therapy should be instituted for these complications. Peritoneal dialysis is not effective, and hemodialysis is only moderately effective in removing sulfonamides.

PATIENT INFORMATION

Sulfamethoxazole is used for the treatment of urinary tract infections caused by sensitive organisms. If this drug is prescribed, it is important that a urine culture be obtained prior to initiating therapy. It is advisable to drink lots of fluids (at least eight glasses of fluids a day) while taking this drug.

AVAILABILITY

Tablets—500 mg
Oral suspension—500 mg/5 mL

The information here is provided as guidance only. Prescribers should always consult the manufacturer's current prescribing information.

SULFASALAZINE (Azulfidine®)

Sulfasalazine, also known as *salicylazosulfapyridine*, is a sulfonamide derivative used in the treatment of ulcerative colitis. The drug is absorbed in its parent form as sulfpuridine, and significant blood levels of the compound may be measurable in patients undergoing therapy for inflammatory bowel disease. There are no oral or intravenous preparations available for clinical use. It is thought that the major activity of sulfasalazine is its anti-inflammatory activity in the distal bowel, which is primarily due to the dissociation of the compound into a salicylate that exerts a local antiprostaglandin effect in the bowel. The drug does not have a specifically demonstrated, clinically relevant antibacterial effect.

Because the drug may be partially absorbed, patients may develop skin eruptions and blood dyscrasias while receiving this medication. However, it is generally not well absorbed, and therefore the most common adverse reactions are anorexia, nausea, vomiting, gastric distress, and, less commonly, headache. When the daily dose reaches 4 g or more and sulfapyridine levels rise above 50 µg/mL, the incidence of adverse reactions tends to increase.

ANTIMICROBIAL ACTIVITY

Sulfamethoxazole exhibits an inhibitory activity against a broad spectrum of gram-positive and gram-negative bacteria, as well as actinomyces, chlamydia, plasmodia, and toxoplasma. However, resistance to sulfamethoxazole is widespread and increasing and is found between one third and more than one half of community and nosocomial strains of bacteria, including Staphylococci, Enterobacteriaceae, *Neisseria meningitidis*, and *Pseudomonas* spp. Susceptibility testing should be performed when using sulfamethoxazole as monotherapy, even for uncomplicated community-acquired infections.

RESISTANCE

Resistance may develop by mutation, either resulting in microbial overproduction of PABA, or a structural change in a folic acid–synthesizing enzyme that has a lowered affinity for sulfonamide. The former mechanism has been implicated in resistant strains of *Neisseria gonorrhea* and *Staphylococcus aureus*, and the latter has been found in strains of *Escherichia coli*. Resistance may also be mediated by plasmids that may code for the production of drug-resistant enzymes such as dihydropteroate synthetase, or it may result in decreased bacterial cell permeability to sulfonamides. More than one mechanism of resistance to sulfonamides may be present in a single bacterial isolate.

SPECIAL PRECAUTIONS

Gastrointestinal effects such as anorexia, nausea, and vomiting may occur after initial doses and are most likely due to mucosal irritation; the intolerance may be alleviated by more even distribution of total daily dose or by administering enteric-coated tablets. If symptoms persist beyond the first few days, the cause may be increased serum levels, and relief may be achieved by halving the dose and then increasing it gradually over a period of several days. If symptoms do not subside, discontinue administration for 5 to 7 days and initiate again with lower daily dose. Continuation of therapy is often necessary even when clinical symptoms, such as diarrhea, are controlled. Dosage may be reduced to a maintenance level after endoscopic examination confirms improvement. Dosage should be increased to previously effective levels if diarrhea or other clinical symptoms recur. Oligospermia and infertility have been reported in male patients who have received sulfasalazine; reversal of effects seems to occur after withdrawal.

INDICATIONS

Ulcerative colitis (unlabeled): ankylosing spondylitis, collagenous colitis, Crohn's disease, rheumatoid arthritis

CONTRAINDICATIONS

Intestinal or urinary obstruction.

Allergy or hypersensitivity to sulfonamides. Patients with documented megaloblastic anemia due to folate deficiency. Patients with severe renal impairment and/or liver parenchymal damage or blood dyscrasias. Gastrointestinal bleeding that is not readily controlled with conservative therapy.

INTERACTIONS

The metabolism of sulfasalazine includes salicylates, therefore patients who have salicylate allergies or porphyria should not take this drug

ADVERSE EFFECTS

Orange–yellow color in urine (when urine is alkaline) or skin.

The most common adverse reactions associated with sulfasalazine include anorexia, headache, nausea, vomiting, gastric distress, and apparently reversible oligospermia. These have been reported in about one third of the patients. Less frequent adverse reactions are skin rash, pruritus, urticaria, fever, anemia, and cyanosis, which may occur at a frequency of one in every 30 patients or less. Experience suggests that with a daily dosage of 4 g or more, or metabolite levels above 50 µg/mL, the incidence of these adverse reactions tends to increase. Other adverse reactions seen with other sulfonamides occur rarely at a level of approximately one per thousand patients or less.

PHARMACOKINETICS AND PHARMACODYNAMICS

Peak serum levels: (therapeutically effective levels range from 5 to 15 mg/dL for most infections)
Serum half-life: no information
Bioavailability: 70% to 100%
Protein binding: no information
Metabolism: in liver by conjugation, acetylation, and other pathways to inactive metabolites
Excretion: renal, by glomerular filtration; tubular reabsorption occurs in varying degrees
Renal impairment: use with caution
Hepatic impairment: use with caution

OVERDOSAGE

There is evidence that the incidence and severity of toxicity are related to the total serum sulfapyridine (a sulfasalazine metabolite) concentration. Symptoms of overdosage may include nausea, vomiting, gastric distress, and abdominal pains. In more advanced cases, central nervous system symptoms such as drowsiness, convulsions, etc., may be observed. Serum sulfapyridine concentrations may be used to monitor the progress of recovery from overdosage. It has not been possible to determine the oral LD_{50} in laboratory animals such as mice, because the highest daily oral dose that can be given (12 g/kg) is not lethal. Doses of sulfasalazine 16 g/d have been given to patients without mortality. *(continued on next page)*

The information here is provided as guidance only. Prescribers should always consult the manufacturer's current prescribing information.

SULFASALAZINE (CONTINUED)

SPECIAL GROUPS

Children: Do not use in infants under 2 months of age unless treating congenital toxoplasmosis as adjunctive therapy with pyrimethamine.
Elderly: May have age-related renal impairment; use with caution.
Renal Impairment: Use with caution; more soluble sulfonamides recommended.
Hepatic impairment: Use with caution.
Pregnancy: Safety not established; sulfonamides cross the placenta, with fetal levels averaging 70% to 90% of maternal levels. Contraindicated at term.
Breast-feeding: Excreted in breast milk; does not pose significant risk to healthy full-term neonates. Do not nurse premature infants or those with hyperbilirubinemia or G-6-PD deficiency.

DOSAGE

Adults: Initially, give 3 to 4 g/d in equally divided doses; initial doses of 1 to 2 g/d may lessen adverse effects (gastrointestinal). Doses of 4 g/d or more increase risk of toxicity. For maintenance, give 2 g/d (500 mg four times daily).
Elderly: May have age-related renal impairment; use with caution.
Children: (over 2 years of age) Initially, give 40 to 60 mg/kg/d in 4 to 6 equally divided doses. For maintenance, give 20 to 30 mg/kg/d in four equal doses. Do not exceed 2 g/d.
Renal impairment: No special dosage given.

OVERDOSAGE *(CONTINUED)*

Gastric lavage or emesis plus catharsis is indicated for overdosage. The urine should be alkalinized. If kidney function is normal, fluids should be forced. If anuria is present, restrict fluids and salt and treat appropriately. catheterization of ureters may be appropriate for complete renal blockage by crystals. The low molecular weight of sulfasalazine and its metabolites may facilitate their removal by dialysis. For agranulocytosis, the drug should be discontinued immediately, the patient should be hospitalized, and appropriate sensitivity should be utilized. For hypersensitivity reactions, the drug treatment needs to be discontinued immediately. Such reactions may be controlled with antihistamines and, if necessary, systemic corticosteroids. If the drug is still needed even after hypersensitivity reactions, desensitization protocols are available and may be undertaken with careful medical supervision.

PATIENT INFORMATION

Sulfasalazine is indicated in the treatment of mild to moderate ulcerative colitis and as adjunctive therapy in severe ulcerative colitis. It is used for the prolongation of remission periods between acute attacks of ulcerative colitis. The dosage should be adjusted to each patient's individual response and tolerance. The drug should be given in evenly divided doses over each 24-hour period; intervals between night time dosage should not exceed 7 hours, with administration after meals recommended as feasible. Experience suggests that daily doses of 4 g or more result in a higher incidence of adverse reactions.

AVAILABILITY

Tablets—500 mg
Enteric-coated tablets—500 mg
Oral suspension—250 mg/5 mL

SULFATHIAZOLE (Sultrin®)

Sulfathiazole is currently used only in combination with sulfacetamide and sulfabenzamide as either an ophthalmologic ointment or for topical vaginal use as a cream or tablet. For ophthalmologic diseases, it has been used most frequently in the management of bacterial conjunctivitis but also has been used as an adjunct in the treatment of trachoma. Because of increasing resistance of many bacteria to sulfonamides, it is recommended that cultures of any drainage from conjunctiva be obtained prior to the initiation of topical therapy with sulfathiazole and other agents. As a cream or vaginal tablet, the combination is used for the treatment of nonspecific vaginitis, particularly that due to *Haemophilus (Gardnerella) vaginalis*.

ANTIMICROBIAL ACTIVITY

Sulfathiazole exhibits an inhibitory activity against a broad spectrum of gram-positive and gram-negative bacteria, as well as actinomyces, chlamydia, plasmodia, and toxoplasma. However, resistance to sulfathiazole is widespread and increasing and is found between one third and more than one half of community and nosocomial strains of bacteria, including Staphylococci, Enterobacteriaceae, *Neisseria meningitidis*, and *Pseudomonas* spp. Susceptibility testing should be performed when using sulfamethoxazole as monotherapy, even for uncomplicated community-acquired infections.

INDICATIONS

Treatment of vaginitis due to *H. (Gardnerella) vaginalis*

CONTRAINDICATIONS

Allergy or hypersensitivity to sulfonamides. Patients with documented megaloblastic anemia due to folate deficiency. Patients with severe renal impairment and/or liver parenchymal damage or blood dyscrasias.

INTERACTIONS

Laboratory test interactions: May interfere with "Uroblisix" test and produce false-positive results with sulfosalicylic acid tests for urinary protein

The information here is provided as guidance only. Prescribers should always consult the manufacturer's current prescribing information.

SULFATHIAZOLE (CONTINUED)

RESISTANCE

Resistance may develop by mutation, either resulting in microbial overproduction of PABA, or a structural change in a folic acid–synthesizing enzyme that has a lowered affinity for sulfonamide. A former mechanism has been implicated in resistant strains of *Neisseria gonorrhea* and *Staphylococcus aureus*, and the latter has been found in strains of *Escherichia coli*. Resistance may also be mediated by plasmids that may code for the production of drug-resistant enzymes such as dihydropteroate synthetase, or it may result in decreased bacterial cell permeability to sulfonamides. More than one mechanism of resistance to sulfonamides may be present in a single bacterial isolate.

SPECIAL PRECAUTIONS

Sulfonamides can be absorbed through vaginal mucosa; therefore, systemic warnings are applicable.
Discontinue treatment if rash or other evidence of systemic toxicity occurs.

SPECIAL GROUPS

Children: Safety and efficacy not established.
Elderly: May have age-related renal impairment (*see* Special Precautions).
Renal impairment: Use with caution (*see* Special Precautions).
Hepatic impairment: Use with caution (*see* Special Precautions).
Pregnancy: Contraindicated at term; in earlier stages, use only when benefits outweigh risk.
Breast-feeding: Discontinue drug or discontinue nursing.

DOSAGE

Adults: One full applicator or one tablet intravaginally twice daily for 4 to 6 days.
Elderly: May have age-related renal impairment; otherwise, same as adults.
Children: Safety and efficacy not established.
Impaired renal or hepatic function: Use with caution.

ADVERSE EFFECTS

Localized irritation or allergic reaction

PHARMACOKINETICS AND PHARMACODYNAMICS

Peak serum levels: not available
Plasma half-life: not available
Bioavailability: not available
Metabolism: in the liver by conjugation, acetylation, and other pathways to inactive metabolites
Excretion: renal, by glomerular filtration; tubular reabsorption occurs in varying degrees
Effect of food: no information
Protein binding: no information
Renal impairment: use with caution
Hepatic impairment: use with caution

OVERDOSAGE

No overdose information is available beyond that known for other sulfa drugs

PATIENT INFORMATION

No additional patient information is necessary beyond that used when prescribing other topical sulfa drugs

AVAILABILITY

Cream—78-g tubes with applicator
Vaginal tablets—package of 20 with applicator

SULFISOXAZOLE (Gantrisin®)

Sulfisoxazole is a highly soluble drug that is particularly useful in the management of urinary tract infections due to susceptible Enterobacteriaceae and, less commonly, *Staphylococcus aureus*. Because of increasing resistance to sulfonamides, it is recommended that urinary tract cultures and susceptibility testing be performed on any isolate from a patient who is being treated with this agent. The drug also is available combined with phenazopyridine, a urinary antiseptic. Thus, common indications for the use of sulfisoxazole include treatment of acute otitis media, chancroid, inclusion conjunctivitis, nocardiosis, and trachoma. Because of the increasing prevalence of resistance, its use in meningitis and rheumatic fever is of historical interest only.

INDICATIONS

Infections of the following types due to susceptible strains of designated organisms:
Meningococcal (when organism is susceptible, used for prophylaxis when sulfonamide-sensitive Group A strains are prevalent)
Otitis media (acute): *H. influenzae* (with erythromycin)
Urinary tract (pyelonephritis or cystitis in absence of uropathy or foreign bodies): *E. coli*, *Klebsiella-Enterobacter*, *P. mirabilis*, and *P. vulgaris*
Chancroid, inclusion conjunctivitis, nocardiosis, rheumatic fever, trachoma

The information here is provided as guidance only. Prescribers should always consult the manufacturer's current prescribing information.

SULFISOXAZOLE (CONTINUED)

ANTIMICROBIAL ACTIVITY

Sulfisoxazole exhibits an inhibitory activity against a broad spectrum of gram-positive and gram-negative bacteria, as well as actinomyces, chlamydia, plasmodia, and toxoplasma. However, resistance to sulfisoxazole is widespread and increasing and is found between one third and more than one half of community and nosocomial strains of bacteria, including Staphylococci, Enterobacteriaceae, *Neisseria meningitidis*, and *Pseudomonas* species. Susceptibility testing should be performed when using sulfamethoxazole as monotherapy, even for uncomplicated community-acquired infections.

RESISTANCE

Resistance may develop by mutation, either resulting in microbial overproduction of PABA, or a structural change in a folic acid–synthesizing enzyme that has a lowered affinity for sulfonamide. A former mechanism has been implicated in resistant strains of *Neisseria gonorrhea* and *Staphylococcus aureus*, and the latter has been found in strains of *Escherichia coli*. Resistance may also be mediated by plasmids that may code for the production of drug-resistant enzymes such as dihydropteroate synthetase, or it may result in decreased bacterial cell permeability to sulfonamides. More than one mechanism of resistance to sulfonamides may be present in a single bacterial isolate.

SPECIAL PRECAUTIONS

Can potentiate blood sugar lowering activity of sulfonylureas, as well as cause hypoglycemia itself.

SPECIAL GROUPS

Children: Do not use in infants under 2 months of age (except for treatment of congenital toxoplasmosis as adjunctive therapy with pyrimethamine).
Elderly: May have age-related renal impairment (*see* Special Precautions).
Renal Impairment: Use with caution (*see* Special Precautions).
Hepatic impairment: Use with caution (*see* Special Precautions).
Pregnancy: Contraindicated at term; in earlier stages, use only when benefits outweigh risk.
Breast-feeding: Contraindicated in nursing infants under 2 months of age; discontinuation of nursing recommended during therapy.

DOSAGE

Adults: (Note: Although recommended, loading dose is not necessary because of the rapid absorption of sulfisoxazole.) Give loading dose of 2 to 4 g, followed by maintenance dose of 4 to 8 g/d in divided doses every 4 to 6 hours.
Elderly: May have age-related renal impairment (*see* Special Precautions); otherwise, same as adults. Elimination is sometimes prolonged without evidence of impairment.
Children: Infants and children over 2 months of age, give initial dose of 75 mg/kg, followed by maintenance dose of 120 to 150 mg/kg/d (4 g/m^2/d) in divided doses every 4 to 6 hours (to a maximum of 6 g/d).
Impaired renal or hepatic function: Usual doses can be given until creatinine clearance exceeds 30 mL/min; one-half daily dose for creatinine clearance 15 to 30 mL/min; do not use if creatinine clearance is less than 15 mL/min; sulfonamides are removed by dialysis. No dosage change is necessary with hepatic insufficiency.

CONTRAINDICATIONS

Allergy or hypersensitivity to sulfonamides. Patients with documented megaloblastic anemia due to folate deficiency. Patients with severe renal impairment and/or liver parenchymal damage or blood dyscrasias.

INTERACTIONS

Laboratory test interactions: May interfere with "Uroblisix" test and produce false-positive results with sulfosalicylic acid tests for urinary protein

ADVERSE EFFECTS

No specific adverse effects have been noted with sulfisoxazole, beyond those noted with other systemically absorbed sulfa drugs (*eg*, sulfamethoxazole)

PHARMACOKINETICS AND PHARMACODYNAMICS

Peak serum levels: 127 to 211 µg/mL from 1 to 4 h after 2-g oral dose
Plasma half-life: 4.6 to 7.8 h
Bioavailability: no information
Metabolism: in liver
Excretion: renal
Effect of food: no information
Protein binding: 85%
Renal impairment: prolonged elimination (*see* Special Precautions)
Hepatic impairment: use with caution (*see* Special Precautions)

OVERDOSAGE

The amount of a single dose that is associated with symptoms of overdosage or is likely to be life threatening has not been reported. Signs and symptoms of overdosage with sulfamethoxazole include anorexia, colic, nausea, vomiting, headache, dizziness, drowsiness, and unconsciousness. Fever, hematuria, and crystalluria may be noted. Blood dyscrasias and jaundice are potential late manifestations of overdosage. General principles of treatment include the immediate discontinuation of the drug, instituting gastric lavage or emesis, forcing oral fluids, and administering intravenous fluids if urine output is low and renal function is normal. The patient should be monitored with blood counts and appropriate blood chemistries, including electrolytes. If the patient becomes cyanotic, the possibility of methemoglobinemia should be considered, and if present, the condition should be treated appropriately with intravenous 1% methaline blue. If significant blood dyscrasia or jaundice occurs, specific therapy should be instituted for these complications. Peritoneal dialysis is not effective, and hemodialysis is only moderately effective in removing sulfonamides.

PATIENT INFORMATION

Sulfisoxazole is used for the treatment of urinary tract infections caused by sensitive organisms. If this drug is prescribed, it is important that a urine culture be obtained prior to initiating therapy. It is advisable to drink lots of fluids (at least eight glasses of fluids a day) while taking this drug.

AVAILABILITY

Tablets—500 mg
Syrup—500 mg acetyl sulfisoxazole/5 mL
Pediatric suspension—500 mg acetyl sulfisoxazole/5 mL

The information here is provided as guidance only. Prescribers should always consult the manufacturer's current prescribing information.

TRIMETHOPRIM (Proloprim®, Trimpex®)

Trimethoprim is a diaminopyrimidine that inhibits bacterial dihydrofolate reductase, resulting in impairment of folic acid biosynthesis in a wide range of bacteria and protozoa. Because of the increasing emergence of resistance to monotherapy and the synergistic effect of combining trimethoprim with sulfonamides that inhibit at a different site in folic acid biosynthesis pathways, the drug is frequently used in combination. Local increases in trimethoprim resistance have been noted in many species of Enterobacteriaceae, including *Shigella* and *Salmonella* in developing countries, limiting its use as monotherapy for traveler's diarrhea. In addition, gram-positive cocci have shown increasing resistance to trimethoprim. Therefore, prior to its use as monotherapy for urinary tract infections, it is recommended that urine cultures and susceptibility testing be performed in order to anticipate whether resistance will pose a problem in clinical management.

In addition to being used as a combination drug with sulfonamides, trimethoprim has been combined with rifampin, polymyxin, amikacin, and metronidazole in the laboratory and in clinical studies overseas. However, it is not approved as a combination drug with any sulfonamide other than sulfamethoxazole.

ANTIMICROBIAL ACTIVITY

Blocks production of tetrahydrofolic acid from dihydrofolic acid by binding to and reversibly inhibiting the required enzyme, dihydrofolate reductase. The binding is much stronger for the bacterial enzyme than for the mammalian. Therefore, trimethoprim interferes with bacterial biosynthesis of nucleic acids and proteins. *In vitro* serial dilution tests have shown that the activity of trimethoprim includes the common urinary tract pathogens, with the exception of *Pseudomonas aeruginosa*.

RESISTANCE

Common non-*Enterobacteriaceae* fecal organisms, *Bacteroides* spp, and *Lactobacillus* species are not susceptible to the recommended levels used in treatment.

SPECIAL PRECAUTIONS

Serious hypersensitivity reactions have been reported rarely with trimethoprim. Trimethoprim rarely has been reported to interfere with hematopoiesis, especially in higher doses and prolonged therapy.

The following symptoms may indicate serious blood disorders requiring immediate blood count evaluations: sore throat, fever, pallor, or purpura. If blood counts are significantly low in any area, discontinue trimethoprim.

Use with caution in patients with possible folate deficiency, impaired renal function, or impaired hepatic function.

SPECIAL GROUPS

Children: Do not use in infants under 2 months of age. Efficacy as a single agent has not been demonstrated in patients under 12 years of age.
Elderly: May have age-related renal impairment (*see* Special Precautions).
Renal Impairment: Use with caution (*see* Special Precautions). Use in patients with creatinine clearance of less than 15 mL/min not recommended.
Hepatic impairment: Use with caution (*see* Special Precautions).
Pregnancy: Use only when benefits outweigh risk.
Breast-feeding: Excreted in breast milk; caution, may interfere with folic acid metabolism.

INDICATIONS

Treatment of initial, uncomplicated urinary tract infections due to susceptible strains of the following organisms:
E. coli, P. mirabilis, Klebsiella pneumoniae, Enterobacter species, coagulase-negative *Staphylococcus* spp (including *S. saprofyticus*)

CONTRAINDICATIONS

Allergy or hypersensitivity to trimethoprim, documented megaloblastic anemia due to folate deficiency

INTERACTIONS

May inhibit hepatic metabolism of phenytoin
Laboratory test interactions: May interfere with serum methotrexate assay as determined by the competitive binding protein technique when a bacterial dihydrofolate reductase is used as the binding protein. No interference occurs if methotrexate is measured by a radioimmunoassay.

ADVERSE EFFECTS

Most common: rash, pruritus
Other: photosensitivity, phototoxicity (and related skin eruptions), gastric distress, nausea, vomiting, glossitis, thrombocytopenia, leukopenia, neutropenia, megaloblastic anemia, methemoglobinemia, fever, increase in blood urea nitrogen, increase in serum creatinine levels
Rare: exfoliative dermatitis, erythema multiforme, Stevens-Johnson syndrome, toxic epidermal necrolysis, anaphylaxis, elevation of serum transaminase and bilirubin, cholestatic jaundice, aseptic meningitis

PHARMACOKINETICS AND PHARMACODYNAMICS

Peak serum levels: 1 µg/mL 1 to 4 h after oral 100-mg dose
Plasma half-life: 8 to 10 h
Bioavailability: readily absorbed
Metabolism: 10% to 20%, in liver
Excretion: renal; by glomerular filtration and tubular secretion
Effect of food: no impairment of absorption
Protein binding: 44%
Renal impairment: prolongs half-life; reduced dosage necessary
Hepatic impairment: use with caution

OVERDOSAGE

Symptoms may include nausea, vomiting, dizziness, headaches, depression, confusion, and bone marrow depression. Treat by gastric lavage and general supportive care. Acidification of the urine will aid in elimination; peritoneal dialysis is not effective, and hemodialysis is only moderately effective.
Chronic overdosage (use of trimethoprim at high doses for prolonged periods) may cause bone marrow depression manifested as thrombocytopenia, leukopenia, or megaloblastic anemia. Discontinue therapy if signs of bone marrow depression occur, and (as some experts recommend) administer leucovorin 5 to 15 mg daily.

The information here is provided as guidance only. Prescribers should always consult the manufacturer's current prescribing information.

TRIMETHOPRIM (CONTINUED)

DOSAGE

Adults: 100 mg every 12 hours or 200 mg every 24 hours, each for 10 days.
Elderly: May have age-related renal impairment; otherwise, same as adults.
Children: Efficacy not established in children under 12 years of age.
Impaired renal function: Creatinine clearance 15 to 30 mL/min, 50 mg every 12 hours. Not recommended for use in patients with creatinine clearance less than 30 mL/min.

PATIENT INFORMATION

Trimethoprim is often given as a combination drug with sulfonamides and can be very effective against a wide range of microbes. However, because of the increasing spread of resistant bacterial strains, it is desirable to have a specimen sent for culture prior to the initiation of treatment. Patients taking trimethoprim should promptly report any new rashes, ulcers, or fevers to their medical providers.

AVAILABILITY

Tablets—100 mg and 200 mg

TRIMETHOPRIM-SULFAMETHOXAZOLE (Bactrim®, Septra®)

Trimethoprim-sulfamethoxazole inhibits bacterial synthesis of dihydrofolic acid by inhibiting the enzyme dihydroptote synthetase by competing with para-aminobenzoic acid. Trimethoprim blocks the production of tetrahydrofolic acid by inhibiting the enzyme dihydrofolate reductase. Together, these agents interact synergistically to block these two consecutive steps in bacterial biosynthesis of extension nucleic acid and proteins, and thus the combination is particularly potent.

The drug is active orally and intravenously against a wide range of bacteria, including Enterobacteriaceae and many gram-positive cocci. However, *Pseudomonas aeruginosa* is intrinsically resistant, and many other gram-negative rods have acquired plasmid- and transposon-mediated resistance in recent years, both in community and nosocomial settings across the globe. Many gram-positive bacteria have acquired resistance to this combination, as well. Therefore, prior to the use of this agent for the management of clinical infections, it is advisable to obtain isolates for susceptibility testing. Trimethoprim-sulfamethoxazole is useful in the management of urinary tract infections, meningitis, osteomyelitis, pulmonary infections, and enteric infections. Allergic reactions, as manifested by maculopapular skin eruptions or leukopenia, are not uncommon, thereby limiting the clinical utility of this versatile agent.

Trimethoprim-sulfamethoxazole also has been extremely effective in the prophylaxis and treatment of *Pneumocystis carinii* pneumonia in patients with AIDS. For treatment of acute infection, intravenous trimethoprim-sulfamethoxazole has been used with great success and is the first-line agent of choice. Prophylaxis against relapse must be lifelong and can be maintained with several oral regimens, including the use of double-strength tablets orally on an every-other-day basis. However, because of an increased incidence of maculopapular eruptions in patients with AIDS, plus the not-infrequent leukopenia, therapy with trimethoprim-sulfamethoxazole in AIDS patients may have to be interrupted. Several investigators have successfully used desensitization protocols and have been able to maintain patients on long-term prophylactic regimens for several years after an initial allergic response. In addition to its activity against *P. carinii* pneumonia, the combination has been used in the treatment (usually in combination with pyrimethamine) and prophylaxis of *Toxoplasma gondii* infection in patients with AIDS.

CONTRAINDICATIONS

Allergy or hypersensitivity to trimethoprim

INTERACTIONS

Trimethoprim may inhibit hepatic metabolism of phenytoin.
Laboratory test interactions: May interfere with serum methotrexate assay as determined by the competitive binding protein technique when a bacterial dihydrofolate reductase is used as the binding protein. No interference occurs if methotrexate is measured by a radioimmunoassay.

ADVERSE EFFECTS

Trimethoprim is generally well tolerated, but uncommon side effects include nausea, diarrhea, skin rashes, oral or genital ulcers, and leukopenia, anemia, or thrombocytopenia

ANTIMICROBIAL ACTIVITY

Bacteria including *Escherichia coli, Klebsiella* spp, *Enterobacter* spp, *Morganella morganii, P. mirabilis*, indole-positive *Proteus* spp including *P. vulgaris, H. influenzae* (including ampicillin-resistant strains), *Streptococcus pneumoniae, Shigella flexneri, Shigella sonnei*, protozoa and fungi including *P. carinii, T. gondii*, and *Isospora belli.*

The information here is provided as guidance only. Prescribers should always consult the manufacturer's current prescribing information.

TRIMETHOPRIM-SULFAMETHOXAZOLE (CONTINUED)

RESISTANCE

Pseudomonas aeruginosa.

SPECIAL PRECAUTIONS

Patients with AIDS may not tolerate or respond to this combination due to their unique immune dysfunction; therefore, its use to treatment *P. carinii* pneumonitis is not recommended. Incidence of side effects, particularly rash, fever, and leukopenia, is significantly increased in this patient group.

Elderly patients may have increased risk of serious adverse effects, especially when complicating conditions exist (*ie*, renal impairment, hepatic impairment, concomitant use of other drugs). Adjustments in dosage should be made in patients with renal impairment. Of the adverse effects, severe skin reactions, bone marrow depression, or decrease in platelets with or without purpura are most frequently reported. Patients receiving certain diuretics, particularly thiazide-type, may have increased incidence of thrombocytopenia with purpura.

SPECIAL GROUPS

Children: Do not use in infants under 2 months of age.

Elderly: May have age-related renal impairment (*see* Special Precautions).

Renal Impairment: Use with caution (*see* Special Precautions).

Hepatic impairment: Use with caution (*see* Special Precautions).

Pregnancy: Contraindicated at term; in earlier stages, use only when benefits outweigh risk.

Breast-feeding: Not recommended for use. Premature infants or those with hyperbilirubinemia or G-6-PD deficiency are especially at risk.

DOSAGE

Adults: For urinary tract infections and shigellosis, 160 mg trimethoprim with 800 mg sulfamethoxazole every 12 hours for 10 to 14 days (5 days for shigellosis). For traveller's diarrhea, same dosage for 5 days. For acute exacerbation of chronic bronchitis, same dosage for 14 days. For *P. carinii* pneumonitis, 20 mg/kg trimethoprim with 800 mg sulfamethoxazole per day in divided doses every 6 hours for 14 days. For chancroid (*Haemophilus ducreyi* infection) as an alternative regimen, 160 mg trimethoprim with 800 mg sulfamethoxazole orally every 12 hours for 7 days. *Intravenous dosage* for adults and children over 2 months of age (normal renal function) for severe urinary tract infections and shigellosis, 8 to 10 mg/kg/d (based on trimethoprim in divided doses every 6 to 12 hours for up to 14 days (urinary tract infection) or 5 days (shigellosis).

Elderly: May have increased risk for serious adverse effects (*see* Special Precautions); reduced dosage may be necessary.

(Continued on next page)

PHARMACOKINETICS AND PHARMACODYNAMICS

Peak serum levels: 1 to 4 h after oral administration; 1 to 1.5 h after intravenous administration

Plasma half-life: trimethoprim 8 to 11 h, sulfamethoxazole 10 to 12 h after oral administration; 11.3 h trimethoprim and 12.8 h sulfamethoxazole for intravenous

Bioavailability: no information

Metabolism: in liver to inactive metabolites

Excretion: renal, by glomerular filtration and tubular secretion

Effect of food: no information

Protein binding: 44% trimethoprim, 70% sulfamethoxazole

Renal impairment: increases half-life; dosage adjustment necessary

Hepatic impairment: use with caution

The information here is provided as guidance only. Prescribers should always consult the manufacturer's current prescribing information.

TRIMETHOPRIM-SULFAMETHOXAZOLE (CONTINUED)

DOSAGE (CONTINUED)

Children: For urinary tract infections and acute otitis media:

Pediatric Dosage of Trimethoprim-Sulfamethoxazole for the Treatment of Urinary Tract Infections and Acute Otitis Media

Weight, kg	Teaspoonfuls, every 12 hours	Tablets, every 12 hours
10	1 (5 mL)	—
20	2 (10 mL)	1
30	3 (15 mL)	1.5
40	4 (20 mL)	2 or 1 double-strength

Pediatric Dosage of Trimethoprim-Sulfamethoxazole for the Treatment of Pneumocystis carinii Pneumonia

Weight, kg	Teaspoonfuls, every 6 hours	Tablets, every 6 hours
8	1 (5 mL)	—
16	2 (10 mL)	1
24	3 (15 mL)	1.5
32	4 (20 mL)	2 or 1 double-strength

Dosage of Trimethoprim-Sulfamethoxazole for Patients With Impaired Renal Function

Creatinine clearance, mL/min	Dosage
> 30	Usual regimen (above)
15–30	1/2 usual regimen
< 15	not recommended

ORAL AND PARENTERAL: Urinary tract infections: *E. coli, Klebsiella, Enterobacter* spp, *M. morganii, P. mirabilis, P. vulgaris*
(Note: Treat initial, uncomplicated urinary tract infections with a single antibacterial agent. Parenteral therapy is indicated in severe or complicated infections when oral therapy is not feasible.)
Shigellosis enteritis: *S. flexneri, S. sonnei*
P. carinii pneumonitis: *ORAL*: Acute otitis media (in children): *H. influenzae, S. pneumoniae*
(Note: Data are limited on the safety of repeated use in children under 2 years of age. Not indicated for prophylactic or prolonged use.)
Acute exacerbations of chronic bronchitis (in adults): *H. influenzae, S. pneumoniae*
Traveler's diarrhea (in adults): enterotoxigenic *E. coli*

OVERDOSAGE

Overdosage with trimethoprim may result in severe rashes, oral or genital ulcerations, or pancytopenia

PATIENT INFORMATION

Trimethoprim is often given as a combination drug with sulfonamides and can be very effective against a wide range of microbes. However, because of the increasing spread of resistant bacterial strains, it is desirable to have a specimen sent for culture prior to the initiation of treatment. Patients taking trimethoprim should promptly report any new rashes, ulcers, or fevers to their medical providers.

AVAILABILITY

Tablets—80 mg trimethoprim and 400 mg sulfamethoxazole
Tablets double-strength—160 mg trimethoprim and 800 mg sulfamethoxazole
Oral suspension—40 mg trimethoprim and 200 mg sulfamethoxazole per 5 mL
Infusion—80 mg trimethoprim and 400 mg sulfamethoxazole per 5 mL

The information here is provided as guidance only. Prescribers should always consult the manufacturer's current prescribing information.

TETRACYCLINES

CLASS DESCRIPTION

The tetracyclines have one of the broadest spectra of any family of antimicrobials: this includes gram-positive, gram-negative, and anaerobic bacteria; spirochetes; mycobacteria; rickettsia; mycoplasma; chlamydiae; and protozoa. There are, however, many newer antimicrobials with a greater degree of activity against specific organisms. Nevertheless, the tetracyclines remain the drugs of choice or effective alternative therapy for a wide and diverse group of infections. Although some of the analogues can be used parenterally, the preferred route of administration for the tetracyclines is by mouth. All are bacteriostatic at therapeutic concentrations. The compounds can be conveniently divided pharmacokinetically into short-, intermediate-, and long-acting analogues (Table 9-1). Among the five major analogues currently available, tetracycline and doxycycline are most useful clinically [1].

CHEMISTRY AND CLASSIFICATION

The first tetracycline, chlortetracycline, was discovered by screening a wide variety of organisms obtained from the soil for antimicrobial

Table 9-1. The Tetracyclines

Agent	Trade Name	Manufacturer	Dosage–Form
Short acting			
Tetracycline	Generic		Suspension—125 mg/5 mL
	Sumycin	Apothecon	Syrup—125 mg/5 mL buffered with potassium phosphate
Tetracycline hydrochloride	Achomycin-V	Lederle	Capsule—100, 250, and 500 mg
	Generic		
	Panmycin	Upjohn	Capsules—250 mg
	Robitet	Robins	Capsules—250, 500 mg
	Sumycin	Apothecon	Capsules or tablets—250 and 500 mg
Oxytetracycline hydrochloride	Generic		Capsules—250 mg
	Terramycin	Pfizer	Capsules—250 mg base
Oxytetracycline* (intramuscular)	Terramycin IM*	Roerig	Intramuscular solution—50 mg/mL with 2% lidocaine; 125 mg/mL with 2% lidocaine
Oxytetracycline* (oral mixture)	Urobiotic-250*	Roerig	Oxytetracycline hydrochloride—250 mg
			Sulfamethizole—250 mg
			Phenazopyridine hydrochloride—50 mg
Intermediate acting			
Demeclocycline hydrochloride	Declomycin	Lederle	Capsules—150 mg
			Tablets—150 and 300 mg
Long acting			
Doxycycline calcium	Vibramycin	Pfizer	Syrup—50 mg base/5 mL
Doxycycline hyclate	Generic		Capsules—50 and 100 mg
			Tablets—100 mg
	Doryx	Parke-Davis	Capsules (coated pellets)—100 mg base
	Doxychel	Rachelle	Capsules—50 and 100 mg base
			Tablets—50 and 100 mg base
	Doxy-Tabs	Barr	Tablets—100 mg base
	Doxy-Caps	Barr	Capsules—50 and 100 mg base
	Vibra-Tabs	Pfizer	Tablets—100 mg base
Doxycycline monohydrate	Monodox	Oclassen	Capsules—50 and 100 mg base
	Vibramycin	Pfizer	Powder equivalent to 25 mg base/5 mL after reconstitution
Doxycycline hyclate (intravenous)	Generic		Intravenous sterile powder—100 and 200 mg
	Doxy	Lyphomed	Powder—100 and 200 mg
	Doxychel	Rachelle	100 and 200 mg
	Vibramycin IV	Roerig	Powder—100 and 200 mg with ascorbic acid 480 or 960 mg, respectively
Minocycline hydrochloride	Generic		Capsules and tablets—50 and 100 mg base
	Minocin	Lederle	Capsules (pellet filled)—50 and 100 mg base
			Oral suspension—50 mg base/5 mg/containing alcohol 5%
Minocycline hydrochloride (intravenous)	Minocin IV	Lederle	Sterile powder—100 mg

*Neither the intramuscular form nor the antibiotic mixture can be recommended.

The information here is provided as guidance only. Prescribers should always consult the manufacturer's current prescribing information.

properties. This compound is no longer available except for topical use. Tetracycline was produced by the catalytic dehalogenation of this compound. Both doxycycline and minocycline were derived semisynthetically. Different compounds and their generic names are derived from the substitutions on the four fused-ring hydronaphthacene nucleus (Fig. 9-1).

MECHANISM OF ACTION

The tetracyclines inhibit protein synthesis by reversibly binding on the $30S$ ribosomal subunit at a position that blocks attachment of the aminoacyl-t-RNA to the acceptor site on the messenger RNA–ribosome complex. This effectively prevents the addition of new amino acids into the growing peptide chain [2].

ANTIMICROBIAL ACTIVITY

The spectra of all the tetracyclines are similar. It follows, therefore, that laboratories usually test susceptibility by class using the tetracycline disk. Organisms are considered susceptible if the minimum inhibitory concentrations (MICs) are 4 µg/mL or less. A moderate susceptibility of 8 µg/mL is useful particularly for treating urinary tract infections. An MIC of 16 µg/mL or more should be considered resistant [3]. Although the spectra are similar, there are differences in degree of susceptibility between the analogues that should be noted. The lipophilic congeners (minocycline followed by doxycycline) are more active than those that are more hydrophilic (oxytetracycline and tetracycline). These differences are frequently two- to fourfold. The activity of doxycycline and tetracycline against many bacteria is found in Table 9-2.

Among gram-positive aerobic bacteria, there is a great deal of variability in susceptibility among the species. In general, *Streptococcus pneumoniae* are susceptible, though pockets of resistance are present [4]. Almost two thirds of the isolates that are resistant to penicillins also are resistant to tetracycline (≥ 8 mcg/mL). The activity against *Streptococcus pyogenes* and *Streptococcus agalactiae* is highly variable, and the *enterococcus* species are resistant, with some exceptions. *Staphylococcus aureus* are often resistant to most analogues, but minocycline can have activity against this organism, including those that are methicillin-resistant. The clinical importance of this remains to be determined [5]. Nocardia is susceptible to minocycline and this is occasionally useful clinically as is erysipelothrix rhusiopathical.

For gram-negative bacteria, the activity of the tetracyclines is also variable. The activity against the Enterobacteriaceae is weak in comparison with newer antimicrobials. *Escherichia coli* acquired in the community frequently can be inhibited by concentrations achieved in the urine. However, the activity for *Vibrio cholerae*, *vulnificus* and other vibrios, *Brucella* spp and *Pseudomonas pseudomallei* is significant and particularly relevant clinically. *Campylobacter* spp are often susceptible, whereas *Shigella* have become increasingly resistant. Most *Helicobacter pylori* are susceptible but additional drugs are necessary to eradicate this organism. *Haemophilus influenzae* are generally susceptible, more so to doxycycline than to tetracycline as is *Branhamella catarrhalis*. Gonococci are also generally susceptible, but those resistant to penicillin G are also found to be resistant to tetracycline. Meningococococci also are sensitive, particularly to minocycline. The MIC$_{90}$ of minocycline for meningococci is 1.6 µg/mL (range 0.8–1.6 µg/mL). This can be important clinically as an alternative form of prophylaxis against this organism. *Legionella* spp are generally resistant. *Calymmatobacterium granulomatis* is susceptible as are many *Eikenella corrodens*, *Pasteurella multocida*, *Yersinia pestis*, and *Y. enterocolitica*. Among anaerobic organisms, the susceptibility of *Actinomyces* spp is extremely important clinically, whereas other gram-positive anaerobes are variable. *Bacillus anthracis*, *Clostridium perfringens*, *Clostridium tetani* are generally susceptible and the tetracyclines may be useful clinically as alternative therapy.

Many spirochetes, including *Borrelia burgdorferi* and *Treponema pallidum*, are highly susceptible. *Mycobacterium marinum* is susceptible and responds clinically to minocycline. The other organisms with susceptibility to the tetracyclines include rickettsia, chlamydiae, mycoplasma, and the protozoa (*Plasmodium malariae*, *Entamoeba histolytica*). Viruses and fungi are uniformly resistant [1].

MECHANISM OF BACTERIAL RESISTANCE

The mechanism of resistance is usually by decreasing the influx of tetracycline into the cell or increasing the ability of the cell to export the antibiotic, thus preventing tetracycline accumulation. The latter method is energy dependent. An additional method of resistance occurs when tetracyclines are unable to prevent attachment of aminoacyl-t-RNA to the ribosomal acceptor site. Tetracyclines are seldom, if ever, inactivated biologically or altered chemically by resistant bacteria. Resistance to one tetracycline usually implies resistance to all, although some exceptions occur, and may be passed by plasmids or within transposable elements [2,4].

PHARMACOKINETICS

The pharmacokinetic parameters of the tetracyclines are shown in Table 9-3 [1]. The antibiotics, when administered orally, reach maximum concentration 1 to 3 hours after administration. Following a 200-mg dose, doxycycline and minocycline achieve serum levels of 2.5 µg/mL, with over 90% absorption. This absorption occurs primarily in the proximal small intestine. The other compounds are less completely absorbed; however, 500 mg of tetracycline gives peak

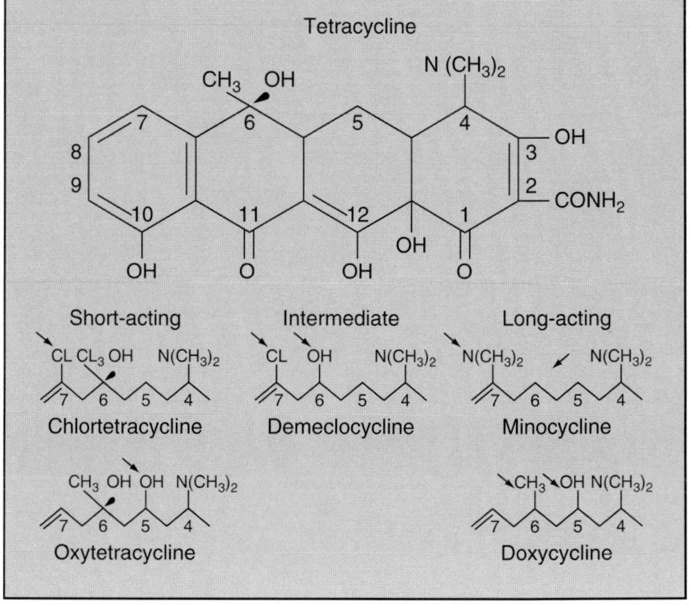

FIGURE 9-1.

The chemical structure of tetracycline.

The information here is provided as guidance only. Prescribers should always consult the manufacturer's current prescribing information.

levels of 4 µg/mL, with about 77% bioavailability. The half-lives of the short-acting analogues tetracycline and oxytetracycline are 8 and 9 hours, respectively, whereas the longer-acting compounds minocycline and doxycycline have half-lives of 16 and 18 hours, respectively. The half-lives for the latter compounds are sufficient for a once daily dosing for the treatment of many minor infections.

Of the available tetracyclines, with the possible exception of minocycline, adequate therapeutic concentrations are obtained in the urine for the treatment of susceptible organisms. Minocycline has the least urinary excretion at 6%.

Protein binding of the analogues is variable but tends to be greater for the intermediate- and long-acting compounds. The

Table 9-2. *In vitro* Activity of Tetracycline and Doxycycline Against Selected Bacteria

Organism	Tetracycline			Doxycycline		
	MIC$_{50}$	MIC$_{90}$	Range	MIC$_{50}$	MIC$_{90}$	Range
Gram-negative aerobes						
Escherichia coli	12.5	> 25	3.1–> 25	12.5	> 25	3.1–> 25
Klebsiella pneumoniae	> 25	> 25	6.3–> 25	> 25	> 25	6.3–> 25
Enterobacter spp	3.1	25	0.8–> 25	25	> 25	6.3–> 25
Shigella spp	3.1	> 25	0.8–> 25			
Campylobacter jejuni	0.8	> 25	0.4–> 25	0.4	12.5	0.4– 25
Proteus mirabilis	> 25	> 25	> 25	> 25	> 25	>25
Proteus spp (indole +)	> 25	> 25	> 25	> 25	> 25	>25
Pseudomonas aeruginosa	> 25	> 25	> 25	> 25	> 25	>25
Haemophilus influenzae	6.3	12.5	3.1–12.5	1.6	3.1	1.6–6.3
Neisseria gonorrhoeae	0.8	6.3	0.4–6.3	0.4	6.3	0.4–6.3
Neisseria meningitidis	0.8	3.1	0.8–3.1	1.6	6.3	1.6–6.3
Pseudomonas pseudomallei	1.6	3.1	1.6–3.1			
Gram-negative anaerobes						
Bacteroides fragilis	16	> 32	0.5–> 32	2.0	16	0.5–32
Bacteroides melaninogenicus	0.5	8.0	0.5–> 32	0.5	2.0	0.5–> 32
Gram-positive aerobes						
Staphylococcus aureus	3.1	> 25	0.8–> 25	1.6	> 25	0.4–> 25
*Streptococcus pneumonia**	0.4	0.8	0.4–3.1	0.4	0.4	0.4
Streptococcus pyogenes†	0.8	6.3	0.4–> 25	0.4	0.8	0.4–25
Streptococcus agalactiae	1.6	> 25	1.6–> 25	0.8	25	0.8–25
Enterococcus spp	> 25	> 25	6.3–> 25	> 25	> 25	6.3–> 25
Gram-positive anaerobes						
Peptococcus	16	32	0.5–> 32	4.0	8.0	0.5–32
Peptostreptococcus	4.0	32	0.5–> 32	2.0	8.0	0.5–16
Clostridium perfringens	2.0	> 32	0.5–> 32	0.5	16	0.5–16

**Some series show S. pneumoniae more resistant.*
†*Some series indicate that 20% to 40% of S. pyogenes have become resistant.*
MIC—minimum inhibitory concentration.

Table 9-3. Pharmacokinetic Properties of the Tetracyclines

Drug	Dose, *mg*	C$_{max}$, *mg/L*	Half-life, *h*	Protein binding, %	Bioavailability, %	VD, *L*	Urinary excretion, %
Short acting							
Oxytetracycline	500	2	9	35	58	128	70
Tetracycline	500	4	8	65	77	108	60
Intermediate							
Demeclocycline	300	2	12	91	66	121	39
Long acting							
Doxycycline	200	2.5	18	93	93	50	42
Minocycline	200	2.5	16	76	95	60	6

The information here is provided as guidance only. Prescribers should always consult the manufacturer's current prescribing information.

protein binding of doxycycline is 93% compared with 65% for tetracycline.

The apparent volume of distribution is greater than extracellular body water, suggesting sequestration in the tissues, presumably the liver. The long-acting compounds doxycycline and minocycline have the highest protein binding, the smallest apparent volume of distribution, and the highest blood levels for the dose administered. Doxycycline hyclate and minocycline hydrochloride also can be administered intravenously. These analogues are less irritating to the veins than tetracycline, which is no longer marketed for this route of administration. Nevertheless, thrombophlebitis may result from prolonged therapy. Serum concentrations of the long-acting compounds are 4 µg/mL after 30 minutes. Once tissue distribution occurs, serum levels are similar to those achieved following oral administration.

The tetracyclines have excellent tissue distribution. The lipid solubility may be an important determinant in diffusion in many tissues. Minocycline followed by doxycycline is more lipophilic than are the other tetracyclines. The tetracyclines obtain levels in cerebrospinal fluid that are 10% to 26% of serum levels and, in unobstructed bile, five to 20 times serum levels. The compounds cross the placenta, are secreted in breast milk, and accumulate in fetal bone and teeth.

DOSAGE ADJUSTMENTS FOR RENAL AND HEPATIC INSUFFICIENCY

Because of toxicity at higher serum levels, none of the tetracyclines, with the exception of doxycycline, should be administered to patients with renal failure. In renal failure, doxycycline is excreted into the gastrointestinal tract, allowing the half-life, and therefore its dose, to be unchanged. Although serum levels are not known to be affected in hepatic disease, these compounds should be used with much caution in such situations because of their inherent hepatic toxicity [1].

INDICATIONS

The tetracyclines are useful in a variety of diseases caused by specific organisms and syndromes (Table 9-4) [1,6]. For most diseases, tetracycline and doxycycline can be used interchangeably. However, doxycycline offers some advantage because of its better gastrointestinal absorption, with less diarrhea and longer half-life, as well as the ability to administer the antibiotic in patients with renal failure. Although at one time the high cost of doxycycline was a consideration, both tetracycline and doxycycline are now available generically, making cost no longer a major consideration. Other analogues, however, can be much more expensive and offer no therapeutic advantage. Oral therapy is the preferred route of administration. Doxycycline is the preferred analogue when intravenous therapy is required. None are recommended for intramuscular administration.

Although minocycline is often slightly more active than doxycycline, the high incidence of vestibular toxicity has limited its usefulness [7]. However, it is still the tetracycline of choice in selected indications, such as for *M. marinum* infections and as an alternative prophylaxis regimen for meningococcal disease.

ADVERSE REACTIONS

The most frequent side effects of the tetracyclines involve the gastrointestinal tract. Anorexia, nausea, vomiting, and epigastric distress are dose related and limit the dose of the analogues. The frequency of gastrointestinal side effects is about 10% for those taking 2 g of tetracycline or its equivalent daily. Food reduces these symptoms but may markedly decrease the absorption of tetracycline and demeclocycline [1].

Other gastrointestinal symptoms from these irritative substances include esophageal ulcerations, which produce retrosternal pain exacerbated by swallowing. Taking capsules with plenty of water and *not* immediately before bedtime may help to prevent this toxicity. Patients with esophageal obstruction or motility disorders are particularly at risk. Whereas upper gastrointestinal side effects are caused by the irritative nature of these compounds, bulky loose stools and diarrhea are caused by alteration in the intestinal flora. These side effects appear to be more common with analogues that are poorly absorbed. Doxycycline produces less of an effect than does tetracycline. Although the diarrhea usually subsides when the antibiotic is stopped, pseudomembranous colitis caused by *Clostridium difficile* has been reported, as have rare cases (reported in the older literature) of fulminating diarrhea caused by *S. aureus*. Other side effects caused by alteration of flora include monilial overgrowth in the oral and anogenital region, including proctitis and pruritic anis and vaginal moniliasis.

One of the most serious side effects caused by the tetracycline family of antibiotics is hepatotoxicity. First described with chlortetracycline, it has been noted with other analogues as well and is associated with a very high mortality. Patients who are pregnant are particularly at risk, as are those who develop high serum levels from renal failure. The compounds are contraindicated in pregnancy, and only doxycycline should be administered to patients with renal impairment. Pancreatitis has been noted with or without overt liver disease.

The tetracyclines aggravate preexisting renal failure by inhibiting protein synthesis, which increases azotemia from amino acid metabolism. Demeclocycline causes nephrogenic diabetes insipidus, a side effect that has been used therapeutically, although renal failure has complicated its use for this purpose in patients with cirrhosis [8]. Outdated tetracycline has produced a Fanconi-like syndrome with renal tubular acidosis; tetracycline formulations producing this syndrome have been modified, making it unlikely that the complication will recur.

With many of the analogues benign intracranial hypertension (pseudotumor cerebra) has been described in infants and adults [9]. Vertigo, however, is a side effect that appears to be unique for minocycline. The symptoms of lightheadedness, loss of balance, dizziness, and tinnitus are more common in women and are reversible but have seriously limited the use of minocycline [7].

The tetracyclines produce a gray–brown to yellow discoloration of the teeth [10,11]. This darkening effect is permanent and is associated with hypoplasia of the enamel and depression of skeletal growth in premature infants. The effect on permanent teeth appears to be related to the total dose of antibiotic administered, but there is some variability in staining with similar tetracycline exposure. Primary teeth generally show the darkening more than the larger, thicker, and more opaque permanent teeth. The tetracyclines should, therefore, not be administered to pregnant women and children under the age of 8 years, the period when tooth enamel is being formed. It occasionally, however, may be necessary to give a single course of tetracyclines to young children when the alternative therapies may be more toxic. Such is the case for the oral treatment of Rocky Mountain spotted fever [12]. Doxycycline combines less with calcium than

The information here is provided as guidance only. Prescribers should always consult the manufacturer's current prescribing information.

Table 9-4. Therapeutic Indications for the Tetracyclines

Therapy of first choice	Effective Alternative Therapy
Gram-negative bacteria	Gram-negative bacteria
Brucella (with gentamicin in seriously ill patients)	*Campylobacter jejuni*
Calymmatobacterium granulomatis (granuloma inguinale)	*Eikenella corrodens*
	Francisella tularensis (tularemia)
Helicobacter pylori (plus metronidazole plus bismuth subsalicylate)	*Pasteurella multocida*
	Pseudomonas pseudomallei (melioidosis) (doxycycline with trimethoprim—sulfamethoxazole and chloramphenicol)
Pseudomonas mallei (glanders) (with streptomycin)	*Spirillum minus* and *Streptobacillus moniliformis* (rat bite fever)
Vibrio cholerae (cholera)	*Rochalimaea henselae* (bacillary angiomatosis)
Vibrio parahaemolyticus	*Yersinia pestis* (plague)
Vibrio vulnificus	*Xanthomonas maltophilia* (minocycline)
Gram-positive bacteria	Gram-positive bacteria
None	*Nocardia* spp (minocycline)
Anaerobes	Anaerobes
None	*Actinomyces israelii* (actinomycosis)
	Bacillus anthracis (anthrax)
	Clostridium tetani
Spirochetes	Spirochetes
Borrelia burgdorferi (Lyme disease, early) (doxycycline)	*Leptospira* spp (leptospirosis)
Borrelia recurrentis (relapsing fever)	*Treponema pallidum* (syphilis)
	Treponema pertenue (yaws, nasopalatal)
Mycobacteria	Mycobacteria
Mycobacterium fortuitum (plus amikacin)	*Mycobacterium leprae* (leprosy) (minocycline)
Mycobacterium marinum (minocycline)	
Rickettsia	
Ehrlichiosis	
Q fever	
Rickettsial pox	
Rocky Mountain spotted fever	
Scrub typhus	
Typhus fever (epidemic, endemic)	
Chlamydiae	Chlamydia
Chlamydia trachomatis (nonspecific urethritis, cervicitis, lympho-granuloma venereum) trachoma	None
Chlamydia pneumoniae (TWAR strain)	
Chlamydia psittaci (psittacosis, ornithosis)	
Mycoplasma	Mycoplasma
None	*Mycoplasma pneumoniae*
	Ureaplasma urealyticum
Protozoa	Protozoa
Balantidium coli (balantidiasis)	*P. falciparum* (chloroquine-resistant) oral therapy with quinine sulfate plus pyrimethamine-sulfadoxine
Syndromes	Syndromes
Epididymitis, acute (sexually transmitted form)	Acne
Pelvic inflammatory disease (doxycycline in combination with other antibiotics)	Chronic bronchitis
Nonspecific urethritis	
Urethral syndrome, acute	
Preventive therapy	Effective alternative preventive therapy
Leptospirosis	Oral bowel preparation for intestinal surgery (tetracycline plus neomycin); (doxycycline)
Borrelia burgdorferi (Lyme disease)	*Neisseria meningitidis* (minocycline)
	Malaria (chloroquine-resistant areas)

Tetracycline and doxycycline can be used interchangeably unless indicated.

The information here is provided as guidance only. Prescribers should always consult the manufacturer's current prescribing information.

other tetracyclines and may produce less dental discoloration than tetracycline [11].

Adverse reactions to the skin may be allergic or toxic. Photosensitivity reactions are probably toxic in nature and consist of a red rash on areas exposed to sunlight; they may be associated with onycholysis. These reactions are seen most commonly with demeclocycline but occur with all analogues. Patients should use protective measures and avoid prolonged exposure to ultraviolet light. An increase in pigmentation of the nail, skin, and sclera has been noted rarely with prolonged administration of minocycline [13]. Hematologic reactions are rare, but hemolytic anemia, thrombocytopenia, thrombocytopenic purpura, neutropenia, and eosinophilia have been reported.

Hypersensitivity reactions, including anaphylaxis, urticaria, periorbital edema, fixed drug eruptions, and morbilliform rashes, are not common but can occur with all the tetracyclines. Exfoliative dermatitis has been reported. Other possible hypersensitivity reactions include exacerbation of lupus erythematosus, polyarthralgia, and serum sickness–like reactions (fever, rash, arthralgia, and pulmonary infiltrates with eosinophilia). When individuals are allergic to one analogue, they should be considered allergic to all.

FOOD INTERACTIONS

Food and some dairy products adversely affect the absorption of tetracyclines. Doxycycline and minocycline are least affected.

DRUG INTERACTIONS

Antacids containing aluminum, zinc, magnesium, or bismuth salts (or other divalent and trivalent cations) impair absorption of tetracyclines because they form poorly soluble chelates. Tetracyclines should be administered at least 2 hours before or after these agents. Colestipol, bismuth subsalicylate, and sodium bicarbonate also interfere with absorption [14,15].

There is *in vitro* antagonism between the bacteriostatic drug tetracycline and bactericidal drugs such as penicillin. An adverse outcome was noted with penicillin and tetracycline for the treatment of pneumococcal meningitis. Care should be exercised in combining penicillin with tetracycline for serious infections.

Methoxyflurane anesthesia may cause nephrotoxicity when administered with tetracyclines. Also, administration of the tetracyclines with diuretics produces an elevated blood urea nitrogen level, although the exact mechanism is not known. Women taking oral contraceptives have become pregnant and had menstrual irregularities while receiving tetracyclines, perhaps caused by the reduction in bacterial hydrolysis of conjugated estrogen in the intestine [15].

The half-life of doxycycline is reduced almost by half by induction of hepatic enzymes by drugs such as carbamazepine, phenytoin, and barbiturates. Similarly, chronic ethanol injection also has resulted in a shorter half-life of doxycycline but not tetracycline. Rifampin also has reduced plasma levels of patients treated for brucellosis, and this may have therapeutic implications [16].

Although theoretically tetracyclines may increase the hypoprothrombinemic response to oral anticoagulants, clinical evidence is lacking. Patients should, however, be monitored when taking tetracyclines. Similarly, digoxin should be monitored because an occasional patient may have increased digoxin levels by eradication of intestinal flora responsible for its metabolism.

PATIENT INFORMATION

Patients should be advised to:
1) drink at least one glass of water (240 cc) while taking tetracyclines;
2) take pills at least 1 hour before bedtime;
3) avoid taking antacids, bismuth subsalicylate, or iron-containing multivitamins within a 2-hour period before or after tetracycline absorption;
4) take pills 1 hour before or 2 hours after meals and dairy products; doxycycline and minocycline are only minimally affected and can be taken with meals;
5) do not take during pregnancy;
6) use additional forms of contraception if oral contraception is used during tetracycline therapy; and
7) avoid prolonged exposure to ultraviolet light.

REFERENCES

1. Standiford HC: Tetracyclines and chloramphenicol. In *Principles and Practice of Infectious Diseases*, edn. 4. Edited by Mandell GL, Bennett JE, Dolin R. New York: Churchill Livingstone Inc; 1995:306–317.

2. Chopra I: Tetracycline analogs whose primary target is not the bacterial ribosome. *Antimicrob Agents Chemother* 1994, 38:637–640.

3. National Committee for Clinical Laboratory Standards, Method for Dilution: *Antimicrobial Susceptibility Tests Fifth Edition: Approved Standard*, edn 2. NCCLS Publications M-1–A2, Villanova PA: NCCLS; 1990.

4. Chopra I, Harkey PM, Hinton M: Tetracyclines: Molecular and clinical aspects. *J Antimicrob Chemother* 1992, 29:245–277. Treatment of prosthetic valve endocarditis due to methicillin-resistant *Staphylococcus aureus* with minocycline. *UID* 1990, 161:812–813.

5. Lawlor MT, Sullivan MC, Levitz RE, *et al.*: Treatment of prosthetic valve endocarditis due to methicillin-resistant *Staphylococcus aureus* with minocycline. *J Infect Dis* 1990, 161:812–813.

6. The Choice of Antimicrobial Drugs. *Med Lett Drugs Ther* 1994, 36:53–60.

7. Fanning WL, Gump DW, Sofferman RA: Side effects of minocycline: A double blind study. *Antimicrob Agents Chemother* 1977, 11:712–717.

8. Forrest JN Jr, Cox M, Hong C, *et al.*: Superiority of demeclocycline over lithium in the treatment of chronic syndrome of inappropriate secretion of antidiuretic hormone. *N Engl J Med* 1978, 298:173–177.

9. Walters BN, Gubbay SS: Tetracycline and benign intracranial hypertension: Report of five cases. *BMJ* 1981, 282:19–20.

10. Grossman ER, Walcheck A, Freedman H: Tetracyclines and permanent teeth: The relationship between doses and tooth color. *Pediatrics* 1971, 47:567–570.

11. Forti G, Benincori C: Doxycycline and the teeth. *Lancet* 1969, i:782.

12. Abramson JS, Givner LB: Should tetracycline be contraindicated for therapy of presumed Rocky Mountain spotted fever in children less than 9 years of age? *Pediatrics* 1990, 86:123–124.

13. Angeloni VL, Salasche SJ, Ortiz R: Nail, skin and scleral pigmentation induced by minocycline. *Cutis* 1987, 40:229–233.

14. Friedman H, Greenblatt DJ, Le Duc BW: Impaired absorption of tetracycline by colestipol is not reversed by orange juice. *J Clin Pharmacol* 1989, 29:748–751.

15. Hansten PD, Horn JR: Tetracycline interactions. In *Drug Interactions and Updates*. Applied Therapeutics Inc.: Vancouver, Washington; 1993:275–281.

16. Colmenero JD, Fernandez-Gallardo LC, Agundez AG, *et al.*: Possible implications of deoxycycline-rifampin interactions for treatment of brucellosis. *Antimicrob Agents Chemother* 1994, 38:2798–2802.

The information here is provided as guidance only. Prescribers should always consult the manufacturer's current prescribing information.

DEMECLOCYCLINE (Declomycin®)

The spectrum of activity of *demeclocycline* is similar to the other tetracycline analogues. There are few, if any, advantages to this analogue. Its half-life of 12 hours makes this tetracycline intermediate, between the short- and long-acting compounds. Its only unique characteristic, producing reversible nephrogenic diabetes insipidus, has been used to treat inappropriate antidiuretic hormone secretion. It is the analogue most frequently associated with photosensitivity reactions. The cost for a therapeutic course is much greater than for tetracycline or doxycycline. It should not be used in patients who are pregnant or breast feeding or in children 8 years of age or younger.

ANTIMICROBIAL ACTIVITY

Microorganisms may be considered susceptible if minimum inhibitory concentration is not more than 4 µg/mL and intermediate if greater than 4 to 12.5 µg/mL. The activity of demeclocycline is similar to tetracycline and doxycycline.

RESISTANCE

If an organism is resistant to tetracycline, it is generally considered to be resistant to demeclocycline as well.

SPECIAL PRECAUTIONS

Phototoxic effects are most common with demeclocycline.
Demeclocycline has caused nephrogenic diabetes insipidus syndrome (polyuria, polydipsia, and weakness) in some patients receiving long-term therapy. The syndrome is dose dependent and reversible on discontinuation of therapy.

INDICATIONS

See Table 9-4 for complete indications for tetrycyclines. Treatment of infections due to susceptible strains of designated organisms: rickettsiae (Rocky Mountain spotted fever, typhus fever and the typhus group, Q fever, rickettsialpox); *Mycoplasma pneumoniae* (PPLO, Eaton agent); agents of psittacosis and ornithosis; agents of lymphogranuloma venereum and granuloma inguinale; *Borrelia recurrentis*; *Hemophilus ducreyi, Yersinia pestis, Francisella tularensis, Bartonella bacilliformis, Bacteroides* species, *Vibrio comma, Vibrio fetus, Brucella* spp (in conjunction with streptomycin)
When penicillin is contraindicated: *Treponema pallidum, Treponema pertenue, Bacillus anthracis, Fusobacterium fusiforme, Actinomyces* spp

CONTRAINDICATIONS

Allergy or hypersensitivity to tetracyclines

INTERACTIONS

Antacids; anticoagulants, oral barbiturates (carbamazepine, hydantoins); cimetidine; digoxin; insulin; iron salts, oral; lithium; methoxyflurane; oral contraceptives; penicillins, sodium bicarbonate
Food interactions: Food and some dairy products inhibit tetracycline absorption. Give tetracycline 1 hour before or 2 hour after meals.

ADVERSE EFFECTS

Central nervous system: transient myopathy
Dermatologic: rash (maculopapular-erythematous), exfoliative dermatitis (infrequent), photosensitivity, onycholysis and discoloration of the nails (rare) (Note: Onycholysis has been reported to occur in up to 25% of patients experiencing phototoxicity.)
Gastrointestinal: *ORAL AND PARENTERAL*: anorexia, nausea, vomiting, diarrhea, epigastric distress, bulky or loose stools, stomatitis, sore throat, glossitis, hoarseness, black hairy tongue, dysphagia, enterocolitis, inflammatory lesions with monilial overgrowth in anogenital region (including proctitis and pruritus ani). *ORAL ONLY*: esophageal ulcers (most often in patients with an esophageal obstructive element or hiatal hernia. (Note: Patient should remain standing for at least 90 seconds after medication is swallowed and should take medication with a full glass of water at least 1 hour before bedtime to minimize the problem.)
Hematologic: hemolytic anemia, thrombocytopenia, thrombocytopenic purpura, neutropenia, eosinophilia
Hepatic: fatty liver, hepatotoxicity (rare), increased liver enzymes, hepatitis (rare), hepatic cholestasis (rare). (Note: Effects usually associated with high doses.)
Hypersensitivity: urticaria, angioneurotic edema, anaphylaxis anaphylactoid purpura, pericarditis, exacerbation of lupus erythematosus, polyarthralgia, serum sickness–like reactions (fever, rash, arthralgia), pulmonary infiltrates with eosinophilia

(Continued on next page)

The information here is provided as guidance only. Prescribers should always consult the manufacturer's current prescribing information.

DEMECLOCYLINE (CONTINUED)

SPECIAL GROUPS

Children: Do not use in children 8 years of age or younger.
Elderly: May have age-related renal impairment; otherwise, same as adults.
Renal impairment: Not to be used in patients with renal impairment (*see* Special Precautions).
Hepatic impairment: Use with caution (*see* Special Precautions).
Pregnancy: Do not use demeclocycline during pregnancy or the postpartum period.
Breast-feeding: Discontinue nursing or discontinue therapy.

DOSAGE

Adults: 150 mg every 6 hours or 300 mg every 12 hours.
Elderly: May have age-related renal impairment; otherwise, same as adults.
Children: (Children older than 8 years of age only), 6 to 12 mg/kg in divided doses every 6 to 12 hours, depending on severity of infection.
Impaired renal function: Contraindicated.

ADVERSE EFFECTS *(CONTINUED)*

Renal: increase in blood urea nitrogen (dose related)
Miscellaneous: pseudotumor cerebri (adults) and bulging fontanels (infants), brown-black microscopic discoloration of thyroid gland (prolonged use only), tooth discoloration (rare in adults)

PHARMACOKINETICS AND PHARMACODYNAMICS

Peak serum levels: approximately 2 µg/mL following a 300-mg dose orally
Plasma half-life: 12 h
Bioavailability: approximately 66%
Metabolism: no information
Excretion: 39% unchanged in urine
Effect of food: inhibits absorption, take on empty stomach
Protein binding: 91%
Renal impairment: contraindicated
Hepatic impairment: use with caution

OVERDOSAGE

Discontinue medication, treat patients symptomatically, and give supportive care. Dialysis does not alter serum half-life.

PATIENT INFORMATION

Take on empty stomach at least 1 hour before or 2 hours after meals. Take with a full glass of water. Avoid simultaneous dairy products, antacids, laxatives, or iron-containing products. If antacid must be taken, take at least 2 hours before or after tetracycline agent. Avoid prolonged exposure to ultraviolet light.

AVAILABILITY

Capsules—150 mg
Tablets—150 mg and 300 mg

DOXYCYCLINE (Doryx®, Monodox®, Vibramycin®)

Doxycycline, a long-acting analogue with a half-life of 18 hours, has emerged as one of the most popular of the tetracyclines. The analogue is one of the most active members of the family *in vitro*, and it can be taken less frequently (once or twice per day), is less affected by food than many of the other analogues, and is the only tetracycline analogue that can be administered in patients with renal failure. The cost of doxycycline is currently similar to tetracycline, as is the adverse reaction profile. Doxycycline is the preferred analogue when intravenous administration is required. It has developed a specific niche for the treatment of many sexually transmitted diseases in which *Chlamydia trachomatis* plays a role. Thus, it is a recommended regimen for the treatment of lymphogranuloma venereum and nongonococcal urethritis. Because of the high prevalence of coinfection with *C. trachomatis* among adults and adolescents with gonococcal infection, presumptive treatment of *Chlamydia* infection for patients being treated for gonorrhea is appropriate with this antibiotic, particularly if no diagnostic test for *C. trachomatis* is available. Because of gonococcal resistance, however, it should not be used alone for gonococcal infections unless the susceptibilities are known.

(Continued on next page)

INDICATIONS

See Table 9-4 for complete indications for tetrycyclines.
Infections of the following types due to susceptible strains of designated organisms:
Rocky Mountain spotted fever, typhus fever (and typhus group), rickettsialpox, and tick fevers due to *Rickettsia*
Respiratory tract: *Mycoplasma pneumoniae* (alternative therapy)
Lymphogranuloma venereum, urethral, endocervical, or rectal infections or trachoma: *C. trachomatis*
Psittacosis: *Chlamydia psittaci*
Urethritis (nongonococcal): *Ureaplasma urealyticum*
Relapsing fever: *Borrelia recurrentis*
Chancroid: *Haemophilus ducreyi*
Plague: *Yersinia pestis* (alternative therapy)
Tularemia: *Francisella tularensis* (alternative therapy)
Cholera: *Vibrio cholerae*
Campylobacter fetus infections: *Campylobacter fetus*
Bartonellosis: *Bartonella bacilliformis*
Granuloma inguinale: *Calymmatobacterium granulomatis*

The information here is provided as guidance only. Prescribers should always consult the manufacturer's current prescribing information.

DOXYCYCLINE (CONTINUED)

This analogue is recommended for both inpatient (intravenous) and outpatient (oral) therapy of pelvic inflammatory disease in association with a cephalosporin as well as for epididymitis in men less than 35 years of age. It also should be considered in a treatment regimen for sexual disease prophylaxis following sexual assault in adults and adolescents. The dose for these indications is 100 mg twice a day. Like other tetracyclines, it should not be used in patients who are pregnant or breast feeding, and it should only be given under extenuating circumstances in children 8 years or younger. Doxycycline does interact with other drugs metabolized by the liver more frequently than do the other analogues, which may result in a shorter half-life. Such is the case when it is administered in patients who also are taking carbamazepine, phenytoin, the barbiturates, or ethanol chronically.

ANTIMICROBIAL ACTIVITY

There can be a great deal of variability in susceptibility for gram-positive and -negative bacteria. The following gram-negative bacteria are frequently susceptible: *Neisseria gonorrhea*, *Calymmatobacterium granulomatis*, *Haemophilus ducreyi*, *Haemophilus influenzae*, *Yersinia pestis*, *Francisella tularensis*, *Vibrio cholerae*, *Bartonella bacilliformis*, and *Brucella* spp. Other organisms that are generally susceptible include: Rickettsiae, *Chlamydia psittaci* and *trachomatis*, *Mycoplasma pneumoniae*, *Ureaplasma urealyticum*, *Borrelia burgdorferi*, *Borrelia recurrentis*, *Treponema pallidum*, *Treponema pertenue*, *Clostridium* spp, *Fusobacterium fusiforme*, *Actinomyces* spp, *Bacillus anthracis*, *Propionibacterium acnes*, *Entamoeba* spp, *Balantidium coli*, and *Plasmodium falciparum*.
Although some strains of *Escherichia coli*, *Klebsiella* spp, *Enterobacter aerogenes*, *Shigella* spp, and *Acinetobacter* spp are susceptible, resistance is common. Some strains of *Streptococcus pyogenes*, *Streptococcus pneumonae*, and enterococci are sensitive, but susceptibility tests should be performed.

RESISTANCE

Up to 44% of strains of *Streptococcus pyogenes* including two thirds of those resistant to penicillan G and 74% of *Streptococcus faecalis* are resistant. Gonococci resistant to penicillin G are usually resistant to doxycycline.

SPECIAL PRECAUTIONS

Only doxycycline should be used in patients with renal function impairment. Monitoring of function is recommended with prolonged therapy.
Antianabolic effect of tetracyclines may cause increased blood urea nitrogen. Patients with significant renal function impairment may exacerbate their azotemia, hyperphosphatemia, or acidosis due to higher serum levels of tetracycline agent. (Effect does not occur with doxycycline.)
Liver toxicity is an increased risk with parenteral administration to pregnant or postpartum patients with pyelonephritis.
Photosensitivity has been observed with tetracycline therapy. Advise patient to use protective measures and to avoid prolonged exposure to ultraviolet light.
Parenteral therapy should be used only when oral therapy is not possible or when high blood levels are needed rapidly. Institute oral therapy as soon as clinically feasible.
Thrombophlebitis may result from prolonged intravenous therapy. Intramuscular administration produces lower blood levels than oral form and is painful.
Doses of intravenous tetracyclines in excess of 2 g/d have been associated with death secondary to liver failure. Serum tetracycline levels should not exceed 15 μg/mL, and other hepatotoxic drugs should not be used concomitantly. The danger is increased in patients with renal or hepatic impairment and pregnant patients; monitor function tests.
Tetracyclines form a stable calcium complex in any bone-forming tissue; a decrease in fibula growth rate has been observed in premature infants given oral tetracycline doses of 25 mg/kg every 6 hours.
Use of tetracyclines during the period of tooth development (from last half of pregnancy through the 8th year of life) may cause permanent discoloration of deciduous and permanent teeth. Enamel hypoplasia also has been reported.

(Continued on next page)

CONTRAINDICATIONS

Allergy or hypersensitivity to tetracyclines

INTERACTIONS

Laboratory test interactions: False elevations of urinary catecholamine levels may occur due to interference with the fluorescence test
Antacids; anticoagulants, oral barbiturates; carbamazepine, hydantoins; cimetidine; digoxin; insulin; iron salts, oral lithium; methoxyflurane; oral contraceptives; penicillins, sodium bicarbonate

ADVERSE EFFECTS

Central nervous system: transient myopathy
Dermatologic: rash (maculopapular-erythematous), exfoliative dermatitis (infrequent), photosensitivity, onycholysis and discoloration of the nails (rare). (Note: Onycholysis has been reported to occur in up to 25% of patients experiencing phototoxicity.)
Gastrointestinal: *ORAL AND PARENTERAL*: anorexia, nausea, vomiting, diarrhea, epigastric distress, bulky or loose stools, stomatitis, sore throat, glossitis, hoarseness, black hairy tongue, dysphagia, enterocolitis, inflammatory lesions with monilial overgrowth in anogenital region (including proctitis and pruritus ani). *ORAL ONLY*: esophageal ulcers (most often in patients with an esophageal obstructive element or hiatal hernia. (Note: Patient should remain standing for at least 90 seconds after medication is swallowed and should take medication with a full glass of water at least 1 hour before bedtime to minimize the problem.)
Hematologic: hemolytic anemia, thrombocytopenia, thrombocytopenic purpura, neutropenia, eosinophilia
Hepatic: fatty liver, hepatotoxicity (rare), increased liver enzymes, hepatitis (rare), hepatic cholestasis (rare). (Note: Effects usually associated with high doses.)
Hypersensitivity: urticaria, angioneurotic edema, anaphylaxis anaphylactoid purpura, pericarditis, exacerbation of lupus erythematosus, polyarthralgia, serum sickness–like reactions (fever, rash, arthralgia), pulmonary infiltrates with eosinophilia
Local: irritation with intramuscular injection
Renal: increase in blood urea nitrogen (dose related)
Miscellaneous: pseudotumor cerebri (adults) and bulging fontanels (infants), brown-black microscopic discoloration of thyroid gland (prolonged use only), tooth discoloration (rare in adults)

PHARMACOKINETICS AND PHARMACODYNAMICS

Peak serum levels: 2.5 μg/mL following a 200-mg dose orally
Plasma half-life: 18 h
Bioavailability: 93%
Excretion: 30% to 42% unchanged in urine
Effect of food: inhibits absorption; take on empty stomach
Protein binding: 80% to 95%
Renal impairment: half-life not affected
Hepatic impairment: use with caution

The information here is provided as guidance only. Prescribers should always consult the manufacturer's current prescribing information.

DOXYCYCLINE (CONTINUED)

SPECIAL PRECAUTIONS *(CONTINUED)*

Pseudotumor cerebri in adults has been associated with tetracycline use. Clinical signs include headache and blurred vision. Bulging fontanels have been associated with tetracycline use in infants. Although conditions and symptoms usually resolve after discontinuation of tetracycline, the possibility for permanent sequelae exists. Do not use outdated tetracycline products under any circumstances. Degradation products of tetracyclines are extremely nephrotoxic and occasionally have produced a Fanconi-like syndrome.

Some products and preparations may contain sulfites, which may cause allergic-type reactions, including anaphylactic and life-threatening asthmatic episodes.

In sexually transmitted infections in which primary or secondary syphilis may be suspected, proper diagnostic procedures are indicated, including darkfield examinations and monthly serologic tests for a minimum of 4 months. Continuation of clinical and serologic examinations every 6 months for 2 to 3 years is recommended for all cases.

Antacids containing aluminum, zinc, magnesium, or bismuth salts (or other divalent and trivalent cations) impair absorption of tetracyclines because they form a poorly soluble chelate, possibly decreasing antimicrobial efficacy. Administer tetracyclines at least 2 hours before or after these agents.

Prolonged or repeated antibiotic therapy may result in bacterial or fungal overgrowth of nonsusceptible organisms, leading to secondary infection.

Avoid rapid intravenous administration. Thrombophlebitis may result from prolonged intravenous therapy.

Continue therapy at least 24 to 48 hours after symptoms and fever have subsided.

SPECIAL GROUPS

Children: Do not use in children 8 years of age or younger.
Elderly: May have age-related renal impairment; otherwise, same as adults.
Renal impairment: Recommended doses safe for use, monitor function.
Hepatic impairment: Use with caution.
Pregnancy: Do not use tetracycline during pregnancy.
Breast-feeding: Discontinue nursing or discontinue therapy.

DOSAGE

Adults: (Note: Therapeutic antibacterial serum activity will ordinarily persist for 24 hours.) *ORAL:* 200 mg on 1st day of treatment (100 mg every 12 hours) followed by a maintenance dose of 100 mg/d, administered as a single dose or as 50 mg every 12 hours. For severe infections, 100 mg every 12 hours. For acute gonococcal infection when the organism is sensitive, 200 mg immediately and then 100 mg at bedtime on the 1st day; follow with 100 mg every 12 hours for 3 days. For primary and secondary syphilis, 100 mg orally two times a day for 2 weeks. For uncomplicated urethral, endocervical, or rectal infections in adults due to *C. trachomatis*, 100 mg every 12 hours for 7 days. For pelvic inflammatory disease, give 100 mg doxycycline intravenously or orally every 12 hours with cefoxitin. *PARENTERAL:* (Do not inject intramuscularly or subcutaneously) 100 to 200 mg/d by intravenous infusion; duration of infusion may vary but is usually 1 to 4 hours; continue therapy for a minimum of 24 to 48 hours after symptoms have subsided.
Elderly: Same as adults.
Children: Do not use in children 8 years of age or younger. *ORAL:* (< 45 kg) 4.4 mg/kg divided doses every 12 hours on 1st day, followed with 2.2 mg/kg given as a single dose or two divided doses on subsequent days. For severe infection, up to 4.4 mg/kg/d may be used. For children over 45 kg, use adult dose. *PARENTERAL:* (< 45 kg) 4.4 mg/kg on the 1st day in one to two infusions, follow with 2.2 to 4.4 mg/kg given as one or two infusions, depending on severity of infection. For children over 45 kg, use adult dose.
Impaired renal function: Normal doses are safe; monitor function.

OVERDOSAGE

Discontinue medication, treat patients symptomatically, and give supportive care. Dialysis does not alter serum half-life.

PATIENT INFORMATION

Take on empty stomach at least 1 hour before or 2 hours after meals. Take with a full glass of water. Avoid simultaneous dairy products, antacids, laxatives, or iron-containing products. If antacid must be taken, take at least 2 hours before or after tetracycline agent.

Avoid prolonged exposure to ultraviolet light.

AVAILABILITY

Capsules—50 mg (as hyclate) and 50 mg (as monohydrate)
Capsules—100 mg (as hyclate) and 100 mg (as monohydrate)
Tablets—50 mg (as hyclate), 100 mg (as hyclate), and 100 mg (as monohydrate)
Capsules coated pellets—100 mg (as hyclate)
Powder for Oral Suspension—25 mg (as monohydrate) per 5 mL when reconstituted
Syrup—50 mg (as calcium)
Powder for Injection—100 mg (as hyclate) and 200 mg (as hyclate)

The information here is provided as guidance only. Prescribers should always consult the manufacturer's current prescribing information.

MINOCYCLINE (Dynacin®, Minocin®)

Minocycline is the most active of all of the currently available tetracyclines. Unfortunately, the vestibular toxicity has reduced its use for many indications. Also, cost is a factor that reduces its popularity relative to the other analogues. Nevertheless, its high degree of activity, long half-life (16 hours), good bioavailability, relative lack of effect by food, and lipophilic characteristics make it the drug of choice for a few selected indications, including infections caused by *Mycobacterium marinum*. It is an alternative therapy for *Xanthomonas maltophilia* and *Mycobacterium leprae* and an alternative prophylaxis for meningococcal disease. It is not recommended for pregnant or breast-feeding women or children 8 years of age or younger.

ANTIMICROBIAL ACTIVITY

The spectrum is similar to the other tetracyclines. This analogue, however, may be slightly more active than the less lipophilic congeners. In some cases, this may be a two- to fourfold increase in activity. The activity of minocycline for *Nocardia* and *Mycobacterium marianum*, *Xanthomonas maltophilia*, and for meningococci are particularly relevant clinically. (*See* Antimicrobial Activity for doxycycline.)

RESISTANCE

Up to 44% of strains of *Streptococcus pyogenes* including two thirds of those resistant to penicillan G and 74% of *Streptococcus faecalis* are resistant. Gonococci resistant to penicillin G are usually resistant to the tetracyclines.

SPECIAL PRECAUTIONS

Unlike most other tetracyclines, minocycline should be taken with food or milk. *See* Special Precautions for doxycycline.

SPECIAL GROUPS

Children: Do not use in children 8 years of age or younger.
Elderly: May have age-related renal impairment.
Renal impairment: Not recommended.
Hepatic impairment: Use with extreme caution.
Pregnancy: Do not use tetracycline during pregnancy.
Breast-feeding: Discontinue nursing or discontinue therapy.

INDICATIONS

See Table 9-4 for complete indications for the tetracyclines.
Rickettsia infection; *Mycoplasma pneumoniae* infection; agents of psittacosis and ornithosis (*Chlamydia psittaci*); agents of lymphogranuloma venereum and granuloma inguinale (*Chlamydia trachomatis* and *Calymmatobacterium granulomatis*, respectively); spirochetal agent of relapsing fever (*Borrelia recurrentis*)
Gram-negative: *Haemophilus ducreyi*, *Yersinia pestis*, *Francisella tularensis*, *Bartonella bacilliformis*, *Bacteroides* spp, *Vibrio comma*, *Vibrio fetus*, *Brucella* spp (in conjunction with streptomycin), *Helicobacter pylori* (plus metronidazole and bismuth subsalicylate), *Pseudomonas mallei* (glanders) (with streptomycin)
Nocardiosis (as an alternative to sulfonamides)
Treatment of asymptomatic carriers of *Neisseria meningitidis* (alternative to rifampin)

CONTRAINDICATIONS

Allergy or hypersensitivity to tetracyclines

INTERACTIONS

Antacids; anticoagulants, oral; barbiturates (carbamazepine, hydantoins); cimetidine; digoxin; insulin; iron salts, oral; lithium; methoxyflurane; oral contraceptives; penicillins, sodium bicarbonate
Food interactions: Food and some dairy products inhibit absorption of most tetracyclines. Minocycline is an exception and can be administered with meals.

ADVERSE EFFECTS

Stevens-Johnson syndrome (rare)
Central nervous system: transient myopathy
Dermatologic: rash (maculopapular-erythematous), exfoliative dermatitis (infrequent), photosensitivity, onycholysis and discoloration of the nails (rare). (Note: Onycholysis has been reported to occur in up to 25% of patients experiencing phototoxicity.)
Gastrointestinal: *ORAL AND PARENTERAL*: anorexia, nausea, vomiting, diarrhea, epigastric distress, bulky or loose stools, stomatitis, sore throat, glossitis, hoarseness, black hairy tongue, dysphagia, enterocolitis, inflammatory lesions with monilial overgrowth in anogenital region (including proctitis and pruritus ani). *ORAL ONLY*: esophageal ulcers (most often in patients with an esophageal obstructive element or hiatal hernia.) (Note: Patient should remain standing for at least 90 seconds after medication is swallowed and should take medication with a full glass of water at least 1 hour before bedtime to minimize the problem.)
Hematologic: Hemolytic anemia, thrombocytopenia, thrombocytopenic purpura, neutropenia, eosinophilia
Hepatic: fatty liver, hepatotoxicity (rare), increased liver enzymes, hepatitis (rare), hepatic cholestasis (rare) (Note: Effects usually associated with high doses.)
Hypersensitivity: urticaria, angioneurotic edema, anaphylaxis anaphylactoid purpura, pericarditis, exacerbation of lupus erythematosus, polyarthralgia, serum sickness–like reactions (fever, rash, arthralgia), pulmonary infiltrates with eosinophilia

(Continued on next page)

The information here is provided as guidance only. Prescribers should always consult the manufacturer's current prescribing information.

MINOCYCLINE (CONTINUED)

DOSAGE

Adults: *ORAL*: 200 mg initially, followed by 100 mg every 12 hours or 100 to 200 mg initially followed by 50 mg every 6 hours. For primary and secondary syphilis, give usual dose over a period of 10 to 15 days, close follow-up and repeated serologic tests recommended. For uncomplicated urethral, endocervical, or rectal infection due to *Chlamydia trachomatis* or *Ureaplasma urealyticum*, 100 mg every 12 hours for a minimum of 7 days. For gonorrhea in patients sensitive to penicillin, 200 mg initially followed by 100 mg every 12 hours for a minimum of 4 days, with repeated cultures within 2 to 3 days after therapy is completed. For meningococcal carrier state, 100 mg every 12 hours for 5 days. For *Mycobacterium marinum* infections, (optimal doses not established) 100 mg every 12 hours for 6 to 8 weeks (successful in limited number of cases). *PARENTERAL*: 200 mg initially followed by 100 mg every 12 hours, do not exceed 400 mg in 24 hours.

Elderly: May have age-related renal impairment; otherwise, same as adults.

Children: Do not use in children 8 years of age or younger. *ORAL*: Give 4 mg/kg initially, followed by 2 mg/kg every 12 hours. *PARENTERAL*: 4 mg/kg initially, followed with 2 mg/kg every 12 hours.

Impaired renal function: Not recommended.

ADVERSE EFFECTS *(CONTINUED)*

Local: irritation with intramuscular injection

Renal: increase in blood urea nitrogen (dose related)

Miscellaneous: pseudotumor cerebri (adults) and bulging fontanels (infants), brown-black microscopic discoloration of thyroid gland (prolonged use only), tooth discoloration (rare in adults)

PHARMACOKINETICS AND PHARMACODYNAMICS

Peak serum levels: 2.5 µg/mL following a 200-mg dose orally.

Plasma half-life: 16 h

Bioavailability: 95%

Metabolism: liver

Excretion: 6% to 12% unchanged in urine

Effect of food: take with food or milk

Protein binding: 70% to 80%

Renal impairment: half-life is prolonged; administration not recommended

Hepatic impairment: use with caution

OVERDOSAGE

Discontinue medication, treat patient symptomatically, and give supportive care. Dialysis does not alter serum half-life.

PATIENT INFORMATION

Avoid activities requiring alertness or coordination; minocycline may cause lightheadedness or dizziness.

Take with a full glass of water. Avoid simultaneous dairy products, antacids, laxatives, or iron-containing products. If antacid must be taken, take at least 2 hours before or after tetracycline agent.

Avoid prolonged exposure to ultraviolet light.

AVAILABILITY

Capsules—50 mg (as hydrochloride) and 100 mg (as hydrochloride)

Capsules, pellet-filled—50 mg (as hydrochloride) and 100 mg (as hydrochloride)

Oral Suspension—50 mg (as hydrochloride) per 5 mL

Powder for Injection—100 mg

The information here is provided as guidance only. Prescribers should always consult the manufacturer's current prescribing information.

OXYTETRACYCLINE (Terra-Cortril®, Terramycin®)

Oxytetracycline was the second of the tetracycline analogues to be developed. It is very similar to tetracycline in regard to *in vitro* activity. Also, like tetracycline, it is in the "short-acting" category. The cost of oxytetracycline, however, is considerably greater than tetracycline, and this has limited its use. There are no significant advantages. Like the other analogues, it should not be used during pregnancy or while breast-feeding. It should not be used in children 8 years of age or younger and is not recommended for parenteral administration.

ANTIMICROBIAL ACTIVITY

Spectrum and activity similar to tetracycline.

RESISTANCE

Up to 44% of strains of *Streptococcus pyogenes* including two thirds of those resistant to penicillan G and 74% of *Streptococcus faecalis* are resistant. Gonococci resistant to penicillin G are usually resistant to the tetracyclines.

SPECIAL PRECAUTIONS

See Special Precautions for doxycycline.

SPECIAL GROUPS

Children: Do not use in children 8 years of age or younger.
Elderly: May have age-related renal impairment.
Renal impairment: Not recommended (*see* Special Precautions).
Hepatic impairment: Use with caution (*see* Special Precautions).
Pregnancy: Do not use tetracycline during pregnancy.
Breast-feeding: Discontinue nursing or discontinue therapy.

INDICATIONS

See Table 9-4 for complete indications for the tetracyclines.
Infections due to susceptible strains of designated organisms: *Escherichia coli, Enterobacter aerogenes, Shigella* spp, *Mima* spp, *Herellea* spp
Respiratory and urinary infections: *Haemophilus influenzae, Klebsiella* spp
Upper respiratory infections: *Streptococcus pneumoniae*
When penicillin is contraindicated: *Neisseria gonorrhoeae, Treponema pallidum, Treponema pertenue* (syphilis and yaws), *Listeria monocytogenes, Clostridium* spp, *Bacillus anthracis, Fusobacterium fusiforme, Actinomyces* spp
Uncomplicated urethral, endocervical, or rectal **infection:** *Chlamydia trachomatis*

CONTRAINDICATIONS

Allergy or hypersensitivity to tetracyclines

INTERACTIONS

Antacids; anticoagulants, oral; barbiturates (carbamazepine, hydantoins); cimetidine; digoxin; insulin; iron salts, oral; lithium; methoxyflurane; oral contraceptives; penicillins, sodium bicarbonate
Food interactions: Food and some dairy products inhibit tetracycline absorption. Give tetracycline 1 hour before or 2 hours after meals.

ADVERSE EFFECTS

Central nervous system: transient myopathy
Dermatologic: rash (maculopapular-erythematous), exfoliative dermatitis (infrequent), photosensitivity, onycholysis and discoloration of the nails (rare). (Note: Onycholysis has been reported to occur in up to 25% of patients experiencing phototoxicity.)
Gastrointestinal: *ORAL AND PARENTERAL*: anorexia, nausea, vomiting, diarrhea, epigastric distress, bulky or loose stools, stomatitis, sore throat, glossitis, hoarseness, black hairy tongue, dysphagia, enterocolitis, inflammatory lesions with monilial overgrowth in anogenital region (including proctitis and pruritus ani). *ORAL ONLY*: esophageal ulcers (most often in patients with an esophageal obstructive element or hiatal hernia.) (Note: Patient should remain standing for at least 90 seconds after medication is swallowed and should take medication with a full glass of water at least 1 hour before bedtime to minimize the problem.)
Hematologic: Hemolytic anemia, thrombocytopenia, thrombocytopenic purpura, neutropenia, eosinophilia
Hepatic: fatty liver, hepatotoxicity (rare), increased liver enzymes, hepatitis (rare), hepatic cholestasis (rare). (Note: Effects usually associated with high doses.)
Hypersensitivity: urticaria, angioneurotic edema, anaphylaxis anaphylactoid purpura, pericarditis, exacerbation of lupus erythematosus, polyarthralgia, serum sickness–like reactions (fever, rash, arthralgia), pulmonary infiltrates with eosinophilia
Local: irritation with intramuscular injection
Renal: increase in blood urea nitrogen (dose related)
Miscellaneous: pseudotumor cerebri (adults) and bulging fontanels (infants), brown-black microscopic discoloration of thyroid gland (prolonged use only), tooth discoloration (rare in adults)

The information here is provided as guidance only. Prescribers should always consult the manufacturer's current prescribing information.

OXYTETRACYCLINE (CONTINUED)

DOSAGE

Adults: *ORAL:* (same as tetracycline) 1 to 2 g in divided doses every 6 to 12 hours, based on severity of infection. For brucellosis, 500 mg every 6 hours for 3 weeks with streptomycin 1 g intramuscularly twice daily for the 1st week and once daily for the 2nd week. For syphilis, give 500 mg every 6 hours for 14 days. For syphilis of greater than 1 year's duration, 4 weeks is recommended length of therapy. Close follow-up is recommended. For uncomplicated urethral, endocervical, or rectal infection in adults due to *Chlamydia trachomatis*, 500 mg orally every 6 hours for a minimum of 7 days. For severe acne (long-term therapy), give 1 g/d initially in divided doses, follow with 125 to 500 mg/d maintenance dose. *PARENTERAL* (for intramuscular use only): 250 mg once every 24 hours or 300 mg in divided doses every 8 to 12 hours. Intramuscular administration may produce lower serum levels than oral administration.

Elderly: May have age-related renal impairment; otherwise, same as adults.

Children: Do not use in children 8 years of age or younger. *ORAL:* (same as tetracycline) 25 to 50 mg/kg in two to four divided doses every 6 to 12 hours, based on severity of infection. *PARENTERAL:* 15 to 25 mg/kg, up to maximum of 250 mg per single daily injection; dosage may be divided and given at intervals of every 8 to 12 hours.

Impaired renal function: Not recommended.

PHARMACOKINETICS AND PHARMACODYNAMICS

Peak serum levels: 2 µg/mL following a 500-mg oral dose
Plasma half-life: 9 h
Bioavailability: 58%
Excretion: 70% unchanged in urine
Effect of food: inhibits absorption; take on empty stomach
Protein binding: 20% to 40%
Renal impairment: prolongs half-life and decreases elimination; not recommended for administration
Hepatic impairment: use with caution

OVERDOSAGE

Discontinue medication, treat patients symptomatically, and give supportive care. Dialysis does not alter serum half-life.

PATIENT INFORMATION

Take on empty stomach at least 1 hour before or 2 hours after meals. Take with a full glass of water. Avoid simultaneous dairy products, antacids, laxatives, or iron-containing products. If antacid must be taken, take at least 2 hours before or after tetracycline agent.

Avoid prolonged exposure to ultraviolet light.

AVAILABILITY

Capsules—250 mg (as hydrochloride)
Injection—50 mg/mL with 2% lidocaine
Injection—125 mg/mL with 2% lidocaine

The information here is provided as guidance only. Prescribers should always consult the manufacturer's current prescribing information.

TETRACYCLINE (Achromycin®, Topicycline®)

Tetracycline has been the most popular member of this family of antimicrobials. The *in vitro* spectrum is typical of most of the early analogues, and the cost is extremely low. Pharmacokinetically, the half-life of approximately 8 hours places this analogue as a "short-acting" tetracycline. The adverse reactions and drug interactions are not unique to this member of the family. Like other tetracyclines, it should never be given to children 8 years of age or younger unless extenuating circumstances prevail. It is contraindicated in women who are pregnant or breast-feeding or in patients with renal impairment. It is not recommended for intramuscular or intravenous administration.

ANTIMICROBIAL ACTIVITY

There can be a great deal of variability in susceptibility for gram-positive and -negative bacteria. The following gram-negative bacteria are frequently susceptible: *Neisseria gonorrhea, Calymmatobacterium granulomatis, Haemophilus ducreyi, Haemophilus influenzae, Yersinia pestis, Francisella tularensis, Vibrio cholerae, Bartonella bacilliformis,* and *Brucella* spp.

Other organisms that are generally susceptible include: Rickettsiae, *Chlamydia psittaci* and *trachomatis, Mycoplasma pneumoniae, Ureaplasma urealyticum, Borrelia burgdorferi, Borrelia recurrentis, Treponema pallidum, Treponema pertenue, Clostridium* spp, *Fusobacterium fusiforme, Actinomyces* spp, *Bacillus anthracis, Propionibacterium acnes, Entamoeba* spp, *Balantidium coli,* and *Plasmodium falciparum.*

Although some strains of *Escherichia coli, Klebsiella* spp, *Enterobacter aerogenes, Shigella* spp, and *Acinetobacter* spp are susceptible, resistance is common. Some strains of *Streptococcus pyogenes, Streptococcus pneumonae,* and enterococci are sensitive, but susceptibility tests should be performed.

RESISTANCE

Up to 44% of strains of *Streptococcus pyogenes* including two thirds of those resistant to penicillan G and 74% of *Streptococcus faecalis* are resistant to the tetracycline agents.

SPECIAL PRECAUTIONS

See Special Precautions for doxycycline.

SPECIAL GROUPS

Children: Do not use in children younger than 8 years of age.
Elderly: May have age-related renal impairment.
Renal impairment: Not recommended.
Hepatic impairment: Use with caution (*see* Special Precautions).
Pregnancy: Do not use tetracycline during pregnancy.
Breast-feeding: Discontinue nursing or discontinue therapy.

INDICATIONS

See Table 9-4 for complete indications for the tetracyclines.

Infections due to designated susceptible strains of organisms:
Escherichia coli, Enterobacter aerogenes, Shigella spp, *Mima* spp, *Herellea* spp

Respiratory and urinary infections: *Haemophilus influenzae, Klebsiella* spp

Upper respiratory infections: *Streptococcus pneumoniae*

When penicillin is contraindicated: *Neisseria gonorrhoeae, Treponema pallidum, Treponema pertenue* (syphilis and yaws), *Listeria monocytogenes, Clostridium* spp, *Bacillus anthracis, Fusobacterium fusiforme, Actinomyces* spp

Uncomplicated urethral, endocervical, or rectal infection: *Chlamydia trachomatis*

CONTRAINDICATIONS

Allergy or hypersensitivity to tetracyclines

INTERACTIONS

Antacids; anticoagulants, oral; barbiturates (carbamazepine, hydantoins); cimetidine; digoxin; insulin; iron salts, oral; lithium; methoxyflurane; oral contraceptives; penicillins, sodium bicarbonate

Food interactions: Food and some dairy products inhibit tetracycline absorption. Give tetracycline 1 hour before or 2 hours after meals.

ADVERSE EFFECTS

Central nervous system: transient myopathy

Dermatologic: rash (maculopapular-erythematous), exfoliative dermatitis (infrequent), photosensitivity, onycholysis and discoloration of the nails (rare). (Note: Onycholysis has been reported to occur in up to 25% of patients experiencing phototoxicity.)

Gastrointestinal: ORAL AND PARENTERAL: anorexia, nausea, vomiting, diarrhea, epigastric distress, bulky or loose stools, stomatitis, sore throat, glossitis, hoarseness, black hairy tongue, dysphagia, enterocolitis, inflammatory lesions with monilial overgrowth in anogenital region (including proctitis and pruritus ani). *ORAL ONLY:* esophageal ulcers (most often in patients with an esophageal obstructive element or hiatal hernia.) (Note: Patient should remain standing for at least 90 seconds after medication is swallowed and should take medication with a full glass of water at least 1 hour before bedtime to minimize the problem.)

Hematologic: hemolytic anemia, thrombocytopenia, thrombocytopenic purpura, neutropenia, eosinophilia

Hepatic: fatty liver, hepatotoxicity (rare), increased liver enzymes, hepatitis (rare), hepatic cholestasis (rare). (Note: Effects usually associated with high doses.)

Hypersensitivity: urticaria, angioneurotic edema, anaphylaxis anaphylactoid purpura, pericarditis, exacerbation of lupus erythematosus, polyarthralgia, serum sickness–like reactions (fever, rash, arthralgia), pulmonary infiltrates with eosinophilia

Local: irritation with intramuscular injection

Renal: increase in blood urea nitrogen (dose related)

Miscellaneous: pseudotumor cerebri (adults) and bulging fontanels (infants), brown-black microscopic discoloration of thyroid gland (prolonged use only), tooth discoloration (rare in adults)

The information here is provided as guidance only. Prescribers should always consult the manufacturer's current prescribing information.

TETRACYCLINE (CONTINUED)

DOSAGE

ORAL: 1 to 2 g in divided doses every 6 to 12 hours, based on severity of infection. For brucellosis, 500 mg every 6 hours for 3 weeks with streptomycin 1 g intramuscularly twice daily for the 1st week and once daily for the 2nd week. For primary and secondary syphilis, give 500 mg every 6 hours for 14 days; close follow-up is recommended. For syphilis of greater than 1 year's duration, 4 weeks is recommended. For uncomplicated urethral, endocervical, or rectal infection in adults due to *Chlamydia trachomatis*, 500 mg orally every 6 hours for a minimum of 7 days. For severe acne (long-term therapy), give 1 g/d initially in divided doses, follow with 125 to 500 mg/d maintenance dose.

Elderly: May have age-related renal impairment; otherwise, same as adults.

Children: (Do not use in children 8 years of age or younger.) *ORAL*: 25 to 50 mg/kg in two to four divided doses every 6 to 12 hours, based on severity of infection. *PARENTERAL*: (Intramuscularly): 15 to 25 mg/kg to a maximum of 250 mg per single daily injection; dose may be divided and given every 8 to 12 hours. (Intravenously): 12 mg/kg/d in divided doses every 12 hours, from 10 to 20 mg/d may be given based on severity of infection.

Impaired renal function: Not recommended.

PHARMACOKINETICS AND PHARMACODYNAMICS

Peak serum levels: 4 µg/mL following a 500-mg dose orally

Plasma half-life: 8 h

Bioavailability: 77%

Metabolism: no information

Excretion: 60% unchanged in urine

Effect of food: decreases absorption

Protein binding: 65%

Renal impairment: prolonged half-life and decreased elimination; should not be used with renal impairment

Hepatic impairment: use with caution

OVERDOSAGE

Discontinue medication, treat patients symptomatically, and give supportive care. Dialysis does not alter serum half-life.

PATIENT INFORMATION

Take on empty stomach at least 1 hour before or 2 hours after meals. Take with a full glass of water. Avoid simultaneous dairy products, antacids, laxatives, or iron-containing products. If antacid must be taken, take at least 2 hours before or after tetracycline agent.

Avoid prolonged exposure to ultraviolet light.

AVAILABILITY

Capsules—100 mg, 250 mg, and 500 mg
Tablets—250 mg and 500 mg
Oral Suspension—125 mg/5 mL
Syrup—135 mg/5mL
Powder for Intramuscular Injection—100 mg and 500 mg in vials (with 40 mg procaine hydrochloride)
Powder for Intravenous Injection—250 mg and 500 mg in vials

The information here is provided as guidance only. Prescribers should always consult the manufacturer's current prescribing information.

CHLORAMPHENICOL

CLASS DESCRIPTION

Chloramphenicol is a broad-spectrum highly effective antibiotic. Its clinical usefulness, however, has decreased over the years because of significant toxicity in the form of aplastic anemia and the availability of newer more active antibiotics. Nevertheless, it remains an important drug for selective indications. A newer derivative, thiamphenicol, has a similar spectrum but has not been reported to cause aplastic anemia. Because this analogue is not available in the United States, it is not discussed in detail.

CHEMISTRY AND CLASSIFICATION

The structure of chloramphenicol is seen in Figure 9-2. Thiamphenicol has the *p*-nitro group on the benzene ring replaced by a methylsulfonyl group. Although initially discovered by screening organisms, chloramphenicol was the first antibiotic whose chemical synthesis was economically and technically practical for large-scale production [1].

MECHANISM OF ACTION

Chloramphenicol enters the cell by an energy-dependent process. The antibiotic blocks protein synthesis by reversibly binding to the $50S$ subunit of the $70S$ ribosome at a position that prevents attachment of the amino acid-containing end of the aminoacyl–tRNA to its binding region. This prevents the association of the amino acid substrate with peptidyl transferase and thereby prevents peptidyl bond formation [2,3], resulting in bacteriostatic activity against most organisms at therapeutic concentrations. However, the antibiotic is bactericidal against some meningeal pathogens, such as *Haemophilus influenzae*, *Streptococcus pneumoniae*, and *Neisseria meningitidis* but not *Streptococcus agalactiae* or enteric gram-negative bacilli [4,5]. The mitochondria of human cells also contain $70S$ ribosomal particles. The effect of chloramphenicol on these cells has been suggested as a cause for the dose-related bone marrow suppression caused by chloramphenicol but not the idiosyncratic aplastic anemia.

IN VITRO ACTIVITY

The antibiotic has significant activity against a wide range of organisms, including gram-positive and gram-negative aerobic bacteria, anaerobes, spirochetes, rickettsiae, chlamydiae, and mycoplasmas. The activity for some of these organisms is seen in Table 9-5. Although many of these organisms are inhibited by concentrations easily achieved in the serum of patients, less toxic antibiotics are available for treatment of most. *Salmonella* generally are susceptible in the United States, but imported strains may be highly resistant [6]. *H. influenzae*, *S. pneumoniae*, and *N. meningitidis* are generally susceptible in the United States. In other countries, such as Spain, however, resistance particularly to *H. influenzae* may be frequent [7]. The antibiotic has activity against

Table 9-5. *In vitro* Activity of Chloramphenicol*

Aerobic	MIC$_{50}$	MIC$_{90}$	Range
Gram-positive aerobes			
Staphylococcus aureus	6.3	12.5	3.1–25
Staphylococcus aureus (methicillin-resistant)	> 25	> 25	> 25
Streptococcus pyogenes	3.1	3.1	1.6–12.5
Streptococcus agalactiae	3.1	6.3	3.1–12.5
Streptococcus viridans	3.1	6.3	3.1–12.5
Group D streptococci (Enterococcus)	> 25	> 25	> 25
Streptococcus pneumonia	3.1	6.3	3.1–6.3
Gram-positive anaerobes			
Peptococcus spp	1.6	3.1	< 0.4–> 25
Peptostreptococcus spp	1.6	3.1	< 0.4–6.3
Propionibacterium acnes	1.6	1.6	< 0.4–3.1
Eubacterium lentum	3.1	6.3	< 0.4–6.3
Clostridium perfringens	3.1	3.1	0.8–3.1
Clostridium spp	1.6	3.1	< 0.4–6.3
Gram-negative aerobes			
Haemophilus influenzae	1.6	3.1	1.6–3.1
Neisseria meningitidis	0.8	3.1	0.8–3.1
Neisseria gonorrhoeae	0.8	1.6	< 0.4–3.1
Escherichia coli	6.3	12.5	1.6–> 25
Klebsiella pneumoniae	3.1	> 25	1.6–> 25
Enterobacter	12.5	> 25	3.1–> 25
Serratia marcescens	25	> 25	6.3–> 25
Proteus mirabilis	6.3	12.5	3.1–> 25
Proteus (indole-positive)	12.5	> 25	3.1–> 25
Salmonella typhosa	3.1	6.3	3.1–> 12.5
Salmonella paratyphi A	6.3	6.3	3.1–> 25
Vibrio cholerae	6.3	6.3	6.3–> 25
Brucella spp	3.1	3.1	1.6–6.3
Pseudomonas aeruginosa	> 25	>25	> 25
Pseudomonas pseudomallei	6.3	12.5	6.3–12.5
Bordetella pertussis	1.6	3.1	< 1.6–12.5
Gram-negative anaerobes			
Veillonella spp	1.6	3.1	< 0.4–3.1
Bacteroides fragilis	6.3	6.3	0.8–12.5
Bacteroides melaninogenicus	1.6	6.3	0.4–6.3
Fusobacterium spp	1.6	6.3	0.4–6.3

* The National Committee for Clinical Laboratory Standards suggests that 4 mg/mL be considered susceptible when testing Haemophilus influenzae and 12 mg/mL or less be considered susceptible when testing other organisms.
MIC—minimum inhibitory concentration (μg/mL).

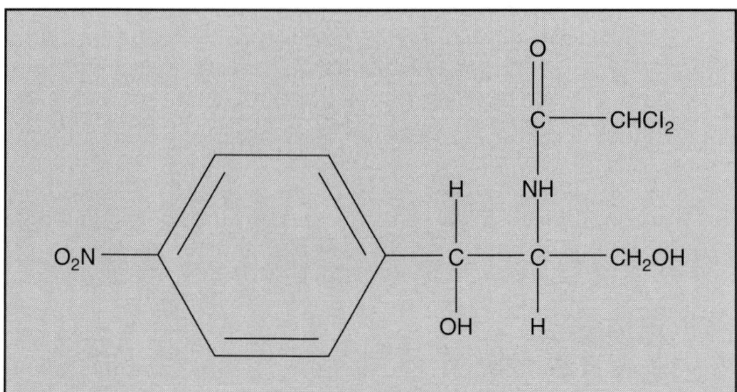

FIGURE 9-2.

The chemical structure of chloramphenicol. For thiamphenicol, the *p*-nitro group on the benzene ring is replaced by a methylsulfonyl group.

The information here is provided as guidance only. Prescribers should always consult the manufacturer's current prescribing information.

many anaerobic bacteria including *Bacteroides fragilis*. Chloramphenicol has activity against rickettsiae, and this has major importance clinically. It has no clinical useful activity against viruses or fungi.

MECHANISMS OF BACTERIAL RESISTANCE

Bacteria develop resistance to chloramphenicol by two major mechanisms: 1) they become impermeable to the antibiotic, and 2) they produce an enzyme, acetyl-transferase, that acetylates the antibiotic to an inactive diacetyl derivative. The resistance by acetyl-transferase has been plasmic-mediated and responsible for a number of chloramphenicol-resistant typhoid and *Shigella* epidemics throughout the world [8,9].

PHARMACOKINETICS

Chloramphenicol is available in an encapsulated form containing the base, a tasteless suspension in the form of chloramphenicol palmitate (used particularly for children), and a chloramphenicol succinate ester for intravenous administration. The oral encapsulated form is well absorbed from the gastrointestinal tract, achieving peak serum levels of 12 mg/mL of active chloramphenicol following a 1-g dose. The chloramphenicol palmitate must be hydrolyzed by pancreatic esterases in the intestine to active chloramphenicol. The bioavailability of this product is approximately 80%, producing peak plasma concentrations in 2 to 3 hours after administration, but this may be very erratic in the newborn [1,10].

The intravenous succinate ester, also a prodrug, must be hydrolyzed within the body to active chloramphenicol. The levels achieved by this preparation are 70% of those obtained after oral administration because of incomplete hydrolysis. This may, however, be quite variable, particularly in newborn infants and young children. One study has shown that serum levels were consistently lower when treating typhoid fever compared with other diseases with this product and suggested increasing the dose to 75 mg/kg/d to compensate [11].

Although the intramuscular route is well tolerated and produces peak serum levels in areas under the serum curve similar to intravenous administration, DuPont *et al.* [12] showed peak concentrations of only one half to two thirds those obtained following intravenous administration because of delayed absorption. This finding was associated with a delayed therapeutic response and increased relapse rate of typhoid fever [12]. This poor response did not occur in the treatment of children with pneumonias and other serious infections [13]. Caution is recommended if this route is contemplated, and measurement of serum levels is advised.

The half-life of chloramphenicol in adults is 4 hours after a single intravenous injection. The antibiotic primarily is conjugated with glucuronic acid by the liver and excreted in this inactive form by the kidney. Only about 0.14% of active chloramphenicol is recovered in the bile. However, about 5% to 10% of the dose is recovered in the urine as active chloramphenicol. This provides urine concentrations of 150 to 200 µg/mL, sufficient to treat urinary tract infections should this be necessary. These levels are markedly diminished, however, in patients with renal failure [14].

The antibiotic is bound to protein from 25% to 50% and has an apparent volume of distribution of 100 L. It has a high degree of lipid solubility and a small molecular size. It is not surprising, therefore, that it diffuses well into many tissues and body fluids. Levels in cerebrospinal fluid are 30% to 50% of serum levels, even without inflammation. Levels in the brain are about 36 µg/mL compared

with corresponding serum levels of 4 µg/mL. Aqueous humor levels are 50% of serum levels, but rabbit studies suggest topical administration may be a more efficient method to produce these high concentrations [1]. Therapeutic concentrations are attained in the synovial, pleural, and acidic fluid. The antibiotic is found intracellularly as well as extracellularly. Chloramphenicol crosses the placenta to the fetal circulation, but there are negligible amounts in the amniotic fluid [15–17].

METABOLISM IN CHILDREN

There is a wide variation in the metabolism and excretion of chloramphenicol in children. Dose requirements may vary three-fold in children of the same age. This variation may be even greater in newborns and young infants in whom the glycuronyl transferase system and renal function are not fully developed. The mean elimination half-life has been reported to be 12 hours in newborns less than 1 week of age compared with 9 hours for neonates from 1 week to 2 months. Thus, the initial dose for newborns less than 1 week old should be 25 mg/kg every 24 hours and for infants 1 to 4 weeks old, 25 mg/kg every 12 hours instead of the usual 50 mg/kg/d divided into 6-hour dosing intervals for older children and adults. *However, the wide variation makes monitoring of serum levels imperative* [18–20].

DOSAGE ADJUSTMENTS FOR RENAL AND HEPATIC INSUFFICIENCY

Renal failure has little effect on the half-life of biologically active chloramphenicol but markedly affects its metabolites. Fortunately, the metabolites do not appear to be as toxic as the parent compound. Therefore, the dose should not be modified to maintain therapeutic levels. Neither peritoneal nor hemodialysis alters serum levels sufficiently to require dose alteration. This is not the case with liver disease: patients with hepatic diseases, as evidenced by jaundice or ascites, conjugate chloramphenicol at a slower rate. Active chloramphenicol levels increase, and bone marrow suppression occurs [21]. A suggested regimen for adult patients with liver disease is a 1-g loading dose followed by 500 mg every 6 hours, limiting the course of therapy, when possible, to 10 to 14 days. Monitoring serum levels in these situations is highly recommended [1].

MONITORING SERUM LEVELS

Because of the narrow therapeutic-to-toxic ratio and the variability of the metabolism of chloramphenicol, it is important to monitor serum levels in newborns and premature infants, in patients with hepatic disease, and in patients taking potentially interacting drugs. To ensure efficacy and prevent toxicity, peak levels should be maintained between 10 and 20 µg/mL and trough concentrations between 5 to 10 µg/mL. Dose-dependent bone marrow depression has been associated with peak serum concentrations above 25 µg/mL [1].

INDICATIONS

The advent of the third-generation cephalosporins and the fluoroquinolones has reduced the indications for chloramphenicol. Nevertheless, it remains a very important therapeutic agent in many areas of the world and for selective alternative indications in the United States (Table 9-6). Chloramphenicol is used as alternative

The information here is provided as guidance only. Prescribers should always consult the manufacturer's current prescribing information.

therapy for bacterial meningitis caused by *H. influenzae*, *S. pneumoniae*, and *N. meningitidis* when the patient is allergic to penicillin. Even here, some prefer a third-generation cephalosporin unless the allergy to the penicillin is of the immediate type (IgE mediated), such as with hives or anaphylaxis. It is seldom useful in pneumococcal diseases resistant to penicillin G. Chloramphenicol is useful for most rickettsial diseases, including Rocky Mountain spotted fever and typhus fever when parenteral therapy is required. Because of its spectrum, which includes *N. meningitidis* and Rocky Mountain spotted fever, it is useful for very sick individuals with fever and a petechial rash in whom these two diseases are in the differential diagnosis [1].

Chloramphenicol is highly active against *Salmonella typhosa* and is very effective for therapy. Although it continues to be used as the drug of choice in many parts of the world, the availability of the quinolones has superseded its use for this indication in the United States. Similarly, for non-*typhosa* strains of *Salmonella*, chloramphenicol is now best described as an effective alternative therapy in the United States [22].

TOXICITY

Hematologic

There are two types of adverse reactions related to the bone marrow caused by chloramphenicol: 1) reversible bone marrow depression, and 2) idiosyncratic aplastic anemia. Reversible bone marrow depression is a direct pharmacologic effect caused by inhibition of mitochondrial protein synthesis. It is manifested by any combination of reticulocytopenia, anemia, leukopenia, and thrombocytopenia. There is an increase in serum iron concentration and reduced uptake of radioactive iron by the erythrocytes, indicating a decrease in hemoglobin synthesis. On bone marrow examination, there is vacuolization of both erythroid and myeloid precursors, which are not unique for chloramphenicol. It is clearly dose related and occurs in patients receiving 4 g or more per day and in patients in whom serum levels are above 25 µg/mL. These levels occur in patients with hepatic disease receiving normal doses. The toxicity is reversible when the antibiotic is discontinued [23].

The second type of adverse reaction, aplastic anemia, is rare, occurring in one in 24,500 to 40,800 patients who receive the antibiotic. This is 13 times the incidence for aplastic anemia in the general population. Chloramphenicol is the most common cause of the syndrome. Although the pathogenesis is not known, it appears to be caused by a mechanism that is different from bone marrow suppression, which is dose related. The aplastic anemia is not dose related and may occur weeks to months after completion of therapy. Although it is more common after oral therapy, it is documented from parenteral chloramphenicol and even following administration of eyedrops [24,25]. Because some of the cases occur concurrently with antibiotic administration, it appears rational to monitor blood counts on a twice-weekly basis [26]. Consider discontinuing the antibiotic. If the leukocytes decrease to 2500/mm in this decision it is important to recognize, that low numbers of leukocytes occur in diseases such as typhoid fever, an illness for which chloramphenicol frequently is prescribed [1].

A more recent report of the association of chloramphenicol with childhood leukemia also is of concern [27]. In a population-based case-control interview study of 309 childhood leukemia cases and 618 age- and sex-matched controls, there was an increase in the relationship between chloramphenicol and the risk of both acute lymphocytic and nonlymphocytic leukemia. This was particularly apparent for children receiving the antibiotic for greater than 10 days. Although leukemia is known to follow aplastic anemia, these children did not have prior aplastic anemia. Until this is more clearly defined, therapy should be stopped or changed as quickly as possible to alternative effective agents when possible [27].

Chloramphenicol also has been associated with hemolytic anemia in patients with the Mediterranean form of glucose-6-phosphate dehydrogenase deficiency. It does not occur with the milder A type, which is the most common form in the black population.

Gray Baby Syndrome

This syndrome, originally noted in neonates, consists of abdominal distention, vomiting, flaccidity, cyanosis, circulatory collapse, and death. It reflects the diminished ability of neonates to conjugate chloramphenicol and excrete the active form in the urine. Although initially recognized in neonates, it has been noted in toddlers and, after accidental overdoses, in adults. It may present with unexplained metabolic acidosis. Serum levels with the syndrome are generally greater than 50 µg/mL. It is due in part to impaired myocardial contractility related to direct interference of myocardial tissue respiration and oxidative phosphorylation. The association with premature infants and neonates makes reduction of the dose to 25 mg/kg/d and the monitoring of serum levels essential in this age group. Large-volume exchange transfusions or charcoal hemoperfusion have been used to accelerate drug removal should the toxicity occur [28,29].

Neurologic Toxicity

There are a number of neurologic sequelae described with chloramphenicol use, including peripheral neuritis, headache, depression, ophthalmoplegia, and mental confusion. Optic neuritis, manifested

Table 9-6. Indications for Chloramphenicol

Indications	Comments
Effective alternative therapy	
Bacterial meningitis	For penicillin-allergic patients
Haemophilus influenzae	
Streptococcus pneumoniae	
Neisseria meningitidis	
Brain abscess	
Chlamydia psittaci	
Clostridium perfringens	
Ehrlichia	
Pseudomonas mallei	With streptomycin
Pseudomonas pseudomallei	With doxycycline
(acute melioidosis)	
Mergon	
Rickettsial infections	Preferred by many physicians when parental therapy is required
Rocky Mountain spotted fever	
Typhus (murine)	
Scrub typhus	
Tick-bite fever	
Q fever	
Typhoid fever and invasive salmonellosis	In some countries, chloramphenicol remains the standard of therapy
Vibrio vulnificus cellulitis or sepsis	

The information here is provided as guidance only. Prescribers should always consult the manufacturer's current prescribing information.

by a decrease in visual acuity, has been described in patients receiving chloramphenicol over a prolonged period of time [1].

Allergic and Other Adverse Effects

Allergic reactions, including anaphylaxis and drug fevers, are rare. However, Herxheimer-like reactions have been reported during therapy for syphilis, brucellosis, and typhoid fever. Gastrointestinal symptoms, including nausea, vomiting, diarrhea, glossitis, and stomatitis, do occur but are not common. A decrease in vitamin K synthesis, resulting in bleeding, has occurred following prolonged administration [1].

DRUG INTERACTIONS

Chloramphenicol is metabolized by the liver. Physicians should be careful when administering other agents metabolized by this route and monitor for possible interactions. Phenytoin, rifampin, and phenobarbital increase the clearance of chloramphenicol and decrease the serum concentration, perhaps by inducing hepatic microsomal enzymes. Monitoring serum levels to assure therapeutic levels is indicated when these drugs are used concurrently [30].

Chloramphenicol, presumably by inhibiting hepatic microsomal enzymes, prolongs the half-life of tolbutamide, chlorpropamide, phenytoin, barbiturates, cyclophosphamide, and warfarin and has resulted in severe toxicity, including death. Chloramphenicol may inhibit the response to iron therapy or vitamin B12 (cyanocobalamin) in patients with anemia. A bacteriostatic drug, such as chloramphenicol, may interfere with the action of a bactericidal agents such as penicillin. This may have clinical relevance in treating *S. agalactiae* or gram-negative meningitis. Where the two agents must be given in combination, it is suggested that the bactericidal agent be administered before chloramphenicol [30].

REFERENCES

1. Standiford HC: Tetracyclines and chloramphenicol. In *Mandell, Douglas and Bennett's Principles and Practice of Infectious Diseases*, edn 4. Edited by Mandell GL, Bennett JE, and Dolin R. New York: Churchill Livingstone; 1995:306–317.

2. Abdel-Sayed S: Transport of chloramphenicol into sensitive strains of *Escherichia coli* and *Pseudomonas aeruginosa*. *J Antimicrob Chemother* 1987, 19:7–20.

3. Turk DC: A comparison of chloramphenicol and ampicillin as bactericidal agents for *Haemophilus influenzae* type B. *J Med Microbiol* 1977, 10:127.

4. Rahal JJ, Simberkoff MS: Bactericidal and bacteriostatic action of chloramphenicol against meningeal pathogens. *Antimicrob Agents Chemother* 1979, 16:13.

5. Weeks JL, Mason EO Jr, Baker CJ: Antagonism of ampicillin and chloramphenicol for meningeal isolates of group B streptococci. *Antimicrob Agents Chemother* 1981, 20:281.

6. Cherubin CE, Neu HC, Rahal JJ, *et al.*: Emergence of resistance to chloramphenicol in *Salmonella*. *J Infect Dis* 1977, 135:807.

7. Kabani A, Joffe A, Jadavji T: *Haemophilus* influenzae Type B resistant to ampicillin and chloramphenicol. *Pediatr Infect Dis J* 1991, 9:681.

8. Editorial: Drug resistance in salmonellas. *Lancet* 1982, i:1391.

9. Spika JS, Waterman SH, Soo Hoo GW, *et al.*: Chloramphenicol-resistant *Salmonella newport* traced through hamburger to dairy farms. *N Engl J Med* 1987, 316:565–570.

10. Ambrose PJ: Clinical pharmacokinetics of chloramphenicol and chloramphenicol succinate. *Clin Pharmacokinet* 1984, 9:222–238.

11. Bhutta ZA, Niazi SK, Suria A: Chloramphenicol clearance in typhoid fever: implications for therapy. *Indian J Pediatr* 1992, 59:213–219.

12. DuPont HL, Hornick RB, Weiss CF, *et al.*: Evaluation of chloramphenicol acid succinate therapy of induced typhoid fever and Rocky Mountain spotted fever. *N Engl J Med* 1970, 282:53.

13. Shann F, *et al.*: Absorption of chloramphenicol sodium succinate after intramuscular administration in children. *N Engl J Med* 1985, 313:410–414.

14. Lindberg AA, Nilsson LH, Bucht H, *et al.*: Concentration of chloramphenicol in the urine and blood in relation to renal function. *BMJ* 1966, 2:724.

15. Woodward TE, Wisseman CL: *Chloromycetin (Chloramphenicol)*. New York: Medical Encyclopedia; 1958.

16. Kramer PW, Griffith RS, Campbell RL, *et al.*: Antibiotic penetration of the brain: A comparative study. *J Neurosurg* 1969, 31:295.

17. George FJ, Hanna C: Ocular penetration of chloramphenicol. *Arch Ophthalmol* 1977, 95:879.

18. Smith AL, Weber A: Pharmacology of chloramphenicol. *Pediatr Clin North Am* 1983, 30:209–236.

19. Kauffman RE, Miceti JN, Strebel L, *et al.*: Pharmacokinetics of chloramphenicol and chloramphenicol succinate in infants and children. *J Pediatr* 1981, 93:315.

20. Kauffman RE, Thirumoorthi MC, Buckley JA, *et al.*: Relative bioavailability of intravenous chloramphenicol succinate and oral chloramphenicol palmitate in infants and children. *J Pediatr* 1981, 99:363.

21. Suhrland LG, Weisberger AS: Chloramphenicol toxicity in liver and renal disease. *Arch Intern Med* 1963, 112:161.

22. The choice of antibacterial drugs. *Med Lett Drugs Ther* 1994, 36:53–60.

23. Scott JL, Finegold SM, Belkin GA, *et al.*: A controlled double-blind study of the hematologic toxicity of chloramphenicol. *N Engl J Med* 1965, 272:1137.

24. Wallerstein RO, Condit PK, Kasper CK, *et al.*: Statewide study of chloramphenicol therapy and fatal aplastic anemia. *JAMA* 1969, 208:2045.

25. Best WR: Chloramphenicol-associated blood dyscrasias: A review of cases submitted to the American Medical Association Registry. *JAMA* 1967, 201:181.

26. Daum RS, Cohen DL, Smith AL: Fatal aplastic anemia following apparent "dose-related" chloramphenicol toxicity. *J Pediatr* 1979, 94:403.

27. Shu XO, Linet MS, Gao RN, *et al.*: Chloramphenicol use and childhood leukaemia in Shanghai. *Lancet* 1987, ii:934–937.

28. Suarez CR, Ow EP: Chloramphenicol toxicity associated with severe cardiac dysfunction. *Pediatr Cardiol* 1992, 13:48–51.

29. Stevens DC, Kleinman MB, Lietman PS, *et al.*: Exchange transfusion in acute chloramphenicol toxicity. *J Pediatr* 1981, 99:651.

30. Chloramphenicol (chloromycetin) Interactions. In *Antibiotic Drug Interactions*. Edited by Hansten PO and Horn JR. Vancouver WA: Applied Therapeutics; 1993:213–216.

The information here is provided as guidance only. Prescribers should always consult the manufacturer's current prescribing information.

CHLORAMPHENICOL (Chloromycetin®)

In vitro, chloramphenicol exerts a bacteriostatic effect on a wide range of gram-negative and gram-positive bacteria and spirochetes; it is also active against rickettsiae, *Chlamydia* and *Mycoplasma* spp. Because of severe toxicity (aplastic anemia) its use is limited in the United States

ANTIMICROBIAL ACTIVITY

Gram-positive: *Streptococcus pyogenes, Streptococcus agalactiae, Streptococcus viridans, Streptococcus pneumoniae, Peptococcus* spp, *Peptostreptococcus* spp, *Propionibacterium acnes, Eubacterium* spp, *Clostridium perfinges,* and *Clostridium* spp. *Staphylococcus aureus is highly variable.*
Gram-negative: *Haemophilus influenzae, Neisseria meningitidis, Neisseria gonorrhoeae, Salmonella typhosa, Vibrio cholera, Brucella* spp, *Pseudomonas pseudomallei, Bordetella pertussis, Veillonella* spp, *Bacteroides melaningenicus, Fusobacterium* spp. Strains of *Escherichia coli, Klebsiella pneumoniae,* and *Proteus mirabilis* can be highly variable.
Other: *Rickettsia* and *Chlamydia* are generally susceptible.

RESISTANCE

Some outbreaks of *Salmonella* have been caused by chloramphenicol-resistant strains. Rare strains of *H. influenzae, N. meningitidis,* and *S. pneumoniae* are resistant. Viruses and fungi are resistant.

SPECIAL PRECAUTIONS

Serious and fatal blood dyscrasias can occur after administration of chloramphenicol in both short- and long-term therapy. Reports of aplastic anemia terminating in leukemia have been made. Do not use if agents with less potential danger can be effective. This agent must not be used to treat trivial infections (*eg*, colds, influenza, infections of the throat) or infections other than those indicated, nor should it be used as a prophylaxis for bacterial infection.
Adequate blood studies must be made before and during therapy. *Be aware* that such studies may reveal early peripheral blood changes (leukopenia, reticulocytopenia, granulocytopenia) before they become irreversible, but *they should not be relied on for detection of bone marrow suppression occurring prior to aplastic anemia.*
Use with caution in patients with acute intermittent porphyria or glucose-6-phosphate dehydrogenase deficiency.
Prolonged or repeated use of antibiotic agents may cause bacterial or fungal overgrowth of nonsusceptible organisms, leading to secondary infection. Appropriate measures should be taken to eliminate superinfection should it occur.
Toxic reactions ("gray syndrome") have occurred in premature infants and neonates, including fatalities (approximately 40%); clinical and laboratory studies give the following information:
Therapy instituted in first 48 hours of life in most cases.
Symptoms appeared after first 3 to 4 days with high doses.
Symptoms in order of appearance include abdominal distension (with or without emesis), progressive pallid cyanosis, vasomotor collapse (often accompanied by irregular breathing), and death within a few hours of onset. Additional initial symptoms may include refusal to suck, loose green stools, flaccidity, ashen color, lowered temperature, and refractory lactic acidosis. Death occurs in approximately 40% of patients within 2 days of initial symptoms.
Progression of symptoms accelerated with higher doses.
Studies of serum levels showed unusually high drug concentrations with doses over 25/mg/kg/d in newborns.
Preexisting liver dysfunction may be a significant risk factor.
Discontinuation of therapy at first sign of associated symptoms frequently reverses process, with complete recovery.

INDICATIONS

(Note: *See* Special Precautions.) Because of toxicity, chlomephenicol is recommended as alternative therapy. Indications for alternative therapy include:
Acute infection due to *S. typhi.* (Note: Recommendations for continued use at therapeutic levels for 8 to 10 days after patient is afebrile [to decrease risk of relapse]. Not recommended for routine treatment of typhoid "carrier" state.)
Bacterial meningitis due to *H. influenzae, S. pneumonia,* and *N. meningitidis*
Brain abscess
Serious infections due to susceptible strains of the following:
Salmonella species, *H. influenzae* (especially meningeal), rickettsiae, lymphogranuloma-psittacosis group, various gram-negative bacteria (bacteremia); susceptible anaerobic organisms, other susceptible organisms that have proven resistant to other appropriate antimicrobial agents, or if *Bacteroides fragilis* is suspected
Pseudomonas mallei, (with streptomycin), *Pseudomonas pseudomallei* (with doxycycline), rickettsial infections (Rocky Mountain spotted fever, murine typhus, scrub typhus, tick-bite fever, Q fever), Ehrlichiosis, *Vibrio vulcificus*
Also used in cystic fibrosis regimens

CONTRAINDICATIONS

Allergy or hypersensitivity to chloramphenicol. Do not use as treatment for trivial infection, in cases where chloramphenicol is not indicated, or as prophylaxis for bacterial infection.

INTERACTIONS

Dicumarol, phenytoin, phenobarbital, tolbutamide, chlorpropamide, cyclophosphamide, acetaminophen, iron salts, vitamin B_{12}, penicillin, rifampin

ADVERSE EFFECTS

Blood dyscrasias (*see* Special Precautions); gray syndrome (*see* Special Precautions); nausea; vomiting; glossitis; stomatitis; diarrhea; headache; mild depression; confusion; delirium; fever; macular rashes; angioedema; urticaria; anaphylaxis; Herxheimer reactions (during therapy for typhoid fever); optic or peripheral neuritis (long-term therapy; discontinuation recommended); enterocolitis

The information here is provided as guidance only. Prescribers should always consult the manufacturer's current prescribing information.

CHLORAMPHENICOL (CONTINUED)

SPECIAL GROUPS

Children: Use with caution in infants and neonates; risk of gray syndrome toxicity. Drug serum levels should be monitored in neonates.
Elderly: No dosage adjustment necessary.
Renal impairment: No dosage adjustment is necessary unless liver impairment also is present.
Hepatic impairment: Inhibits metabolism and excretion; reduced dosage necessary.
Pregnancy: Use with caution; studies indicate the potential for harm to fetus.
Breast-feeding: Use with caution; weigh benefits against risk.

DOSAGE

(Note: Chloramphenicol sodium succinate is for intravenous administration only; it is ineffective if given intramuscularly.)
Adults: For rickettsial infection or typhoid fever, 50 mg/kg/d in divided doses every 6 hours. For serious infection (*eg*, meningitis or brain abscess) or for infections due to moderately resistant organisms, up to 100 mg/kg/d decreasing as soon as possible.
Elderly: Same as adults unless liver impairment exists.
Children: Neonates, 25 mg/kg/d in four divided doses every 6 hours; any increased dosage should only be given to maintain blood concentration in effective range. Beyond 2 weeks of age, full-term infants may be given up to 50 mg/kg/d in four doses every 6 hours. Neonates under 2 kg, 25 mg/kg once a day. Neonates from birth to 7 days and over 2 kg, 25 mg/kg once a day. Neonates over 7 days and over 2 kg, 50 mg/kg/d in divided doses every 12 hours.
(Note: The above recommendations are very important because blood concentration in all infants [premature and full-term] under 2 weeks of age differs from that of other infants because of the maturity of the metabolic functions of the liver and kidneys. When functions are immature [or severely impaired in adults], high concentrations are found and tend to increase with successive doses.)
For infants and children with immature metabolism, 25 mg/kg/d, monitor serum levels carefully.
Impaired renal or hepatic function: For impaired hepatic function adjust dosage based on drug concentration in the blood. In the adult, an initial loading dose of 1 g followed with a dosage of 500 mg every 6 hours is recommended until levels are obtained. No dose adjustment is required for renal impairment.

PHARMACOKINETICS AND PHARMACODYNAMICS

Peak serum levels: 12 µg/mL 1 h after first 1-g dose orally
Plasma half-life: (elimination half-life) 4 h
Bioavailability: 80%; may be erratic in newborns
Metabolism: inactive prodrug is rapidly hydrolyzed to active chloramphenicol base
Excretion: total urinary excretion, 68% to 99%; 5% to 10% as free chloramphenicol; remainder as inactive metabolites excreted by liver
Protein binding: 25% to 50%
Renal impairment: little effect on biologically active chloramphenicol but decreased excretion of metabolites, however, no reduction of dose required.
Hepatic impairment: protein binding and clearance decreased; dosage reduction is required

OVERDOSAGE

Large volume exchange transfusions or charcoal hemoperfusion have been used to accelerate drug removal in babies with gray baby syndrome and high serum levels of chloramphenicol

AVAILABILITY

Capsules—250 mg
Oral Suspension—150 mg/5 mL
Powder for Injection—100 mg/mL (reconstituted)

The information here is provided as guidance only. Prescribers should always consult the manufacturer's current prescribing information.

CLASS DESCRIPTION

Antimicrobial agents for therapy for mycobacterial infections comprise a diverse group of agents. Twenty-five drugs having activity against mycobacteria are alluded to herein, including 11 that are described in detail because of their primary roles against mycobacteria. Therapeutic agents within this group can differ markedly from one another in chemistry, pharmacokinetics, adverse reactions, mechanisms of action, and in bacteristatic versus bactericidal effects. These agents variously may affect cell wall synthesis, often involving an essential mycobacterial lipid–mycolic acid; oxygen-dependent metabolic pathways; protein synthesis; folate metabolism; or nucleic acid synthesis.

In this section, antimycobacterial agents are considered in four subgroups according to their activity principally for either: 1) *Mycobacterium tuberculosis*, 2) *Mycobacterium avium* complex (MAC), 3) various nontuberculous mycobacterial species (excluding MAC and *Mycobacterium leprae*), or 4) *M. leprae*.

ANTITUBERCULOUS AGENTS

Traditionally, drugs for treatment of tuberculosis have been categorized by the terms *first-line* or *primary* (characterized by greater efficacy and lesser toxicity) and *second-line*, also termed *secondary* or *re-treatment* agents (having less efficacy and a tendency to greater toxicity) [1]. Table 10-1 lists first-line agents and daily dosages for adults. The Advisory Council for the Elimination of Tuberculosis–recommended twice and thrice weekly dosage regimens and dosages for children have been published by the Centers for Disease Control and Prevention (CDC) [2]. Because of characteristic slow growth, tubercle bacilli can approach near dormancy so that long courses of treatment—measured in months—are necessary for successful antituberculous therapy.

Second-line antituberculous agents are administered when resistance to first-line agents is encountered, in retreatment regimens following relapse, or when intolerance to first-line agents exists. A cardinal rule when adding antituberculous agents to a failed regimen is to **add two second-line agents concurrently**, so that rapidly acquired resistance to a lone additional agent can be avoided [4]. Second-line antituberculous agents are reviewed in Table 10-2. Amikacin, a congener of kanamycin with the potential for nephrotoxicity and ototoxicity characteristic of the aminoglycosides, possesses considerable activity against *M. tuberculosis in vitro* and in animals. Lack of clinical experience and expense preclude its elevation to first-line antituberculous status. Administered parenterally, amikacin provides alternative therapy in resistant cases. Kanamycin's only advantage over amikacin is lower price.

Two agents that are sometimes listed as second-line antituberculous agents are not discussed: Amithiazone (thiocetazone) is not available in the United States and causes an unacceptable frequency of toxic reactions in persons who are HIV-infected; viomycin is unavailable in the United States.

Table 10-1. First-line Agents Approved for Treatment of Tuberculosis

Generic name	Trade name	Route of administration	Usual adult daily dosage* (maximum dose)
Ethambutol	Myambutol	Oral	15–25 mg/kg (1.6 g)
Isoniazid	Generic	Oral	5 mg/kg (300 mg)
	Nydrazide	Intramuscular	5 mg/kg (300 mg)
	Rifamate†	Oral	2 capsules
Pyrazinamide	Generic	Oral	15–30 mg/kg (2 g)
Rifampin	Rifadin	Oral, Intramuscular	10 mg/kg (600 mg)
	Rimactane	Oral	10 mg/kg (600 mg)
	Rifamate†	Oral	2 capsules
Streptomycin sulfate	Generic	Intramuscular	15 mg/kg (1 g)

*Recommendations of Advisory Council for the Elimination of Tuberculosis; see reference [2] for twice and thrice weekly regimens and for dosages for children.
†Isoniazid–rifampin combination.

Table 10-2. Second-line Agents Approved for Treatment of Tuberculosis

Generic name	Trade name	Route of administration	Usual recommended adult daily dosage
Amikacin*	Amikin	Intramuscular, Intravenous	10–15 mg/kg (maximum 1 g)
Capreomycin	Capastat	Intramuscular	7.5–15 mg/kg (maximum 1 g)
Cycloserine	Seromycin	Oral	0.5–1.0 g (often 0.5 g)
Ethionamide	Trector SC	Oral	0.5–1.0 g (often 0.5–0.75 g)
Para-aminosalicyclic acid†	Generic	Oral	6.0–12.0 g

*Basic pharmacologic information about amikacin is found in the section on aminoglycoside antibiotics.
†Available in the United States from the Centers for Disease Control and Prevention.

The information here is provided as guidance only. Prescribers should always consult the manufacturer's current prescribing information.

Mechanisms of Resistance to Antituberculous Agents

Genetically determined heterosusceptibility exists among *M. tuberculosis* organisms such that therapy with any single drug will result in selection and overgrowth of subpopulations of tubercle bacilli resistant to that agent. Thus, **a cornerstone of successful antituberculous treatment is multiple drug therapy to prevent emergence of resistance** and subsequent clinical relapse. Currently recommended regimens include three- or four-drug combinations [2].

Multiple Drug Resistance

Given the requirement for multidrug treatment over a long period of time, the major determinant of outcome of antituberculous therapy is compliance through patient education and, at times, by directly supervised drug administration [5]. Over the years, inadequate therapy has favored selection of numerous strains of tubercle bacilli having resistance to multiple drugs.

(Multidrug-resistant *M. tuberculosis*) (MDR-TB) strains are generally characterized by resistance to at least isoniazid and rifampin [6]. MDR-TB strains are especially prone to flourish in disadvantaged populations—particularly where poverty, crowding, illicit drug use, and HIV infection coexist. Clinical presentations of MDR-TB infection in patients with AIDS can be very atypical [7].

However, MDR-TB infection can be controlled by properly designed and supervised multidrug regimens. Agents useful against MDR-TB are indicated in Table 10-3; none are FDA-approved for this indication, but consensus guidelines for therapeutic and preventive regimens have been published by the CDC [8].

AGENTS FOR *MYCOBACTERIUM AVIUM* COMPLEX

Mycobacterium avium complex, classified among the nontuberculous mycobacteria, formerly caused nondisseminated pulmonary infections mainly due to *M. intracellulare* subspecies occurring in persons with chronic obstructive lung disease. Now MAC (*M. avium* subspecies) is recognized as a particular threat to patients with AIDS, in whom disseminated infection is the rule. Marginal drug activity and propensity for MAC infections in persons with compromised host defenses have dictated prolonged multidrug therapy—even for life in persons with AIDS. The risk for MAC infection is so great late in the course of AIDS that preventive therapy should be considered. Drugs for MAC are listed in Table 10-4. Only rifabutin is FDA-approved for prophylaxis of MAC. Only clarithromycin is FDA-approved for treatment of MAC. Clarithromycin by itself has produced gratifying clinical and microbiologic responses in disseminated MAC infections in

Table 10-3. Additional Agents for Treatment of Multiple Drug–resistant Tuberculosis

Generic name	Trade name	Route of administration	Usual adult daily dosage
Azithromycin*	Zithromax	Oral	250–500 mg
Ciprofloxacin*	Cipro	Oral, Intravenous	1.0–1.5 g
Clarithromycin*	Biaxin	Oral	1.0 g
Ofloxacin^	Floxin	Oral, Intravenous	800 mg
Rifabutin	Mycobutin	Oral	300 mg
Sparfloxacin†	—	—	—

Pharmacologic information about these agents is found in sections dealing with their usage in bacterial infections.
†*Investigational.*

Table 10-4. Agents for Treatment of *Mycobacterium avium* Complex

Generic name	Trade name	Route of administration	Usual adult daily dosage
Amikacin*	Amikin	Intramuscular, Intravenous	7.5–15 mg/kg (maximum 1 g)
Azithromycin*	Zithromax	Oral	250–500 mg
Ciprofloxacin*	Cipro	Oral, Intravenous	1.0–1.5 g
Clarithromycin*	Biaxin	Oral	1.0 g
Clofazimine	Lamprene	Oral	50–300 mg (usually 100–200 mg)
Ethambutol	Myambutol	Oral	15–25 mg/kg (25 mg/kg not for > 60 d)
Ofloxacin*	Floxin	Oral, Intravenous	800 mg
Rifampin	Rifadin Rimactane	Oral, Intravenous Oral	600 mg
Rifabutin	Mycobutin	Oral	300 mg
Sparfloxacin†	—	—	—

Additional information about these agents is found in sections dealing with their usage in bacterial infections.
†*Investigational.*

The information here is provided as guidance only. Prescribers should always consult the manufacturer's current prescribing information.

AIDS. Because of concern regarding emergence of resistance [9], many authorities now recommend clarithromycin in combination with one or two additional drugs active against MAC, such as clarithromycin plus rifabutin; clarithromycin plus rifampin and ethambutol; or clarithromycin plus rifampin and clofazimine [10].

AGENTS FOR NONTUBERCULOUS MYCOBACTERIA OTHER THAN *MYCOBACTERIUM AVIUM* COMPLEX AND *MYCOBACTERIUM LEPRAE*

The ecology and growth characteristics of nontuberculous mycobacteria (also termed *mycobacteria other than tuberculosis* [MOTT] and previously termed *atypical* mycobacteria) are diverse, as is their susceptibility to antimycobacterial drugs. Nontuberculous mycobacteria can even be susceptible to conventional antibacterial agents. **Whenever possible, selection of agents for nontuberculous mycobacteria should be guided by susceptibility testing**, especially in infections caused by *Mycobacterium fortuitum*, *Mycobacterium abcessus*, or *Mycobacterium chelonae* [14]. A compilation of agents for treating nontuberculous mycobacteria appears in Table 10-5. None of these agents have FDA on-label indications for these relatively infrequent infections. Opportunistic pathogens included among nontuberculous mycobacteria generally infect through environmental exposure, including direct inoculation, which can result in localized infection. Progressive disease usually occurs in persons having impaired host defenses (*eg*, malnutrition, emphysema, foreign body, or immunosuppression including those having AIDS). Therapy for mycobacterial infections in AIDS may be confounded by malabsorption that attends AIDS-related diarrhea [15,16].

Nontuberculous mycobacteria and their commonly recommended initial therapies include 1) *Mycobacterium kansasii*—isoniazid, rifampin, and ethambutol. Isoniazid has long been included in regimens for *M. kansasii* despite lack of *in vitro* activity. Clarithromycin is a promising new agent for *M. kansasii*; 2) *Mycobacterium marinum*—rifampin plus either doxycycline (or minocycline), trimethoprim-sulfamethoxazole, clarithromycin, or ethambutol. A combination of clarithromycin and ethambutol was bactericidal *in vitro* [17]; 3) *Mycobacterium scrofulaceum*—no consensus therapy exists. Agents having activity are amikacin, erythromycin, and rifampin; 4) *M. fortuitum*—cefoxitin and amikacin usually have been recommended. Beta-lactams (cefmetazole, imipenem-cilastatin), quinolones (ciprofloxacin, ofloxacin), and trimethoprim-sulfamethoxazole provide other, including oral, alternatives; 5) *M. chelonae*—clarithromycin (or azithromycin) plus tobramycin; 6) *M. abscessus*—amikacin, cefoxitin, and clarithromycin; 7) *Mycobacterium haemophilum*—several agents including ciprofloxacin, clarithromycin, clofazimine, and rifampin are active, but no consensus regimen exists. Authoritative references should be consulted whenever selecting therapy or determining dosage for nontuberculous mycobacterial infections [14].

AGENTS FOR LEPROSY

Therapy for infection with *M. leprae* (Hansen's bacillus) over many years consisted principally of monotherapy with dapsone. Both the prolonged clinical responses to treatment with dapsone and the relative success of worldwide monotherapy depended on the remarkably slow growth of Hansen's bacillus. However, over time the consequence of monotherapy is the widespread emergence of resistance among strains of *M. leprae*. Thus, the presently recommended therapy for leprosy (Hansen's disease) consists of multidrug regimens given over long periods of time. Table 10-6 lists drugs that have been combined in multidrug regimens. Dapsone and clofazimine are FDA-approved for treatment of leprosy. Investigational therapies have included clarithromycin [18], minocycline [19], and sparfloxacin [20].

Clinical subtleties of the disease combined with immunologically and drug-mediated toxic reactions during therapy require familiarity with leprosy for effective treatment. Because leprosy is encountered infrequently in the United States, its treatment here is best undertaken in consultation with specialists familiar with the condition, such those at the Gillis W. Long Hansen's Disease Center in Carville, LA.

Table 10-5. Agents for Treatment of Nontuberculous Mycobacteria Other Than *Mycobacterium avium* Complex

Generic name	Trade name	Routes of administration
Amikacin*	Amikin	Intramuscular, Intravenous
Azithromycin*	Zithromax	Oral
Cefmetazole*	Zefazone	Intramuscular
Cefoxitin*	Mefoxin	Intramuscular, Intravenous
Clarithromycin*	Biaxin	Oral
Clofazimine	Lamprene	Oral
Cycloserine	Seromycin	Intramuscular
Doxycycline*	Generic	Oral, Intravenous
Erythromycin*	Generic	Oral, Intravenous
Ethambutol	Myambutol	Oral
Ethionamide	Trecator SC	Oral
Imipenem-cilastatin*	Primaxin	Intramuscular, Intravenous
Isoniazid	Generic	Oral
Minocycline*	Generic	Oral
	Minocin	Intravenous
Rifabutin	Mycobutin	Oral
Rifampin	Rifadin	Oral, Intravenous
	Rimactane	Oral
Streptomycin	Generic	Intramuscular
Tobramycin*	Nebcin	Intramuscular, Intravenous
Trimethoprim-sulfamethoxazole*	Generic	Oral, Intravenous

*Additional information about these agents is found in sections dealing with their usage in bacterial infections.

Table 10-6. Agents for Treatment of Leprosy

Generic name	Trade name	Route of administration
Clarithromycin	Biaxin	Oral
Clofazimine	Lamprene	Oral
Dapsone	Generic	Oral
Rifampin	Rifadin	Oral, Intravenous
	Rimactane	Oral

The information here is provided as guidance only. Prescribers should always consult the manufacturer's current prescribing information.

REFERENCES

1. Alford RH, Wallace RJ, Jr: Antimycobacterial agents. In *Principles and Practice of Infectious Diseases*, edn 4. Edited by Mandell GL, Bennett JE, Dolin R. New York: Churchill Livingstone; 1995:387–399.

2. CDC: Initial therapy for tuberculosis in the era of multidrug resistance: Recommendations of the Advisory Council for the elimination of tuberculosis. *MMWR* 1993, 42(RR-7):1–8.

3. Bocherding SM, Baciewicz AM, Self TH: Update on rifampin drug interactions II. *Arch Intern Med* 1992, 152:711–716.

4. Mahmoudi A, Iseman MD: Pitfalls in the care of patients with tuberculosis: Common errors and their association with the acquisition of drug resistance. *JAMA* 1993, 270:65–68.

5. Weiss SE, Slocum PC, Blaise FX, *et al.*: The effect of directly observed therapy on the rates of drug resistance and relapse in tuberculosis. *N Engl J Med* 1994, 330:1179–1184.

6. Goble M, Iseman MD, Madsen LA, *et al.*: Treatment of 171 patients with pulmonary tuberculosis resistant to isoniazid and rifampin. *N Engl J Med* 1993, 328:527–532.

7. Fischl MA, Daikos GL, Uttamchandani RB, *et al.*: Clinical presentation and outcome of patients with HIV infection and tuberculosis caused by multiple-drug-resistant bacilli. *Ann Intern Med* 1992, 117:184–190.

8. CDC: Management of persons exposed to multidrug-resistant tuberculosis. *MMWR* 1992, 41(RR-11):61–71.

9. Wolinsky E: *Mycobacterium avium* strains resistant to clarithromycin and azithromycin. *Antimicrob Agents Chemother* 1994, 38:635.

10. Benson CA: Treatment of disseminated disease due to the *Mycobacterium avium* complex in patients with AIDS. *Clin Infect Dis* 1994, 18(Suppl 3):S237–S242.

11. Woodley CL, Kilburn JO: *In vitro* susceptibility of *Mycobacterium avium* complex and *Mycobacterium tuberculosis* strains to a spiro-piperidyl rifamycin. *Am Rev Respir Dis* 1992, 126:586–587.

12. Nightingale SD, Cameron DW, Gordon FM, *et al.*: Two controlled trials of rifabutin prophylaxis against *Mycobacterium avium* complex infection in AIDS. *New Engl J Med* 1993, 329:828–833.

13. Frank MO, Graham MB, Wispelway B: Rifabutin and uveitis. *N Engl J Med* 1994, 330:868.

14. Wallace RJ, O'Brian K, Glassroth J, *et al.*: Diagnosis and treatment of disease caused by nontuberculous mycobacteria (official statement of the American Thoracic Society). *Am Rev Respir Dis* 1990, 142:940–953.

15. Peloquin CA, MacPhee AA, Berning SE: Malabsorption of antimycobacterial medications. *N Engl J Med* 1993, 329:1122–1123.

16. Gordon SM, Horsburgh CR Jr, Peloquin CA, *et al.*: Low serum levels of oral antimycobacterial agents in patients with disseminated *Mycobacterium avium* complex disease. *J Infect Dis* 1993, 168:1559–1562.

17. Bonnett E, Debat-Zoguereh D, Petit N: Clarithromycin: A potent agent against infections due to *Mycobacterium marinum. Clin Infect Dis* 1994, 18:664–666.

18. Chan GP, Garcia-Ignacio BY, Chavez VE, *et al.*: Clinical trial of clarithromycin for lepromatous leprosy. *Antimicrob Agents Chemother* 1994, 38:515–517.

19. Ji B, Jamet P, Perani EG, *et al.*: Powerful bactericidal activities of clarithromycin and minocycline against *Mycobacterium leprae* in lepromatous leprosy. *J Infect Dis* 1993, 168:188–190.

20. Chan GP, Garcia-Ignacio BY, Chavez VE, *et al.*: Clinical trial of sparfloxicin for lepromatous leprosy. *Antimicrob Agents Chemother* 1994, 38:61–65.

The information here is provided as guidance only. Prescribers should always consult the manufacturer's current prescribing information.

CAPREOMYCIN (Capastat®)

A polypeptide antibiotic, *capreomycin* shares many characteristics with the amino-glycosides, including a requirement for intramuscular injection. Because of activity against many resistant strains of tubercle bacilli, it may emerge as a first-line agent, especially when resistance to streptomycin is encountered. After an initial 2 to 4 months of dosing of 1 g given five times weekly, capreomycin subsequently can be administered 1 g two to three times weekly.

ANTIMICROBIAL ACTIVITY

Active against human strains of *Mycobacterium tuberculosis*.

RESISTANCE

Cross-resistance has occurred in varying degrees between capreomycin, kanamycin, and neomycin. (No cross-resistance has been reported between capreomycin, isoni-azid, aminosalicylate sodium, cycloserine, streptomycin, ethionamide, or ethambutol.) Most strains of multidrug–resistant *M. tuberculosis* are susceptible to capreomycin.

SPECIAL PRECAUTIONS

Eighth cranial nerve toxicity is associated with capreomycin; use extreme caution in ad-ministering this agent to patients with renal impairment or preexisting auditory impair-ment. Weigh potential benefits of use against potential risks. Perform audiometric measurements of vestibular function before beginning therapy and at regular intervals during treatment. (Note: Because other parenteral antituberculosis agents (*eg*, strepto-mycin) have had similar, sometimes irreversible, toxic effects, simultaneous administra-tion of these agents with capreomycin is not recommended. Use other ototoxic or neph-rotoxic agents only with great caution.) Dosage reduction is necessary if renal function is impaired. Hypersensitivity reactions have occurred with capreomycin. Nephrotox-icity: elevation of blood urea nitrogen (in 36% of 722 patients > 20 mg/dL, 10% > 30 mg/dL), depression of creatinine clearance and abnormal urine sediment. Toxic neph-ritis was reported in one patient with tuberculosis and portal cirrhosis who received capreomycin (1 g) and aminosalicylate sodium daily for 1 month. This patient developed renal insufficiency and oliguria and died; autopsy showed subsiding acute tubular necrosis. Electrolyte disturbances resembling Bartter's syndrome occurred in one patient. Hypokalemia may occur with capreomycin therapy; determine serum potassium levels frequently.

SPECIAL GROUPS

Children: Safety and efficacy not established.
Elderly: Caution in presence of preexisting auditory or renal impairment.
Renal impairment: Reduced dosage necessary (*see* Special Precautions).
Hepatic impairment: No specific information.
Pregnancy: Safety not established; use only if benefits outweigh risk.
Breast-feeding: Use caution; not known whether excreted in breast milk.

DOSAGE

Adults: Administer by intramuscular injection into deep muscle mass; superficial injections may be associated with increased pain and sterile abscesses. (Note: Administer with at least two other antituberculous agents to which the patient's strain of bacilli is susceptible.) Usual dose is 1 g daily intramusculary (do not exceed 20 mg/kg/d) for 60 to 120 days, followed by 1 g antimusculary 2 to 3 times weekly. Therapy for tuberculosis should be maintained for 12 to 24 months. If facilities for intramusculary administration are not available, a change to oral therapy is indicated.
Elderly: May have age-related renal impairment; otherwise, same as adult.
Children: Safety not established; however, a dosage of 15 mg/kg/d (maximum 1 g) has been recommended.
Renal impairment: Reduce dosage based on creatinine clearance.

INDICATIONS

Concomitant use with other antituberculous agents in pulmonary infections due to capreomycin-suscepti-ble strains of *M. tuberculosis* when primary agents (isoniazid, rifampin) have proved ineffective or cannot be used because of toxicity or presence of resistant tubercle bacilli

CONTRAINDICATIONS

Allergy or hypersensitivity to capreomycin

INTERACTIONS

Aminoglycosides (additive nephro- and ototoxicity)
Nondepolarizing neuromuscular blocking agents

ADVERSE EFFECTS

Nephrotoxicity, ototoxicity, hypersensitivity
Hepatic changes: decreased excretory function with-out change in aspartate aminotransferase or alanine aminotransferase in presence of preexisting liver disease; abnormal results in liver function tests have occurred
Hematologic: leukocytosis, leukopenia, thrombocy-topenia (rare); the majority of patients receiving capreomycin have had eosinophilia exceeding 5% while undergoing daily injections; these effects subsided with reduction of capreomycin dosage to 2 to 3 g weekly

PHARMACOKINETICS AND PHARMACODYNAMICS

Peak serum levels: at 1 to 2 h following 1 g intramuscu-lar dose
Plasma half-life: no information
Bioavailability: not absorbed orally in significant quantities
Metabolism: no information
Excretion: unaltered, 52% in urine within 12 h
Protein binding: no information
Renal impairment: reduced dosage necessary (*see* Special Precautions)
Hepatic impairment: no information

OVERDOSAGE

Any adverse effects listed may be seen as effects of overdose. Supportive therapy is indicated, and hemodialysis may be useful in patients with signifi-cant renal impairment.

AVAILABILITY

Powder for injection—1 g (as sulfate) per 10-mL vial

The information here is provided as guidance only. Prescribers should always consult the manufacturer's current prescribing information.

CLOFAZIMINE (Lamprene®)

An orally administered dye, *clofazimine* accumulates within macrophages, persists over long periods of time, colors tissues from yellow to red, and appears to affect oxygen-dependent mycobacterial metabolic pathways. Its tolerance and dosage have varied widely from 50 to 300 mg daily, with a usual dosage of 100 mg.

ANTIMICROBIAL ACTIVITY

Mycobacterium leprae; *Mycobacterium avium* complex.

RESISTANCE

Does not show cross-resistance with dapsone or rifampin.

SPECIAL PRECAUTIONS

Clofazimine has been associated with severe gastrointestinal effects. Rare reports include splenic infarction, bowel obstruction, and gastrointestinal bleeding. Death has been reported following severe abdominal symptoms, and autopsies have revealed crystalline deposits of clofazimine in intestinal mucosa, liver, gallbladder, bile, spleen, adrenals, subcutaneous fat, mesenteric lymph nodes, muscles, bone, and skin. Use with caution in patients predisposed to gastrointestinal problems or those who have preexisting problems such as pain or diarrhea. Dosages exceeding 100 mg should be given for minimal periods under close supervision only. If patient complains of colicky-burning pain, nausea, vomiting, or diarrhea, reduce dose or increase dosage interval or discontinue drug altogether.

Reactive depression may result due to skin discoloration caused by clofazimine (two suicides have been reported); keep patient under close supervision and give supportive care. Oil may be applied to the skin to alleviate dryness and ichthyosis. Sun exposure accentuates skin pigmentation.

SPECIAL GROUPS

Children: Safety and efficacy not established.
Elderly: No specific information.
Renal impairment: No information.
Hepatic impairment: No information.
Pregnancy: Use only when benefit is greater than risk. Adequate studies not performed. Crosses placenta.
Breast-feeding: Do not use unless benefit is greater than risk; excreted in breast milk.

INDICATIONS

1) *Treatment of lepromatous leprosy*, including dapsone-resistant lepromatous leprosy and lepromatous leprosy complicated by erythema nodosum leprosum
(Note: Combination drug therapy is recommended for initial treatment of multibacillary leprosy to prevent the development of drug resistance.)
2) *Treatment of M. avium complex* infections in combination with other agents

CONTRAINDICATIONS

None known

INTERACTIONS

Dapsone

ADVERSE EFFECTS

Pigmentation of skin (pink to brownish black; 75% to 100% of patients), gastrointestinal intolerance, ichthyosis or dryness of skin, rash, pruritis, phototoxicity, erythroderma, acneiform eruptions, monilial cheilosis, abdominal pain, diarrhea, nausea, vomiting, bowel obstruction, gastrointestinal bleeding, anorexia, constipation, weight loss, hepatitis, jaundice, eosinophilic enteritis, enlarged liver, conjunctival or corneal pigmentation, dryness or burning or irritation of eyes, discolored urine, feces, sputum, sweat, elevated blood sugar or erythrocyte sedimentation rate, splenic infarction, thromboembolism, anemia, cystitis, bone pain, edema, fever, lymphadenopathy, vascular pain, diminished vision, dizziness, drowsiness, fatigue, headache, giddiness, neuralgia, taste disorder, and depression
Laboratory effects: Elevated albumin, serum bilirubin, aspartate aminotransferase, eosinophilia, hypokalemia

The information here is provided as guidance only. Prescribers should always consult the manufacturer's current prescribing information.

CLOFAZIMINE (CONTINUED)

DOSAGE

1) *For leprosy*—**Adults:** (Note: Clofazimine should be used in combination with one or more other antileprosy agents to prevent emergence of drug resistance.) For dapsone-resistant leprosy, 100 mg clofazimine per day in combination with one or more other antileprosy drugs for 3 years, followed by monotherapy with 100 mg clofazimine per day; clinical improvement should be detected between first and third months of treatment and is usually clearly evident by the sixth month.

For dapsone-sensitive multibacillary leprosy, combination therapy with one or two other antileprosy drugs is recommended, giving the triple-drug regimen for a minimum of 2 years and continuing until negative skin smears are obtained; follow by monotherapy with an appropriate antileprosy agent.

2) *For erythema nodosum leprosum*—treatment is based on severity of symptoms; basic antileprosy therapy is used, and if nerve or skin ulceration is threatened, corticosteroids may be given. Clofazimine 100 to 200 mg/d for up to 3 months may be useful in eliminating or reducing corticosteroid requirements. Dosages over 200 mg/d are generally not recommended; dose should be tapered to 100 mg as soon as possible after reactive episode is controlled. Patient should be under medical supervision at all times.

Elderly: No special dosage given.

Children: Safety and efficacy not established.

3) *For M. avium complex (MAC)*—used in multidrug regimens, usually with clarithromycin or rifampin or rifabutin customarily at a dose of 100 mg daily.

PHARMACOKINETICS AND PHARMACODYNAMICS

Peak serum levels: 0.7 µg/mL and 1 µg/mL after 100-mg and 300-mg doses

Plasma half-life: 70 d

Bioavailability: highly lipophilic; deposited primarily in fatty tissue and in reticuloendothelial system

Metabolism: no metabolites

Excretion: negligible; retained in body for long periods

Effect of food: take with meals

Protein binding: deposited primarily in fatty tissue; taken up by macrophages

Renal impairment: no information

Hepatic impairment: no information

OVERDOSAGE

No specific data available. Empty stomach by inducing vomiting or gastric lavage. Employ usual supportive measures.

AVAILABILITY

Capsules—50 mg and 100 mg

The information here is provided as guidance only. Prescribers should always consult the manufacturer's current prescribing information.

CYCLOSERINE (Seromycin®)

Providing alternative oral therapy for resistant infections, *cycloserine* unfortunately has limited activity against *Mycobacterium tuberculosis* (MDR-TB) strains. Because essentially no cycloserine blood–brain barrier exists, central nervous system dysfunction and organic depression can develop. Dosage of 500 mg to 1 g is usually divided into two portions.

ANTIMICROBIAL ACTIVITY

Mycobacterium tuberculosis.

RESISTANCE

Not predictably active against multiply drug–resistant *M. tuberculosis.*

SPECIAL PRECAUTIONS

Central nervous system (CNS) toxicity is associated with cycloserine. Discontinue if patient develops allergic dermatitis, seizures, convulsions, psychosis, somnolence, depression, confusion, hyperreflexia, headache, tremor, vertigo, paresis, or dysarthria. Risk of convulsions is increased in chronic alcoholics. (Anticonvulsants or sedatives may be helpful in control of symptoms of CNS toxicity; patients receiving > 500 mg/d for such symptoms should be observed carefully.)
Toxicity is related to excessive blood levels (> µg/mL) due to high dosage or inadequate renal clearance.
Monitoring of hematologic, renal, and hepatic function should be performed regularly.
Patients with significant renal function impairment should not receive cycloserine. Dosage must be reduced in patients with renal insufficiency to avoid accumulation and toxicity.
Cultures should be obtained to determine susceptibility before treatment begins. Cycloserine has been associated with a few cases of vitamin B_{12} (or folic acid) deficiency, megaloblastic anemia, or sideroblastic anemia. If evidence of anemia manifests, appropriate tests and therapies should be performed.
Weekly blood level determinations should be made in patients with renal impairment receiving doses > 500 mg/d.

SPECIAL GROUPS

Children: Safety and efficacy not established.
Elderly: May have age-related renal impairment.
Renal impairment: Reduced dosage necessary; contraindicated in severe impairment.
Hepatic impairment: Use with caution.
Pregnancy: Use only if clearly needed; potential for harm not known.
Breast-feeding: Discontinue drug or discontinue nursing.

DOSAGE

Adults: 500 mg to 1 g daily in divided doses, with simultaneous monitoring of blood levels. Usual initial dosage is 250 mg twice daily every 12 hours for the first 2 weeks; do not exceed 1 g/d. Pyridoxine 200 to 300 mg/d may prevent or treat neurotoxic effects.
Elderly: May have age-related renal impairment; otherwise, same as adults.
Children: Safety not established; however, a dose of 10 to 20 mg/kg/d (maximum 0.75 to 1 g/d) has been recommended.
Renal impairment: No data to indicate appropriate dosage in renal dysfunction.

INDICATIONS

Treatment of active pulmonary and extrapulmonary tuberculosis when organisms are susceptible; after failure of treatment with primary antituberculous drugs. Administer in combination with other effective agents.

CONTRAINDICATIONS

Allergy or hypersensitivity to cycloserine, epilepsy, depression, severe anxiety or psychosis, severe renal insufficiency, and excessive concurrent use of alcohol or chronic alcoholism

INTERACTIONS

Alcohol, isoniazid

ADVERSE EFFECTS

Central nervous system (*see* Special Precautions), sudden development of congestive heart failure, skin rash, and elevated transaminase (especially in patients with liver disease)

PHARMACOKINETICS AND PHARMACODYNAMICS

Peak serum levels: 3 to 8 h
Plasma half-life: no information
Bioavailability: no percentage given; widely distributed
Metabolism: 35%
Excretion: 50% unchanged in urine in first 12 h; 65% in 72 h
Effect of food: no information
Protein binding: no information
Renal impairment: leads to toxic accumulation
Hepatic impairment: no information

OVERDOSAGE

Symptoms can occur if > 1 g is ingested. Chronic toxicity can occur if > 500 mg/d is administered. Effects include CNS depression with accompanying drowsiness, mental confusion, headache, vertigo, hyperirritability, paresthesia, dysarthrias, and psychosis. Paresis, convulsions, and coma may occur with larger doses.
Management includes supportive care; charcoal may be more effective than emesis or lavage. Hemodialysis removes cycloserine from the blood but should be used only in cases of life-threatening toxicity. Pyridoxine 200 to 300 mg/d may treat neurotoxic effects.

AVAILABILITY

Capsules—250 mg

The information here is provided as guidance only. Prescribers should always consult the manufacturer's current prescribing information.

DAPSONE

Administered orally, *dapsone* is effective in reducing the systemic burden of *Mycobacterium leprae* over a period of months. Unfortunately, when administered alone, secondary resistance of *M. leprae* can be expressed years later. Toxic reactions can complicate dapsone therapy; because it is an oxidant drug, dapsone can result in dose-dependent hemolysis in susceptible persons.

ANTIMICROBIAL ACTIVITY

Mycobacterium leprae.

RESISTANCE

Resistance encouraged by use of dapsone in single-drug regimen.

SPECIAL PRECAUTIONS

Deaths from agranulocytosis, aplastic anemia, and other blood dyscrasias associated with dapsone have been reported. Weekly blood counts are recommended for the first month of therapy, and monthly counts should be made for 6 months and semiannually thereafter. Discontinue dapsone if decrease in leukocytes or platelets or hematopoiesis occurs, and observe patient intensively.

Anemia existing prior to therapy should be treated before therapy is instituted. Hemoglobin should be monitored. Hemolysis and methemoglobin may be poorly tolerated by patients with severe cardiopulmonary disease.

Hypersensitivity reactions, including cutaneous reactions (bullous eruption, exfoliative dermatitis, toxic erythema, erythema multiforme, toxic epidermal necrolysis, morbilliform and scarlatiniform reactions, urticaria, and erythema nodosum), are directly due to drug sensitization. If new or toxic reactions occur, discontinue dapsone and treat appropriately.

Sulfone syndrome, an unusual and potentially fatal hypersensitivity reaction, may occur. Symptoms include fever, malaise, hepatitis with hepatic necrosis, exfoliative dermatitis, lymphadenopathy, methemoglobinemia, and hemolytic anemia.

Leprosy reactional states are not hypersensitivity reactions and do not require discontinuation of dapsone but may be confused with dapsone reactions.

Hemolysis–Heinz body formation may be exaggerated in patients with glucose-6-phosphate dehydrogenase (G-6-PD) deficiency, methemoglobin reductase deficiency, or hemoglobin M; the reaction is frequently dose related. Use caution in administering dapsone to such patients or to patients exposed to other agents or conditions that may produce hemolysis (eg, infection or diabetic ketosis).

Toxic hepatitis and cholestatic jaundice have been reported early in dapsone therapy. Hyperbilirubinemia occurs more often in G-6-PD–deficient patients. Baseline and subsequent monitoring of liver function are recommended; if abnormalities are detected, discontinue dapsone until their source is established. Dapsone has been found to be carcinogenic in small animals.

Dapsone levels are affected by acetylation rates. Patients with high acetylation rates or who are receiving treatment affecting acetylation may require dosage adjustment.

INDICATIONS

All types of leprosy except for cases where dapsone resistance is proven. Also alternative agent for prevention or therapy of *Pneumocystis carinii* infections in AIDS patients.

CONTRAINDICATIONS

Allergy or hypersensitivity to dapsone or its derivatives

INTERACTIONS

Rifampin
Folic acid antagonists
Para-aminobenzoic acid
Activated charcoal

ADVERSE EFFECTS

Hematologic: The most common effect is dose-related hemolysis including hemolytic anemia, which can be most serious in persons with preexisting anemia. Almost all patients demonstrate a loss of 1 to 2 g hemoglobin, an increase in reticulocytes (2%–12%), shortened red cell life span, and a rise in methemoglobin; G-6-PD–deficient patients have a greater response. Hypoalbuminemia without proteinuria has occurred. Other adverse effects include nausea, vomiting, abdominal pain, anorexia, headache, insomnia, vertigo, phototoxicity, blurred vision, tinnitus, fever, lupus erythematosus, paresthesia, tachycardia, infectious mononucleosis-like syndrome, male infertility, and peripheral neuropathy.

PHARMACOKINETICS AND PHARMACODYNAMICS

Peak serum levels: 4 to 8 h
Plasma half-life: 10 to 50 h
Bioavailability: when given orally, is rapidly and almost completely absorbed
Metabolism: acetylated in liver
Excretion: 70% to 85% in urine as conjugates and unidentified metabolites
Effect of food: does not block absorption
Protein binding: 70% to 90%; major metabolites, 99%
Renal impairment: no information
Hepatic impairment: dapsone levels are affected by acetylation rates (*see* Special Precautions)

The information here is provided as guidance only. Prescribers should always consult the manufacturer's current prescribing information.

DAPSONE (CONTINUED)

SPECIAL GROUPS

Children: No special information provided.
Elderly: No special information provided.
Renal impairment: No special information provided.
Hepatic impairment: Toxic hepatitis and cholestatic jaundice have occurred.
Pregnancy: Use only when necessary.
Breast-feeding: Excreted in breast milk; hemolytic reactions can occur in neonates; discontinue drug or discontinue nursing.

DOSAGE

Adults: For leprosy (Note: To reduce secondary dapsone resistance, the World Health Organization [WHO] Expert Committee on Leprosy recommends therapy be commenced and maintained at full dosage without interruption.): 50 to 100 g daily. For bacteriologically negative tuberculoid and indeterminate type leprosy, 100 mg/d with 6 months of rifampin 600 mg/d is recommended. Continue dapsone therapy for minimum of 3 years after all signs of clinical activity are controlled for tuberculoid and indeterminate patients. For lepromatous and borderline patients, give dapsone therapy in full dosage (100 mg/d) for many years, perhaps for life. The WHO Committee recommends administration for at least 10 years after the patient is bacteriologically negative. More than 5 years of continuous therapy is required to render most patients with lepromatous leprosy bacteriologically negative.
Elderly: Same as adults.
Child: Use adult regimens as guidelines, giving correspondingly smaller doses.
(Note: Secondary dapsone resistance should be suspected whenever a lepromatous or borderline lepromatous patient receiving dapsone relapses clinically and bacteriologically. If such cases demonstrate no response to regular and supervised dapsone therapy within 3 to 6 months, consider the resistance confirmed clinically. Treat with other agents.)

OVERDOSAGE

Symptoms include nausea, vomiting, and hyperexcitability and can appear after a few minutes or up to 24 hours after ingestion. Methemoglobin-induced depression, convulsions, and severe cyanosis require prompt treatment. Headache, hemolysis, and permanent retinal damage have occurred.
Treat by stomach evacuation, by aspiration and lavage. In normal methemoglobin reductase–deficient patients, methylene blue 1 to 2 mg/kg given slowly intravenously is the treatment of choice. Effect is complete at 30 min but may require repeating if methemoglobin reaccumulates. For nonemergencies, if necessary, methylene blue may be given orally in doses of 3 to 5 mg/kg every 4 to 6 hours. Do not give to fully expressed G-6-PD–deficient patients. Hemolysis may be treated by transfusion. Oxygen, intravenous fluids, and other supportive measures also may be helpful.

AVAILABILITY

Tablets–25 mg and 100 mg

The information here is provided as guidance only. Prescribers should always consult the manufacturer's current prescribing information.

ETHAMBUTOL (Myambutol®)

Having bacteriostatic activity, *ethambutol* is a well-tolerated oral "companion" drug used to diminish the likelihood of resistance emerging during therapy for tuberculosis. Its principal toxicity, which can be especially subtle in the elderly, is optic—affecting color perception and acuity. Regular visual testing is thus recommended. Ethambutol generally is not recommended for children less than 6 years of age whose visual acuity can not be monitored reliably [2].

ANTIMICROBIAL ACTIVITY

Effective against most strains of *Mycobacterium tuberculosis*.

RESISTANCE

Poor activity against most multidrug–resistant *M. tuberculosis* strains.

SPECIAL PRECAUTIONS

Optic neuritis has been associated with ethambutol; use of this agent may have adverse effects on vision, generally reversible when promptly discontinued (in rare cases, recovery may be delayed up to 1 year or more). Acuity changes may be unilateral or bilateral, and testing on both eyes should be performed before and periodically during treatment. Testing should include ophthalmoscopy, finger perimetry, and testing of color discrimination. In patients with preexisting visual defects, consideration of benefits versus risks of use should be made.
Renal function impairment requires reduced dosages; ethambutol is excreted by the kidneys.
Periodic monitoring of renal, hepatic, and hematopoietic systems is recommended during prolonged therapy.

SPECIAL GROUPS

Children: Not recommended for use in children under 6 years of age.
Elderly: May have age-related renal impairment and may be more susceptible to optic neuropathy.
Renal impairment: Reduced dosage necessary.
Hepatic impairment: May cause transient impairment of function or abnormal function.
Pregnancy: Use when clearly indicated; weigh benefits against risk.
Breast-feeding: No information.

DOSAGE

Adults: (Note: Do not use ethambutol alone. Administer once every 24 hours only. Continue treatment until bacteriologic conversion is permanent and maximal improvement has occurred.) For initial treatment (patients who have not received previous antituberculous therapy), give 15 mg/kg as a single dose once every 24 hours; isoniazid has been given concurrently in a single daily dose by mouth. For re-treatment (patients who have received previous therapy), give 25 mg/kg as a single oral dose once every 24 hours (monthly eye examinations are recommended). Concurrent administration of at least two other antituberculous drugs that demonstrate efficacy should be used (usually those not previously used in the patient). Decrease dose after 60 days to 15 mg/kg and give as a single dose once every 24 hours.
Elderly: May have age-related renal impairment; otherwise, same as adults.
Children: Safety not established in children under 6 years of age who are not able to have visual function assessed accurately.
Renal impairment: Reduce dosage proportionally to reduction in renal function.

INDICATIONS

Pulmonary tuberculosis, as treatment in combination with at least two other antituberculous agents
(Note: In patients who have received previous therapy, mycobacterial resistance to other drugs used in initial therapy is frequent. In re-treatment, combine ethambutol with at least two of the second-line drugs not previously administered to the patient and to which bacterial susceptibility has been proved.)

CONTRAINDICATIONS

Allergy or hypersensitivity to ethambutol
Known optic neuritis (unless clinical judgment determines use to be indicated)

INTERACTIONS

Aluminum salts

ADVERSE EFFECTS

Ophthalmic: may produce decrease in visual acuity (*see* Special Precautions). Other adverse effects include anaphylactoid reactions, rash, nausea, anorexia, vomiting, abdominal pain, fever, malaise, headache, dizziness, confusion, elevated serum uric acid levels, precipitation of acute gout, transient impairment of liver function, toxic epidermal necrolysis, thrombocytopenia, and joint pain.

PHARMACOKINETICS AND PHARMACODYNAMICS

Peak serum levels: 2 to 5 µg/mL 2 to 4 h after 15- to 25-mg dose
Plasma half-life: no information
Bioavailability: no information
Metabolism: by liver, 20% in 24 h
Excretion: 50% unchanged in urine (8% to 15% as metabolites), 20% to 25% in feces
Effect of food: not affected; take with food
Protein binding: no information
Renal impairment: marked accumulation may occur
Hepatic impairment: transient impairment due to drug has little effect

OVERDOSAGE

No information

AVAILABILITY

Tablets—100 mg and 400 mg

The information here is provided as guidance only. Prescribers should always consult the manufacturer's current prescribing information.

ETHIONAMIDE (Trecator-SC®)

Ethionamide may be employed for supervised therapy for resistant infections. However, gastrointestinal intolerance is likely to produce poor compliance or drug discontinuation.

ANTIMICROBIAL ACTIVITY
Mycobacterium tuberculosis.

RESISTANCE
Approximately one half of multidrug–resistant *M. tuberculosis* strains will be resistant to ethionamide.

SPECIAL PRECAUTIONS
Gastrointestinal intolerance is the the most frequent adverse effect associated with ethionamide; 50% of patients are unable to tolerate doses > 500 mg.
Hepatic toxicity is a rare effect.
Pretreatment examinations should be made and should include *in vitro* susceptibility tests of *M. tuberculosis.*
Serum transaminase (aspartate aminotransferase, alanine aminotransferase) monitoring should be performed every 2 to 4 weeks during therapy.
Diabetes mellitus may become more difficult to manage during ethionamide therapy.

SPECIAL GROUPS
Children: Optimum dosage not established; this does not preclude use when essential.
Elderly: No special information given.
Renal impairment: No special information given.
Hepatic impairment: Hepatic toxicity occurs rarely; contraindicated in severe hepatic damage.
Pregnancy: Use only when clearly indicated; when benefits are greater than risk.
Breast-feeding: No information.

DOSAGE
Adults: (In combination with at least two other antituberculous drugs) 0.5 to 1 g/d in divided doses.
Elderly: No special dosage given.
Children: A dose of 15 to 20 mg/kg/d (maximum 1 g) has been recommended. Concomitant administration of pyridoxine also is recommended.

INDICATIONS
Treatment of any form of active tuberculosis when treatment with first-line agents (isoniazid, rifampin) has failed. Use only in combination with other antituberculous agents.

CONTRAINDICATIONS
Allergy or hypersensitivity to ethionamide, severe hepatic damage

INTERACTIONS
No information

ADVERSE EFFECTS
Drowsiness and asthenia (common), anorexia, nausea, vomiting, diarrhea, metallic taste, rash, acne, neurotoxicity, depression, convulsions, peripheral neuritis and neuropathy, olfactory disturbances, blurred vision, diplopia, optic neuritis, dizziness, headache, restlessness, tremors, psychosis, postural hypotension, alopecia, thrombocytopenia, pellagra-like syndrome, gynecomastia, impotence, menorrhagia, hepatitis, and jaundice

PHARMACOKINETICS AND PHARMACODYNAMICS
Peak serum levels: 3 h
Plasma half-life: no information
Bioavailability: 75% to 85% of oral dose is absorbed
Metabolism: by liver
Excretion: metabolites excreted in urine
Effect of food: no information
Protein binding: no information
Renal impairment: no information
Hepatic impairment: no information

OVERDOSAGE
No information

AVAILABILITY
Tablets—250 mg

The information here is provided as guidance only. Prescribers should always consult the manufacturer's current prescribing information.

ISONIAZID (Nydrazid®, Rifamate®)

Since its introduction in 1952, *isoniazid* has provided the mainstay of antituberculous therapy. Well absorbed orally, distributed throughout the body, and generally well tolerated, limitations to its use relate mainly to emergence of resistance, which in certain populations has become a serious concern, and to infrequent but potentially serious hepatotoxicity, especially in the elderly (limiting its role in preventive therapy in this age group). Supervised administration in combination regimens can serve to preserve isoniazid's life-saving role in treatment of tuberculosis.

ANTIMICROBIAL ACTIVITY

Active against actively growing tubercle bacilli.

RESISTANCE

Resistance to isoniazid often, in combination with resistance to rifampin (multi-drug–resistant *M. tuberculosis* has emerged as a significant concern worldwide).

SPECIAL PRECAUTIONS

Warning: Hepatic toxicity resulting in severe and sometimes fatal hepatitis has been associated with isoniazid use and may occur even after many months of treatment. Risk is age related and also is increased with daily consumption of alcohol. Careful monthly monitoring (especially interview) is recommended. Serum transaminase concentrations become elevated in 10% to 20% of patients (usually during the first months of therapy but can occur at any time), and enzyme levels generally return to normal despite continuing therapy, but in a few cases progressive liver dysfunction may occur. Patients should be advised to contact physician immediately if symptoms of hepatitis occur (fatigue, weakness, malaise, anorexia, nausea, or vomiting). Discontinue isoniazid in presence of hepatic damage and do not reinstitute until symptoms and laboratory abnormalities have returned to normal. Preventive treatment should be deferred in patients with acute hepatic disease.

Neurologic toxicity: Neuropathy related to pyridoxine (vitamin B_6) deficiency is sometimes observed in adults receiving high doses of isoniazid. Supplementation with pyridoxine is recommended in patients likely to develop peripheral neuropathies secondary to isoniazid therapy; doses of 6 to 50 mg/d have been recommended. Stop all drugs and make complete systematic evaluations in the event of hypersensitivity reaction. Reinstitute isoniazid therapy in small doses and increase gradually. If symptoms recur, withdraw therapy.

INDICATIONS

All forms of tuberculosis due to susceptible organisms; also recommended for preventive therapy in specific cases

CONTRAINDICATIONS

Patients who have previous isoniazid-associated hepatic injury or other severe adverse reactions to isoniazid

INTERACTIONS

Alcohol, aluminum salts, oral anticoagulants, benzodiazepines, carbamazepine, cycloserine, disulfiram, enflurane, halothane, hydantoins, ketoconazole, meperidine, and rifampin

Drug–food interactions: Isoniazid has some monoamine oxidase inhibitor activity, and an interaction may occur with tyramine-containing foods. Diamine oxidase also may be inhibited, which may cause exaggerated response (headache, palpitations, sweating, hypotension, flushing, diarrhea, itching) to foods containing histamine (tuna, sauerkraut juice, yeast extract).

ADVERSE EFFECTS

(Note: Most frequent effects are those involving the central nervous system and hepatic systems; toxic effects are usually dose-related.)

Central nervous system: Peripheral neuropathy

Gastrointestinal: Nausea, vomiting, epigastric distress

Hepatic: Elevated serum transaminase, bilirubinemia, bilirubinuria, jaundice, severe and sometimes fatal hepatitis

Hematologic: Agranulocytosis; hemolytic, sideroblastic, or aplastic anemia; thrombocytopenia; eosinophilia

Hypersensitivity: Fever, rash, lymphadenopathy, vasculitis

Metabolic: Pyridoxine deficiency, pellagra, hyperglycemia, metabolic acidosis, gynecomastia, hypocalcemia, hypophosphatemia

Miscellaneous: Rheumatic syndrome and systemic lupus erythematosus–like syndrome, local irritation at injection site

PHARMACOKINETICS AND PHARMACODYNAMICS

Peak serum levels: 1 to 2 h

Plasma half-life: variable; depends on acetylator status

Bioavailability: well absorbed from gastrointestinal tract or intramuscularly

Metabolism: acetylated by the liver (approximately 50% of blacks and whites are "slow acetylators"

Excretion: 50% to 70% as unchanged drug and metabolites by kidneys in 24 h

Effect of food: decreases rate and extent of absorption

Protein binding: no information

Renal impairment: minor effect on elimination

Hepatic impairment: prolongs half-life

The information here is provided as guidance only. Prescribers should always consult the manufacturer's current prescribing information.

ISONIAZID (CONTINUED)

SPECIAL GROUPS

Children: No special information given.
Elderly: Risk of hepatotoxicity increases with age (50 or more years).
Renal impairment: Elimination is independent of renal function; no special dosage required.
Hepatic impairment: Use extreme caution; contraindicated in severe impairment.
Pregnancy: Use only when clearly necessary; weigh benefits against risk to fetus.
Breast-feeding: Isoniazid is excreted in breast milk; observe for adverse effects.

DOSAGE

Adults: For tuberculosis (in combination with other effective antituberculous agents), 5 mg/kg/d (up to 300 mg total) in a single dose orally or intramuscularly. For preventive treatment, 300 mg/d in single oral dose.
Elderly: May be more susceptible to hepatic toxicity.
Children: For tuberculosis (in combination with other effective antituberculous agents), 10 to 20 mg/kg/d (300 mg total) in a single dose, depending on severity of infection. For preventive treatment, 10 mg/kg/d (up to 300 mg total) in a single dose.

OVERDOSAGE

Symptoms occur in 30 minutes to 3 hours and may include nausea, vomiting, dizziness, slurring of speech, blurring of vision, and hallucinations. Extreme overdose is marked by respiratory distress, central nervous system depression, progressing rapidly from stupor to profound coma, and possibly severe, intractable seizures. Ingestion of 80 to 150 mg/kg will result in generalized seizures and a high possibility of fatality.

Secure airway and establish respiration. Gastric lavage is recommended in the first 2 to 3 hours but not until convulsions are controlled. Administration of a short-acting barbiturate intravenously or diazepam followed by pyridoxine intravenously (usually 1 mg per 1 mg of isoniazid ingested) may be used to control convulsions. Blood samples should be taken for immediate measurement of gases, electrolytes, blood urea nitrogen, glucose, and so forth, and to type and crossmatch blood in the event of hemodialysis becoming necessary. Rapid control of metabolic acidosis is crucial to management. Give sodium bicarbonate intravenously immediately and repeat as needed, adjusting subsequent dosage based on laboratory findings (serum sodium, pH). Begin forced osmotic diuresis early and continue for hours after clinical improvement has been remarked to hasten renal clearance of the drug and thus help prevent relapse. Monitor fluid input and output.

Hemodialysis is recommended for severe cases, and if not available, peritoneal dialysis may be used concomitantly with forced diuresis. Protect against hypoxia, hypotension, aspiration pneumonitis, and so forth.

AVAILABILITY

Tablets—50 mg, 100 mg, 300 mg
Syrup—50 mg/5 mL
Injection—100 mg/mL

The information here is provided as guidance only. Prescribers should always consult the manufacturer's current prescribing information.

PARA-AMINOSALICYLIC ACID

With limited application as an alternative oral component of multidrug regimens, *para-aminosalicylic acid* (PAS) has long been out of favor in the United States because of gastrointestinal intolerance. Daily dosage is divided into three to four portions taken with food. PAS may be obtained in the United States from the Centers for Disease Control and Prevention (CDC).

ANTIMICROBIAL ACTIVITY
Mycobacterium tuberculosis.

RESISTANCE
Approximately one half of multidrug–resistant *M. tuberculosis* strains are para-aminosalicylate susceptible.

SPECIAL PRECAUTIONS
Gastrointestinal intolerance—best administered after meals.

SPECIAL GROUPS
Elderly: Sodium salt may cause fluid retention, aggravating congestive heart failure.
Renal impairment: Dosage reduction or avoid because gastrointestinal symptoms and acidosis may be aggravated.
Hepatic impairment: May cause toxic hepatitis; use with caution.

DOSAGE
Adults: 200 mg/kg every 6 hours (to maximum of 12 g).
Elderly: No information.
Children: 150 to 200 mg/kg/d (to maximum of 12 g).

INDICATIONS
Rarely used (in the United States) in combination regimens for treatment of tuberculosis infections

CONTRAINDICATIONS
Allergy or hypersensitivity to para-aminosalicylic acid

INTERACTIONS
Isoniazid—Inhibits acetylation of isoniazid, increasing its serum concentrations, especially in "slow" acetylators

ADVERSE EFFECTS
Gastrointestinal intolerance may be so severe as to preclude its usage in some individuals
Other adverse effects include lymphoid hyperplasia; mononucleosis-like syndrome with fever, adenopathy, rash, and hepatosplenomegaly; and hypersensitivity and drug-induced lupuslike syndrome

PHARMACOKINETICS AND PHARMACODYNAMICS
Peak serum levels: 7 to 8 µg/mL
Bioavailability: well absorbed and distributed widely except central nervous system
Metabolism: acetylated in the liver
Excretion: promptly in urine as metabolites principally
Effect of food: minor; necessary for tolerance
Protein binding: 60% to 70%
Renal impairment: accumulation of metabolites; probenecid blocks tubular secretion

OVERDOSAGE
Discontinue drug; consider hemodialysis

AVAILABILITY
In United States from CDC Drug Service ([404] 639-3670)

The information here is provided as guidance only. Prescribers should always consult the manufacturer's current prescribing information.

PYRAZINAMIDE

Lowered dosage from that used in initial trials has allowed *pyrazinamide* to be used safely. Administered orally and as infrequently as once weekly in multidrug regimens, it now enjoys first-line status. The drug's acid stability gives it a special role against tubercle bacilli within macrophages, increasing efficacy of short-course regimens.

ANTIMICROBIAL ACTIVITY

Active against *Mycobacterium tuberculosis*, especially at acid pH based on the concentration of the drug attained at the site of infection.

RESISTANCE

Approximately one half of multidrug–resistant *M. tuberculosis* strains are susceptible to pyrazinamide.

SPECIAL PRECAUTIONS

Use only in combination with other appropriate antituberculous drugs. Pyrazinamide inhibits renal excretion of urates, often results in hyperuricemia (usually asymptomatic). Those patients already undergoing therapy should have baseline serum uric acid determinations. If signs of hyperuricemia accompanied by acute gouty arthritis appear, discontinue treatment.

Patients undergoing treatment with pyrazinamide should have baseline liver function determinations. Closely observe patients with preexisting liver disease or those with increased risk for drug-related hepatitis (*ie*, alcohol abusers). If signs of hepatocellular damage appear, discontinue pyrazinamide and do not resume.

Clinical data are limited on the use of pyrazinamide in patients 65 years of age and over; start dosage at lower end of range when treating this age group.

Patients infected with HIV may require a longer course of therapy. Be alert to any Centers for Disease Control and Prevention (CDC) updates in recommendations for these patients.

Diabetes mellitus may become more difficult to manage during therapy with pyrazinamide.

SPECIAL GROUPS

Children: Appears to be well tolerated.
Elderly: Use caution and lower doses; experience is limited.
Renal impairment: No dosage reduction required, but dosages in the lower range are recommended.
Hepatic impairment: Use with extreme caution and monitor closely; contraindicated in severe hepatic damage.
Pregnancy: Use only when clearly indicated.
Breast-feeding: Use with caution.

DOSAGE

Adults: (In combination with other antituberculous drugs only.) Usual dose is 15 to 30 mg/kg once daily. (CDC recommendations do not exceed 2 g/d as daily regimen.) Alternative dosage is twice weekly, 50 to 70 mg/kg based on lean body weight; developed to promote patient compliance with outpatient basis (evaluation finds this often exceeds the 3-g daily allowance, but no increase in adverse effects has been reported). Patients with HIV infection may require an extended course of therapy.
Elderly: Doses given from the lower end of the adult regimen are recommended.
Children: No specific dosages given.

INDICATIONS

Initial treatment of active tuberculosis in adults and children, combined with other antituberculous drugs
Also used after treatment failure of other primary agents for any form of active tuberculosis

CONTRAINDICATIONS

Allergy or hypersensitivity to pyrazinamide, severe hepatic damage, and acute gout

INTERACTIONS

Laboratory test interactions: Pyrazinamide has been reported to interfere with *Acetest* and *Ketostix* urine tests by producing a pink-brown color

ADVERSE EFFECTS

Hepatic abnormalities, mild arthralgia and myalgia, nausea, vomiting, anorexia, hypersensitivity reactions, rash, fever, porphyria, gout, hyperuricemia, thrombocytopenia, sideroblastic anemia with erythroid hyperplasia, vacuolation of erythrocytes, increased serum iron concentration, dysuria (rare), and adverse effects on clotting mechanisms (rare)

PHARMACOKINETICS AND PHARMACODYNAMICS

Peak serum levels: 2 h; range from 30 to 50 µg/mL with doses of 20 to 25 mg/kg
Plasma half-life: 9 to 10 h
Bioavailability: well absorbed from the gastrointestinal tract; widely distributed
Metabolism: hydrolyzed in liver to active metabolite
Excretion: glomerular filtration; approximately 70% of oral dose in 24 h
Effect of food: no information
Protein binding: no information
Renal impairment: half-life may be prolonged; no significant effect
Hepatic impairment: half-life may be prolonged (*see* Special Precautions)

OVERDOSAGE

Experience is limited, therefore employ clinical monitoring, paying special attention to hepatic function, and institute supportive therapy; pyrazinamide is dialyzable

AVAILABILITY

Tablets—500 mg

The information here is provided as guidance only. Prescribers should always consult the manufacturer's current prescribing information.

RIFABUTIN (Mycobutin®)

Formerly termed *ansamycin*, *rifabutin*, a rifamycin antibiotic, is active against 90% of *Mycobacterium avium* complex strains at concentrations achievable orally [11] and has shown promise clinically [12]. Toxicity resembles that of rifampin except for the occurrence of uveitis [13] and a serum sickness–like syndrome when doses exceed 300 mg daily; this also often occurs when given in combination with either fluconazole or clarithromycin, which apparently increase plasma rifabutin concentrations.

ANTIMICROBIAL ACTIVITY

Demonstrated *in vitro* activity against *Mycobacterium avium* complex (MAC) organisms isolated from both HIV-positive and HIV-negative patients. Rifabutin is active *in vitro* against many strains of *Mycobacterium tuberculosis*.

RESISTANCE

Cross-resistance between rifampin and rifabutin commonly is observed with *M. tuberculosis* and *M. avium* complex isolates; isolates of *M. tuberculosis* that are resistant to rifampin are usually resistant to rifabutin.

SPECIAL PRECAUTIONS

Do not administer to patients with active tuberculosis. Immediately evaluate patients with complaints consistent with active tuberculosis who are receiving rifabutin prophylaxis. Those with active disease should be given an effective combination regimen. Administration of single-agent rifabutin to patients with active tuberculosis may lead to development of tuberculosis that is resistant to both rifabutin and rifampin. There are no data to support rifabutin as an effective prophylaxis against *M. tuberculosis*. When prophylaxis is required, a combination of isoniazid and rifabutin may be given concurrently.

Fertility was impaired in male rats given 160 mg/kg, 32 times the human dose. Rifabutin may be associated with neutropenia and thrombocytopenia (rarely); periodic hematologic studies should be considered in patients receiving prophylaxis. Rifabutin has liver enzyme–inducing properties, and rifampin, a related drug, is known to reduce the activity of certain other drugs. Rifabutin may be expected to have similar interactions, and dosage adjustment for other drugs may be necessary if they are given concurrently with rifabutin.

Rifabutin can be mixed with foods such as applesauce if necessary to facilitate administration.

Rifabutin has caused a syndrome of uveitis and arthralgias when dosage has exceeded 300 mg per day or when combined with clarithromycin or ketoconazole, which apparently interfere with rifabutin's metabolism.

SPECIAL GROUPS

Children: Safety and efficacy not established (limited data available for use in HIV-positive children).
Elderly: Steady-state pharmacokinetics are more variable (70 years and older).
Renal impairment: No information.
Hepatic impairment: Pharmacokinetics modified only slightly.
Pregnancy: Use only if benefit greater than risk.
Breast-feeding: Discontinue drug or discontinue nursing.

DOSAGE

Adults: 300 mg once a day. If gastrointestinal sensitivity is significant, doses of 150 mg twice daily may be given with food.
Elderly: No information.
Children: Safety and efficacy not established.

INDICATIONS

Prevention of disseminated MAC disease in patients with advanced HIV infection

CONTRAINDICATIONS

Allergy or hypersensitivity to rifabutin or any other rifamycins

INTERACTIONS

Zidovudine, didanosine, and clarithromycin or ketoconazole (*see* Special Precautions)
Food interactions: High-fat meals inhibit rate of absorption but do not affect overall absorption; rifabutin may be mixed with foods such as applesauce

ADVERSE EFFECTS

Discolored urine, rash, nausea, abdominal pain, increased aspartate aminotransferase (> 150 U/L), increased alanine aminotransferase (> 150 U/L), vomiting, headache, fever, diarrhea, dyspepsia, eructation, anorexia, flatulence, flulike syndrome, hepatitis, hemolysis, arthralgia, myositis, chest pressure or pain with dyspnea, skin discoloration, seizure, paresthesia, aphasia, confusion, nonspecific T-wave changes on electrocardiogram, myalgia, uveitis, insomnia, and increased alkaline phosphatase
Hematologic: Neutropenia, leukopenia, anemia, thrombocytopenia, eosinophilia

PHARMACOKINETICS AND PHARMACODYNAMICS

Peak-serum levels: 375 ng/mL at 3.3 h after a 300-mg dose
Plasma half-life: 45 h
Bioavailability: 20%
Metabolism: five metabolites identified, 25-*O*-desacetyl and 31-hydroxy most predominant
Excretion: 53% in urine; primarily as metabolites
Effect of food: high-fat meals slow absorption; do not affect overall
Protein binding: 85%
Renal impairment: reduced drug distribution and faster elimination
Hepatic impairment: pharmacokinetics modified only slightly

OVERDOSAGE

No experience exists with overdose of rifabutin; however, clinical experience with rifamycins indicates gastric lavage within a few hours of overdose, followed by instillation of an activated charcoal slurry into the stomach; neither hemodialysis or forced diuresis is expected to enhance systemic elimination

AVAILABILITY

Capsules—150 mg

The information here is provided as guidance only. Prescribers should always consult the manufacturer's current prescribing information.

RIFAMPIN (Rifadin®, Rimactane®)

Known as *rifampicin* in the United Kingdom, *rifampin* is well absorbed orally and distributed throughout the body, including the central nervous system, as evidenced by orange discoloration of body fluids. Rifampin's bactericidal activity has been pivotal in reducing the duration of antituberculous therapy. Resistance, which is becoming increasingly prevalent, can emerge quickly unless rifampin is part of a multidrug regimen. Gastrointestinal irritation is frequent but usually tolerable; hepatotoxicity is also rather prevalent but seldom serious and generally reversible. Rifampin stimulates cytochrome P-450–mediated enzymatic hepatic metabolism of many substances, including therapeutic agents, so that familiarity with the most important of the more than 100 potential rifampin-related drug interactions is advisable [3].

ANTIMICROBIAL ACTIVITY

In vitro activity against the following organisms: *Mycobacterium leprae*, *Mycobacterium tuberculosis*, and many nontuberculous mycobacteria.

RESISTANCE

Used alone, resistance to rifampin occurs predictably despite its bactericidal action. Rifampin-resistant *M. tuberculosis* isolates are often resistant to other drugs as well. Strict adherence to multidrug regimens, which may include directly observed dosing, is the best means to prevent rifampin resistance.

SPECIAL PRECAUTIONS

Hepatic toxicity and fatalities associated with jaundice in patients with liver disease and in patients receiving rifampin concomitantly with other hepatotoxic agents have been reported. Weigh benefits against risks when considering use in hepatic impairment. Monitor liver function prior to therapy and every 2 to 4 weeks during therapy. If symptoms or signs of hepatocellular damage manifest, withdraw rifampin immediately.

Dosage adjustment necessary in hepatic impairment.

Hyperbilirubinemia may occur in early days of treatment. Make decision to discontinue therapy based on patient's condition and repeat tests.

Porphyria exacerbation has occurred with rifampin.

Hypersensitivity reactions have occurred during intermittent therapy and even after therapy was resumed after accidental interruption; reversible with discontinuation of rifampin.

Accelerated growth of lung carcinoma has occurred in humans taking rifampin; no relationship has yet been established.

Intermittent therapy may be used with close monitoring.

Urine, feces, saliva, sputum, sweat, semen, and tears may be red-orange; soft contact lenses may be permanently discolored. Rifampin also may color cerebrospinal fluid yellow.

Intravenous preparation is for intravenous infusion only. Do not administer intramuscularly or subcutaneous.

Complete blood count should be done prior to start of therapy and periodically during treatment, if clinically indicated; recommendation is to take sample before daily dosing.

Hematologic effects, most notably thrombocytopenia, have occurred primarily with high-dose intermittent therapy and are reversible if rifampin is discontinued as soon as purpura occurs. Cerebral hemorrhage and fatalities have occurred when rifampin administration has continued or resumed after appearance of purpura.

INDICATIONS

1) Tuberculosis—pulmonary and extrapulmonary forms. *ORAL:* Treatment of tuberculosis (all forms) in combination with at least two other antituberculous agents. *INTRAVENOUS:* Initial treatment and re-treatment of tuberculosis when oral form is not possible or not tolerated.
2) Combination therapy for several nontuberculous mycobacteria
3) Combination therapy of leprosy

CONTRAINDICATIONS

Allergy or hypersensitivity to any rifamycin

INTERACTIONS

Digoxin, enalapril, halothane, isoniazid, ketoconazole, others

Laboratory test interactions: Therapeutic levels of rifampin inhibit standard assays for serum folate and vitamin B_{12}

Rifampin drug interactions (due to hepatic microsomal enzyme induction): Acetaminophen, oral anticoagulants, barbiturates, benzodiazepines (metabolized by oxidation), beta-blockers, chloramphenicol, clofibrate, oral contraceptives, corticosteroids, cyclosporine, digitoxin, disopyramide, estrogens, hydantoins, methadone, mexiletine, quinidine, sulfones, sulfonylureas, theophyllines (dyphylline most likely does not interact), tocainide, and verapamil

ADVERSE EFFECTS

Flulike symptoms (dose related), asymptomatic elevations of liver enzymes, rash, heartburn, epigastric distress, anorexia, nausea, vomiting, gas, abdominal pain, headache, fatigue, drowsiness, flushing, ataxia, osteomalacia, weakness, myopathy, urticaria, pruritis, dizziness, confusion, visual disturbances, exudative conjunctivitis, peripheral neuropathy, menstrual disturbances, fever, edema of face and extremities, and shortness of breath or wheezing

Hematologic effects: Eosinophilia, transient leukopenia, hemolytic anemia, decreased hemoglobin, hemolysis, thrombocytopenia

Renal: Hemoglobinuria, hematuria, renal insufficiency, acute renal failure (interstitial nephritis)

Hepatic: Hepatitis, shocklike syndrome with hepatic involvement (rare), abnormal liver function tests

Other: Deep vein thrombosis has been reported

PHARMACOKINETICS AND PHARMACODYNAMICS

Peak serum levels: in 1 to 4 h; range, 4 to 32 µg/mL (3.5 to 15µg/mL in children)

Plasma half-life: mean, 3 h

Bioavailability: no percentage given; lipid soluble and widely distributed

Metabolism: in liver by deacetylation

Excretion: 40% in bile; 6% to 30% in urine (30%–60% deacetylated; 50% unchanged)

Effect of food: inhibits absorption

Protein binding: 80%

Renal impairment: dosage adjustment not necessary

Hepatic impairment: dosage adjustment necessary

The information here is provided as guidance only. Prescribers should always consult the manufacturer's current prescribing information.

RIFAMPIN (CONTINUED)

SPECIAL GROUPS

Children: No specific information.
Elderly: May be more sensitive to adult dose.
Renal impairment: No information.
Hepatic impairment: Dosage adjustment necessary.
Pregnancy: Do not use.
Breast-feeding: Discontinue drug or discontinue nursing.

DOSAGE

Adults: *Oral*: (Take on empty stomach 1 hour before or 2 hours after meals).
ORAL and *INTRAVENOUS*: For tuberculosis, 600 mg once daily in combination with at least two other antituberculous agents according to the CDC guidelines.
Elderly: May be more sensitive to higher doses.
Children: For tuberculosis 10 to 20 mg/kg (do not exceed 600 mg/d).

OVERDOSAGE

Symptoms include nausea, vomiting, and increased lethargy—all a short time after ingestion. Other less serious adverse effects may manifest and be more significant. Liver enlargement, possibly with tenderness, may develop within a few hours after severe overdosage; jaundice may develop quickly. Direct and total bilirubin levels may increase rapidly with severe overdosage; hepatic enzyme levels may be affected. Nonfatal overdoses as high as 12 g have been reported. Treat with gastric lavage (preferable to emesis) and instill activated charcoal slurry following evacuation of stomach. Antiemetic medication may be necessary to control nausea and vomiting. Forced diuresis, with measured intake and output, will promote excretion of the drug. Bile drainage may be indicated in the presence of serious hepatic impairment (lasting more than 24–48 hours), or extracorporeal hemodialysis may be necessary.

AVAILABILITY

Capsules—150 mg and 300 mg
Powder for injection—600 mg

The information here is provided as guidance only. Prescribers should always consult the manufacturer's current prescribing information.

STREPTOMYCIN

Introduced over 50 years ago, *streptomycin* provided the first really effective antituberculous therapy within the limitations imposed by intramuscular injection, vestibular toxicity, and emergence of resistance if given alone. Streptomycin has reemerged as a useful agent in multidrug regimens, especially when resistance to isoniazid and rifampin is encountered or likely.

ACTIVITY

Most strains of *Mycobacterium tuberculosis*, *M. kansasii*, *M. scrofulaceum*, and *M. ulcerans*.

SPECIAL PRECAUTIONS

Generally avoid or use special caution in combination with other aminoglycosides or capreomycin.

SPECIAL GROUPS

Children: Reduce dosage based on body weight.
Elderly: Increased risk for toxicity. May have age-related renal impairment; reduced dosage or lengthened dosage intervals may be necessary.
Renal impairment: Use extreme caution. A single dose may produce high blood levels for several days in patients who are severely uremic; cumulative effect may produce ototoxic sequelae.
Hepatic impairment: No information.
Pregnancy: Use with caution; potential for harm to fetus.
Breast-feeding: Not recommended. Potential for serious adverse reactions in nursing infant.

DOSAGE

Generally, 0.5 to 1.0 g 5 days per week is recommended.
(Note: Use intramuscular route only. If toxic symptoms occur, discontinue streptomycin or reduce dosage to 1 g 2 to 3 times a week. Streptomycin may be stopped when toxic symptoms appear, impending toxicity is suspected, organisms become resistant, or full therapeutic effect is reached.)
Adults: For combination therapy, give 0.5 to 1 g streptomycin with appropriate doses of combinations of antitubercular drugs (*eg*, isoniazid, ethambutol, rifampin, pyrazinamide).
Elderly: Reduce daily dosage of streptomycin according to age, renal function, and eighth nerve function.
Children: 20 to 40 mg/kg/d; maximum dose is 0.75 to 1 g.
Renal impairment: Reduce dosage according to degree of impairment.

INDICATIONS

Treatment of all forms of *M. tuberculosis* when due to susceptible organisms; used only in combination with other antituberculous agents; selected infections with nontuberculous mycobacteria having demonstrated susceptibility to streptomycin

CONTRAINDICATIONS

Hypersensitivity to streptomycin

INTERACTIONS

Ototoxic potential of streptomycin may be increased in combination with furosemide or ethacrynic acid. Nephrotoxic potential may be accentuated by nonsteroidal anti-inflammatory drugs.

ADVERSE EFFECTS

Neuromuscular blockade, urticaria, anaphylaxis, paresthesia of face, angioneurotic edema, exfoliative dermatitis, azotemia, pancytopenia, muscular weakness, and amblyopia

PHARMACOKINETICS AND PHARMACODYNAMICS

Peak serum levels: 25 to 50 μg/mL within 1 h after injection of 1 g
Plasma half-life: normal renal function, 2.5 h; end-stage renal disease, 100 h
Excretion: renal, by glomerular filtration; with normal renal function, 29% to 89% in 24 h
Effect of food: not applicable
Renal impairment: reduction in glomerular function results in decreased excretion and increased serum and tissue levels

OVERDOSAGE

No specific treatment for vestibular toxicity; early discontinuation may facilitate recovery. Dialysis is rarely necessary for reversible renal failure.

PATIENT INFORMATION

Patients should be advised and interviewed about vestibular symptoms and advised against concurrent furosemide, ethycrinic acid, or receiving other aminoglycosides for intercurrent infections

AVAILABILITY

Intramuscular injection, 1 g in 2.5 mL ampules (requires refrigeration)

The information here is provided as guidance only. Prescribers should always consult the manufacturer's current prescribing information.

CLASS DESCRIPTION

Until recently, fungal infections were not considered a major health problem. Consequently, limited resources and effort were expended by the pharmaceutical industry to discover new agents. Furthermore, because the differences between fungal cells and mammalian cells are less than those between bacterial cells and mammalian cells, agents that damage or kill fungal cells are more likely to have toxic effects on mammalian cells as well—a problem that does not exist for many antibacterial agents. A number of agents with substantial antifungal activity were discarded because of toxicity. For these reasons, progress in antifungal therapy has been slow, and only a few antifungal agents are available.

The number of drugs available for the treatment of systemic fungal infections is limited, although there are additional drugs available for topical applications only (and not included in this chapter). Three of the antifungal drugs are antibiotics: griseofulvin and the polyene antibiotics nystatin and amphotericin B. The remaining agents are chemically synthesized and include the antimetabolite flucytosine (5-fluorocytosine) and the azole compounds miconazole, clotrimazole, ketoconazole, fluconazole, and itraconazole. The azole compounds are divided into two groups based on the number of nitrogen atoms in the azole ring. Miconazole, clotrimazole, and ketoconazole are imidazoles, containing two nitrogens, whereas fluconazole and itraconazole are triazoles, containing three nitrogens in the azole ring.

Although some antifungal agents have been available for many years, information on their clinical efficacy against some fungal infections is sparse, and optimum dosing schedules of amphotericin B for the treatment of cryptococcosis and candidiasis are still debated. Although the combination of amphotericin B and 5-fluorocytosine is synergistic *in vitro* and in experimental animal models, no study has determined whether the combination is superior to amphotericin B alone for the treatment of candidiasis. Some of the deficiencies in adequate information reflect the less rigorous requirements for release of new drugs in the past, especially when only a few agents were available. Other contributing factors include the limited number of cases of some fungal infections, such as pseudallescheriasis or even aspergillosis, and the difficulty of conclusively establishing the diagnosis ante mortem in some fungal infections, such as disseminated candidiasis and aspergillosis. A further difficulty in evaluating efficacy of antifungal agents is the occurrence of some fungal infections (eg, aspergillosis and trichosporonosis) almost exclusively in immunocompromised patients in whom recovery is more often related to improvements in host defenses than in the efficacy of antifungal therapy.

GRISEOFULVIN

Griseofulvin is a fungistatic antibiotic produced by several species of *Penicillium*. Because of its poor solubility, it is available as oral preparations only.

Efficacy and Use

Griseofulvin is active *in vitro* against the dermatophytes *Trichophyton*, *Microsporum*, and *Epidermophyton*. It has no activity against yeasts or molds. This drug is effective for the treatment of tinea infections. It is not active against tinea versicolor, which is caused by *Malassezia furfur*. Because skin and nail infections can be caused by other fungi, it is important to identify the infecting organisms before instituting therapy with griseofulvin. Because hygienic factors play an important role in the acquisition and recurrence of dermatophyte infections, attention to good hygienic practices is an important component of successful therapy.

Mode of Action

The major effect of griseofulvin is to cause metaphase arrest of cell division by disrupting the mitotic spindle. It also causes the production of defective DNA that is unable to replicate.

Pharmacokinetics

Griseofulvin is absorbed predominantly from the duodenum [1]. There are two types of preparations, microsize and ultramicrosize. Absorption of the microsize preparations is unreliable and can vary from 25% to 70% of the dose administered. Absorption of the ultramicrosize preparation is more reliable, and peak serum concentrations of 0.4 to 2 µg/mL can be obtained 4 to 8 hours after administration of a 250-mg dose. The drug is concentrated in skin, hair, and nails but also in other organs including the liver, fat, and skeletal muscles. The drug is tightly bound to newly formed keratin, thus providing an unfavorable environment for infection. The drug is converted in the liver to an inactive metabolite; about 30% to 50% of this metabolite is excreted in the urine. Some of the drug is excreted in the perspiration, which may enhance its deposition in the skin. The elimination half-life varies from 9 to 24 hours.

Indications

As a general rule, griseofulvin therapy should be reserved for those patients whose infection fails to respond to topical agents. Although patients may note improvement in symptoms after several days of therapy, the drug should be continued for 2 to 4 weeks to avoid relapses. Nail infections are slow to resolve and may require therapy for more than 1 year.

Adverse Reactions and Contraindications

The most frequent side effect is headache, which may be severe but usually disappears during continued therapy. Some patients may develop gastrointestinal disturbances. Hypersensitivity and photosensitivity reactions may occur and require discontinuation of therapy. Renal, hepatic, and hematologic parameters should be determined during prolonged administration, and the drug should be discontinued if the patient develops neutropenia. Griseofulvin should not be given to patients with porphyria, lupus erythematosus, or severe liver disorders or during pregnancy.

Patient Information

Patients should be advised to follow good hygienic practices to optimize therapeutic outcome. They should avoid intense exposure to sunlight during therapy. Women of childbearing potential should be advised regarding use of contraceptive measures because of the potential fetal toxicity of this drug.

POLYENE ANTIBIOTICS

Amphotericin B and nystatin are polyene macrolide antibiotics produced by *Streptomyces nodosus* and *Streptomyces noursei*, respectively. Both drugs are poorly soluble in water. Nystatin is available as oral and topical preparations only [2]. The commercial preparation of amphotericin B for intravenous use is a complex with sodium

The information here is provided as guidance only. Prescribers should always consult the manufacturer's current prescribing information.

desoxycholate that is dispersed as a colloid in water. Both of these drugs are considered fungicidal agents. Emergence of resistance has been determined infrequently during therapy with these drugs.

Efficacy and Use

Nystatin is used for the treatment of superficial infections caused by *Candida* spp. *Candida rugosae*, a rare cause of infection, is inherently resistant to nystatin. Topical applications are effective for the treatment of cutaneous infections such as perlèche, intertriginous infection, paronychia, and diaper rash. Tablets are available for treatment of vaginitis. An oral suspension is available for the treatment of thrush and *Candida* esophagitis. Although it is effective for the treatment of esophagitis, responses occur less frequently and more slowly than treatment with systemic agents.

Amphotericin B is the antifungal agent with the broadest spectrum of activity. It is effective for the treatment of candidiasis, aspergillosis, coccidioidomycosis, cryptococcosis, histoplasmosis, blastomycosis, and phycomycosis. It is an alternative therapy for the cutaneous and mucocutaneous forms of leishmaniasis caused by *Leishmania braziliensis* or *mexicana*. It also is used to treat meningitis caused by *Naegleria* species. Emergence of resistance has been rare, but *Candida lusitaniae*, an uncommon pathogen, may be inherently resistant or develop resistance during therapy. The azole compounds are the preferred treatment for pseudallescheriasis and trichosporonosis. Recent studies also have demonstrated occasional therapeutic failures due to resistant strains in patients with aspergillosis and candidiasis.

Mechanism of Action

The polyene antibiotics exert their antifungal effect by binding to sterol compounds in the fungal cell membrane. This binding alters membrane permeability and causes leakage of cytoplasmic constituents out of the cell. Amphotericin B binds preferentially to ergosterol, a major component of the fungal cell wall. Because cholesterol is a major component of the mammalian cell wall, the drug has a differential effect between these cells. Resistance to amphotericin B appears to be caused by loss of ergosterol from the fungal cell membrane.

Pharmacokinetics

Nystatin is not absorbed from intact skin or the gastrointestinal tract. Although amphotericin B has been available for about 30 years, little is known about its pharmacokinetics [3]. The mean peak serum concentration is about 1 µg/mL after 30 mg is administered intravenously over several hours and about 2 µg/mL after 50 mg is administered. The average steady-state concentration of the drug in plasma is about 0.5 µg/mL. The initial serum half-life is about 24 hours, and the terminal half-life is about 15 days. When administered over 45 minutes, the serum concentration 1 hour after completion is nearly twice as high as when administered over 5 hours. At 18 hours and thereafter, the differences are minimal. When a double dose is administered every other day, the peak serum concentration is 80% to 100% higher, however, there is no close correlation between the dose administered and the serum concentration. Furthermore, serum concentrations do not appear to increase with increasing doses above 50 mg. The trough concentrations with the every-other-day schedule usually are similar to those achieved with the daily dose schedule.

After intravenous infusion, no more than 40% of the dose can be accounted for in the serum and extracellular fluid. Ten percent is strongly bound to plasma proteins. Concentrations of amphotericin B in fluids from inflamed pleura, peritoneum, synovium, and aqueous humour are about two thirds of trough concentrations in plasma. The drug does not penetrate the blood–brain barrier adequately; apparently a major portion of the drug is bound to tissues and released slowly.

About 2.5% to 13% appears in the urine within 24 hours after a single dose, and 40% appears after 7 days. Following multiple doses, on the other hand, only 2% to 5% can be detected in the urine. Low levels can be detected in the urine for at least 7 weeks after cessation of therapy. The fraction of drug excreted in the urine is so low that reduced renal function has little effect on the serum concentration. The drug is not removed during dialysis procedures. Animal studies have suggested that the biliary route may be important in the excretion of amphotericin B. The major excretory pathway of amphotericin B remains unknown.

Indications

Nystatin is available for the treatment of superficial forms of candidiasis, including cutaneous infection, thrush, vaginitis, and esophagitis. There are a variety of topical preparations that appear to be as efficacious as nystatin for vaginitis. Women with recurrent vaginitis usually require systemic therapy. Patients with chronic mucocutaneous candidiasis require systemic therapy. Nystatin is the most widely used agent for thrush, but clotrimazole is better tolerated. Further, the orally absorbable agents are often more effective (but more expensive).

Amphotericin B is indicated for the treatment of serious systemic infections, but its potential toxicity mitigates against its use for minor to moderately severe infections [4]. Its indications and dosage schedules are listed in Table 11-1.

Adverse Reactions

The toxicities of amphotericin B are of such great magnitude that they (rather than the response to therapy) frequently dictate the dose and schedule of drug administration. Amphotericin B causes acute toxicities that may be idiosyncratic or dose related; it also causes chronic toxicities [5]. Idiosyncratic reactions include flushing, anaphylactic shock, acute liver failure, thrombocytopenia, vertigo, generalized pain, grand mal convulsions, ventricular fibrillation and cardiac arrest, rash, and hearing loss.

Fever and chills occur in virtually all patients. Headache occurs in 45% of patients; anorexia in 50%; and vomiting in 20%. Acute symptoms usually can be controlled with drugs such as hydrocortisone, phenothiazines, and meperidine.

Amphotericin B is a local irritant, causing pain at the infusion site and phlebitis. Heparin (5 to 50 mg) mixed in the infusion may diminish the phlebitis. Extravasation causes local irritation.

Nephrotoxicity is the most serious side effect of amphotericin B therapy, and virtually every patient develops some manifestations of renal damage. The usual side effects include urinary abnormalities, hyposthenuria, azotemia, hypokalemia, renal tubular acidosis, and nephrocalcinosis. Proteinuria is uncommon, but hyaline and granular casts and pyuria are common. Approximately 90% of patients develop an increase in blood urea nitrogen or creatinine. There is no correlation between the degree of azotemia and the total dose of amphotericin B administered. Renal tubular acidosis and renal potassium loss may result in hypokalemia; supplemental potassium can diminish this problem. Amphotericin B suppresses production of erythrocytes, possibly by reducing erythropoietin production, and causes a normocytic, normochromic anemia.

The information here is provided as guidance only. Prescribers should always consult the manufacturer's current prescribing information.

FLUCYTOSINE

Flucytosine is a chemically synthesized fluorinated pyrimidine related to 5-fluorouracil and floxuridine.

Efficacy and Use

Flucytosine is active against *Cryptococcus neoformans*, *Candida* spp, *Torulopsis glabrata*, and some fungi that cause chromoblastomycosis. About 5% to 10% of strains of *Candida* spp and *C. neoformans* are inherently resistant to flucytosine, and about 5% develop resistance during therapy. Consequently, flucytosine should not be used alone, except for the treatment of candida urinary tract infections. Because *in vitro* studies have demonstrated synergistic interactions between flucytosine and amphotericin B, the combination is used for treatment of cryptococcosis and candidiasis. Sporadic reports suggest that the combination may be beneficial against aspergillosis. The only clinical trial that demonstrated greater efficacy for flucytosine plus amphotericin B than for amphotericin B alone was in patients with cryptococcal meningitis. There are some experimental and clinical data that suggest it may enhance the efficacy of amphotericin B in aspergillosis, but this has never been well substantiated. Flucytosine's potential for causing myelosuppression has limited its use because many fungal infections occur in patients with already compromised bone marrow.

Mode of Action

Flucytosine interferes with pyrimidine metabolism and, ultimately, RNA and protein synthesis. The drug enters the fungal cell and is deaminated to 5-fluorouracil, which is incorporated into RNA. It also is converted to fluorodeoxyuridine monophosphate, which inhibits thymidylate synthetase and DNA synthesis. Mammalian cells do not convert large amounts of flucytosine to 5-fluorouracil (hence its selective toxicity against fungi). Resistance to flucytosine may occur at any enzymatic step associated with the drug's entry into the cell, its deamination, or its incorporation into RNA.

Pharmacokinetics

Flucytosine is available as an oral preparation only. About 75% to 90% is absorbed from the gastrointestinal tract [6]. Ingestion with a meal or antacids decreases the rate of absorption during the 1st hour but not its total absorption. It is widely distributed into body tissues, peritoneal fluid, bronchial secretions, and aqueous humor. The drug readily crosses the blood–brain barrier, and about 65% to 90% of the simultaneous plasma concentration is achieved in the cerebrospinal fluid. Administration of the recommended dose provides serum concentrations ranging from a peak of about 70 μg/mL to a trough of about 35 μg/mL. The serum half-life is 3 to 6 hours in normal individuals. Flucytosine binds minimally to serum proteins. About 80% of the drug is excreted unchanged into the urine by glomerular filtration. Urine concentrations are about 10 times higher than serum concentrations.

Indications

Flucytosine is indicated as combination therapy with amphotericin B for the therapy of serious candida and cryptococcal infections. The combination may occasionally be beneficial in patients with aspergillosis who are failing to respond to amphotericin B alone. The drug can be used alone for the treatment of candida urinary tract infections.

Adverse Reactions and Warnings

Side effects occur in about 5% of patients and generally involve the bone marrow, liver, and gastrointestinal tract. The most common gastrointestinal toxicities are nausea, vomiting, and diarrhea [7]. A few cases of severe enterocolitis and perforation have occurred. Hepatic toxicities consist of elevated serum transaminases and alkaline phosphatase that are reversible, but, rarely, patients have developed hepatomegaly or patchy hepatic necrosis. Bone marrow toxicity is manifested by anemia, leukopenia, and thrombocytopenia. Rare toxicities include rashes, confusion, hallucinations, headaches, and vertigo.

It is advisable to monitor serum concentration even in patients without renal impairment because myelosuppression is more common if the concentration exceeds 100 μg/mL, and it is prudent to maintain serum concentrations above 25 μg/mL to prevent emergence of resistance. Hemograms and liver and renal function studies should be monitored two to three times a week during therapy.

Table 11-1. Indications for Amphotericin B Therapy*

Disease	Dose	Duration
Aspergillosis and phycomycosis	1.0–1.5 mg/kg/d until renal impairment requires modification	Depends on response
Blastomycosis (severe)	50 mg 3 × weekly	13–20 weeks
Candidiasis	0.5–0.7 mg/kg/d	At least 2 weeks after resolution of all signs and symptoms of infection
Candidemia	25–50 mg/d	Total dose, 250–500 mg
Coccidioidomycosis	1.0–1.5 mg/kg/d to toxicity, then 1.0–1.5 mg/kg 3 × weekly	Pulmonary: 0.5–1.5 g total dose Disseminated: 2.5–3.0 g total dose
Cryptococcosis	0.6–1.0 mg/kg/d	Depends on underlying condition (*eg*, AIDS), extent of infection, and rapidity of response
Histoplasmosis (severe)	0.5–0.6 mg/kg/d	Acute: 500 mg total dose Chronic pulmonary: 1.5–3.5 g total dose Disseminated: 10 weeks
Sporotrichosis	0.5 mg/kg/d	1.5–2.5 g total dose

Alternative regimens have been suggested for some of these diseases.

The information here is provided as guidance only. Prescribers should always consult the manufacturer's current prescribing information.

Because the drug is excreted primarily in the urine, dosage must be adjusted according to renal function. One method is to administer 12.5 to 37.5 mg/kg at intervals equal to twice the serum half-life of flucytosine (approximately five to six times the serum creatinine concentration). Obviously the most reliable method is to measure serum concentrations and adjust the dose accordingly. And, because amphotericin B alters renal function, it is especially important to monitor renal function when administering the combination.

AZOLE ANTIFUNGAL AGENTS

Azoles that are available for the treatment of fungal infections include the imidazoles and the triazoles (Fig. 11-1). Imidazoles are five-membered ring structures containing two nitrogen atoms with a complex side chain attached to one of the nitrogen atoms. Triazoles are similar structures, containing three nitrogen atoms in the five-membered ring. The imidazoles used for systemic therapy are keto-conazole and miconazole. Clotrimazole is used for superficial infections such as thrush. There are several other similar agents that are available for topical use only, including econazole, butoconazole, and oxicona-zole. The triazoles available for systemic therapy are fluconazole and itraconazole. Terconazole is a triazole available for topical use only. The topical antifungals are not included in this discussion.

Efficacy and Use

The activity of the various azole compounds against the more common fungal infections is shown in Table 11-2. All of the azole compounds are active against candida infections. Only fluconazole has been shown to be as effective as amphotericin B in hematoge-nously disseminated infection. Clotrimazole use is limited to oropha-ryngeal candidiasis. There is some evidence to suggest that ketoconazole has limited efficacy against *Candida tropicalis* and

Candida krusei is inherently resistant against fluconazole. Itraconazole is very effective for the treatment of histoplasmosis and blastomycosis. Ketoconazole and fluconazole are also active against these infections, but itraconazole appears to be the superior agent. Fluconazole is effective for the treatment of cryptococcosis, including meningitis, and is considered the drug of choice for maintenance therapy for cryptococcal meningitis in AIDS patients. Although itraconazole has activity against cryptococcal infections, its role in the treatment of cryptococcal meningitis is uncertain.

Although all four systemic azoles are purported to have activity against coccidioidomycosis, including meningitis, recent data suggest that fluconazole and itraconazole are superior to miconazole and ketoconazole. Miconazole is considered the drug of choice for the treatment of pseudallescheriasis. Other azoles are probably also effective, but experience with them is limited. The azole compounds are probably superior to amphotericin B for the treatment of trichosporonosis. The limited number of patients with this infection precludes a comparative trial, but some strains are resistant to amphotericin B. Itraconazole is the only azole compound with activity against aspergillosis. Its activity in neutropenic patients is not well demonstrated, and its relative efficacy compared with amphotericin B has not been determined. Azole compounds also have activity against paracoccidioidomycosis, chromomycosis, and sporotrichosis.

Mechanism of Action

The principal mechanism of action of the azole compounds is to preferentially inhibit cytochrome P-450 enzymes in fungal organisms [8]. The major enzyme inhibited by the azoles is the 14alpha-demethylase that is responsible for the conversion of lanosterol to ergosterol, which is the major component of the fungal cell membrane. To a lesser extent, these compounds interfere with the mammalian enzyme that converts lanosterol to cholesterol, which is a

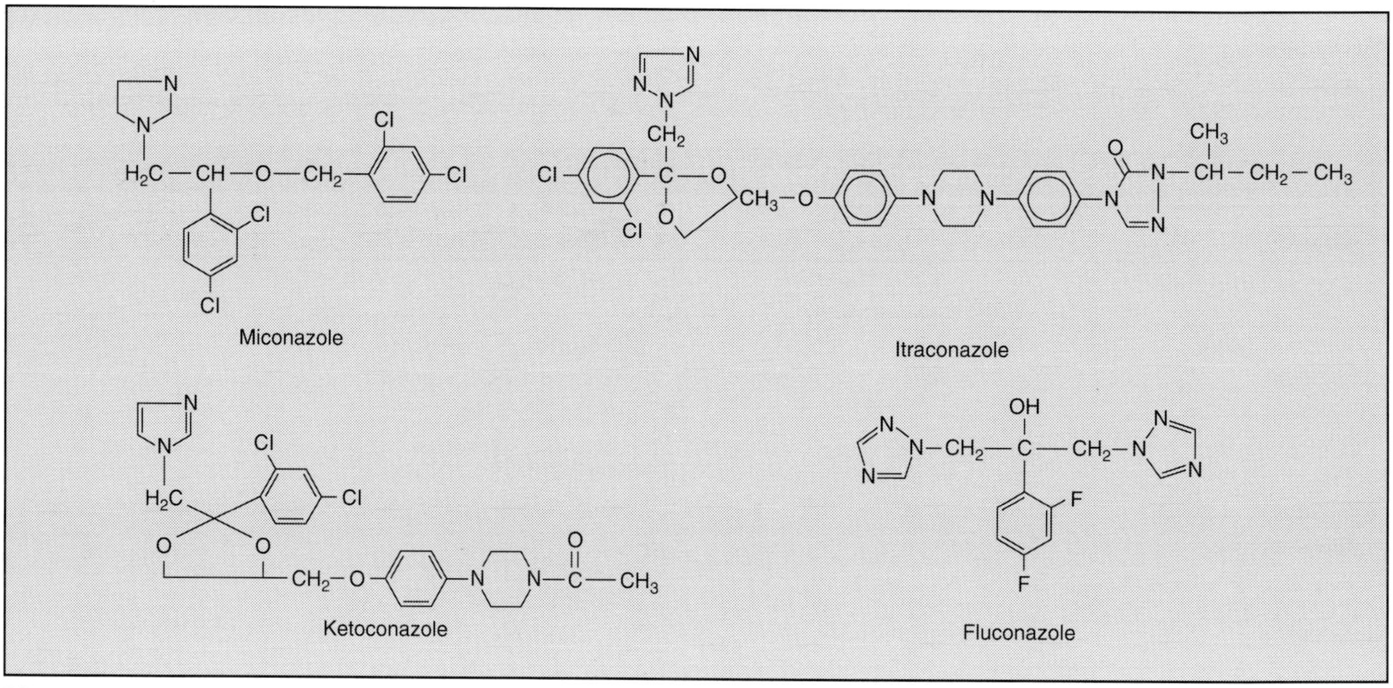

FIGURE 11-1.

Chemical structures of systemic azole compounds.

The information here is provided as guidance only. Prescribers should always consult the manufacturer's current prescribing information.

major component of membranes and a hormone precursor. Ketoconazole can also inhibit $C_{17,20^-}$ desmolase, an enzyme responsible for steroid synthesis. The selective inhibition of fungal enzyme versus mammalian enzyme may impact on the frequency and severity of adverse effects. For example, the concentrations of ketoconazole and fluconazole required for inhibition of the cytochrome oxidase of *Candida albicans* are comparable. Approximately 200 times more fluconazole than ketoconazole is required for inhibiting the rat liver cytochrome oxidase.

Interference with the synthesis of ergosterol leads to the production of a defective cell membrane with altered permeability. Azole compounds also may have a direct effect on the fatty acids of cell membranes, causing leakage of proteins and amino acids and interference with uptake of essential nutrients. They also may inhibit catalase systems, decrease fungal adherence, and inhibit formation of germ tube and mycelia. Azole compounds generally are considered to be fungistatic against most organisms, but differentiation between fungistatic and fungicidal activity often depends on laboratory methodology.

Pharmacokinetics

The azole antifungal agents differ substantially in their pharmacokinetic properties [9]. Clotrimazole is provided as a troche that requires 15 to 30 minutes for dissolution in the mouth. Concentrations sufficient to inhibit most *Candida* spp are detected in the saliva for up to 3 hours thereafter. Table 11-3 provides information regarding the pharmacokinetic properties of the other four agents.

Miconazole is available only as an intravenous preparation. Because of its limited solubility in water, the intravenous preparation contains lactic acid and Cremophor EL (polyethylene glycol, castor oil, and parabens). Intravenous doses of 600 to 1000 mg produce peak serum concentrations of 7.5 to 10 µg/mL, but the serum concentrations fall to less than 1 µg/mL within 2 hours; this may be of considerable importance because the minimal inhibitory concentration required for most fungi is 0.1 to 1.0 µg/mL. Miconazole disappears from the plasma in a triphasic pattern, with a terminal half-life of about 24 hours. Over 90% of the drug is bound to plasma proteins. It readily penetrates into inflamed joints, vitreous humor, and the peritoneal cavity but not into sputum and saliva. The

Table 11-2. Uses for Azole Compounds

	Azole Compound				
	Clotrimazole	**Miconazole**	**Ketoconazole**	**Fluconazole**	**Itraconazole**
Blastomycosis	-	-	+	±	+
Candidiasis	+	±	+	+	+
Cryptococcosis	-	±	-	+	±
Coccidioidomycosis	-	±	±	+	+
Histoplasmosis	-	-	+	±	+
Pseudallescheriasis	-	+	Unknown	Unknown	Unknown
Aspergillosis	-	-	-	-	+
Trichosporonosis	-	+	+	+	Unknown

+—active; - —inactive; ±—limited activity.

Table 11-3. Pharmacokinetic Properties of Azole Antifungal Agents

Property	Miconazole	Ketoconazole	Fluconazole	Itraconazole
Route	Intravenous	Oral	Intravenous, oral	Oral
Usual dose	0.6–1.8 g	200–400 mg	100–400 mg	200 mg
Peak serum concentration, µg/mL*	7.5–10.0	1.7–3.6	2.5–6.7	0.1
Terminal half-life, *h*	24, triphasic	8, biphasic	20–30	15–40, triphasic
Protein binding, %	90	99	11	99.8
CSF and serum concentration	< 10	< 10	> 60	< 10
Excretion	Liver	Liver	Kidney	Liver
Absorption, %	50	75	85	99
Active drug in urine, %	1	2	65	< 1

*Following the administration of usual doses.
CSF—cerebrospinal fluid.

The information here is provided as guidance only. Prescribers should always consult the manufacturer's current prescribing information.

concentration in cerebrospinal fluid is low and unpredictable. The drug is metabolized in the liver by destruction of the imidazole ring. About 15% to 20% is excreted in the urine as inactive metabolites. Serum concentrations are not affected by renal impairment, hemodialysis, or continued drug administration.

The absorption of ketoconazole depends on acid in the stomach because it must be converted to the hydrochloride salt [10]. The administration of antacids or H_2 blocking agents greatly reduces its absorption. For example, the mean peak serum concentrations (µg/mL) of ketoconzaole following 200 mg alone and in combination with 400 mg of cimetidine were 4.5 and 1.3, respectively. Administration with food enhances absorption. Ketoconazole disappears from the serum in a biphasic manner. The initial serum half-life is 1.5 to 2 hours; the terminal half-life is nearly 4 hours after a 400-mg dose. More than 90% of circulating ketoconazole is bound to serum albumin. The drug penetrates the blood–brain barrier very poorly. Limited data suggest that the pharmacokinetics of ketoconazole are not altered substantially in patients with hepatic or renal impairment. The drug is metabolized in the liver by degradation of the imidazole ring, and the inactive metabolites are excreted via the bile. About 15% of ketoconazole is excreted in the urine but with only a small amount as active drug. Its absorption in patients undergoing continuous peritoneal dialysis is greatly reduced, and distribution into peritoneal fluid is negligible. Eighty-five percent of ketoconazole is bound to plasma proteins, and 15% is bound to blood cells, mainly membranes and probably also to hemoglobulin. About 70% of a dose is excreted over 4 days; 57% in feces and 13% in urine.

Fluconazole is rapidly and completely absorbed from the gastrointestinal tract; hence serum concentrations are similar following oral and intravenous administration [11]. Gastrointestinal absorption is not greatly affected by gastric acidity. Food does not impact substantially on absorption. Steady-state serum concentrations of fluconazole are attained within 5 to 10 days, and an initial loading dose is recommended (twice the usual daily dose). The drug is evenly distributed in body tissues, crosses the blood–brain barrier, and penetrates into the vitreous and aqueous humors of the eye. The drug is only minimally metabolized in the liver and excreted largely unchanged in the urine. Consequently, dosage schedules must be adjusted in patients with renal impairment.

Itraconazole is a highly lipophilic compound that is almost insoluble in water and dilute acids [12]. It is ionized only at low pH, as in gastric juice. The bioavailability of itraconazole after a single oral dose is approximately 55% and varies depending on the formulation (capsules versus solution). Absorption is enhanced by the presence of food in the stomach. Absorption also depends on the presence of acid in the stomach. The serum elimination half-life is 15 to 25 hours after the first dose but increases to 34 to 42 hours after 2 weeks of administration. Itraconazole plasma concentrations are quite low, but tissue concentrations are two to three times higher than plasma concentrations, with adipose tissue concentrations 20 times higher. Circulating drug is almost entirely bound to plasma proteins, primarily albumin. Concentrations in eye fluid, cerebrospinal fluid, and saliva are negligible. The drug may persist in tissues for long periods. The drug is highly metabolized in the liver, with 54% excreted in the feces and 35% in the urine as metabolites.

Indications

The use of azole compounds is changing since fluconazole and itraconazole became available. Clotrimazole remains an effective and well-tolerated topical agent for oropharyngeal candidiasis. Its disad-

vantage is the dosage schedule of five times daily. Oral absorbable agents are more effective, but ketoconazole and itraconazole are unreliable in some patient populations (*eg*, AIDS, bone marrow transplant) because of unreliable absorption. Fluconazole is effective for treatment of oropharyngeal and esophageal candidiasis, but breakthrough infection in patients with far-advanced AIDS receiving fluconazole prophylaxis has raised concerns about the emergence of resistance. Recent prospective comparative studies of fluconazole versus amphotericin B for treatment of hematogenous infection indicate that the two agents are equally effective, and fluconazole is less toxic [13]. Fluconazole appears to be more effective than amphotericin B for treatment of the chronic disseminated candidiasis that occurs in leukemic patients. Single oral doses of fluconazole (150–200 mg) recently have been approved for candida vaginitis.

Itraconazole is the most appropriate therapy for blastomycosis and histoplasmosis, except for those patients who are acutely ill and have rapidly disseminated infection or meningitis [14]. Fluconazole is effective therapy for cryptococcal infection, including meningitis. Amphotericin B should be given initially to patients who are seriously ill, with substitution of fluconazole as the patient stabilizes. Fluconazole is the drug of choice for maintenance therapy in AIDS patients with cryptococcal meningitis. Itraconazole may be used for treatment of aspergillosis, but amphotericin B should be used for initial therapy in most cases [15]. Both fluconazole and itraconazole have been shown to be effective in coccidioidomycosis, but their efficacy compared with amphotericin B has not been ascertained. Miconazole is considered the drug of choice for pseudallescheriasis, although other azoles may be equally effective. Azoles appear to be more effective than amphotericin B for treatment of trichosporonosis.

Special Groups

Absorption of ketoconazole and itraconazole is unreliable in patients with achlorhydria. Miconazole, ketoconazole, and itraconazole should be administered with caution in patients with hepatic impairment. Fluconazole dosage must be adjusted in patients with renal impairment.

Drug interactions have been described with the azole compounds, most often with ketoconazole. This drug must not be given to patients taking terfenadine or astemizole because of the possibility of fatal cardiac arrhythmias. Other important interactions are listed in Table 11-4. Some of these interactions also have been described to a lesser extent with other azole compounds.

In children, experience with the azoles is limited. Recent pharmacokinetic data indicate that neonates have a lower peak serum concentration but a longer serum half-life of fluconazole. The pharmacokinetics approach that of the adult by about 2 months of age. These drugs should be avoided in pregnant and nursing women. Patients with known allergies to any azole probably should not be given these drugs except under special circumstances.

Patient Information

Patients should be warned about use of other medications while taking azole compounds. Mothers requiring an azole compound should not breast-feed, and pregnant women should avoid these drugs.

Warnings and Adverse Reactions

The potential toxicities of azole compounds are gastrointestinal, hepatic, endocrinologic, metabolic, hematologic, and carcinogenic and also occur as the result of drug–drug interactions. At conventional doses these compounds have been very well tolerated, even

The information here is provided as guidance only. Prescribers should always consult the manufacturer's current prescribing information.

when administered for prolonged periods of time. Nausea and vomiting have been reported in 2% to 10% of patients. Other general adverse effects include headache, fever, fatigue, abdominal pain, and diarrhea. Hypersensitivity reactions, consisting of pruritus, rash, and eosinophilia occur rarely. Urticaria, exfoliative dermatitis, and anaphylaxis have been reported, but none has been fatal.

A major concern with azole compounds is the potential for hepatic toxicity. During the first 2 weeks transient elevations in transaminase and alkaline phosphatase occur in approximately 10% of patients receiving ketoconazole; these usually return to normal with continued treatment. Clinical hepatitis is estimated to occur in one in 1500 patients receiving long-term therapy. It is usually reversible when the drug is discontinued, but recovery may take several months. A few patients have died of fulminant hepatic failure. Transient liver abnormalities have been described in about 3% of patients receiving fluconazole or itraconazole.

Ketoconazole has a direct effect on steroidogenesis by the adrenal gland in humans. There have been no cases of clinical adrenal insufficiency, but this could be a problem in patients receiving high doses for prolonged durations. Ketoconazole also appears to depress serum testosterone concentrations, resulting in increased estradiol-to-testosterone ratios. Within 6 weeks of therapy, about 5% of men develop bilateral gynecomastia, which may persist until therapy is discontinued. There is some information to indicate that at higher dosage (600 mg/d) itraconazole causes endocrinologic toxicities that

are presumably due to the accumulation of steroid precursors with aldosterone-like effects. These adverse effects have been manifested as hypokalemia and hypertension. Patients also have rarely developed hypokalemia, presumably related to fluconazole administration.

A wide variety of side effects have been reported with miconazole. In 30% to 35% of patients, it causes local phlebitis, which can be reduced by using a central venous catheter. About 20% to 35% of patients complain of pruritus, but only 10% develop a rash. In some cases the pruritus may be sufficiently intense to require discontinuation of therapy. Nausea occurs in 20% to 45% of patients, but vomiting occurs in less than 10%. Fever and chills have been observed in 10% of patients. Miconazole causes rouleau formation of erythrocytes, which probably is clinically unimportant. About 45% of patients develop a transient normocytic or microcytic anemia; as many as 30% develop thrombocytosis, although thrombocytopenia also has been reported.

Hyponatremia may occur in up to 45% of patients. Hyperlipidemia and increased serum triglycerides with or without elevated serum cholesterol occur during therapy. These side effects do not appear to be dose related and resolve when the drug is discontinued. Transient tachycardia, cardiac arrhythmias, anaphylaxis, cardiac arrest, and respiratory arrest occasionally have occurred. These side effects have been attributed to the use of overly concentrated preparations or overly rapid infusions of drug; hence, the drug must be given cautiously. Some side effects, such as pruritus, hyperlipidemia, and cardiopulmonary arrest may be due to Cremophor EL rather than to miconazole.

Table 11-4. Drug–Drug Interactions With Ketoconazole

Effector drug	Drug affected	Effect
Rifampin	Ketoconazole	Reduces serum concentrations
Isoniazid	Ketoconazole	Additive effect on rifampin reduction of serum concentrations
Ketoconazole	Coumarin	Enhances anticoagulation
Ketoconazole	Cyclosporine	Increases serum concentrations and serum creatinine concentrations
Ketoconazole	Phenytoin	Increases serum concentrations; can affect both drugs
Ketoconazole	Theophylline	Decreases serum concentrations
Ketoconazole	Oral antidiabetic agents	May cause hypoglycemia
Ketoconazole	Terfenadine	Increases serum concentrations; rarely causes fatal arrhythmias
Ketoconazole	Astemizole	Increases serum concentrations; rarely causes fatal arrhythmias

REFERENCES

1. Lin C, Symchowicz S: Absorption, distribution, metabolism, and excretion of griseofulvin in man and animals. *Drug Metab Reb* 1975, 4:75–94.

2. Author ?: Nystatin. In *The Use of Antibiotics: A Comprehensive Review With Clinical Emphasis*, edn 4. Edited by Kucers A, Bennett N. Philadelphia: JB Lippincott; 1987:1478–1480.

3. Atkinson AJ Jr, Bennett JE: Amphotericin B pharmacokinetic in humans. *Antimicrob Agents Chemother* 1985, 13:371–376.

4. Utz JP: Chemotherapy of the systemic mycoses. *Med Clin North Am* 1986, 66:221–230.

5. Clements JS Jr, Peacock JE Jr: Amphotericin B revisited: Reassessment of toxicity. *Am J Med* 1990, 88:5-22N–5-27N.

6. Cutler RE, Blair AD, Kelly MR: Flucytosine kinetics in subjects with normal and impaired renal function. *Clin Pharmacol Ther* 1978, 24:333–342.

7. Stamm AM, Diasio RB, Dismukes WE, *et al.*: Toxicity of amphotericin B plus flucytosine in 194 patients with cryptococcal meningitis. *Am J Med* 1987, 83:236–242.

8. Van den Bossche H, Willemsens G, Cools W, Lauwers WFJ, Le Jeune L: Biochemical effects of miconazole on fungi. II. Inhibitions of ergosterol

biosynthesis in *Candida albicans. Chem Bio Interact* 1978, 21:59–78.

9. Bodey GP: Azole antifungal agents. *Clin Inf Dis* 14(Suppl 1):S161–169.

10. Bodey GP: Topical and systemic antifungal agents. In *Update on Antibiotics II. Medical Clinics of North America*. Edited by Neu H. Philadelphia: WB Saunders; 1988:637–659.

11. Brammer KW, Farrow PF, Faulkner JK: Pharmacokinetics and tissue penetration of fluconazole in humans. *Rev Infect Dis* 1990, 12(Suppl 3):S318–326.

12. Grant SM, Clissold SP: Itraconazole: A review of its pharmacodynamic and pharmacokinetic properties, and therapeutic use in superficial and systemic mycoses. *Drugs* 1989, 37:310–344.

13. Rex JH, Bennett JE, Sugar AM, *et al.*: A randomized trial comparing fluconazole with amphotericin B for treatment of candidemia in patients without neutropenia. *N Engl J Med* 1994, 331:1325–1130.

14. Dismukes WE, Bradsher RW, Cloud GC, *et al.*: Itraconazole therapy for blastomycosis and histoplasmosis. *Am J Med* 1992, 93:489–497.

15. Denning DW, Tucker RM, Hanson LH, Stevens DA: Treatment of invasive aspergillosis with itraconazole. *Am J Med* 1989, 86:791–800.

The information here is provided as guidance only. Prescribers should always consult the manufacturer's current prescribing information.

AMPHOTERICIN B (Fungizone®)

Amphotericin B is a polene antibiotic produced by a strain of *Streptomyces nodosus*. The drug is considered to be a fungicidal agent, based on *in vitro* studies. It should be used primarily for patients with progressive, potentially fatal fungal infections; it should not be used to treat common, clinically inapparent types of fungal disease showing only positive skin or serologic tests.

ANTIMICROBIAL ACTIVITY

INTRAVENOUS: Active against *Histoplasma capsulatum*, *Coccidioides immitis*, *Candida* spp, *Blastomyces dermatitidis*, *Rhodotorula* spp, *Cryptococcus neoformans*, *Sporothrix schenckii*, *Mucor* spp, *Aspergillus* spp. No activity against bacteria, rickettsiae, or viruses.
TOPICAL: May be used for treating candida infections.

SPECIAL PRECAUTIONS

INTRAVENOUS: Balance possible lifesaving effect against dangerous adverse effects when using amphotericin B, considering it is the only effective treatment for many potentially fatal fungal diseases.
Nephrotoxic effect is a limiting factor for use; some permanent impairment often occurs, especially with large doses (> 5 g). Dysfunction usually improves with interruption of therapy, dose reduction, or prolonged dosage intervals; sodium loading may help reduce nephrotoxicity in sodium-depleted patients but may also be a problem in patients with cardiac or hepatic disease. Note that decreased glomerular filtration rate and renal blood flow, increased serum creatinine and renal tubular dysfunction are important side effects.
Prolonged therapy is most often necessary, adverse reactions are common, and some reactions are potentially dangerous. Use only in patients who are hospitalized or who are under close medical supervision. Use only in patients for whom a diagnosis of progressive, potentially fatal types of mycotic infection has been clinically established, preferably by positive culture or histologic study. It is an accepted practice to administer empirically to neutropenic patients with prolonged fever (3–7 days) that is of undetermined origin and fails to respond to broad-spectrum antibacterial antibiotics.
Pulmonary effects such as acute dyspnea, hypoxemia, and interstitial infiltrates have occurred in patients with neutropenia who received amphotericin B and leukocyte transfusions. These effects can occur with the therapy alone, but they may be more common when the two therapies are administered concurrently.
This potential problem may be avoided by increasing the time interval between the administration of amphotericin B and leukocyte transfusions.
TOPICAL: For external use only; contact with eyes should be avoided. If hypersensitivity occurs, discontinue use.

INDICATIONS:

INTRAVENOUS: Treatment of cryptococcosis; North American blastomycosis; disseminated forms of candidiasis, coccidioidomycosis, and histoplasmosis; mucormycosis (phycomycosis) due to species of the genera *Mucor*, *Rhizopus*, *Absidia*, *Entomophthora*, and *Basidiobolus*; sporotrichosis (*S. schenckii*); and aspergillosis. May also be useful in the treatment of American mucocutaneous leishmaniasis but is not the drug of choice in primary therapy. (Note: For use in patients with progressive and potentially fatal infections only [*see* Special Precautions].)
TOPICAL: Treatment of cutaneous and mucocutaneous mycotic infection due to *Candida* spp

CONTRAINDICATIONS

INTRAVENOUS: Hypersensitivity to amphotericin B, except in cases where condition requiring treatment is life-threatening and amenable only to amphotericin B
TOPICAL: Hypersensitivity to any of the preparation components

INTERACTIONS

INTRAVENOUS: Corticosteroids, cyclosporine
Due to its hypokalemic effect, amphotericin B may potentiate the effects of *digitalis glycosides* and *neuromuscular blocking agents*; however, drug interactions have not been documented

ADVERSE EFFECTS

INTRAVENOUS: General toxic reactions: fever (with or without shaking, chills), headache, anorexia, malaise, generalized pain (including muscle and joint)
Gastrointestinal: nausea, vomiting, dyspepsia, diarrhea, cramping, epigastric pain; rare: melena, hemorrhagic gastroenteritis, acute liver failure
Hematologic: normochromic and normocytic anemia; rare: coagulation defects, thrombocytopenia, leukopenia, agranulocytosis, eosinophilia, leukocytosis
Local: venous pain at injection site with phlebitis and thrombophlebitis
Renal: hypokalemia, azotemia, hyposthenuria, nephrocalcinosis, renal tubular acidosis; rare: anuria, oliguria; permanent damage is often related to a large total dose (> 5 g)
Miscellaneous: weight loss; rare: anaphylactoid reactions, flushing, dyspnea
Cardiovascular: rare: arrhythmias, ventricular fibrillation, cardiac arrest, hypertension, hypotension
Dermatologic: maculopapular rash, pruritus (without rash)
Special senses: hearing loss, tinnitus, transient vertigo, blurred vision, diplopia
(Note: Most patients demonstrate some tolerance, usually at less than full therapeutic dosages. Administration of aspirin, antipyretics [*eg*, acetaminophen], antihistamines, and antiemetics before infusion and maintenance of sodium balance may lessen severity of reactions. Anorexia and phlebitis may be diminished by administering on alternate days. Febrile reactions may be decreased by giving small doses of intravenous adrenal corticosteroids just prior to infusion [keep dosage and duration of corticosteroids to a minimum].

(Continued on next page)

The information here is provided as guidance only. Prescribers should always consult the manufacturer's current prescribing information.

SPECIAL GROUPS

INTRAVENOUS:

Children: Safety and efficacy not established; however, systemic fungal infections have been treated without reports of usual side effects. Use lowest possible dose.

Elderly: May have age-related renal impairment.

Renal impairment: Use with extreme caution.

Hepatic impairment: No information.

Pregnancy: Use only when clearly indicated; adequate human studies not performed.

Breast-feeding: Not known whether excreted; consider discontinuing nursing or eliminating intravenous amphotericin B.

DOSAGE

INTRAVENOUS:

Adults: A test dose of 1 mg in 20 mL of dextrose solution 5% should be given over a 20- to 30-minute period and temperature, pulse, respirations, and blood pressure should be monitored. If the test dose is tolerated, an initial therapeutic dose should be given the same day. For serious infections, the initial dose should be 0.25 to 0.3 mg/kg, with gradual escalation to maximum intended dose within 2 to 3 days. The maximum tolerated dose seldom exceeds 1 mg/kg/d, although occasional patients may tolerate up to 1.5 mg/kg. Lower doses of 0.3 to 0.6 mg/kg/d may be used for treating some infections, such as candidiasis. Patients developing a serum creatinine level exceeding 2.5 to 3.0 mg/dL should have the drug withheld for several days until the creatinine level stabilizes. Therapy can then be reinstituted at a lower dose or on an every-other-day schedule. It is customary to administer infusions over a 2- to 6-hour period. Rapid infusions (45–60 minutes) may be hazardous in patients with renal impairment. A minimum of several months of therapy is usually necessary; shorter durations may lead to relapse. *Do not exceed total daily dose of 1.5 mg/kg.* For sporotrichosis, usual dose per injection is 20 mg; therapy range is up to 9 months. For aspergillosis, may be treated up to 11 months with total doses of 3.6 g. For rhinocerebral phycomycosis (usually follows a rapidly fatal course; therapy must be more aggressive than that for more indolent mycoses; pulmonary phycomycosis is often an incidental finding at autopsy), diabetic control must be instituted before treatment with amphotericin B can be achieved. A minimum cumulative dose of at least 3 g of amphotericin B is recommended; however, although a total dose of 3 to 4 g will infrequently cause permanent renal impairment, it is reasonable to consider when clinical evidence of deep tissue invasion exists.

Elderly: May have age-related renal impairment requiring extra caution.

Children: No special dosage given (*see* Special Precautions).

Renal Impairment: No special dosage given; use extreme caution (*see* Special Precautions).

TOPICAL: Apply liberally to candidal lesions two to four times a day. Duration of therapy depends on patient response. Intertriginous lesions often respond in several days, and treatment may be complete in 1 to 3 weeks. Candidiasis of the diaper area, perlèche, and glabrous skin lesions usually resolve in 1 to 2 weeks. Interdigital lesions may need 2 to 4 weeks of intensive therapy, and paronychias also may require prolonged therapy. Onychomycoses that respond may need several months of treatment or more. (Note: Relapses are frequent in the latter three conditions.)

ADVERSE EFFECTS *(CONTINUED)*

Intravenous meperidine usually controls the rigors induced by amphotericin B. Dantrolene was successful in three patients for prophylaxis [50 mg orally] and treatment [50 mg intravenous] of amphotericin B–induced rigors. Thrombophlebitis may be lessened by adding a small amount of heparin to infusion [500–2000 units], rapid infusion rate, removal of needle after infusion, rotation of infusion sites, administration through large central vein or distal veins, and use of pediatric scalp–vein needle. Chemical irritation may occur from extravasation.)

TOPICAL: *Cream* may have a drying effect on skin of some patients; local irritation (erythema, pruritus, or burning sensation) may occur, especially in intertriginous areas.

Lotion use has had rare local intolerance, including increased pruritus; allergic contact dermatitis is rare.

Ointment may occasionally cause irritation when applied to moist intertriginous areas.

PHARMACOKINETICS AND PHARMACODYNAMICS

Peak serum levels: *INTRAVENOUS*—0.5–2 µg/mL after initial intravenous infusion of 1 to 5 mg/d, gradually increased to 0.4–0.6 mg/kg/d

Serum half-life: *INTRAVENOUS*—initial phase, 24 h; second phase, 15 d

Bioavailability: *INTRAVENOUS*—no information

Metabolism: metabolic pathways not known

Excretion: *INTRAVENOUS*—cumulative urinary output over 7 days is approximately 40% of drug infused

Renal impairment: use with extreme caution (*see* Special Precautions)

Hepatic impairment: no information

OVERDOSAGE

INTRAVENOUS: Large doses (> 5 g cumulative) can cause permanent renal impairment

PATIENT INFORMATION

INTRAVENOUS: No information

TOPICAL: For external use only. Avoid contact with eyes. Cleanse affected areas prior to application unless otherwise directed.

Liberal application with gentle rubbing distribution recommended.

Cream may cause drying and slight discoloration of skin; lotion or ointment may cause staining of nail lesions (not skin) if thoroughly rubbed in. Itching, redness, or burning may also occur, especially in folds of skin; contact physician if these symptoms become intolerable, if rash develops, or if condition being treated worsens.

Discoloration of fabrics may be removed by hand-washing with soap and warm water for cream or lotion and with standard cleaning fluid for ointment.

AVAILABILITY

Injection—50 mg per vial (with 41 mg sodium desoxycholate) Sterile lyophilized cake (may partially reduce to powder after manufacture)

Cream—3% in 20 g (aqueous vehicle)

Lotion—3% in 30 mL (aqueous vehicle)

Ointment—3% in 20 g (polyethylene and mineral oil gel base with titanium dioxide)

The information here is provided as guidance only. Prescribers should always consult the manufacturer's current prescribing information.

CLOTRIMAZOLE (Lotrimin®, Lotrisone®, Mycelex®)

Clotrimazole is a broad-spectrum antifungal agent available in oral, vaginal, and topical preparations.

ANTIMICROBIAL ACTIVITY

ORAL, VAGINAL TABLETS, and *VAGINAL CREAM*: Fungicidal *in vitro* against *Candida albicans* and other *Candida* spp.
TOPICAL PREPARATIONS (CREAM, SOLUTION, and *LOTION)*: Inhibits growth of pathogenic dermatophytes, yeasts, and *Malassezia furfur*; exhibits fungistatic and fungicidal activity *in vitro* against isolates of *Trichophyton rubrum*, *Trichophyton mentagrophytes*, *Epidermophyton floccosum*, *Microsporum canis*, and *Candida* spp (including *Candida albicans*).
(Note: No resistance [single- or multiple-step] has developed during successive passages of *C. albicans* and *T. mentagrophytes*.)

SPECIAL PRECAUTIONS

ORAL: Not indicated for treatment of systemic mycoses.
Abnormal liver function tests occurred in clinical trials; approximately 15% of patients had minimally elevated levels. Periodic assessment of hepatic function is recommended, especially in patients with preexisting impairment.
TOPICAL PREPARATIONS (CREAM, SOLUTION, and *LOTION)*:
For external use only; avoid contact with eyes.
If irritation or sensitivity occurs, discontinue use and treat appropriately.

SPECIAL GROUPS

Children: *ORAL:* Safety and efficacy not established for children under 3 years of age.
Elderly: No information.
Renal impairment: No information.
Hepatic impairment: *ORAL:* Periodic evaluation of liver function recommended (*see* Special Precautions).
Pregnancy: *ORAL:* Adequate human studies not performed; use only when clearly indicated and when benefits outweigh risks. *TOPICAL PREPARATIONS* (*CREAM, SOLUTION*, and *LOTION):* Adequate human studies not performed; use only if clearly indicated during first trimester.
Breast-feeding: *ORAL*: No information. *TOPICAL PREPARATIONS (CREAM, SOLUTION*, and *LOTION):* Not known whether excreted, use with caution.

DOSAGE

Adult: *ORAL:* Give one troche five times daily for 14 days. Data are limited concerning safety and efficacy following prolonged administration.
VAGINAL TABLETS: Insert one 100-mg tablet intravaginally at bedtime for seven nights or two 100-mg tablets intravaginally for three nights.
VAGINAL CREAM: Use one applicatorful intravaginally per day, preferably at bedtime, for 7 to 14 days. (Note: Patients treated for 14 days had significantly higher cure rates.)
TOPICAL PREPARATIONS (CREAM, SOLUTION, and *LOTION)*:
Massage gently into affected area and surrounding skin two times a day (morning and evening). Improvement usually occurs within 1 week. If no improvement has been demonstrated after 4 weeks, reevaluate condition.
Elderly: No information.
Children: *ORAL:* Use in children under 3 years of age not recommended; no special dosage given.
Renal impairment: No information.

INDICATIONS

ORAL: Treatment of oropharyngeal candidiasis
TOPICAL PREPARATIONS (CREAM, SOLUTION and *LOTION)*: (*Over-the-counter products*) Topical treatment of tinea pedis, tinea cruris, and tinea corporis due to *T. rubrum*, *T. mentagrophytes*, *E. floccosum*, and *M. canis*
(Mycelex® and Lotrimin® prescription) Treatment of candidiasis due to *C. albicans* and tinea versicolor due to *M. furfur*; in addition, Mycelex® is effective for over-the-counter indications

CONTRAINDICATIONS

Allergy or hypersensitivity to clotrimazole or any product component

INTERACTIONS

No information

ADVERSE EFFECTS

ORAL: Nausea, vomiting
Laboratory test abnormalities: Liver function tests; elevated AST levels reported in approximately 15% of patients in clinical trials
TROPICAL PREPARATIONS (CREAM, SOLUTION, and *LOTION)*: Erythema, stinging, blistering, peeling, pruritis, urticaria, burning

PHARMACOKINETICS AND PHARMACODYNAMICS

Very limited absorption; basically a topical agent

OVERDOSAGE

No information

PATIENT INFORMATION

ORAL: Dissolve troche slowly in mouth
VAGINAL TABLETS or *CREAM*: Use at bedtime
TOPICAL PREPARATIONS (CREAM, SOLUTION, and *LOTION)*: For external use only; avoid contact with eyes.
Cleanse affected area before each application unless otherwise directed. Continue medication for full treatment period even if condition resolves; if no improvement occurs within 4 weeks or if irritation occurs contact physician.

AVAILABILITY

Troches—10 mg
Vaginal tablets—100 mg, 500 mg, and 100 mg with lactose
Vaginal cream—1%
Vaginal inserts—100 mg
Vulvar cream—1%
Topical cream—1%
Topical solution—1%
Topical lotion—1%

The information here is provided as guidance only. Prescribers should always consult the manufacturer's current prescribing information.

FLUCONAZOLE (Diflucan®)

Fluconazole is a synthetic, broad-spectrum, *bis*-triazole antifungal agent for oral and intravenous administration.

ANTIMICROBIAL ACTIVITY

Active *in vitro* against *Cryptococcus neoformans* and *Candida* spp. Fungistatic activity has been demonstrated in both normal and immunocompromised animal models for systemic and intracranial fungal infections due to *C. neoformans* and for systemic infections due to *Candida albicans*.

SPECIAL PRECAUTIONS

Liver function test abnormalities developed during therapy indicate need for monitoring of liver function for more severe hepatic damage. If clinical signs and symptoms of liver disease develop, discontinue fluconazole.

Renal impairment significantly affects pharmacokinetics; an inverse relationship exists between elimination half-life and creatinine clearance. Three-hour hemodialysis session decreases plasma concentrations by approximately 50%. Patients with immunodeficiency who develop rashes should be monitored closely; drug should be discontinued if lesions progress.

Male rats treated with 5 and 10 mg/kg/d had increased incidence of hepatocellular adenomas.

SPECIAL GROUPS

Children: There is limited information on the use of fluconazole in children. The serum concentration in neonates is one half that of adults, but the mean serum half-life is prolonged to 89 hours. The serum half-life is 56 hours at 2 weeks of age and equivalent to adults by 6 to 8 weeks of age. Therapeutic efficacy appears to be comparable to that in adults.

Elderly: May have age-related renal impairment requiring reduced dosage.

Renal impairment: Reduced dosage necessary (*see* Special Precautions).

Hepatic impairment: Monitoring of functions recommended (*see* Special Precautions).

Pregnancy: Adequate human studies not performed; animal studies show possible significant risk to fetus. Use only when clearly indicated and when benefits outweigh risks.

Breast-feeding: Not known whether excreted; use with caution.

DOSAGE

Adults: (Note: Oral absorption is rapid and nearly complete, thus daily dosing is the same for oral and intravenous forms.) Dosage should be individualized; patients with AIDS, cryptococcal meningitis, or recurrent oropharyngeal candidiasis often require maintenance therapy to prevent relapse.

For oropharyngeal candidiasis, 200 mg on 1st day followed by 100 mg once a day for 1 week. Higher doses given for shorter durations have been effective.

For esophageal candidiasis, 200 mg on 1st day followed by 100 mg once a day for at least 2 weeks after symptoms have cleared. Doses up to 400 mg/d may be used based on patient response.

Fluconazole recently has been approved for the treatment of vaginal candidiasis with a single dose of 150–200 mg orally.

For systemic candidiasis, 400 mg on 1st day followed by 200–400 mg once a day for a minimum of 2 weeks, and for at least 2 weeks after symptoms have cleared.

For cryptococcal meningitis, 400 mg on 1st day followed by 200 mg once a day for 10 to 12 weeks after cerebrospinal fluid is culture-negative. Higher doses (up to 800 mg/d) may be more effective. Patients with AIDS require 200 mg once a day for suppression of relapse.

(Continued on next page)

INDICATIONS

Treatment of oropharyngeal and esophageal candidiasis and for serious systemic candidal infections, including urinary tract infection, peritonitis, and pneumonia. Also used for treatment of cryptococcal meningitis when causative organisms are confirmed by serology or histopathology prior to therapy; treatment may be initiated before results are confirmed, and dosage should be adjusted accordingly as necessary. Limited information suggests that fluconazole may be useful for management of serious coccidioidal infection and trichosporonosis. It appears to be less effective than itraconazole for the treatment of histoplasmosis in patients with AIDS.

CONTRAINDICATIONS

Allergy or hypersensitivity to fluconazole or product components (Note: Data regarding cross-sensitivity among other azole antifungal drugs are not available.)

INTERACTIONS

Cimetidine, cyclosporine, hydrochlorothiazide, oral contraceptives, phenytoin, rifampin, sulfonylureas, and warfarin

ADVERSE EFFECTS

(Note: In combined clinical trials, patients with underlying serious disease such as AIDS or malignancy rarely developed severe hepatic reactions or exfoliative skin disorders. Two hepatic reactions and one skin reaction were associated with fatalities. Because many factors were present, causal association with fluconazole is uncertain. Clinical adverse effects were more frequent in patients with HIV; however, patterns were similar to that of other patients.)

Nausea, headache, skin rash, vomiting, abdominal pain, and diarrhea

Laboratory test abnormalities: significant increase in AST levels in patients with serious underlying disease (incidence was greater in patients undergoing concomitant therapy with rifampin, phenytoin, isoniazid, valproic acid, and oral sulfonylurea hypoglycemic drugs)

PHARMACOKINETICS AND PHARMACODYNAMICS

Peak serum levels: 6.72 µg/mL between 1 to 2 h after single 400-mg oral dose

Serum half-life: 30 h

Bioavailability: oral, > 90% compared with intravenous administration

Protein binding: 11% to 12%

Metabolism: 11% of excreted dose as metabolites

Excretion: primarily renal; approximately 80% of dose unchanged in urine

Renal impairment: significantly affects pharmacokinetics; inverse relationship between elimination half-life and creatinine clearance

Hepatic impairment: close monitoring of function recommended

The information here is provided as guidance only. Prescribers should always consult the manufacturer's current prescribing information.

FLUCONAZOLE (CONTINUED)

DOSAGE (CONTINUED)

Elderly: May have age-related renal impairment; otherwise, same as adults.
Children: Neonates (< 2 weeks of age): 3 to 12 mg/kg every 72 hours.
Neonates (2–4 weeks of age): 3 to 12 mg/kg every 48 hours.
Older infants: 3 to 12 mg/kg every day.
Dosage depends on severity of infection.
Renal impairment: Give initial loading dose of 50 to 400 mg. Subsequent daily dose should be based on the following guidelines:

Dosage of Fluconazole Related to Renal Function

Creatinine clearance, mL/min	Normal dosage recommended, %
> 50	100
21–50	50
11–20	25
Patients on regular hemodialysis	One normal dose after each dialysis

OVERDOSAGE

In animal studies, symptoms included decreased motility and respiration, ptosis, lacrimation, salivation, urinary incontinence, loss of righting reflex, cyanosis, and death—sometimes preceded by clonic convulsions
Treatment should be symptomatic and supportive, including gastric lavage if clinically indicated

PATIENT INFORMATION

No information

AVAILABILITY

Tablets—50 mg, 100 mg, and 200 mg
Injection—200 mg/100 mL in 100 mL vials and 400 mg/200 mL in 200 mL vials

FLUCYTOSINE (5-FC OR 5-FLUOROCYTOSINE) (Ancobon®)

Flucytosine is rarely used alone; it is usually used in combination with amphotericin B (*see* Interactions).

ANTIMICROBIAL ACTIVITY

Active *in vitro* and *in vivo* against *Candida* and *Cryptococcus*.

SPECIAL PRECAUTIONS

Determine status of renal and hepatic function, hematology, and electrolytes. Close monitoring of renal, hematologic, and hepatic status of all patients is absolutely necessary during therapy. If blood urea nitrogen or serum creatinine is elevated, or if other signs of renal impairment exist, reduce dosage. Renal impairment: use extreme caution.
Bone marrow depression: use caution; patients who may be at greater risk for bone marrow depression include those with hematologic disease, those undergoing radiation or marrow-suppressant drug therapy, or those with a history of radiation or treatment with such drugs.

SPECIAL GROUPS

Children: Safety and efficacy not established.
Elderly: May have age-related renal impairment (*see* Special Precautions).
Renal impairment: Use extreme caution.
Hepatic impairment: Monitor function closely.
Pregnancy: Adequate human studies not performed; use only when benefits outweigh risks.
Breast-feeding: Not known whether excreted; however, due to potential for serious adverse effects, decision to discontinue therapy or discontinue nursing must be made.

INDICATIONS

Treatment of severe infections due to susceptible strains of *Candida* (septicemia, endocarditis, urinary tract infection) or *Cryptococcus* (meningitis, pulmonary infection; good response also occurred in septicemias and urinary tract infections)
May be used for treatment of chromocycosis

CONTRAINDICATIONS

Allergy or hypersensitivity to flucytosine

INTERACTIONS

Amphotericin B (may increase therapeutic action and toxicity of flucytosine) and cytosine
Laboratory test interactions: interferes with creatinine value determinations by the dry-slide enzymatic method (Jaffé method is recommended)

ADVERSE EFFECTS

Central nervous system: ataxia, hearing loss, headache, paresthesia, parkinsonism, peripheral neuropathy, pyrexia, vertigo, sedation, confusion, hallucinations, psychosis
Dermatologic: rash, pruritus, urticaria, photosensitivity
Genitourinary: azotemia, creatinine and blood urea nitrogen elevation, crystalluria, renal failure
Gastrointestinal: nausea, emesis, abdominal pain, diarrhea, anorexia, dry mouth, duodenal ulcer, gastrointestinal hemorrhage, hepatic dysfunction, jaundice, ulcerative colitis, bilirubin elevation, elevation of hepatic enzymes
Hematologic: anemia (occasionally aplastic), agranulocytosis, eosinophilia, leukopenia, pancytopenia, thrombocytopenia
Respiratory: respiratory arrest, chest pain, dyspnea
Miscellaneous: cardiac arrest, fatigue, hypoglycemia, hypokalemia, weakness

PHARMACOKINETICS AND PHARMACODYNAMICS

Peak serum levels: within 2 h
Serum half-life: 2 to 5 h with normal renal function

(Continued on next page)

The information here is provided as guidance only. Prescribers should always consult the manufacturer's current prescribing information.

FLUCYTOSINE (5-FC OR 5-FLUOROCYTOSINE) (CONTINUED)

DOSAGE

Adults: 50 to 150 mg/kg/d in divided doses at 6-hour intervals. Capsules should be taken a few at a time over a period of 15 minutes to reduce nausea and vomiting.
Elderly: May have age-related renal impairment; otherwise, same as adults.
Children: Safety and efficacy not established.
Renal impairment: Dose at lower levels (*see* Special Precautions).

PHARMACOKINETICS AND PHARMACODYNAMICS *(CONTINUED)*

Bioavailability: no percentage given; well absorbed and well distributed after oral administration, cerebrospinal fluid concentrations approximate 65% to 90% of serum levels
Protein binding: no information
Metabolism: no information
Excretion: 80% to 90% excreted unchanged in urine by glomerular filtration
Renal impairment: half-life significantly increases
Hepatic impairment: no information

OVERDOSAGE

No experience with overdose. Pronounced manifestations of known clinical adverse effects would be expected. Prolonged serum concentrations exceeding 100 µg/mL may be associated with greater incidence of toxicity, especially gastrointestinal, hematologic, and hepatic. Treatment would include immediate gastric lavage or emesis. Adequate fluid intake should be maintained, by intravenous administration if necessary. Hematologic, renal, and hepatic function should be closely monitored, and therapeutic measures should be taken to treat any abnormalities. Hemodialysis rapidly reduced serum concentrations in anuric patients and should be considered.

PATIENT INFORMATION

Take capsules a few at a time over a period of 15 minutes to reduce gastrointestinal upset; contact physician if these effects become intolerable

AVAILABILITY

Capsules—250 mg and 500 mg

GRISEOFULVIN (Fulvicin®, Grifulvin V®, Gris-PEG®, Grisactin®)

Griseofulvin is an antibiotic derived from a species of *Penicillium*. Available for oral administration in regular and ultramicrosize forms. The ultramicrosize form has a gastrointestinal absorption efficiency approximately 1.5 times that of conventional microsized griseofulvin, permitting the oral ingestion of two thirds as much drug per dose; however, clinical evidence does not exist to suggest that this has any advantage in regard to safety or efficacy.

ANTIMICROBIAL ACTIVITY

Active (fungistatic) *in vitro* against species of *Microsporum*, *Epidermophyton*, and *Trichophyton*. Griseofulvin has no effect on bacteria or other fungi.

SPECIAL PRECAUTIONS

Safety and efficacy not established for use as prophylaxis of fungal infections. Hypersensitivity reactions may occur and sometimes require withdrawal of therapy. Chronic use in mice at levels ranging from 0.5% to 2.5% of daily diet resulted in increased incidence of liver tumors; thyroid tumors manifested in male rats receiving levels of 2%, 1%, and 0.2% of daily diet.
Prolonged therapy requires close observation and periodic monitoring of renal, hepatic, and hematopoietic function. *(Continued on next page)*

INDICATIONS

Treatment of ringworm infection of skin, hair, and nails; particularly tinea corporis, tinea pedis, tinea cruris, tinea barbae, tinea capitis, and tinea unguium (onychomycosis) when due to one or more of the following fungi: *Trichophyton rubrum, Trichophyton tonsurans, Trichophyton mentagrophytes, Trichophyton interdigitalis, Trichophyton verrucosum, Trichophyton mengnini, Trichophyton gallinae, Trichophyton crateriform, Trichophyton sulphureum, Trichophyton schoenleini, Microsporum audouini, Microsporum canis, Microsporum gypseum,* and *Epidermophyton floccosum*

CONTRAINDICATIONS

Allergy or hypersensitivity to griseofulvin, porphyria, hepatocellular failure

INTERACTIONS

Anticoagulants, barbiturates, oral contraceptives

The information here is provided as guidance only. Prescribers should always consult the manufacturer's current prescribing information.

GRISEOFULVIN (CONTINUED)

SPECIAL PRECAUTIONS (CONTINUED)

Possible cross-sensitivity with penicillin may exist; however, known penicillin-sensitive patients have been treated effectively and without difficulty.
Lupus erythematosus–like syndromes or exacerbation of lupus has occurred.
Photosensitivity may occur; advise patients to take protective measures and to avoid prolonged exposure.

SPECIAL GROUPS

Children: Safe for use. (Dosage not established for those 2 years of age and younger.)
Elderly: No special information given.
Renal impairment: Monitor function periodically.
Hepatic impairment: Monitor function periodically (*see* Special Precautions); contraindicated in hepatocellular failure.
Pregnancy: Do not use in pregnant women or in women who are contemplating pregnancy.
Breast-feeding: No information.

DOSAGE

(Note: Confirmed, accurate diagnosis of causative organism is essential. Therapy should be continued until complete eradication of organism is demonstrated by clinical or laboratory examinations [general treatment periods are 4–6 weeks for tinea capitis; 2–4 weeks for tinea corporis; 4–8 weeks for tinea pedis; and 4 months (fingernails) and 6 months (toenails) for tinea unguium, depending on rate of growth]. Good hygiene should be observed to control sources of infection or rein-fection, and concomitant use of appropriate topical agents is usually necessary, especially in tinea pedis. In some forms of athlete's foot, yeasts and bacteria may be involved in addition to fungi; griseofulvin will not eradicate bacterial or candidal infection.)
Adults: For tinea corporis, tinea cruris, and tinea capitis: give single or divided daily dose of 500 mg microsize (330–375 mg ultramicrosize).
For tinea pedis and tinea unguium, five 0.75–1 g microsize (660–750 mg ultrami-crosize) per day in divided doses.
Elderly: Same as adults.
Children: (Note: Dosage not established for children 2 years of age or younger.)
Give 11 mg microsize per kg per day or 7.3 mg ultramicrosize per kg per day. The following guidelines are suggested:

Griseofulvin Dosage in Children

Weight, *lb*	Weight, *kg*	Daily dose, *mg*	
		Microsize	Ultramicrosize
30–50	13.6–23	125–250	82.5–165
> 50	> 23	250–500	165–330

Renal impairment: No special dosage given.

ADVERSE EFFECTS

Hypersensitivity: skin rash, urticaria, angioneurotic edema (rare)
Gastrointestinal: oral thrush, nausea, vomiting, diarrhea, epigastric distress
Miscellaneous: headache, fatigue, dizziness, insomnia, mental confusion, impaired performance of routine activities; rare: interference with porphyrin metabo-lism, proteinuria, leukopenia, hepatic toxicity, gastrointestinal bleeding, menstrual irregularities, paresthesias of hands and feet (after prolonged therapy)
(Note: If granulocytopenia occurs, discontinue use. Serious reactions are usually associated with high doses or longer periods of therapy.)

PHARMACOKINETICS AND PHARMACODYNAMICS

Peak serum levels: 0.5 to 2 μg/mL approximately 4 h after 0.5 g microsize; serum levels may be increased in patients with impaired absorption by administering with a high-fat meal
Serum half-life: no information
Bioavailability: no information
Protein binding: no information
Metabolism: no information
Excretion: no information
Renal impairment: monitor function periodically
Hepatic impairment: contraindicated in hepatocellular failure

OVERDOSAGE

No information

PATIENT INFORMATION

Continue medication for entire course of therapy; positive effects may not be noticed for some time.
Avoid prolonged exposure to sunlight or ultraviolet light; wear protective clothing and sunscreen.
If fever, sore throat, or skin rash occurs, contact physician immediately.
Oral suspension should be stored in a light-resistant container.

AVAILABILITY

Tablets (microsize)—250 mg and 500 mg
Capsules (microsize)—125 mg and 250 mg
Oral suspension (microsize)—125 mg/5 mL
Tablets (ultramicrosize)—125 mg, 165 mg, 250 mg, and 330 mg

The information here is provided as guidance only. Prescribers should always consult the manufacturer's current prescribing information.

ITRACONAZOLE (Sporanox®)

Itraconazole is a synthetic triazole antifungal agent for oral administration.

ANTIMICROBIAL ACTIVITY

Active *in vitro* against *Blastomyces dermatitidis*, *Histoplasma capsulatum* and *duboisii*, *Aspergillus flavus* and *fumigatus*, and *Cryptococcus neoformans*. Also demonstrates variable *in vitro* activity against *Sporothrix schenckii*, *Trichophyton* spp, *Candida albicans*, and *Candida* spp.

SPECIAL PRECAUTIONS

Coadministration of terfenadine with itraconazole is contraindicated. Serious cardiovascular effects, including death, ventricular tachycardia, and torsade de pointes, have been documented because of increased terfenadine concentrations induced by itraconazole.

Hepatic toxicity: if signs or symptoms of liver disease or dysfunction develop, discontinue itraconazole.

Patients infected with HIV usually require maintenance therapy to prevent relapse of histoplasmosis. Studies investigating safety and efficacy of this agent for patients with HIV are ongoing. Additionally, because hypochlorhydria has occurred in these patients, absorption of itraconazole may be decreased.

In trials with male rats given 3.1 times the maximum recommended human dose of itraconazole, the rats had a slightly higher incidence of soft-tissue sarcoma; female rats treated with 6.25 times the maximum human dose had increased incidence of squamous cell carcinoma of the lung. Preexisting hepatic impairment warrants monitoring of hepatic enzyme test values.

SPECIAL GROUPS

Children: Safety and efficacy are not established; however, a small group of patients aged 3 to 16 years have been treated with 100 mg/d with no serious adverse effects.

Elderly: No information.

Renal impairment: No information.

Hepatic impairment: Monitor hepatic enzyme test values.

Pregnancy: Pregnancy category C. Possible significant risk to fetus has been demonstrated in animal studies; use only if benefits outweigh risks.

Breast-feeding: Excreted in breast milk; do not use in a patient who is nursing.

DOSAGE

Adults: (Note: Take with full meal for maximal absorption.) Recommended dose is 200 mg once a day; if no improvement occurs or fungal disease progresses, increase dose in 100-mg increments to a maximum of 400 mg/d (doses > 200 mg should be given in two divided doses).

For life-threatening conditions, give loading dose of 200 mg three times a day (600 mg/d) for the first 3 days. Continue treatment for minimum of 3 months and until clinical evidence and laboratory tests indicate that fungal infection has subsided; treatment periods that are too short may result in recurrence of active infection.

Elderly: No information.

Children: Dosage not established.

Renal impairment: No information.

INDICATIONS

Itraconazole has been approved for the management of blastomycosis (pulmonary and extrapulmonary) and histoplasmosis (including chronic cavitary pulmonary disease and disseminated nonmeningeal histoplasmosis). Published studies indicate that it is effective for the management of aspergillosis, paracoccidioidomycosis, and coccidioidomycosis. It may also be useful for therapy of sporotrichosis, chromomycosis, and cutaneous leishmaniasis. Although candida infections have been treated successfully with itraconazole, its efficacy compared with that of amphotericin B and fluconazole has not been established. Dosage is usually 100 to 400 mg/d and duration of therapy varies depending on causative organism, severity, and promptness of response. Dosage is usually 50 to 400 mg/d and duration of therapy varies from 1 day to over 6 months, depending on condition and mycological response.

CONTRAINDICATIONS

Coadministration of terfenamide (*see* Special Precautions)
Allergy or hypersensitivity to itraconazole or other azole agents
Astemizole, cisapride, and oral triazolam

INTERACTIONS

Cyclosporine, digoxin, H_2 antagonists, isoniazid, phenytoin, rifampin, oral hypoglycemics, terfenadine, warfarin, astemizole, tacrolimus, cisapride, lovastatin, simvastatin, quindine, dihydropyridine calcium channel blockers

ADVERSE EFFECTS

Central nervous system: headache, dizziness, insomnia
Dermatologic: rash (more frequent in patients being treated concomitantly for immunodeficiency), pruritus
Gastrointestinal: nausea, vomiting, diarrhea, abdominal pain, anorexia, flatulence
Psychiatric: decreased libido, somnolence, depression
Systemic: edema, fatigue, fever, malaise
Miscellaneous: hypertension, abnormal hepatic function, hypokalemia, albuminuria, impotence, tinnitus, adrenal insufficiency, gynecomastia, breast pain (male)

PHARMACOKINETICS AND PHARMACODYNAMICS

Peak serum levels: 239 ng/mL (after 200-mg single dose); 2282 ng/mL (200 mg daily at steady-state); absorption may be variable and depends on gastric acidity, hence, serum concentration may be reduced in patients who have fasted and those taking antacids or H_2 blockers
Serum half-life: 21 h (after 200-mg single dose); 64 h (200 mg daily at steady-state)
Bioavailability: 55%
Protein binding: 99.8%
Metabolism: by liver, extensive, to large number of metabolites including hydroxyitraconazole, the major metabolite
Excretion: fecal excretion of parent drug between 3% to 18%; renal, < 0.03%
Renal impairment: no information
Hepatic impairment: monitor hepatic enzyme values (*see* Special Precautions)

OVERDOSAGE

Not removable by dialysis. Employ supportive measures, including gastric lavage with sodium bicarbonate.

PATIENT INFORMATION

Take medication with a full meal; contact physician if symptoms or signs of liver dysfunction occur, such as unusual fatigue, anorexia, nausea, vomiting, jaundice, dark urine, or pale stool

AVAILABILITY

Capsules—100 mg

The information here is provided as guidance only. Prescribers should always consult the manufacturer's current prescribing information.

KETOCONAZOLE (Nizoral®)

Ketoconazole is an imidazole, broad-spectrum, antifungal agent for oral and topical administration.

ANTIMICROBIAL ACTIVITY

ORAL: Active against *Blastomyces dermatitidis*, *Candida* spp, *Coccidioides immitis*, *Histoplasma capsulatum*, *Paracoccidiodes brasiliensis*, *Phialophora* spp, *Trichophyton* spp, *Epidermophyton* spp, and *Microsporum* spp. Activity has been demonstrated in animal models against *Malassezia furfur* and *Cryptococcus neoformans*.
TOPICAL: Inhibits growth of the following dermatophytes and yeast by altering permeability of cell membranes: *Trichophyton rubrum*, *Trichophyton mentagrophytes*, *Trichophyton tonsurans*, *Microsporum canis*, *Microsporum audouini*, *Microsporum gypseum*, *Epidermophyton floccosum*, *Candida albicans*, *Candida tropicalis*, *Phialophora ovale (Malassezia ovale)*, and *Phialophora orbiculare (Malassezia furfur)*.

SPECIAL PRECAUTIONS

ORAL: Hepatic toxicity (primarily hepatocellular), including some fatalities, has been associated with ketoconazole. Monitor liver function carefully during therapy and advise patients of the risk.
High doses of ketoconazole are known to suppress adrenal corticosteroid secretion. In clinical trials with 350 patients with metastatic prostatic cancer, 11 fatalities were reported within 2 weeks of beginning high-dose ketoconazole (1200 mg/d); it is unknown whether deaths were related to therapy.
Hypersensitivity reactions have been reported; anaphylaxis occurs rarely after the first dose; have epinephrine 1:1000 readily available.
Serum testosterone levels are lowered by ketoconazole (impaired with doses of 800 mg/d and abolished by doses of 1600 mg/d); levels return to baseline values once therapy is discontinued. Follow recommended dosage guidelines.
Gastric acidity is necessary for ketoconazole dissolution and absorption. If patient requires antacids, anticholinergics, or H_2 blockers, administer at least 2 hours after ketoconazole. In achlorhydria, dissolve each tablet in 2 mL aqueous solution of 0.2 M HCl; use straw to prevent contact with teeth and follow with a glass of water.
TOPICAL: For external use only; contact with eyes is to be avoided.
If sensitivity or chemical irritation occurs, discontinue use.
Cream preparation contains sulfites that may cause allergic-type reactions in some patients, including anaphylactic symptoms and life-threatening asthmatic episodes.

SPECIAL GROUPS

Children: *ORAL*: Do not use in pediatric patients unless benefits clearly outweigh risk. Safety not established for use in children under 2 years of age.
TOPICAL: Safety and efficacy not established.
Elderly: No information.
Renal impairment: No information.
Hepatic impairment: *ORAL*: Use extreme caution (*see* Special Precautions).
Pregnancy: *ORAL* and *TOPICAL*: Pregnancy category C. Adequate human studies not performed; animal studies suggest possible risk to fetus. Use only if benefits outweigh risk.
Breast-feeding: *ORAL*: Mothers being treated with ketoconazole should not nurse. *TOPICAL*: Safety not established; use caution.

INDICATIONS

ORAL: Treatment of systemic infections of the following types: candidiasis, chronic mucocutaneous candidiasis, oral thrush, blastomycosis, coccidioidomycosis, histoplasmosis, chromomycosis, and paracoccidioidomycosis. Also used to treat severe recalcitrant cutaneous dermatophyte infections unresponsive to topical therapy or to oral griseofulvin or in patients unable to take griseofulvin.
(Unlabeled:) Treatment of onychomycosis due to *Trichophyton* spp and *Candida* spp; pityriasis versicolor (tinea versicolor); tinea pedis, corporis, and cruris (200–400 mg/d); tinea capitis (3.3–6.6 mg/kg/d); and vaginal candidiasis
Alternative therapy for prostate cancer with doses of 400 mg every 8 hours (*see* Special Precautions)
Treatment of Cushing's syndrome with 800 to 1200 mg/d
TOPICAL CREAM: Tinea corporis, tinea cruris, and tinea pedis due to *T. rubrum*, *T. mentagrophytes*, and *E. floccosum*; tinea (pityriasis) versicolor due to *P. orbiculare* (*M. furfur*); cutaneous candidiasis due to *Candida* spp; and seborrheic dermatitis
TOPICAL SHAMPOO: Reduction of scaling due to dandruff

CONTRAINDICATIONS

Allergy or hypersensitivity to ketoconazole
Terfenadine, astemizole, and cisapride

INTERACTIONS

ORAL: Antacids, anticoagulants (oral), antihistamines (astemizole, terfenadine), corticosteroids, cyclosporine, histamine H_2 antagonists, isoniazid, rifampin, theophyllines, phenytoin, oral hypoglycemics, lorafadine, and methylprednisolone

ADVERSE EFFECTS

ORAL: *Central nervous system*: headache, dizziness, somnolence, photophobia (rare)
Gastrointestinal: nausea or vomiting, abdominal pain, diarrhea, hepatoxicity
Neuropsychiatric: suicidal tendencies, severe depression (rare)
Other: pruritus, fever, chills, impotence, gynecomastia, thrombocytopenia, leukopenia, hemolytic anemia, bulging fontanelles (rare), hypersensitivity including urticaria (*see* Special Precautions), oligospermia (at dosages higher than recommended)
TOPICAL CREAM: Severe irritation, pruritus, stinging, painful allergic reaction (one patient)
TOPICAL SHAMPOO: Increase in normal hair loss, irritation (rare), abnormal hair texture, scalp pustules, mild dryness of skin, itching, oiliness or dryness of hair and scalp

The information here is provided as guidance only. Prescribers should always consult the manufacturer's current prescribing information.

KETOCONAZOLE (CONTINUED)

DOSAGE

ORAL: (Note: Minimum treatment period for candidiasis is 1 to 2 weeks; for other indicated systemic mycoses, duration is 6 months. Chronic mucocutaneous candidiasis usually requires maintenance therapy. Recalcitrant dermatophyte infections require 4 weeks when glabrous skin is present; palmar and plantar infections respond more slowly, and apparent cures may remanifest after discontinuation of therapy. Inadequate duration of treatment may result in recurrence of active condition.)

Adults: *ORAL*: Give initial dose of 200 mg once a day; if clinical response is poor, or in more serious infections, increase dose to 400 mg once a day.

TOPICAL CREAM: For cutaneous candidiasis, tinea corporis, tinea cruris, and tinea (pityriasis) versicolor, apply to affected area and surrounding areas once a day for a minimum of 2 weeks (6 weeks with tinea pedis). For seborrheic dermatitis, apply to affected area two times a day for 4 weeks or until condition is cleared.

TOPICAL SHAMPOO: After thoroughly moistening hair and scalp with water, apply enough shampoo to produce lather sufficient for hair and scalp. Massage gently over entire scalp for approximately 1 minute and rinse thoroughly with warm water. Repeat and leave shampoo on scalp for an additional 3 minutes, rinse, and dry. Use shampoo twice a week for 4 weeks, with a minimum of 3 days between each shampooing. Thereafter, intermittent use is recommended to maintain control.

Elderly: No information.

Children: *ORAL*: (over 2 years of age) 3.3 to 6.6 mg/kg/d as a single daily dose (not approved).

Renal impairment: No information.

PHARMACOKINETICS AND PHARMACODYNAMICS

Peak serum levels: 3.5 µg/mL in 1 to 2 h after 200-mg oral dose with meal

Serum half-life: 2 h during first 10 h; 8 h thereafter

Bioavailability: no information

Protein binding: 99%, mainly to albumin

Metabolism: in liver, to inactive metabolites

Excretion: enterohepatic; major route of excretion through the bile into the intestinal tract, 13% in urine with 2% to 4% unchanged

Renal impairment: no dosage adjustment necessary

Hepatic impairment: monitor function carefully (*see* Special Precautions)

OVERDOSAGE

ORAL: Use supportive and symptomatic care, including gastric lavage with sodium bicarbonate. Ketoconazole is not dialyzable.

TOPICAL SHAMPOO: If ingested, use supportive measures, including gastric lavage with sodium bicarbonate

PATIENT INFORMATION

ORAL: Take with food to minimize gastrointestinal upset and enhance absorption. Do not take with antacids; if antacids are needed, wait 2 hours to take medication.

Headache, dizziness, and drowsiness may occur; therefore, use caution when driving or performing other activities requiring alertness and coordination

If signs or symptoms of liver dysfunction (unusual fatigue, anorexia, nausea, vomiting, jaundice, dark urine, pale stools), abdominal pain, fever, or diarrhea occur, contact physician

TOPICAL: For external use only; avoid contact with eyes

SHAMPOO: Diminishing of curls from permanently waved hair may occur

AVAILABILITY

Tablets—200 mg

Cream—2% in aqueous vehicle (with sodium sulfite), 15 g, 30 g, and 60 g

Shampoo—2% in aqueous suspension, 120 mL

The information here is provided as guidance only. Prescribers should always consult the manufacturer's current prescribing information.

MICONAZOLE (Monistat®)

Miconazole is an imidazole derivative available in systemic, topical, and vaginal forms. The intravenous preparation contains a cremophor vehicle.

ANTIMICROBIAL ACTIVITY

SYSTEMIC: Active against a broad range of fungi *in vitro*. Clinical efficacy has been demonstrated against *Coccidiodes immitis*, *Candida albicans*, *Cryptococcus neoformans*, *Pseudoallescheria boydii* (*Petriellidium boydii*, *Allescheria boydii*), and *Paracoccidioides brasiliensis*.
TOPICAL PREPARATIONS: Inhibits growth of common dermatophytes *Trichophyton rubrum*, *Trichophyton mentagrophytes*, *Epidermophyton floccosum*, *Cryptococcus albicans*, and the active organism in tinea versicolor, *Malassezia furfur*.

SPECIAL PRECAUTIONS

SYSTEMIC: Cardiorespiratory arrest or anaphylaxis has occurred (possibly due to too rapid administration in some cases); rapid injection of undiluted miconazole may cause transient tachycardia or arrhythmia.
Administer by intravenous infusion only, beginning in the hospital only. Later treatment may be continued under ambulatory conditions with suitable patients and close clinical monitoring.
Monitor hemoglobin, hematocrit, electrolytes, and lipids. Cultures are recommended as *Pseudoallescheria* is difficult to distinguish from *Aspergillus* spp.
Drugs with cremophor-type vehicles (such as PEG 40, castor oil) can cause electrophoretic abnormalities of the lipoprotein; effects are reversible on discontinuation but not an indication for discontinuation of themselves.
TOPICAL PREPARATIONS: For external use only; avoid contact with eyes. If sensitivity or irritation occurs, discontinue use.

SPECIAL GROUPS

Children: Safety for use in children under 1 year of age not extensively studied; however, 21 neonates were reported to be treated with no unanticipated adverse reactions (seven of 11 evaluable patients recovered or improved).
Elderly: No information.
Renal impairment: No information.
Hepatic impairment: No information.
Pregnancy: Adequate studies not performed; use only when benefits outweigh risk.
Breast-feeding: No information.

INDICATIONS

SYSTEMIC: Treatment of the following severe systemic fungal infections: coccidioidomycosis, candidiasis, cryptococcosis, pseudallescheriasis, and paracoccidioidomycosis
(Note: For fungal meningitis or *Candida* urinary bladder infections, intravenous infusion alone is not sufficient. Supplementation with intrathecal administration or bladder irrigation is necessary.)
TOPICAL: Over-the-counter and prescription: Treatment of tinea pedis, tinea cruris, and tinea corporis due to *T. rubrum*, *T. mentagrophytes*, and *E. floccosum*
Prescription only: Cutaneous candidiasis (moniliasis): tinea versicolor

CONTRAINDICATIONS

SYSTEMIC: Allergy or hypersensitivity to miconazole

INTERACTIONS

SYSTEMIC: Amphotericin B, anticoagulants, phenytoin
(Note: Because of its structural similarities with ketoconazole, the possibility of similar drug interactions with miconazole should be considered [*see* ketoconazole profile].)

ADVERSE EFFECTS

SYSTEMIC: *Gastrointestinal*: nausea, vomiting, diarrhea, anorexia
Hematologic: transient decreases in hematocrit, thrombocytopenia, aggregation of erythrocytes or rouleau formation on blood smears
Integumentary: phlebitis at infusion site, pruritus, rash (if severe, discontinuation may be necessary)
Miscellaneous: fever or chills, drowsiness, flushes, transient decreases in serum sodium, anaphylaxis, hyperlipemia (due to vehicle, Cremophor EL [PEG 40, castor oil])

PHARMACOKINETICS AND PHARMACODYNAMICS

Peak serum levels: doses > 9 mg/kg produce levels > 1 µg/mL in most cases
Serum half-life: (terminal elimination) 20 to 25 h
Bioavailability: no percentage given
Protein binding: over 90%
Metabolism: rapid metabolism in liver
Excretion: 14% to 22% in urine, mostly as active metabolites
Renal impairment: does not alter pharmacokinetics
Hepatic impairment: no information

OVERDOSAGE

SYSTEMIC: No information

The information here is provided as guidance only. Prescribers should always consult the manufacturer's current prescribing information.

DOSAGE

Adults: *SYSTEMIC*: The following guidelines are recommended:

Daily Dose of Miconazole for Systemic Fungal Infections

Infection	Total daily dosage range, *mg**	Duration, *wks*
Coccidioidomycosis	1800–3600	3–> 20
Cryptococcosis	1200–2400	3–> 12
Pseudoallescheriasis	600–3000	5–> 20
Candidiasis	600–1800	1–> 20
Paracoccidioidomycosis	200–1200	2–> 16

May be divided over three infusions.
(Note: Courses may need to be repeated due to relapse or reinfection.)

VAGINAL: If using Monistat 3® (Ortho Pharmaceutical, Raritan, NJ), insert one suppository intravaginally once daily at bedtime for 3 days.
If using Monistat 7®, insert one applicatorful of cream or one suppository intravaginally once a day at bedtime for 7 days; repeat course if necessary (after other pathogens have been ruled out).
TOPICAL: If using cream, cover affected areas two times a day, in morning and evening (once daily only for tinea versicolor). (Note: Lotion is preferred in intertriginous areas; when using cream, apply sparingly to avoid maceration.)
If using powder or spray sprinkle liberally over affected area in morning and evening.
Early relief occurs in most patients (within 2–3 days; 2 weeks with tinea versicolor); however, treatment of *Candida*, tinea cruris, and tinea corporis is for 2 weeks and tinea pedis is for 1 month to reduce risk of recurrence. If no improvement after 1 month, reevaluate diagnosis.
Elderly: No information.
Children: *SYSTEMIC*: (under 1 year of age) 15 to 30 mg/kg/d; (1–12 years of age) 20 to 40 mg/kg/d. Do not exceed 15 mg/kg/dose.
Renal impairment: No information.
(Note: *SYSTEMIC*: For doses of 2400 mg/d or less, dilute in at least 200 mL of fluid per amp; diluent of choice is 0.9% sodium chloride for injection, and alternatively, 5% dextrose injection. Use infusion rate of approximately 2 h/amp. For doses over 2400 mg/d, infusion rate and diluent should be chosen according to patient tolerability. For intrathecal administration [20 mg/dose] as an adjunct to intravenous treatment in fungal meningitis, succeeding intrathecal injections may be alternated between lumbar, cervical, and cisternal punctures every 3–7 days. For bladder instillation, use 200 mg diluted solution for *Candida* in the urinary bladder.)

PATIENT INFORMATION

SYSTEMIC: No information
TOPICAL: For external use only
Contact physician if condition worsens or if irritation occurs
Complete full course of therapy, even if symptoms subside; contact physician if no improvement occurs after 2 weeks (*Candida* infections, tinea cruris, and tinea corporis) or 4 weeks (tinea pedis)

AVAILABILITY

Injection—10 mg/mL in 20 mL amps (with PEG 40, castor oil, and parabens)
Vaginal suppositories (3-day)—200 mg
Vaginal suppositories (7-day)—100 mg
Vaginal cream (7-day)—2%
Combination (3-day) suppositories—200 mg and (7-day) cream 2%
Topical cream—2% in 15- and 30-g tubes
Topical powder—2% in 90-g bottle
Topical spray—2% in 105-mL can

The information here is provided as guidance only. Prescribers should always consult the manufacturer's current prescribing information.

NYSTATIN (Mycostatin®)

Nystatin is a polyene antibiotic with antifungal activity; it is available in oral (tablets, suspension, and troches), vaginal, and topical preparations.

ANTIMICROBIAL ACTIVITY

TABLETS, SUSPENSION, and *TROCHES*: Fungistatic and fungicidal *in vitro* against a wide range of yeasts and yeastlike fungi.

SPECIAL PRECAUTIONS

TABLETS: None given for this form.
SUSPENSION and *TROCHES*: None given for this form.
TOPICAL PREPARATIONS: For external use only.
If hypersensitivity irritation occurs, withdraw agent.

SPECIAL GROUPS

Children: *TABLETS, SUSPENSION,* and *TROCHES*: No information.
Elderly: *TABLETS, SUSPENSION,* and *TROCHES*: No information.
Renal impairment: *TABLETS, SUSPENSION,* and *TROCHES*: No information.
Hepatic impairment: *TABLETS, SUSPENSION,* and *TROCHES*: No information.
Pregnancy: *TABLETS*: No adverse effects have been observed in infants born to women treated with nystatin.
SUSPENSION and *TROCHES*: Safety for use not established; use only if clearly indicated.
Breast-feeding: *TABLETS, SUSPENSION,* and *TROCHES*: No information.

DOSAGE

Adults: *ORAL*: 500,000 to 1,000,000 units three times a day; continue for a minimum of 48 hours to prevent relapse.
SUSPENSION: 400,000 to 600,000 units four times a day; placing one-half dose in each side of mouth and retaining as long as possible in mouth before swallowing.
TROCHES: 200,000 to 400,000 units four to five times a day for up to 14 days; do not swallow or chew.
POWDER FOR EXTEMPORANEOUS COMPOUNDING: Add one eighth of a teaspoon (approximately 500,000 units) to one-half cup of water and mix well; continue for minimum of 48 hours after perioral symptoms have cleared and cultures are normal.
(Note: To improve oral retention of nystatin, the drug has been given in form of flavored frozen popsicles.)
VAGINAL TABLETS: One tablet (100,000 units) intravaginally daily for 2 weeks; continue for full course of treatment even though symptoms will subside earlier.
TOPICAL PREPARATIONS: Apply to affected area two to three times a day (or as indicated) until healing is complete. For fungal infection of the feet due to *Candida*, dust powder liberally on feet, shoes, and socks. Cream form is preferred for candidiasis in intertriginous areas; however, moist lesions are best treated with powder.
Elderly: *TABLETS, SUSPENSION,* and *TROCHES*: No information.
Children: *TABLETS*: No information. *SUSPENSION, TROCHES,* and *POWDER*: Same as adults.
SUSPENSION: For infants who are premature or who have low birth weight, limited clinical studies show that 100,000 units four times a day is effective.
Renal impairment: *TABLETS, SUSPENSION,* and *TROCHES*: No information.

INDICATIONS

TABLETS: Treatment of intestinal candidiasis
SUSPENSION and *TROCHES*: Treatment of oral candidiasis
TOPICAL PREPARATIONS: Treatment of cutaneous or mucocutaneous mycotic infection due to *Candida albicans* and other *Candida* spp

CONTRAINDICATIONS

TABLETS, SUSPENSION, and *TROCHES*: Allergy or hypersensitivity to nystatin
TOPICAL PREPARATIONS: Allergy or hypersensitivity to any component (Note: Not for ophthalmic use.)

INTERACTIONS

No information

ADVERSE EFFECTS

TABLETS, SUSPENSION, and *TROCHES*: Nystatin is essentially nontoxic and nonsensitizing and is thus well tolerated by all patient groups, including debilitated infants, even on prolonged administration. Large oral doses have occasionally produced diarrhea, gastrointestinal distress, nausea, and vomiting. However, oral suspension has a taste that makes it unpleasant for some patients.

PHARMACOKINETICS AND PHARMACODYNAMICS

Peak serum levels: sparingly absorbed after oral administration; no detectable blood levels when used within recommended parameters
Serum half-life: no information
Bioavailability: no information
Protein binding: no information
Metabolism: no information
Excretion: majority as unchanged in feces
Renal impairment: no information
Hepatic impairment: no information

OVERDOSAGE

No information

PATIENT INFORMATION

TABLETS: Continue treatment for minimum of 2 days after symptoms have cleared.
SUSPENSION and *TROCHES*: Retain drug in mouth as long as possible. Continue treatment for minimum of 2 days after symptoms have cleared.
TOPICAL PREPARATIONS: For external use only; avoid contact with eyes. Cleanse affected area before each application, unless otherwise directed. Discontinue use and contact physician if irritation occurs.

AVAILABILITY

Tablets—500,000 units
Oral suspension—100,000 units per mL in 5, 60, and 480 mL
Troches—200,000 units
Powder for extemporaneous preparation of oral suspension—50,000,000 units; 100,000,000 units; 1,000,000,000 units; 2,000,000,000 units; and 5,000,000,000 units
Vaginal tablets—100,000 units
Oral/vaginal pack—42 oral tablets (500,000 units) and 14 vaginal tablets (100,000 units)
Topical cream—100,000 units per g in 15- and 30-g tubes
Topical ointment—100,000 units per g in 15- and 30-g tubes
Topical powder—100,000 units per g in talc 15 g

The information here is provided as guidance only. Prescribers should always consult the manufacturer's current prescribing information.

INTRODUCTION

Therapy for human viral infections has evolved slowly over the past 30 years since the original demonstration that idoxuridine was effective treatment of herpes simplex virus (HSV) keratoconjunctivitis. Early development of antiviral chemotherapeutics progressed in parallel with the development of drugs to treat human malignancies. Thus, the initial drugs (idoxuridine and cytosine arabinoside), which were developed as antiviral chemotherapeutics, failed to have selective mechanisms of action that allowed differentiation from host cell functions usually inhibited by antitumor agents. The development of idoxuridine for topical treatment of HSV keratoconjunctivitis provided the first demonstration that human viral diseases were amendable to treatment.

During the 1960s and early 1970s, two other antiviral compounds underwent extensive evaluation for prevention and treatment of human viral diseases. Amantadine, a rigid tricyclic amine, initially, was developed for purposes of prevention of influenza A infections in high-risk elderly patients and, subsequently, the treatment of influenza pneumonia in targeted populations. Although efficacy for amantadine was established, acceptance of this medication for routine prevention of influenza infections was, and is to this day, not uniform among practicing physicians in developed countries. During the late 1960s and 1970s, vidarabine was evaluated for the treatment of human herpes virus infections. The development of vidarabine was a landmark in antiviral chemotherapy. With this medication, it was possible to prove without doubt that patients derived clinical benefit from intravenous therapy for the management of herpes simplex encephalitis, neonatal HSV infections, and varicella-zoster virus (VZV) infections in the immunocompromised host. This medication provided the first demonstration that the parenteral administration of an antiviral drug significantly improved the clinical events of healing.

In the 1980s, medical practitioners had several compounds licensed for the treatment of viral diseases. Among these compounds, acyclovir is the most important. The discovery, evaluation, and impact of acyclovir therapy on human herpes virus infections is unparalleled in the development of not only antiviral drugs but also of other antimicrobial agents. This therapeutic agent provides for selective and specific inhibition of viral replication. It is converted by virus-encoded thymidine kinase to its monophosphate derivative, an event that does not occur to any substantial extent in uninfected cells [1]. Subsequent dephosphorylation and triphosphorylation are catalyzed by cellular enzymes, resulting in acyclovir triphosphate concentrations that are 40 to 100 times higher in HSV-infected cells than in uninfected cells. Acyclovir triphosphate inhibits viral DNA synthesis by competing with deoxyguanosine triphosphate as a substrate for viral DNA polymerase [2]. Because acyclovir triphosphate lacks the 3' hydroxyl group required to elongate the DNA chain, the synthesis of viral DNA is terminated. Viral DNA polymerase is tightly associated with the terminated DNA chain and is functionally inactivated [3]. In addition, the viral polymerase has greater affinity for acyclovir triphosphate than does cellular DNA polymerase, resulting in little incorporation of acyclovir into cellular DNA [4]. These observations have defined the required properties for future antiviral drugs, demanding that new drugs be selective and specific inhibitors of viral replication. As such, safety of therapy is mandatory. Importantly, acyclovir has proved effective as both a therapy for and suppression of reactivation of latent genital HSV infections. Treatment of primary infection does not prevent the establishment of latency.

Ribavirin, a guanosine analogue, was the first drug licensed for the treatment of respiratory syncytial virus (RSV) infections. This compound has a broad spectrum of *in vitro* antiviral activity, including activity against both RNA and DNA viruses. However, because of systemic toxicity following parenteral administration, treatment is usually by aerosol administration. Exceptions to aerosol therapy include measles pneumonia, Lassa fever, and some exotic arboviral diseases.

As the 1980s progressed with the development of the AIDS epidemic (as caused by HIV infection) the first of a series of dideoxynucleoside analogues was licensed, ie, azidothymidine (zidovudine). This drug, as with other dideoxynucleoside analogues, is converted to its triphosphate metabolite, which functions as an inhibitor of HIV reverse transcriptase. Therapy slows disease progression but does not cure AIDS. Importantly, therapy significantly decreases the rate of transmission of infection from HIV-infected women to their offspring.

The 1990s have witnessed the appearance of several new medications for the treatment of viral disease. Didanosine and zalcitabine joined zidovudine as therapeutics for HIV infection. Their mechanism of action is similar to zidovudine; however, neither has replaced zidovudine as the initial treatment of choice. Ganciclovir and foscarnet have been licensed as therapies for cytomegalovirus infections in immunosuppressed patients, particularly those with cytomegalovirus retinitis. Famciclovir (Famvir® for herpes zoster) and D4T (stavudine for HIV infection) recently have been licensed in the United States and Europe.

Compounds that modulate the immune response and therefore have the potential of acting synergistically with antiviral drugs are in clinical trials. Such approaches include the use of hyperimmune globulin and human or humanized monoclonal antibodies. New therapeutics for HIV infection are being evaluated in clinical trials as well. These drugs have different sites or mechanisms of action as compared with the dideoxynucleoside analogues. Such drugs include the nonnucleoside reverse transcriptase inhibitors (*eg*, nevarapine) and numerous protease inhibitors.

A fundamental observation in the development of all antiviral drugs is the development of resistance. Although recognized *in vitro* for some time, it was only in the mid 1980s that clinical resistance was established and associated with progressive disease [5]. These observations were made for acyclovir treatment of HSV infections in patients with AIDS. In the intervening decade, antiviral resistance has been recognized for *all* antiviral drugs; however, for nucleoside analogues, resistance has been limited to the immunocompromised host.

CHEMISTRY

Antiviral agents that have been approved to date are in one of four classes: nucleoside analogues (idoxuridine, ribavirin, vidarabine, acyclovir, ganciclovir, zidovudine, famciclovir, didanosine, zalcitabine, and stavudine), pyrophosphate analogues (foscarnet), tricyclic amines, or interferon. Structural similarities are shared by some of the nucleoside analogues, ie, acyclovir, famciclovir (the prodrug for penciclovir), and ganciclovir but certainly not by all. The 3' hydroxyl group on the ribose ring of penciclovir and ganciclovir provides an additional site for phosphorylation that, as a consequence, makes these drugs competitive inhibitors of deoxyguanosine but *not* obligatory DNA chain terminators.

The information here is provided as guidance only. Prescribers should always consult the manufacturer's current prescribing information.

Amantadine and rimantadine are tricyclic amine derivatives. The structure, when relevant, of each of these compounds is presented with a discussion of each drug.

MECHANISM OF ACTION

The mechanism of action of acyclovir is the best described of all the antiviral compounds to date. It is detailed on the previous page. Ganciclovir and penciclovir, drugs licensed for the treatment of other herpes virus infections, act through their triphosphate metabolites as well, functioning as competitive inhibitors of deoxyguanosine. Neither penciclovir nor ganciclovir is an obligate DNA chain terminator.

Foscarnet is a pyrophosphate analogue. It directly binds to guanosine in DNA chain elongation. Thus, it has a mechanism of action that is significantly different from other members of this class of compounds, which have activity against herpesviruses.

The dideoxynucleoside analogues (zidovudine, didanosine, and dideoxycitosine) all presumably work through their triphosphate derivatives, serving as inhibitors of reverse transcriptase. It should be noted that a class of nonnucleoside reverse transcriptase inhibitors (in some cases peptidomimetics), tat inhibitors, and inhibitors of protease expression are all in various stages of development for the treatment of HIV infection.

Both amantadine and rimantadine act on messenger RNA expression for influenza A virus as well as block viral uncoating in the cytoplasm. Because absorption and penetration of the virus occur, the host develops an immune response to the infecting organism.

GENERAL CONSIDERATIONS

Because each of the aforementioned antiviral drugs has different spectrums of activity, pharmacokinetics, pharmacodynamics, and adverse reactions, they are discussed specifically in each area of consideration.

REFERENCES

1. Fyfe JA, Keller PM, Furman PA, *et al.*: Thymidine kinase from herpes simplex virus phosphorylates the new antiviral compound, 9-(2-hydroxyethoxymethyl)guanine. *J Biol Chem* 1978, 253:8721–8727.

2. Derse D, Chang Y-C, Furman PA, Elion GB: Inhibition of purified human and herpes simplex virus–induced DNA polymerase by 9-(2-hydroxyethoxymethyl)guanine [acyclovir] triphosphate: Effect on primer-template function. *J Biol Chem* 1981, 256:11447–11451.

3. Furman PA, St Clair MH, Spector T: Acyclovir triphosphate is a suicide inactivator of the herpes simplex virus DNA polymerase. *J Biol Chem* 1984, 259:9575–9579.

4. Furman PA, St Clair MH, Fyfe JA, *et al.*: Inhibition of herpes simplex virus induced DNA polymerase activity and viral DNA replication of 9-(2-hydroxyethoxymethyl)guanine and its triphosphate. *J Virol* 1979, 32:72–77.

5. Erlich KS, Mills J, Chatis P, *et al.*: Acyclovir resistant herpes simplex virus infections in patients with acquired immunodeficiency syndrome. *N Engl J Med* 1989, 320:293–296.

6. Whitley RJ, Gnann J: Acyclovir: A decade later. *N Engl J Med* 1992, 327:782–789.

The information here is provided as guidance only. Prescribers should always consult the manufacturer's current prescribing information.

ACYCLOVIR (Zovirax®)

Acyclovir represents the first of the truly selective and specific inhibitions of viral replication. As discussed previously, acyclovir is activated by herpes simplex virus (HSV) or varicella-zoster virus (VZV) thymidine kinase. The monophosphate derivative is then converted to the active metabolite, acyclovir triphosphate, which is then a competitive and selective inhibitor of HSV and VZV DNA polymerase. It is an obligate DNA chain terminator. The structure of this drug is illustrated in Fig. 12-1. Currently, it is the treatment of choice for HSV and VZV.

The clinical uses and dosages of administration are summarized in Table 12-1 [6]. Today, acyclovir is the most widely used drug to treat HSV and VZV infections.

Acyclovir is a synthetic acyclic purine nucleoside analogue, available for oral and parenteral use.

INDICATIONS

PARENTERAL: Treatment of initial and recurrent mucosal and cutaneous HSV-1 and HSV-2 and varicella-zoster (chickenpox and shingles) infection in immunocompromised patients.

Herpes simplex encephalitis in patients over 6 months of age.

Severe clinical episodes of genital herpes in patients with normal immunity.

ORAL: Treatment of initial episodes and management of recurrent episodes of genital herpes in certain patients.

Acute treatment of herpes zoster (shingles) and chickenpox (varicella).

Unlabeled: Cytomegalovirus and HSV infection following bone marrow or renal transplantation

Disseminated primary eczema herpeticum

Herpes simplex–associated erythema multiforme

Herpes simplex labialis

Herpes simplex ocular infections

Herpes simplex proctitis

Herpetic whitlow

Herpes zoster encephalitis

Infectious mononucleosis

Varicella pneumonia

Neonatal herpes simplex infections

FIGURE 12-1.

The chemical structure of acyclovir.

Table 12-1. Indications for Acyclovir Therapy

Type of Infection	Route and Dosage*	Comments
Genital HSV		
Initial episode	200 mg orally 5 times/d for 10 d	Preferred route in normal host
	5 mg/kg IV every 8 h for 5 d	Reserved for severe cases
	5% ointment topically every 6 h for 7 d	Less effective than oral therapy
Recurrent episode	200 mg orally 5 times/d for 5 d	Limited clinical benefit
Suppression	400 mg orally twice daily	Titrate dose as required
Mucocutaneous HSV in an	200–400 mg orally 5 times/d for 10 d	
immunocompromised patient	5mg/kg IV every 8 h for 7–10 d†	
	5% ointment topically every 6 h for 7 d	For minor lesions only
HSV encephalitis	10 mg/kg IV every 8 h for 10–14 d‡	Alternative therapy: vidarabine
Neonatal HSV§	10 mg/kg IV every 8 h for 10–14 d‡	Alternative therapy: vidarabine
Varicella		
Normal host	20 mg/kg orally 4 times/d for 5 d (maximal dose, 800 mg 4–5 times/d)	
Immunocompromised patient	10 mg/kg IV every 8 h for 7–10 d‡	
Herpes zoster		
Normal host	800 mg orally 5 times/d for 7 d	Initiate within 48 h of onset of rash
Immunocompromised patient	10 mg/kg IV every 8 h for 7–10 d	Alternative therapy: vidarabine

*The doses are for adults with normal renal function unless otherwise noted.
†A dose of 250 mg per square meter of body surface area should be given to children under 12 years of age.
‡A dose of 500 mg per square meter of body surface area should be given to children under 12 years of age.
§Acyclovir has not been approved by the Food and Drug Administration for this indication.
HSV—herpes simplex virus; IV—intravenously.

The information here is provided as guidance only. Prescribers should always consult the manufacturer's current prescribing information.

ACYCLOVIR (CONTINUED)

MICROBIOLOGY

Active *in vitro* against herpes simplex virus (HSV) types 1 and 2, varicella-zoster, Epstein-Barr, and cytomegalovirus. However, concentrations of drug required to inhibit either of these latter two viruses *in vivo* cannot be achieved.

SPECIAL PRECAUTIONS

Testicular atrophy has occurred in rats given acyclovir intraperitoneally at doses of 320 or 80 mg/kg/d for 1- and 6-month periods, respectively. There was some recovery of sperm production 30 days following the dosage.

Viral isolation and identification in tissue culture are essential to prove HSV infection.

Patients should be advised to avoid sexual intercourse when visible lesions are present due to risk of infecting partners as are good "safe sex" practices as well. Adults aged 50 years or more have increased severity of shingles; treatment with acyclovir showed greater benefit for patients who are elderly. In studies, treatment was begun within 72 hours of rash onset, and resulted in accelerated cutaneous healing and loss of pain.

Treatment of chickenpox in adolescents and adults in controlled studies was initiated within 24 hours of onset of typical rash; no information exists regarding effects of treatment begun in later stages of disease. Early (24 hours or less) therapy accelerates healing. There is no evidence to suggest that acyclovir treatment of chickenpox would have any effect on either decreasing or increasing incidence or severity of recurrent herpes zoster (shingles) later in life. Note that intravenous acyclovir is indicated for treatment of varicella-zoster infection in immunocompromised patients. The American Academy of Pediatrics Redbook Committee recommends therapy of children aged 2 to 12 years who are at increased risk for severe disease (*eg*, atopic dermatitis, etc.) and postpubertal individuals.

Do not exceed recommended dosage, frequency, or duration of treatment. Dosage adjustments should be based on creatinine clearance.

Acyclovir crystals can precipitate in renal tubules if maximum solubility of free drug is exceeded or if administered by bolus injection. Serum creatinine and blood urea nitrogen rise, while creatinine clearance decreases. Bolus administration causes a 10% incidence of renal dysfunction; infusion of 5 mg/kg over 1 hour was associated with a lower frequency (4.6%) of altered renal function. Factors that make further renal impairment more likely include concomitant use of other nephrotoxic drugs, preexisting renal disease, and dehydration. In most cases, changes in renal function are transient and resolve spontaneously or with improvement of water and electrolyte balance, with dosage adjustments, or with discontinuation. However, changes in renal function may progress to acute renal failure.

Intravenous infusion should be accompanied by adequate hydration. Because maximum urinary concentrations occur within the first 2 hours after infusion, sufficient urine outflow should be established during that time to prevent precipitation in renal tubules. Encephalopathic changes characterized by either lethargy, obtundation, tremors, confusion, hallucinations, agitation, seizures, or coma have occurred in approximately 1% of patients receiving high-dose acyclovir (more than 60 mg/kg/d intravenously). Use with caution in patients with underlying neurologic abnormalities, serious renal, hepatic, or electrolyte abnormalities, significant hypoxia, or earlier neurologic reactions to cytotoxic agents.

Resistance, or the emergence of less-sensitive viruses, can occur due to exposure of HSV isolates to acyclovir *in vitro*. In patients with serious immunodeficiency undergoing prolonged or repeated therapy, resistant viruses may result and may not respond fully to further acyclovir therapy. However, resistant viruses can be treated with foscarnet.

CONTRAINDICATIONS

Allergy of hypersensitivity to acyclovir or any product components.

INTERACTIONS

Probenecid

ADVERSE EFFECTS

PARENTERAL (> 1%): Inflammation or phlebitis at injection site, transient elevation of serum creatinine or blood urea nitrogen (usually after too rapid intravenous infusion), nausea or vomiting, itching or rash or hives, elevation of transaminases, encephalopathic changes (*see* Special Precautions)

(< 1%): Anemia, anuria, hematuria, hypotension, edema, anorexia, light-headedness, thirst, headache, diaphoresis, fever, neutropenia, thrombocytopenia, abnormal urinalysis, pain when urinating, pulmonary edema with cardiac tamponade, abdominal pain, chest pain, thrombocytosis, leukocytosis, neutrophilia, ischemia of digits, hypokalemia, purpura fulminans, pressure when urinating, hemoglobinemia, rigors

ORAL: (Treatment of herpes simplex):

Central nervous system: headache, dizziness, fatigue (short-term therapy); headache (long-term and intermittent therapy)

Dermatologic: skin rash (short- and long-term and intermittent therapy)

Gastrointestinal: nausea or vomiting, diarrhea (short-term therapy); nausea, diarrhea (long-term and intermittent therapy)

Other: anorexia, edema, inguinal adenopathy, leg pain, medication taste, sore throat (short-term therapy); asthenia, paresthesia (long-term therapy)

(Treatment of herpes zoster and chickenpox): Malaise, nausea, headache, vomiting, diarrhea, constipation, abdominal pain, rash, flatulence

The information here is provided as guidance only. Prescribers should always consult the manufacturer's current prescribing information.

ACYCLOVIR (CONTINUED)

SPECIAL GROUPS

Children: Safety and efficacy of oral acyclovir in children under 2 years of age not established.

Elderly: May have age-related renal impairment requiring reduced dosage.

Renal impairment: Reduced dosage necessary; monitor function.

Hepatic impairment: No changes required.

Pregnancy: Adequate human studies not performed; animal studies indicate potential risk to fetus. Use only when benefits outweigh risk, *ie*, in life-threatening situations.

Breast-feeding: Excreted in breast milk in levels that can potentially expose infant to dose levels; use with caution.

DOSAGE

Adults: *PARENTERAL*: (Note: For intravenous infusion only. Avoid rapid or bolus intravenous, intramuscular, or subcutaneous injection. Therapy should be initiated as soon as possible following onset of symptoms. Administer over period of at least 1 hour to prevent renal tubular damage.)
The following guidelines are recommended:

Therapeutic Indications and Dosing Regimens of Acyclovir

Indication	Dosage, adults	Dosage, children
Mucosal and cutaneous HSV infections in patients with immunodeficiency	5 mg/kg infused at constant rate over period of 1 h every 8 h for 7 days* (15 mg/kg/d)	250 mg/m² infused at a constant rate over period of 1 h every 8 h for 7 days* (750 mg/m²/d)
Varicella-zoster infections (shingles) in patients with immunodeficiency†	10 mg/kg infused at a constant rate over period of 1 h every 8 h for 7 days‡	500 mg/m² infused at a constant rate over period of at least 1 h every 8 h for 7 days‡
Herpes simplex encephalitis	10 mg/kg infused at a constant rate over at least 1 h every 8 h for 10 days	500 mg/m² infused at a constant rate over period of at least 1 h every 8 h for 10 day§

For severe initial clinical cases of herpes genitalis, use same dose for 5 days.
†Base dosage on ideal body weight (10 mg/kg) for obese patients.
‡Do not exceed 500 mg/m² every 8 hours.
§For patients more than 6 months of age only.

ORAL: For herpes simplex (initial genital herpes), 200 mg every 4 hours (five times a day) for 10 days; patients with extremely severe episodes or inability to take oral medication require hospitalization and more aggressive management (initial intravenous therapy). For chronic suppressive therapy of recurrent disease, 400 mg twice daily for up to 12 months; follow with reevaluation of frequency and severity of HSV to assess the need for more therapy. Alternative regimens include dose ranges from 200 mg three times a day to 200 mg five times a day. Intermittent therapy, 200 mg every 4 hours (five times a day) for 5 days; initiate therapy at first symptom of recurrence.
For acute treatment of herpes zoster, 800 mg every 4 hours (five times a day) for 7 to 10 days.
For chickenpox, 20 mg/kg (do not exceed 800 mg) four times a day for 5 days, initiated at first symptom.

Elderly: *PARENTERAL* and *ORAL*: May have age-related renal impairment; otherwise, same as adult.

Children: *PARENTERAL*: *See* above table. *ORAL*: No information.

(continued on next page)

PHARMACOKINETICS AND PHARMACODYNAMICS

Peak serum levels: 9.8 µg/mL after 1-h infusion of 5 mg/kg dose, 1.5 to 2 h afterward

Serum half-life: 2.5 h

Bioavailability: 15% to 30%, decreases with increasing doses

Protein binding: 9% to 33%

Metabolism: major urinary metabolite is 9-carboxy-methlyguanine, possibly accounting for up to 14% of dose in patients with normal renal function

Excretion: renal, by glomerular filtration and tubular secretion, 62% to 91% of dose

Renal impairment: half-life prolonged and excretion reduced

Hepatic impairment: no information

OVERDOSAGE

Symptoms of overdosage include precipitation of acyclovir in renal tubules (when solubility [2.5 mg/mL] is exceeded in intratubular fluid). Can evolve to acute tubular necrosis.

PARENTERAL: Overdosage has occurred with bolus injections, inappropriately high doses, and in patients whose fluid and electrolyte balance was not properly monitored; elevations in blood urea nitrogen, serum creatinine, and subsequent renal failure resulted.

ORAL: Doses as great as 800 mg six times a day for 5 days have been used without acute adverse effects; however, this should not be used as a recommended dosage.

Treatment of overdosage may include dialysis. Six-hour hemodialysis produces a 60% decrease in plasma acyclovir concentrations; peritoneal dialysis is less efficient.

The information here is provided as guidance only. Prescribers should always consult the manufacturer's current prescribing information.

ACYCLOVIR (CONTINUED)

DOSAGE *(CONTINUED)*

Renal impairment: *PARENTERAL*: The following guidelines are recommended:

Guidelines for Acyclovir Administration With Renal Impairment (Intravenous)

Creatinine clearance, mL/min/1.73 m²	Percent of recommended regular dose	Dosing interval, h
> 50	100	8
25–50	100	12
10–25	100	24
0–10	50	24

For patients on hemodialysis, the mean plasma half-life of acyclovir during hemodialysis is approximately 5 hours; a 60% decrease in plasma concentrations follows a 6-hour dialysis period. Administer a dose after each dialysis.

Guidelines for Acyclovir Administration With Renal Impairment (Oral)

Normal dosage regimen, five times/d	Creatinine clearance, mL/min/1.73 m²	Adjusted dosage regimen	
		Dose, mg	Interval
200 mg every 4 h	> 10	200	Every 4 h, 5 times/d
	0–10	200	Every 12 h
400 mg every 12 h	> 10	400	Every 12 h
	0–10	200	Every 12 h
800 mg every 4 h	> 25	800	Every 4 h, 5 times/d
	10–25	800	Every 8 h
	0–10	800	Every 12 h

For patients on hemodialysis, adjust dosing schedule for dose to be administered after each dialysis; no supplemental dose necessary following peritoneal dialysis.

PATIENT INFORMATION

Avoid sexual intercourse when herpes lesions are present.
Oral acyclovir does not eliminate latent HSV virus and is not a cure.
Do not exceed recommended dosage; do not share medication.
If frequency or severity of recurrences do not improve, contact physician.

AVAILABILITY

Tablets—800 mg
Capsules—200 mg
Suspension—200 mg/5 mL
Powder for injection—500 mg/vial and 1000 mg/vial

The information here is provided as guidance only. Prescribers should always consult the manufacturer's current prescribing information.

AMANTADINE (Symmerrel®)

Amantadine has established value in the prophylaxis and treatment of influenza A infections. This drug, as shown in Fig. 12-2, is a tricyclic amine. It has a rigid structure. Its mechanism of action is that of blocking uncoating of the virus in the cytoplasm as well as inhibition of messenger RNA expression. Because of the mechanism of action of this compound, a host's antibody response will develop to viral infection. Rimantadine has replaced amantadine as the treatment of choice for influenza A infections because of decreased adverse clinical effects. Although the drug has been evaluated for many years and has proved efficacious in the prevention of influenza infection, it is not routinely used because of adverse clinical events. Furthermore, cultural practices, *ie*, the lack of interest in prevention of disease by many Americans, have led to the failure of acceptance of this medication.

Amantadine hydrochloride is available for oral use in capsule and syrup form.

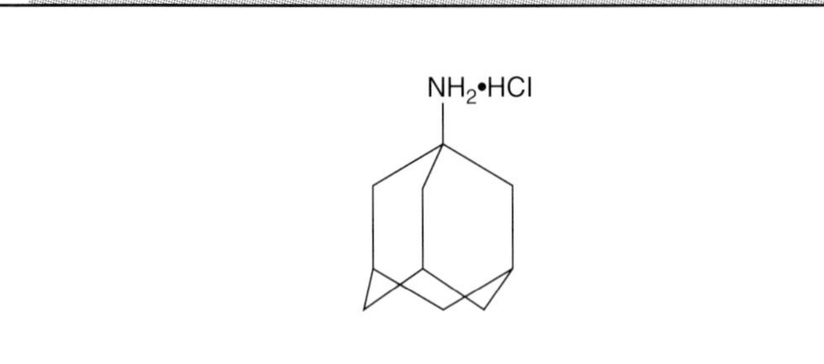

FIGURE 12-2. The chemical structure of amantadine.

MICROBIOLOGY

Amantadine is 70% to 90% effective in preventing conditions caused by circulating strains of type A influenza viruses (not effective against type B influenza). It does not appear to interfere with the immunogenicity of inactivated influenza A virus vaccine.

SPECIAL PRECAUTIONS

Patients with epilepsy, history of epilepsy, or other seizures are at risk for increased seizure activity and should be observed closely during therapy. Dosage reduction is recommended.

Patients with liver disease, history of recurrent eczematoid rash, psychosis, or severe psychoneurosis not controlled by chemotherapeutic agents require extra care when receiving amantadine.

Congestive heart failure has occurred during amantadine use; patients with congestive heart failure or peripheral edema require careful observation and dosage titration.

Physicians should educate elderly and high-risk patients (*eg*, cystic fibrosis, chronic lung disease, smoking) as to the value of prophylactic therapy during influenza season.

SPECIAL GROUPS

Children: Safety and efficacy in infants under 1 year of age not established.
Elderly: Patients aged 65 years and over require reduced dosage.
Renal impairment: Requires reduced dosage; amantadine is not metabolized and is excreted primarily in the urine. Renal impairment leads to accumulation of drug in plasma.
Hepatic impairment: Use caution.
Pregnancy: Adequate human studies not performed; animal studies suggest potential for harm to fetus. Use only when benefits outweigh risk.
Breast-feeding: Excreted in breast milk; use with caution.

INDICATIONS

Prophylaxis or treatment of respiratory illness due to strains of influenza A virus; especially in high-risk patients (those with underlying cardiovascular, pulmonary, metabolic, neuromuscular, or immuno-deficiency disease). When immunization is contra-indicated or unavailable, amantadine may be used as chemoprophylaxis.

CONTRAINDICATIONS

Allergy or hypersensitivity to amantadine

INTERACTIONS

Anticholinergic agents, hydrochlorothiazide plus triamterene

ADVERSE EFFECTS

Most frequent: nausea, dizziness, lightheadedness, insomnia
Less frequent: depression, anxiety, irritability, halluci-nations, confusion, anorexia, dry mouth, constipa-tion, ataxia, livedo reticularis, peripheral edema, orthostatic hypotension, headache
Infrequent: congestive heart failure, psychosis, urinary retention, dyspnea, fatigue, skin rash, vomiting, weakness, slurred speech, visual disturbance
Rare: convulsions, leukopenia, neutropenia, eczematoid dermatitis, oculogyric episodes

PHARMACOKINETICS AND PHARMACODYNAMICS

Peak serum levels: no values given; reached about 4 h after 100-mg dose
Serum half-life: mean half-life of excretion rate is 15 h
Bioavailability: no information
Protein binding: no information
Metabolism: not metabolized
Excretion: in urine
Renal impairment: significantly reduces clearance and increases plasma levels
Hepatic impairment: no information

The information here is provided as guidance only. Prescribers should always consult the manufacturer's current prescribing information.

AMANTADINE (CONTINUED)

DOSAGE

Adults: For influenza A prophylaxis, begin in anticipation of contact or as soon as possible after exposure and continue daily for minimum of 10 days following known exposure. Prophylaxis should be instituted at the onset of reporting influenza cases in the community. If vaccine is unavailable or contraindicated, give for up to 90 days in case of possible repeated and unknown exposures. May be used in addition to inactivated influenza virus A vaccine until antibody responses develop; give for up to 2 weeks after vaccine was administered.

For symptomatic management, begin as soon as possible after onset of symptoms, continuing for minimum of 24 to 48 hours after symptoms clear. Give 200 mg/d as a single dose or 100 mg two times a day (splitting dose may reduce central nervous system adverse effects).

Elderly: *See* table below.

Children: For symptomatic management, (9–12 years of age) 100 mg twice a day; (1–9 years of age) 2 to 4 mg/kg/d once a day or divided and two times a day. Do not exceed 150 mg/d.

Renal impairment: *See* table below.

Amantadine Dose by Age and Degree of Renal Function

Renal function	Dosage*
No apparent renal disease	
1–9 years of age †	4.4–8.8 mg/kg/d in single dose once a day or in divided doses twice a day Do not exceed 150 mg/d
10–64 years of age‡	200 mg once a day or in divided doses twice a day
65 years of age or over	100 mg once a day§
Renal function impairment based on creatinine clearance, *ml/min/1.73 m²*	
30–50	200 mg 1st day; 100 mg/d thereafter
15–29	200 mg 1st day; 100 mg on alternate days
<15	200 mg every 7 days
Patients on hemodialysis	200 mg every 7 days

*As prophylaxis, take every day for duration of influenza A activity in the community (6–12 weeks). As therapy, begin as soon as possible after onset of symptoms and continue for minimum of 24 to 48 hours after symptoms clear (5–7 days).
†Safety in children under 1 year of age not established.
‡For patients with active seizure disorder, reduce dosage to 100 mg/d.
§Recommended to minimize toxicity effects, which are more frequent in elderly patients due to normal renal function decline.

OVERDOSAGE

Symptoms of overdosage include nausea, vomiting, anorexia, and central nervous system effects, such as hyperexcitability, tremors, ataxia, blurred vision, lethargy, depression, slurred speech, and convulsions. Ventricular arrhythmias manifested by torsades de pointes and ventricular fibrillation were observed in a patient who ingested 2.5 g amantadine, and death has occurred from a major overdose. There is no specific treatment or antidote. For central nervous system toxicity, intravenous physostigmine 1 to 2 mg administered slowly every 1 to 2 hours for adults or 0.5 mg at 5- to 10-minute intervals up to a maximum of 2 mg/h for children. For acute overdosage, general supportive measures including immediate gastric lavage or induction of emesis are recommended. Forcing of fluids (using intravenous if necessary) and urinary acidification may increase elimination. Blood pressure, pulse, respiration, temperature, electrolytes, urine pH, and urinary output should be monitored. If hyperactivity or convulsions occur, sedatives or anticonvulsants may be required. Appropriate antiarrhythmic and vasopressor therapy may be given when warranted. Hemodialysis does not remove significant amounts of the drug.

PATIENT INFORMATION

Blurred vision may occur; use caution when driving or performing other tasks requiring good vision and alertness.

If dizziness or lightheadedness occurs, contact physician immediately and avoid sudden changes in posture.

If mood or mental changes, swelling of extremities, difficult urination, or shortness of breath occurs, contact physician immediately.

AVAILABILITY

Capsules—100 mg
Syrup—50 mg/5 mL

The information here is provided as guidance only. Prescribers should always consult the manufacturer's current prescribing information.

DIDANOSINE (Videx®)

Didanosine is a dideoxynucleoside (Fig. 12-3), which when phosphorylated is a reverse transcriptase inhibitor. It was the second compound licensed for treatment of HIV infection. Unlike zidovudine, didanosine is not toxic for hematopoietic precursor cells. As such, it is recommended for patients who have failed on zidovudine or who are intolerant to this medication. Didanosine is a second line of therapy for HIV infections. Painful peripheral neuropathy and pancreatitis are the major dose-limiting toxicities: both usually develop in the first 3 to 6 months of therapy.

Didanosine is a synthetic purine nucleoside analogue of deoxyadenosine. It is available for oral administration.

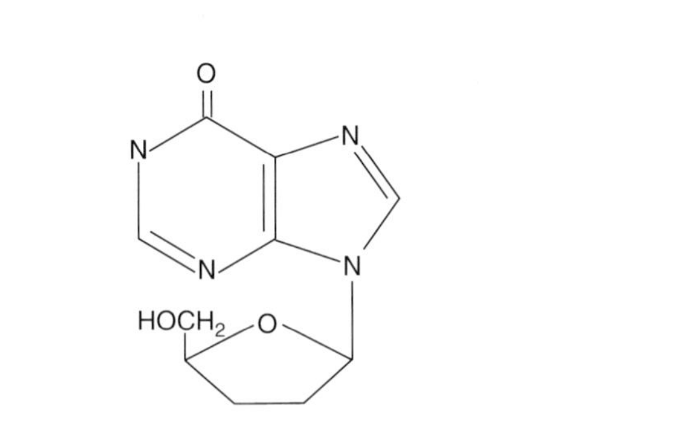

FIGURE 12-3.
The chemical structure of didanosine.

MICROBIOLOGY

Didanosine has *in vitro* antiviral activity in a number of HIV-infected T cell and monocyte-macrophage cell cultures. (Note: As yet, there is no established relationship between *in vitro* susceptibility of HIV to didanosine and the inhibition of HIV replication in humans or in clinical response to therapy.)
Didanosine also inhibits human hepatitis B virus replication *in vitro*; however, the clinical significance is unknown.

SPECIAL PRECAUTIONS

Pancreatitis is the primary clinical toxicity of didanosine therapy and has been fatal in some cases. Pancreatitis should be considered in the event of abdominal pain, nausea, vomiting, or elevated biochemical values (amylase). Didanosine should be discontinued until a diagnosis of pancreatitis is ruled out.
Patients receiving antiretroviral therapy may continue to develop opportunistic infections and other complications of HIV infection; they should remain under close clinical observation of physicians experienced in the management of HIV-associated diseases.
Currently, no data from controlled studies are available concerning the effect of didanosine therapy (such as incidence of opportunistic infection and survival rates) on clinical progression of HIV infection.
Peripheral neuropathy occurring with didanosine use appears to be dose related; patients should be monitored for manifestations of neuropathy, usually characterized by distal numbness, tingling, and pain in the feet or hands. Incidence is more frequent in patients with a history of neuropathy or neurotoxic drug therapy. Dose modification may be necessary in severe cases.
Hepatic failure has occurred with didanosine use, and fatal liver failure of unknown etiology occurred during didanosine therapy in one of 170 patients in phase I studies and in 14 of 7806 in the Expanded Access Program.

(continued on next page)

INDICATIONS

Treatment of adult patients with advanced HIV infection who have already received prior prolonged therapy with zidovudine. Zidovudine remains superior to didanosine for HIV-infected patients who are antiretroviral therapy naive.
Treatment of adults and children over 6 months of age with advanced HIV infection who have demonstrated intolerance or significant clinical or immunologic deterioration during therapy with zidovudine.
(Note: Because zidovudine prolongs survival and decreases incidence of opportunistic infection in patients with advanced HIV infection, zidovudine should be considered as initial treatment unless contraindicated.)

CONTRAINDICATIONS

Allergy or hypersensitivity to didanosine or any preparation components

INTERACTIONS

Fluoroquinolones, tetracyclines

ADVERSE EFFECTS

(Adults)
Body as a whole: chills or fever, asthenia, pain, infection, sarcoma, myopathy, anorexia, allergic reaction, abscess, cellulitis, cyst, dehydration, flu syndrome, hernia, neck rigidity, numbness of hands or feet
Cardiovascular: chest pain, hypotension, hypertension, migraine, palpitation, peripheral vascular disorder, syncope
Central nervous system: neuropathy (all grades), headache, convulsion, abnormal thinking, anxiety or nervousness or twitching, confusion, depression, acute brain syndrome, amnesia, aphasia, ataxia, convulsion (grand mal), dizziness, hyperesthesia, hypertonia, ileus, incoordination, intracranial hemorrhage, malaise, paralysis, paranoid reaction, psychosis, sleep disorder, speech disorder, tremor
Dermatologic: rash or pruritus, herpes simplex, skin disorder, sweating
Gastrointestinal: diarrhea, abdominal pain, nausea or vomiting, pancreatitis, dry mouth, colitis, constipation, eructation, flatulence, gastroenteritis, gastrointestinal hemorrhage, moniliasis (oral), sialadenitis, stomach ulcer hemorrhage
Genitourinary: impotence, kidney calculus, failure or abnormal function, nocturia, urinary frequency, vaginal hemorrhage
Hemic or lymphatic: hemorrhage, lymphoma-like reaction, microcytic anemia
Metabolic or nutritional: anomaly, arthralgia, arthritis, edema (peripheral), hemiparesis, hypokalemia, joint disorder, leg cramp
Respiratory: pneumonia, dyspnea, asthma, bronchitis, increased cough, epistaxis, laryngitis, decreased lung function, pharyngitis, pneumonia (interstitial), respiratory disorder
Special senses: blurred vision, conjunctivitis, diplopia, dry eye, ear disorder, glaucoma, otitis (externa and media), retinitis

(continued on next page)

The information here is provided as guidance only. Prescribers should always consult the manufacturer's current prescribing information.

DIDANOSINE (CONTINUED)

SPECIAL PRECAUTIONS (CONTINUED)

Retinal depigmentation occurred in four pediatric patients; children receiving didanosine should receive dilated retinal examinations every 6 months or if any change in vision occurs.

Myopathy has occurred in mice and rats (but not in dogs) following long-term (more than 90 days) therapy with didanosine at levels 1.2 to 12 times estimated human exposure. Human events have been associated with other nucleoside analogues.

Patients with renal function impairment may be at increased risk of toxicity due to decreased drug clearance. Dosage reduction should be considered.

Patients with hepatic impairment may be at increased risk of toxicity due to altered metabolism; dosage reduction may be required.

In vitro cytogenic study revealed that high concentrations of didanosine (500 μg/mL and over) increased the frequency of cells with chromosome aberrations. A different study showed that didanosine produced such aberrations at 500 μg/mL after 48 hours of exposure; similar chromosomal aberration effects were induced by the natural nucleoside of didanosine, 2′-deoxyinosine and suggest that such effects were not due to a direct genotoxic interaction.

Phenylketonuria alert: didanosine tablets contain 22.5 mg phenylalanine (33.7 mg in the 150-mg tablet).

Sodium restriction alert: didanosine buffered tablets contain 264.5 mg sodium, and each single-dose packet of buffered powder for oral solution contains 1380 mg sodium.

Didanosine has been associated with asymptomatic hyperuricemia; suspension of treatment should be considered if clinical attempts to reduce uric acid levels fail. Diarrhea occurred in 34% of patients in the phase I adult studies with buffered powder for oral solution. If diarrhea occurs, consider trial of chewable or dispersible buffered tablets.

SPECIAL GROUPS

Children: *See* Indications, Special Precautions, and Dosage.
Elderly: May have age-related renal impairment.
Renal impairment: Increased risk for toxicity.
Hepatic impairment: Increased risk for toxicity.
Pregnancy: Adequate human studies not performed; use only if clearly indicated.
Breast-feeding: Not known whether excreted; however, because of the potential for serious adverse effects, decision must be made to discontinue nursing or discontinue didanosine.

DOSAGE

(Note: Use 12-hour dosing interval; administer all formulations on an empty stomach.)
Adults: Two tablets are to be used at each dose to provide buffering and prevent gastric degradation of didanosine. Recommended beginning adult doses are weight dependent; use the following guidelines:

Didanosine Dosing

Patient weight, *kg*	Tablets	Buffered powder
60 or over	200 mg twice a day	250 mg twice a day
Under 60	125 mg twice a day	167 mg twice a day

Elderly: May have age-related renal impairment; otherwise, same as adults.
Children: For prevention of gastric acid degradation, children over 1 year of age should receive a two-tablet dose; children under 1 year of age should receive a one-tablet dose.
(continued on next page)

ADVERSE EFFECTS (CONTINUED)

Laboratory test abnormalities: leukopenia, amylase increase, granulocytopenia, thrombocytopenia, ALT increase, AST increase, alkaline phosphatase increase, hemoglobin decrease, bilirubin increase, uric acid increase

Children:

Body as a whole: chills or fever, anorexia, asthenia, pain, malaise, failure to thrive, weight loss, flu syndrome, change in appetite, alopecia, dehydration, increased appetite

Cardiovascular: vasodilation, arrhythmia

Central nervous system: headache, nervousness, insomnia, dizziness, poor coordination, lethargy, neurologic effects, seizure

Dermatologic: rash or pruritus, skin disorder, eczema, sweating, impetigo, excoriation, erythema

Gastrointestinal: diarrhea, nausea or vomiting, liver abnormalities, abdominal pain, stomatitis or mouth sores, pancreatitis, constipation, oral thrush, melena, dry mouth

Hematologic or lymphatic: ecchymosis, hemorrhage, petechiae

Musculoskeletal: arthritis, myalgia, muscle atrophy, decreased strength

Respiratory: cough, rhinitis, dyspnea, asthma, rhinorrhea, epistaxis, pharyngitis, hypoventilation, sinusitis, rhonchi or rales, congestion, pneumonia

Special senses: ear pain or otitis, photophobia, strabismus, visual impairment

Other: urinary frequency, diabetes mellitus, diabetes insipidus

Laboratory abnormalities: leukopenia, granulocytopenia, thrombocytopenia, anemia, ALT increase, AST increase, alkaline phosphatase increase, bilirubin increase, uric acid increase, amylase increase

PHARMACOKINETICS AND PHARMACODYNAMICS

Peak serum levels: 1.6 μg/mL
Serum half-life: 1.6 h after oral administration
Bioavailability: average, 33%; 20% to 25% greater with tablet than solution
Protein binding: no information
Metabolism: not evaluated in humans; extensive in dogs
Excretion: renal clearance represented approximately 50% of total body clearance; active tubular secretion and glomerular filtration
Renal impairment: limited data; consider reduced dosage
Hepatic impairment: limited data; consider reduced dosage

OVERDOSAGE

No known antidote. Phase I study demonstrated complications to include pancreatitis, peripheral neuropathy, diarrhea, hyperuricemia, and possibly hepatic dysfunction. No information exists to show whether didanosine is dialyzable.

The information here is provided as guidance only. Prescribers should always consult the manufacturer's current prescribing information.

DIDANOSINE (CONTINUED)

DOSAGE (CONTINUED)

Recommended pediatric dosage is dependent on body surface area; use the following guidelines (based on 200 mg/m^2/d average dose):

Didanosine Dosing in Pediatric Patients

Body surface area, m^2	Tablets	Dose pediatric powder	Vol/10 mg/mL admixture
1.1–1.4	100 mg twice a day	125 mg twice a day	12.5 mL twice a day
0.8–1	75 mg twice a day	94 mg twice a day	9.5 mL twice a day
0.5–0.7	50 mg twice a day	62 mg twice a day	6 mL twice a day
< 0.4	25 mg twice a day	31 mg twice a day	3 mL twice a day

Renal impairment: There are insufficient data to recommend dosage adjustment for patients with impaired renal or hepatic function; consider reducing dosage in these patients.

PATIENT INFORMATION

No information

AVAILABILITY

Tablets (buffered and chewable or dispersable)—
  25 mg, 50 mg, 100 mg, and 150 mg
Powder for oral solution (buffered)—100 mg,
  167 mg, 250 mg, and 375 mg
Pediatric powder for oral solution—2 g and 4 g

FAMCICLOVIR (Famvir®)

Famciclovir was licensed in June 1994 by the Food and Drug Administration (FDA) for the treatment of herpes zoster infection and immunocompetent adults. Famciclovir is the first prodrug licensed by the FDA. It is the prodrug of penciclovir, the plasma metabolite that is subsequently taken up by infected cells and converted to the monophosphate derivative. After phosphorylation by cellular kinases, the triphosphate derivative functions as an inhibitor of herpes simplex virus (HSV) and varicella-zoster virus (VZV) DNA polymerase. At dosages of 500 mg three times per day, this drug accelerates cutaneous healing (placebo-controlled studies) and is as effective as acyclovir for the resolution of acute neuritis and chronic pain.

Famciclovir is a guanosine analogue with a similar structure to acyclovir. It is indicated in therapy for uncomplicated herpes zoster infection.

MICROBIOLOGY

Famciclovir is metabolized to penciclovir, which is active against HSV, VZV, and hepatitis B viruses.

SPECIAL PRECAUTIONS

Drug interactions with digoxin (increased plasma concentration), allopurinol

SPECIAL GROUPS

Children: No information.
Elderly: No dosage adjustment necessary.
Renal impairment: Reduced dosing frequency necessary.
Hepatic impairment: No dosage adjustment necessary in well-compensated hepatic impairment; no data for uncompensated hepatic impairment.
Pregnancy: No adequate studies; use only if benefits outweigh risk.
Breast-feeding: Not known whether excreted in human milk; decision should be made whether to discontinue nursing or discontinue drug, taking into account the importance of the drug to the mother.

DOSAGE

Adults: 500 mg three times a day for 7 days.
Elderly: No dosage adjustment necessary.
Children: No information.
Renal impairment: No information.

INDICATIONS

Famciclovir is indicated for the management of acute herpes zoster (shingles)

CONTRAINDICATIONS

Famciclovir is contraindicated in patients with known hypersensitivity to famciclovir

INTERACTIONS

No clinically significant alterations in penciclovir pharmacokinetics were observed following single-dose administration of 500-mg famciclovir after pretreatment with multiple doses of cimetidine, allopurinol, or theophylline.
Concurrent use with probenecid or other drugs significantly eliminated by active renal tubular secretion may result in increased plasma concentrations of penciclovir.
The conversion of 6-deoxy penciclovir to penciclovir is catalyzed by aldehyde oxidase. Interactions with other drugs metabolized by this enzyme could potentially occur.

ADVERSE EFFECTS

Headache, nausea, and fatigue

PHARMACOKINETICS AND PHARMACODYNAMICS

Peak serum levels: achieved between 0.5 and 1.5 h after administration
Serum half-life: 7.2 h
Bioavailability: 70%
Protein binding: < 20% bound to plasma proteins
Metabolism: converted to penicillin
Excretion: rapid and complete via urine (73%) and feces (27%)
Renal impairment: none known
Hepatic impairment: none known

OVERDOSAGE

No information

PATIENT INFORMATION

Gatrointestinal headache 10%

AVAILABILITY

Licensed in the US for herpes zoster and in the UK for herpes zoster and genital herpes

The information here is provided as guidance only. Prescribers should always consult the manufacturer's current prescribing information.

FOSCARNET (Foscavir®)

Foscarnet is a pyrophosphate analogue as shown in Fig. 12-4. In that it is a nonnucleoside analogue, its mechanism of action is different from that of other compounds licensed for the treatment of herpes virus infections. Specifically, drug reversibility blocks the pyrophosphate binding site of viral polymerase. Although the drug has activity against all members of the herpesvirus family, significant nephrotoxicity, acute tubercular necrosis, and interstitial nephritis (alterations of blood urea nitrogen, creatinine, and metabolic abnormalities [calcium, phosphorus, and potassium]) associated with its administration limit the clinical use of this compound. Currently, it is licensed for the treatment of cytomegalovirus retinitis in individuals with HIV infection as well as resistant herpes simplex virus (HSV) or varicella-zoster virus (VZV) infections in the immunocompromised host. Caution should be used in the intravenous administration of this medication because of renal and metabolic toxicity.

Foscarnet is an organic analogue of inorganic pyrophosphate. It is available for intravenous infusion only.

FIGURE 12-4.
The chemical structure of foscarnet.

MICROBIOLOGY

Inhibits replication of all herpes viruses, including cytomegalovirus, herpes simplex types 1 and 2, human herpes virus 6, Epstein-Barr virus, and VZV.

SPECIAL PRECAUTIONS

Renal impairment occurs to some degree in all patients treated with foscarnet—it is the primary toxicity of this agent. Continual monitoring of renal function throughout therapy is indicated, as are dosage adjustments for any changes in function. For patients with existing renal function prior to therapy, reduced dosage is necessary, and adequate hydration before each dosing is recommended.

Alterations in plasma minerals (Ca^2, Mg^2, PO_4) and electrolytes due to foscarnet have led to seizures; patients should be monitored often for any plasma changes.

Seizures have been associated with foscarnet; in most cases, patients had an active central nervous system (CNS) condition or history of CNS condition. Associated risk factors include low baseline absolute neutrophil count, impaired baseline renal function, and low serum calcium. Three seizures were associated with foscarnet overdose, and several with death.

Safety and efficacy are not established for treatment of other cytomegalovirus infections such as pneumonitis or gastroenteritis, congenital or neonatal cytomegalovirus disease, or nonimmunocompromised patients.

Diagnosis of cytomegalovirus retinitis should be made by an ophthalmologist familiar with its presentation and by indirect ophthalmoscopy. In our clinical trial performed by Studies of the Ocular Complications of AIDS, foscarnet and ganciclovir were equally efficacious for therapy of cytomegalovirus retinitis, but foscarnet provided a survival advantage.

Maximum single dose is 120 mg/kg by intravenous infusion over 2 hours; larger doses or more rapid infusions are likely to result in increased toxicity.

(continued on next page)

INDICATIONS

Treatment of cytomegalovirus retinitis in patients with AIDS

CONTRAINDICATIONS

Allergy or hypersensitivity to foscarnet

INTERACTIONS

Nephrotoxic agents, pentamidine, zidovudine

ADVERSE EFFECTS

Most frequent: fever (65%), nausea (47%), anemia (33%), diarrhea (30%), abnormal renal function (27%), vomiting, and headache (26%)

Most severe: death (14%)*, abnormal renal function (14%), marrow suppression (10%), anemia (9%), seizures (7%)

**Death was attributed to foscarnet directly in only one case; however, other effects of foscarnet may have contributed to patient deaths.*

Administration: pain or inflammation at injection site

Body as a whole: fever, fatigue, rigors, asthenia, malaise, pain, infection, sepsis, death, back or chest pain, edema, influenza-like symptoms, bacterial or fungal infection, moniliasis, abscess, hypothermia, syncope, ascites, abnormal crying, malignant hyperplexia, herpes simplex, viral infection, toxoplasmosis

Cardiovascular: hypertension, palpitations, electrocardiogram, abnormalities including sinus tachycardia, first-degree atrioventricular block and nonspecific ST–T segment changes, hypotension, flushing cerebrovascular disorder, cardiomyopathy, cardiac failure or arrest, bradycardia, extrasystole, arrhythmias, atrial arrhythmias or fibrillation, phlebitis, thrombophlebitis

Central nervous system: headache, paresthesia, dizziness, involuntary muscle contractions, hypoesthesia, neuropathy, seizures (including grand mal), tremor, ataxia, dementia, stupor, generalized spasms, sensory disturbances, meningitis, aphasia, abnormal coordination, leg cramps, electroencephalogram abnormalities, vertigo, coma, encephalopathy, abnormal gait, hyperesthesia, hypertonia, visual field defects, dyskinesia, extrapyramidal disorders, hemiparesis, hyperkinesia, vocal cord paralysis, paralysis, paraplegia, speech disorders, tetany, hyporeflexia, hyperreflexia, neuralgia, neuritis, peripheral neuropathy, cerebral edema, nystagmus

Dermatologic: rash, increased sweating, skin ulceration, seborrhea, erythematous rash, maculopapular rash, skin discoloration, facial edema, acne, alopecia, dermatitis, anal pruritus, genital pruritus, aggravated psoriasis, psoriaform rash, skin disorders, dry skin, urticaria, verruca

Endocrine: antidiuretic hormone disorders, decreased gonadotropins, gynecomastia

(continued on next page)

The information here is provided as guidance only. Prescribers should always consult the manufacturer's current prescribing information.

FOSCARNET (CONTINUED)

SPECIAL PRECAUTIONS *(CONTINUED)*

Local irritation and ulceration of penile epithelium have been reported in male patients probably due to presence of drug in urine (one case of vulvovaginal ulceration has occurred); ensuring adequate hydration and daily personal hygiene are recommended.

Anemia occurred in 33% of patients and was usually manageable with transfusions; discontinuation was required in less than 1% of patients. Granulocytopenia occurred in 17% and neutropenia in only 1%.

Foscarnet has a propensity to chelate divalent metal ions and alter serum levels of electrolytes; patients should be monitored carefully for such changes.

Can be used to treat acyclovir-resistant herpes simplex virus disease and ganciclovir cytomegalovirus retinitis failures.

SPECIAL GROUPS

Children: Safety and efficacy not established.

Elderly: May have age-related renal impairment; special care must be taken to assess renal function prior to therapy and during administration.

Renal impairment: Reduced dosage and continual monitoring necessary (*see* Special Precautions).

Hepatic impairment: No information.

Pregnancy: Adequate human studies not performed; use only if clearly indicated.

Breast-feeding: Not known whether excreted; use with caution.

DOSAGE

(Note: Caution. Do not administer by rapid or bolus intravenous injection. Toxicity may be increased due to excessive plasma levels. Carefully control rate of infusion to avoid unintentional overdose; an infusion pump must be used. Use either a central venous line or peripheral venous line. Standard 24 mg/mL solution may be used undiluted if using a central venous catheter for infusion; if a peripheral vein catheter is used, solution must be diluted to 12 mg/mL with 5% Dextrose in Water or with normal saline solution prior to administration to prevent local irritation of peripheral veins. All doses must be individualized based on renal function. Do not exceed recommended dosage or frequency.)

Adults: The indications for use are cytomegalovirus retinitis in HIV infected individuals and acyclovir resistant HSV and VZV infections. Induction treatment (normal renal function) is 60 mg/kg intravenously at a constant rate over a minimum of 1 hour every 8 hours for 2 to 3 weeks. For maintenance treatment, 90 to 120 mg/kg/d as intravenous infusion over a 2-hour period; 90 mg/kg/d is recommended for most patients beginning maintenance therapy.

Elderly: May have age-related renal impairment; otherwise, same as adults.

Children: No dosage established.

Renal impairment: Use with caution. Reduced plasma clearance results in increased plasma foscarnet levels. Foscarnet has nephrotoxic potential. Studies in patient with creatinine clearance less than 50 mL/min or serum creatinine greater than 2.8 mg/dL have not been performed. Monitor renal function at baseline and during induction and maintenance therapy and adjust dosage accordingly. If creatinine clearance drops below limits of dosing nonograms (0.4 mL/min/kg) during treatment, discontinue foscarnet and monitor patient daily until resolution of renal impairment is established.

(continued on next page)

ADVERSE EFFECTS *(CONTINUED)*

Gastrointestinal: anorexia, nausea, diarrhea, vomiting abdominal pain, constipation, dysphagia, dyspepsia, rectal hemorrhage, dry mouth, melena, flatulence, ulcerative stomatitis, pancreatitis, enteritis, enterocolitis, glossitis, proctitis, stomatitis, tenesmus, increased amylase, pseudomembranous colitis, gastroenteritis, oral leukoplakia, oral hemorrhage, rectal disorders, colitis, duodenal ulcer, hematemesis, paralytic ileus, esophageal ulceration, ulcerative proctitis, tongue ulceration

Hematologic: anemia, granulocytopenia, leukopenia, thrombocytopenia, platelet abnormalities, thrombosis, leukocyte cell abnormalities, lymphadenopathy, pulmonary embolism, coagulation disorders, decreased coagulation factors, epistaxis, decreased prothrombin, hypochromic anemia, pancytopenia, hemolysis, leukocytosis, cervical lymphadenopathy, lymphopenia

Hepatic or biliary: abnormal A-G ratio, abnormal hepatic function, increased AST and ALT, cholecystitis, cholelithiasis, hepatitis, cholestatic hepatitis, hepatosplenomegaly, jaundice

Metabolic: mineral or electrolyte imbalances (including hypokalemia, hypocalcemia, hypomagnesemia, hypo- or hyperphosphatemia), hyponatremia, decreased weight, increased alkaline phosphatase, lactic acid dehydronase, and blood urea nitrogen, acidosis, cachexia, thirst, hypercalcemia, dehydration, glycosuria, increased creatinine phosphokinase, diabetes mellitus, abnormal glucose tolerance, hypervolemia, hypochloremia, periorbital edema, hypoproteinemia

Musculoskeletal: arthralgia, myalgia, arthrosis, synovitis, torticollis

Neoplasms: lymphoma-like disorder, sarcoma, malignant lymphoma, skin hypertrophy

Psychiatric: depression, confusion, anxiety, insomnia, somnolence, nervousness, amnesia, agitation, aggressive reaction, hallucination, impaired concentration, emotional lability, psychosis, suicide attempts, delirium, personality disorders, sleep disorders

Reproductive: perineal pain in women, penile inflammation

Respiratory: coughing, dyspnea, pneumonia, sinusitis, pharyngitis, rhinitis, respiratory disorders or insufficiency, pulmonary infiltration, stridor, pneumothorax, hemoptysis, bronchospasm, bronchitis, laryngitis, respiratory depression, abnormal chest roentgenogram, pleural effusion, pulmonary hemorrhage, pneumonitis

Special senses: vision abnormalities, taste perversions, eye abnormalities, eye pain, conjunctivitis, diplopia, blindness, retinal detachment, mydriasis, photophobia, deafness, ear ache, tinnitus, otitis

Genitourinary: alterations in renal function (including serum creatinine, decreased creatinine clearance, and abnormal renal function), albuminuria, dysuria, polyuria, urethral disorder, urinary retention, urinary tract infection, acute renal failure, nocturia, hematuria, glomerulonephritis, micturition disorders or frequency, toxic nephropathy, nephrosis, urinary incontinence, renal tubular disorders, pyelonephritis, urethral irritation, uremia

The information here is provided as guidance only. Prescribers should always consult the manufacturer's current prescribing information.

FOSCARNET (CONTINUED)

DOSAGE (CONTINUED)

Use the following guideline when dosing; actual 24-hour creatinine clearance (mL/min) must be divided by body weight (kg), or estimated creatinine clearance in mL/min/kg may be calculated from serum creatinine using the formula:

Males: $\dfrac{140 - \text{age}}{\text{Serum creatinine} \times 72 + \text{creatinine clearance}}$

Females: $0.85 \times$ above value

Foscarnet Dosing Guidelines With Renal Impairment

Creatinine clearance, mL/min/kg	Equivalent to 60 mg/kg dose every 8 h
1.6 or > 1.6	60
1.5	57
1.4	53
1.3	49
1.2	46
1.1	42
1.0	39
0.9	35
0.8	32
0.7	28
0.6	25
0.5	21
0.4	18

Maintenance Dosing for Foscarnet

Creatinine clearance, mL/min/kg	Equivalent to 90 mg/kg dose every 24 h	Equivalent to 120 mg/kg dose every 24 h
1.4 or > 1.4	90	120
1.2–1.4	78	104
1.0–1.2	75	100
0.8–1.0	71	94
0.6–0.8	63	84
0.4–0.6	57	76

(Note: Other drugs and supplements may be administered to a patient receiving foscarnet; however, care should be taken to administer foscarnet with normal saline or 5% Dextrose Solution only and to avoid administering other drugs or supplements concurrently using the same catheter. Foscarnet is chemically incompatible with 30% dextrose, amphotericin B, and solutions containing calcium, such as Lactated Ringer's and total parental nutrition; it is physically incompatible with acyclovir sodium, ganciclovir, trimetrexate, pentamidine, vancomycin, trimethroprim-sulfamethoxazole, diazepam, midazolam, digoxin, phenytoin, leucovorin, and prochlorperazine.)

PHARMACOKINETICS AND PHARMACODYNAMICS

Peak serum levels: 573 μm 0.9 to 2.4 h after start of infusion of 57 mg/kg every 8-h dose
Serum half-life: 3 h (normal renal function) on days 1 and 3 of therapy (may be underestimated due to limited observation period)
Bioavailability: no percentage given; variable penetration into cerebrospinal fluid observed
Protein binding: 14% to 17%
Metabolism: no information
Excretion: in urine, 80% to 90% unchanged; by glomerular filtration and tubular secretion
Renal impairment: significantly prolongs half-life and increases plasma levels
Hepatic impairment: no information

OVERDOSAGE

In clinical trials, overdosage has been reported in 10 patients; all had adverse effects and all but one recovered completely. One patient died after receiving a total daily dose of 12.5 g for 3 days rather than the intended 10.9 g. The patient experienced a grand mal seizure, became comatose, and died several days later (cause of death listed as respiratory-cardiac arrest). No specific antidote exists. Hemodialysis and hydration may be of benefit but have not been evaluated in clinical trials. Patient should be observed carefully for signs of renal impairment and electrolyte imbalance and should be treated symptomatically.

PATIENT INFORMATION

Because foscarnet is not a cure for cytomegalovirus retinitis, progression of condition may occur during or following treatment.
Regular ophthalmic examinations are necessary, as is close monitoring. Primary toxicities include renal impairment, electrolyte changes, and seizures; dosage adjustments or discontinuation of therapy may become necessary.
Adequate hydration may minimize potential for renal impairment.

AVAILABILITY

Injection—24 mg/mL

The information here is provided as guidance only. Prescribers should always consult the manufacturer's current prescribing information.

GANCICLOVIR (Cytovene®)

Ganciclovir is an acyclic nucleoside analogue licensed for the treatment of cytomegalovirus disease in the immunocompromised host, particularly cytomegalovirus retinitis in HIV-infected individuals and cytomegalovirus infections in high-risk organ transplant recipients. As shown in Fig. 12-5, this compound has two hydroxyl groups on the ribose ring. As a consequence, the 3′ hydroxyl group provides a site for phosphorylation, potentially resulting in significant toxicity. This drug is not an obligate DNA chain terminator. Myelosuppression is the principal dose-limiting toxicity.

This compound has routinely been used as first-line therapy for the treatment of cytomegalovirus retinitis, although some centers use foscarnet for initial induction therapy. Therapy is associated with induction of quiescence of lesions in a majority of patients; however, only for finite periods of time. The drug also has been used as preemptive therapy for cytomegalovirus disease in organ transplant recipients. Disease rates are decreased, but survival is not enhanced. Recent clinical trials have used this medication for oral maintenance therapy for cytomegalovirus retinitis and in prophylactic studies to prevent disease occurrence.

Ganciclovir sodium is an antiviral agent available for parenteral use.

FIGURE 12-5.
The chemical structure of ganciclovir.

MICROBIOLOGY

Active against cytomegalovirus and all other herpesviruses *in vitro* as well; however, clinical use is restrictive to cytomegalovirus disease.

SPECIAL PRECAUTIONS

Safety and efficacy not established for use as treatment for congenital or neonatal cytomegalovirus disease nor for the treatment of cytomegalovirus disease other than retinitis.

Granulocytopenia occurs in approximately 40% of patients with immunodeficiency who receive intravenous ganciclovir. Use with caution in patients with preexisting cytopenias or with histories of cytopenic reactions to other therapies.

Retinal detachment and hemorrhage have occurred both before and after initiation of ganciclovir therapy; association is unknown. Frequent ophthalmic examinations are recommended.

Renal function should be carefully monitored during therapy, especially in patients receiving concomitant agents with nephrotoxic potential.

Doses and infusion rates greater than those recommended most likely will result in increased toxicity.

Phlebitis and pain at injection site are a frequent occurrence; infuse ganciclovir solutions into veins with adequate blood flow only to allow rapid dilution and distribution.

Administration of intravenous infusion should be accompanied by adequate hydration to ensure adequate renal function and normal clearance.

(continued on next page)

INDICATIONS

Treatment of cytomegalovirus retinitis in patients with immunodeficiency, including those with AIDS.

Prevention in transplant patients at risk for cytomegalovirus disease.

Unlabeled: May be useful in treatment of other cytomegalovirus infections in immunocompromised patients, such as pneumonitis, gastroenteritis, or hepatitis.

Oral formulation is under investigation for prophylactic and maintenance therapy. A new drug application is pending review at the Food and Drug Administration.

CONTRAINDICATIONS

Allergy or hypersensitivity to ganciclovir or acyclovir

INTERACTIONS

Cytotoxic agents, imipenem-cilastatin, nephrotoxic agents, probenecid, zidovudine

ADVERSE EFFECTS

Cardiovascular: arrhythmia, hypertension, hypotension
Central nervous system: headache, confusion, abnormal thoughts or dreams, ataxia, coma, dizziness, nervousness, paresthesia, psychosis, somnolence, tremor
Dermatologic: rash, alopecia, pruritus, urticaria
Gastrointestinal: nausea, vomiting, anorexia, diarrhea, hemorrhage, abdominal pain
Genitourinary: hematuria, increased serum creatinine
Hematologic: granulocytopenia, thrombocytopenia* (can occur in up to 40% of patients)
Injection site: inflammation, pain, phlebitis
Laboratory test abnormalities: abnormal liver function values, decreased blood glucose
Miscellaneous: sepsis, fever, chills, edema, infection, malaise, dyspnea, retinal detachment

*Withdrawal of ganciclovir resulted in increased neutrophil-platelet counts in most cases. Although granulocytopenia was reversible in most cases with discontinuation of treatment, irreversible neutropenia occurred in some patients and caused deaths due to severe bacteriologic or fungal infections during neutropenic episodes.

PHARMACOKINETICS AND PHARMACODYNAMICS

Peak serum levels: 8.3 μg/mL after 1-h infusion of 5 mg/kg dose
Serum half-life: 2.9 h
Bioavailability: no percentage given; limited data
Protein binding: 1% to 2%
Metabolism: no information
Excretion: renal, by glomerular filtration; 90% recovered unmetabolized in urine
Renal impairment: excretion significantly reduced
Hepatic impairment: no information

The information here is provided as guidance only. Prescribers should always consult the manufacturer's current prescribing information.

GANCICLOVIR (CONTINUED)

SPECIAL PRECAUTIONS (CONTINUED)

Neutrophil and platelet counts should be performed every 2 days during twice-daily dosing regimens and at least once per week thereafter. Daily monitoring is required in patients who have had previous leukopenia from other nucleoside analogues or in whom neutrophil counts are less than $1000/mm^3$ at start of therapy.

Serum creatinine or creatinine clearance should be monitored a minimum of once every 2 weeks; patients with renal impairment require modified dosage.

SPECIAL GROUPS

Children: Safety and efficacy not established.

Elderly: May have age-related renal impairment; assessment of renal status before and during therapy is necessary.

Renal impairment: Modified dosage necessary.

Hepatic impairment: No information.

Pregnancy: Adequate human studies not performed; animal tests indicate potential for harm to fetus. Use only if benefits outweigh risk.

Breast-feeding: Not known whether excreted. Because of the potential for serious adverse effects in the infant, do not nurse while receiving ganciclovir. Do not resume nursing until at least 72 hours after last dose.

DOSAGE

(Note: Administer intravenously only. Administration by intramuscular or subcutaneous routes may cause severe tissue irritation due to high pH of agent. Do not administer by rapid or bolus intravenous injection; risk of toxicity may be increased due to excessive plasma levels.)

Adults: For induction treatment of cytomegalovirus retinitis, 5 mg/kg intravenous (at a constant infusion rate of 1 hour) every 12 hours for 14 to 21 days. For maintenance, 5 mg/kg intravenous once daily (at a constant infusion rate of 1 hour) for 7 days each week or 6 mg/kg once daily for 5 days each week. For prophylaxis of disease in transplant recipients, initial dose is 5 mg/kg once daily for 7 days each week or 6 mg/kg once daily for 5 days each week; duration depends on degree of immunosuppression.

Elderly: May have age-related renal impairment; adequate assessment of renal status must be made before treatment is initiated.

Children: Safety and efficacy not established.

Renal impairment: Adjust dosage based on the following guidelines:

Ganciclovir Dosing Guidelines With Renal Impairments

Creatinine clearance, mL/min/1.73m^2	Dose, mg/kg	Interval, h
80 or > 80	5.0	12
50–79	2.5	12
25–49	2.5	24
< 25	1.25	24

Creatinine clearance may be related to serum creatinine by using the following formula:

$$\text{Males:} \quad \frac{\text{Weight (kg)} \times (140 - \text{age})}{72 \times \text{serum creatinine (mg/dL)} \times 1.73/\text{body surface area (m}^2)}$$

Females: $0.85 \times$ above value

(Note: Optimal maintenance dose for patients with renal impairment is not known. Dosage may be reduced to 50% of induction dose and the patient monitored for disease progression. For patients undergoing hemodialysis [limited data available], do not exceed 1.25 mg/kg/24 h; on days when hemodialysis is performed, administration should be instituted soon after hemodialysis session ends. Neutrophil and platelet counts should be monitored daily.)

OVERDOSAGE

Data from overdosage in 11 patients showed no adverse effects in three of the patients, reversible neutropenia in three patients (one with a history of bone marrow suppression), irreversible pancytopenia and abdominal pain in one patient, and worsening of hematuria in one patient with preexisting hematuria and renal impairment.

Treatment may include hydration and hemodialysis to reduce drug plasma levels. Hemodialysis may reduce plasma levels by approximately 50%.

PATIENT INFORMATION

Because ganciclovir is not a cure for cytomegalovirus, progression of retinitis may occur during or following treatment. Regular ophthalmic examinations (every 6 weeks) are recommended.

Monitoring of blood counts is extremely important during therapy; granulocytopenia and thrombocytopenia are major toxicities of ganciclovir. Adjustments in dosage or discontinuation may be necessary.

Zidovudine is used commonly in patients with AIDS, and concomitant use with ganciclovir may result in severe granulocytopenia.

Ganciclovir produced decreased sperm production in animals and therefore may cause infertility in humans. The drug has caused birth defects in animals and should not be used by women of childbearing potential; likewise, men should practice barrier contraception during therapy and for 90 days thereafter.

Transplant recipients should know of the high incidence of renal impairment, especially in patients receiving concomitant nephrotoxic agents (*eg*, cyclosporine and amphotericin B).

AVAILABILITY

Powder for injection (lyophilized)—500 mg/vial

The information here is provided as guidance only. Prescribers should always consult the manufacturer's current prescribing information.

IDOXURIDINE (Stoxil®)

Idoxuridine was the first of the nucleoside analogues licensed for the treatment of viral disease. Synthesized by Dr. William Prusoff and subsequently evaluated by Dr. Herbert Kaufman, the compound was proven efficacious for the treatment of herpes simplex keratoconjunctivitis in the early 1960s. Now, over 30 years later, the compound still has a place in the armamentarium of physicians who manage herpetic eye disease. As indicated in Fig. 12-6, idoxuridine is a thymidine analogue. As a consequence, it substitutes for thymidine in DNA synthesis. The resulting DNA is fragile and shears, accounting for the compound's mechanism of action.

Idoxuridine is an antiviral agent exclusively for ophthalmic use.

FIGURE 12-6.
The chemical structure of idoxuridine.

MICROBIOLOGY

Idoxuridine blocks replication of herpes simplex by altering normal DNA synthesis.

SPECIAL PRECAUTIONS

Sensitization may occur; however, it tends to be more common in dermal rather than ophthalmic areas.

Idoxuridine should be considered potentially carcinogenic, although data are limited. Resistance can occur in some strains of herpes; if no response is demonstrated in epithelial infections after 14 days, other forms of therapy should be considered. Continuation of medication for 5 to 7 days after epithelial lesion is healed is necessary to prevent recurrence.

SPECIAL GROUPS

Children: No information.
Elderly: No information.
Renal impairment: No information.
Hepatic impairment: No information.
Pregnancy: Ophthalmic application produced fetal malformations in rabbits; use with caution in women of childbearing potential.
Breast-feeding: Not known whether absorbed after eye application and excreted; do not use when nursing.

DOSAGE

(Note: For best results, infected tissue should be kept saturated with idoxuridine. Continue therapy at latter dosage for 5 to 7 days after healing appears complete to minimize risk of recurrence.)

(continued on next page)

INDICATIONS

Treatment of herpes simplex keratitis; should be prescribed under the care of an ophthalmologist (Note: Epithelial infections [especially initial] respond better than stromal infections. Recurrences are common, and although idoxuridine will control the infection, it will have no effect on scarring, vascularization, or resultant progressive loss of vision.)

CONTRAINDICATIONS

Allergy or hypersensitivity to idoxuridine or any preparation components.
(Note: Because herpes infects and destroys nerves, a sterile trophic ulcer may occur and may not heal with continued idoxuridine therapy. Discontinuation of therapy is often required to stop epithelial toxicity and allow for healing.)

INTERACTIONS

Boric acid–containing solutions

ADVERSE EFFECTS

Irritation, pain, pruritus, inflammation, edema, allergic reactions, photophobia, corneal clouding, stippling, punctate defects in corneal epithelium, follicular conjunctivitis (prolonged use), punctal occlusion (prolonged use), conjunctival scarring (prolonged use), squamous cell carcinoma

PHARMACOKINETICS AND PHARMACODYNAMICS

Not given parenterally

OVERDOSAGE

Local overdosage due to too frequent administration may cause small defects (pseudodendrites) on epithelium of the cornea. If such effects occur, discontinue therapy either temporarily or permanently as indicated by careful observation of the progress of the infection. Systemic overdosage would require a quantity many times greater than that found in the commercial bottle or tube.

PATIENT INFORMATION

Sensitivity to bright light may occur and can be minimized by wearing sunglasses. If no improvement is noted in 7 to 8 days, if condition worsens, or if adverse effects (pain, decreased vision, itching or swelling of eye) occur, contact physician.

AVAILABILITY

Ophthalmic solution—0.1% in 15-mL dropper bottles
Ophthalmic ointment—0.5% (petroleum base) in 4-g tube

The information here is provided as guidance only. Prescribers should always consult the manufacturer's current prescribing information.

IDOXURIDINE (CONTINUED)

DOSAGE (CONTINUED)

Adults: For solution, initially place one drop into each eye every hour during the day and every 2 hours in the evening, continuing until improvement occurs (lack of staining with fluorescein). Dosage is then reduced to one drop every 2 hours during the day and one drop every 4 hours in the evening.

For ointment, place inside of infected conjunctival sac using five instillations per day every 4 hours, with last dose at bedtime.

Concomitant therapy with topical corticosteroids may be used in management of herpes simplex with stromal lesions, corneal edema, or iritis; antibiotics may be used to control secondary infections, and atropine also may be used adjunctively if necessary.
Elderly: Same as adults.
Children: No special dosage given.
Renal impairment: No information.

INTERFERON ALFA (Intron®, Roferon-A®)

Interferon alfa is a small–molecular weight glycoprotein, currently licensed for the treatment of chronic hepatitis B, chronic hepatitis C, and human papillomavirus infections (anogential warts). Studies of interferon alfa (2a or 2b) indicate clinical benefit, albeit limited in duration and not without frequent relapse.

Administration of interferon alfa is associated with a high incidence of adverse clinical events. Tachyphylaxis, which subsequently develops, leads to amelioration of clinical symptomatology.

Interferon alfa is licensed for the treatment of condyloma acuminatum, hepatitis B, and hepatitis C. This agent is under investigational use as a cytokine type to be used in combination with zalcitabine for non-AIDS HIV infection; one formulation is currently classified as being in Food and Drug Administration status phase II/III under the name of *Wellferon* (Burroughs Wellcome, Research Triangle Park, NC). Additionally, Interferon alfa-NL, an orphan drug under the same trade name and sponsor, has proposed use for treatment of AIDS-related Kaposi's sarcoma and human papillomavirus in severe recurrent or resistant respiratory (laryngeal) papillomatosis. Further data are not yet publicly available for either of these uses. Interferon alfa-2a and interferon alfa-2b are presently marketed as antineoplastic agents and, although their (unlabeled) indications listed here are found in the sources, no dosage or other information is published for other uses (*eg*, antiviral).

MICROBIOLOGY

Interferon alfa is broadly capable of inhibiting replication of both RNA and DNA viruses *in vitro*.

SPECIAL PRECAUTIONS

Associated with flulike symptoms until tachyphylaxis develops.

SPECIAL GROUPS

Children: Only used for juvenile laryngeal papillomatosis.
Elderly: No information.
Renal impairment: No information.
Hepatic impairment: No information.
Pregnancy: No information.
Breast-feeding: No information.

DOSAGE

Adults: Three to 6 MU three times weekly to daily for 4 months.
Elderly: No information.
Children: As above.
Renal impairment: No information.

INDICATIONS

For interferon alfa-2a/2b (unlabeled): Chronic non-A, non-B hepatitis, cutaneous warts, herpes simplex, rhinoviruses, vaccinia virus, varicella-zoster, hepatitis B and hepatitis C, multiple sclerosis
Labeled: Condyloma acuminatum

CONTRAINDICATIONS

Allergy or hypersensitivity to interferon or any product components

INTERACTIONS

Aminophylline

ADVERSE EFFECTS

Fever, malaise, chills, flulike symptoms until tachypylois develops pain at injection site. With high dose: neutropenia, bone marrow suppression, fatigue, neurotoxicity, and possible cardiotoxicity.

PHARMACOKINETICS AND PHARMACODYNAMICS

Peak serum levels: no information
Serum half-life: no information
Bioavailability: no information
Protein binding: no information
Metabolism: no information
Excretion: no information
Renal impairment: no information
Hepatic impairment: no information

OVERDOSAGE

No information

PATIENT INFORMATION

Do not change brands of interferon because it may result in alteration of dosage.
Use administration technique as directed by physician.
Drink plenty of fluids, especially at beginning of therapy.

AVAILABILITY

Injection solution—3 and 6 million IU/mL in 1-mL vials
Injection solution—36 million IU/mL in 1-mL vials
Powder for injection—6 million IU/mL (reconstituted)

The information here is provided as guidance only. Prescribers should always consult the manufacturer's current prescribing information.

RIBAVIRIN (Virazole®)

Ribavirin is the only licensed drug for the treatment of respiratory syncytial virus (RSV) infections in high-risk infants. The compound is a nucleoside analogue, as illustrated in Fig. 12-7. Ribavirin is administered as an aerosol to babies with proven (immunofluorescence staining of nasopharyngeal cells with monoclonal antibodies) teratogenicity RSV infection. Because of concern for potential toxicity of free ribavirin in the air, a scavenger system must be employed to retrieve ribavirin administered to the patient. Systemic use is associated with myelosuppression.

Ribavirin is an antiviral agent that is administered by aerosol; however, oral and intravenous formulations exist for compassionate plea therapies (*eg*, lassa fever and hantavirus disease).

FIGURE 12-7.
The chemical structure of ribavirin.

INDICATIONS
Treatment of especially selected hospitalized infants and young children with severe lower respiratory tract infection due to RSV. (Presence of underlying conditions such as prematurity or cardiopulmonary disease may increase the severity of the infection and its risk to the patient. High-risk infants and young children with such conditions may benefit from treatment. Treatment with ribavirin aerosol must be accompanied by, and does not replace, standard supportive respiratory and fluid management.)

CONTRAINDICATIONS
Women of childbearing age or women who are pregnant

INTERACTIONS
None known

ADVERSE EFFECTS
Cardiovascular: cardiac arrest, hypotension, digitalis toxicity
Hematologic: anemia has not been reported with use of aerosol but occurs frequently with oral and intravenous ribavirin; most infants treated with aerosol are not evaluated 1 to 2 weeks after treatment when anemia is most likely to occur; reticulocytosis has been reported with oral use
Pulmonary: worsening of respiratory status, bacterial pneumonia, pneumothorax, apnea, ventilator dependence
Miscellaneous: rash, conjunctivitis

PHARMACOKINETICS AND PHARMACODYNAMICS
Peak serum levels: range after 3 days of therapy (2.5 h per day) was 0.44 to 1.55 µg/mL
Serum half-life: 9.5 h
Bioavailability: unknown (may depend on route of aerosol administration)
Protein binding: no information
Metabolism: no information
Excretion: no information
Renal impairment: no information
Hepatic impairment: no information

MICROBIOLOGY
Ribavirin *in vitro* inhibits RSV, influenza virus, and herpes simplex virus, among many other viruses.

SPECIAL PRECAUTIONS
Can be used in infants who require assisted ventilation.
Chronic obstructive lung disease or asthma increases risk for possible deterioration of respiratory function associated with ribavirin use. Respiratory function should be monitored carefully during treatment. If sudden deterioration occurs, stop treatment. Reinstitute with extreme caution only while monitoring continuously.
Ribavirin has had toxic effects in animals, producing cardiac lesions in mice and monkeys and inflammatory changes in the lungs of developing ferrets. Significance of these effects to human dosing is unknown.
Carcinogenicity *in vivo* studies are incomplete; however, ribavirin produces cell transformation *in vitro* in mammalian systems and has produced benign tumors in rats.
Patients with lower respiratory tract infections due to RSV must have optimum monitoring of respiratory and fluid status.
Testicular lesions (tubular atrophy) have occurred in adult rats at oral dose levels as low as 16 mg/kg/d; effect on fertility is unknown.

The information here is provided as guidance only. Prescribers should always consult the manufacturer's current prescribing information.

RIBAVIRIN (CONTINUED)

SPECIAL GROUPS

Children: Can be used in children with severe, confirmed RSV infection.
Elderly: No information.
Renal impairment: No information.
Hepatic impairment: No information.
Pregnancy: Contraindicated.
Breast-feeding: Not indicated for use in nursing mothers because RSV infection is self-limiting in this population. However, ribavirin is toxic to lactating animals and their offspring, and it is unknown whether the drug is excreted in human breast milk.

DOSAGE

(Note: For aerosol use only. Effective when instituted within the first 3 days of RSV lower respiratory tract infection.)
Adults: *See* child dosage information below.
Elderly: No information.
Children: Treatment is continued for 12 to 18 hours per day for a minimum of 3 days and a maximum of 7. Aerosol is delivered to an infant oxygen hood via the SPAG-2 aerosol generator. Salvage of aerosolized drug is mandatory. Do not administer ribavirin with any other aerosol generating device or with other aerosolized medications. Solubilize drug with sterile USP water for injection or inhalation in the 100-mL vial.

Transfer to clean, sterilized 500-mL wide-mouth Erlenmeyer flask (SPAG-2 Reservoir) and further dilute to final volume of 300 mL with sterile USP water for injection or inhalation. Final concentration should be 20 mg/mL.

(Note: It is of extreme importance that the water used does not have any anti-microbial agent or other substance added. Solutions in the SPAG-2 unit should be discarded at least every 24 hours and whenever the liquid level is low before adding freshly reconstituted solution. The average aerosol concentration for a 12-hour period is 190 μg/L of air.)
Renal impairment: No information.

OVERDOSAGE

No information

PATIENT INFORMATION

No information

AVAILABILITY

Powder for reconstitution for aerosol—6 g powder per 100-mL vial

---

The information here is provided as guidance only. Prescribers should always consult the manufacturer's current prescribing information.

RIMANTADINE (Flumadine®)

Rimantadine was the second compound licensed for prevention and treatment of influenza A infections. The structure of rimantadine is shown in Fig. 12-8. This drug is preferred to amantadine because of a lower incidence of adverse clinical events. Resistant variants have been recovered from 30% of treated children and adults by the 5th day of therapy. Apparent transmission of these variants has led to failure of prophylaxis.

Rimantadine is an antiviral agent that is structurally related to amantadine.

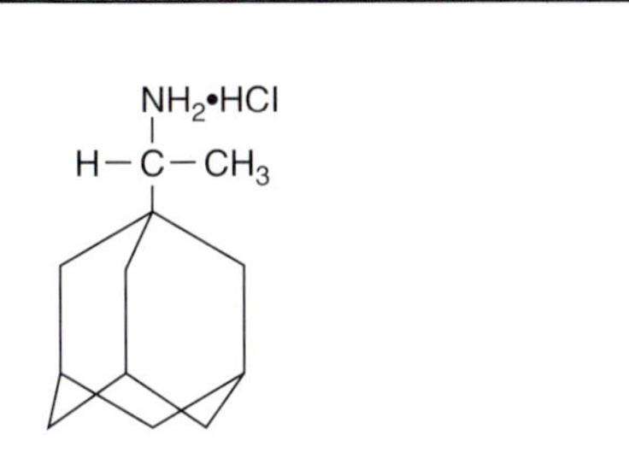

FIGURE 12-8.
The chemical structure of rimantadine.

MICROBIOLOGY

Inhibits replication of all human subtypes of influenza virus (H1N1, H2N2, and H3N2).

SPECIAL PRECAUTIONS

Rimantadine is less toxic than amantadine for prophylaxis and treatment of influenza.

SPECIAL GROUPS

Children: Safer than amantadine.
Elderly: May be more sensitive to effects of drug.
Renal impairment: No information.
Hepatic impairment: Reduced dosage not necessary in less-severe impairment.
Pregnancy: No information.
Breast-feeding: No information.

DOSAGE

Adults: 100 mg twice daily.
Elderly: 100 mg once daily in elderly nursing home patients.
Children: (9 years of age or younger): 5 mg/kg/d in one or two divided doses given orally (not to exceed 150 mg/d); (older children weighing 40 kg or more): 200 mg/d in one or two divided doses; (children older than 9 years but weighing less than 40 kg): 5 mg/kg/d in one or two divided doses.
Renal impairment: Dosage should be reduced if creatinine clearance $\leq$ 10 mL/min.

INDICATIONS

Treatment and prophylaxis of infections caused by influenza A viruses

CONTRAINDICATIONS

No information

INTERACTIONS

No information

ADVERSE EFFECTS

Nervousness, lightheadedness, difficulty in concentration, sleep disturbances, fatigue, vomiting, diarrhea, headache

PHARMACOKINETICS AND PHARMACODYNAMICS

Peak serum levels: no values given; 3 to 6 h after oral administration
Serum half-life: 33 h
Bioavailability: unobtainable due to lack of intravenous form of drug
Protein binding: 40%
Metabolism: in liver; three metabolites (ortho-, para-, and metahydroxylated forms)
Excretion: in urine, less than 1% of parent compound unchanged
Renal impairment: no information
Hepatic impairment: dosage reduction not necessary in less-severe forms of disease

OVERDOSAGE

No information

PATIENT INFORMATION

No information

AVAILABILITY

Recommended for approval October 27, 1987 as *Flumadine* by Forest
Approved 1993, commercially available

The information here is provided as guidance only. Prescribers should always consult the manufacturer's current prescribing information.

TRIFLURIDINE (Viroptic®)

Trifluridine is the treatment of choice for herpes simplex keratoconjunctivitis. The structure of triflurothymidine is illustrated in Fig. 12-9. Currently, frequent administration to the eye is required for control of herpes simplex infections at this site. Nevertheless, clinical efficacy appears to be satisfactory for the management of this disease. The compound is under evaluation for topical treatment of acyclovir-resistant genital herpetic infection in individuals with HIV infection.

Trifluridine is a fluorinated pyrimidine nucleoside exclusively for ophthalmic use.

FIGURE 12-9.
The chemical structure of trifluridine.

MICROBIOLOGY

Active *in vitro* and *in vivo* against herpes simplex virus types 1 and 2; also shows some activity against some strains of adenovirus *in vitro*.

SPECIAL PRECAUTIONS

Do not exceed recommended dosage or frequency.

Mutagenic activity (as well as DNA-damaging and cell-transforming activity) has been observed with trifluridine in various standard *in vitro* test systems. The significance of these findings is not known; however, the potential exists for mutagenic agents to cause damage in humans.

Cross-sensitivity with idoxuridine and trifluridine is rare despite structural similarities.

Transient, mild local irritation of conjunctiva and cornea may occur with use.

Possibility for viral resistance exists; no reports have been made following multiple exposure to trifluridine, but resistance has been documented *in vitro*.

Normal eye can hold approximately 10 μL of fluid, adjusted for effect of blinking, and the average dropper delivers 25 to 50 μL/drop. The value of using more than one drop per dose is questionable.

Compress lacrimal sac for 3 to 5 minutes following placement of drops to minimize systemic absorption.

Topical anesthesia will increase bioavailability of ophthalmic drugs by decreasing blink reflex and production of tears.

SPECIAL GROUPS

Children: No information, especially for the newborn.
Elderly: May have lax eyelids, which may lead to increased retention or absorption.
Renal impairment: No information.
Hepatic impairment: No information.
Pregnancy: Safety not established; use only when clearly indicated and when benefits outweigh risk.
Breast-feeding: Do not prescribe unless benefits outweigh risk.

INDICATIONS

Treatment of primary keratoconjunctivitis and recurrent epithelial keratitis due to herpes simplex virus types 1 and 2. Also used for treatment of epithelial keratitis unresponsive to topical idoxuridine or in cases of ocular toxicity or hypersensitivity to idoxuridine. Trifluridine also has been effective in a small number of patients resistant to topical vidarabine.

CONTRAINDICATIONS

Allergy or hypersensitivity to trifluridine

INTERACTIONS

No information

ADVERSE EFFECTS

Burning or stinging with application, palpebral edema, superficial punctate keratopathy, epithelial keratopathy, hypersensitivity reaction, stromal edema, irritation, keratitis sicca, hyperemia, increased intraocular pressure

PHARMACOKINETICS AND PHARMACODYNAMICS

Not given parenterally

OVERDOSAGE

Overdose from topical application is unlikely; ingestion of entire contents of bottle will most likely result in no adverse effects

PATIENT INFORMATION

Do not discontinue use without advising physician. Stinging may occur momentarily during application. If improvement does not occur within 7 days, if condition gets worse, or if irritation occurs, contact physician.

AVAILABILITY

Ophthalmic solution—1%

The information here is provided as guidance only. Prescribers should always consult the manufacturer's current prescribing information.

TRIFLURIDINE (CONTINUED)

DOSAGE

Adults: Place one drop onto cornea of affected eye every 2 hours during waking hours for maximum of nine drops/d until corneal ulcer has re-epithelialized completely; continue treatment with one drop every 4 hours during waking hours for maximum of five drops/d for 7 additional days. If no improvement occurs after 7 days of treatment or if complete re-epithelialization has not occurred after 14 days of therapy, other forms of treatment should be considered. Periods longer than 21 days should be avoided because of potential for ocular toxicity.

Elderly: No information.

Children: No information.

Renal impairment: No special dosage given.

VIDARABINE (ARABINOSIDE; ARA-A) (Vira-A®)

Vidarabine was the first licensed compound for parenteral administration to patients with life-threatening herpes virus infections (eg, herpes simplex virus [HSV] encephalitis, neonatal HSV infections, and varicella zoster virus [VZV] infections in the immunocompromised host). Its structure is illustrated in Fig. 12-10. The compound is no longer available for intravenous administration; however, the topical formulation remains available for treatment of HSV keratoconjunctivitis. It should be considered a second-line treatment to triflurothymidine.

Vidarabine is a purine nucleoside obtained from fermentation of cultures of *Streptomyces antibioticus*.

FIGURE 12-10.
The chemical structure of vidarabine.

MICROBIOLOGY

Active *in vitro* and *in vivo* against HSV types 1 and 2, and varicella zoster virus.

INDICATIONS

Herpes simplex keratoconjunctivitis

CONTRAINDICATIONS

Allergy or hypersensitivity to vidarabine

INTERACTIONS

Allopurinol

ADVERSE EFFECTS

Central nervous system: tremor, dizziness, headache, hallucinations, confusion, psychosis, ataxia, malaise, fatal metabolic encephalopathy

Gastrointestinal: anorexia, nausea, vomiting, diarrhea; elevated AST and bilirubin, hematemesis

Hematologic: decreased reticulocyte count, hemoglobin, leukocyte hematocrit, leukocyte count, platelet count

Miscellaneous: weight loss, pruritus, rash, pain at injection site

PHARMACOKINETICS AND PHARMACODYNAMICS

Peak serum levels: 0.2 to 0.4 µg/mL after dose of 10 mg/kg; (ara-hx, major metabolite, 3-6 µg/mL)

Serum half-life: 1 h (ara-hx, 3.3 h)

Bioavailability: no information

Protein binding: no information

Metabolism: no route given; major metabolite, arabinosyl hypoxanthine (ara-hx) has approximately 1/10 the activity of vidarabine

Excretion: via kidneys; 41% to 53% recovered in urine

Renal impairment: ara-hx may accumulate

Hepatic impairment: no information

SPECIAL PRECAUTIONS

No data exist to suggest efficacy in treatment of encephalitis due to varicella zoster or vaccinia viruses. Not effective against infections due to adenovirus or RNA viruses, bacteria, or fungi. No data exist to suggest efficacy against cytomegalovirus or smallpox. Early diagnosis and treatment of HSV encephalitis are essential (studies may include cerebrospinal fluid examination and localization of intracerebral lesion by brain scan, electroencephalogram, or computed tomograph; brain biopsy is necessary to confirm etiologic diagnosis by viral isolation in cell cultures or by specific fluorescent antibody techniques).

(continued on next page)

The information here is provided as guidance only. Prescribers should always consult the manufacturer's current prescribing information.

VIDARABINE (ARABINOSIDE; ARA-A) (CONTINUED)

SPECIAL PRECAUTIONS (CONTINUED)

Evidence of neurologic abnormalities at 1 year of age was 44% following vidarabine therapy in infants treated for localized central nervous system infection and 67% of those treated for disseminated infection.

Patients with renal function impairment may have slower rate of excretion of major metabolite of vidarabine (ara-hx) and may require dosage adjustment.

Patients with hepatic impairment should be observed for possible adverse effects.

Carcinogenesis (liver tumors, kidney neoplasia) has occurred in rodents treated with vidarabine. Hepatic megalocytosis also has been found in rodent studies but has not yet been clearly understood as preneoplastic change.

Vidarabine *in vivo* may produce mutagenic effects in male germ cells and can incorporate into mammalian DNA and induce mutation in mammalian cells *in vitro*.

To be effective in treatment of herpes zoster, vidarabine therapy must begin as soon as possible (but no later than 72 hours) after vesicular lesions appear.

Vidarabine is relatively insoluble and therefore often requires large amounts of fluid during administration. Use caution in patients susceptible to fluid overloading or cerebral edema (*ie*, patients with central nervous system infection or impaired renal function).

Hemoglobin, hematocrit, white blood cells, and platelets may be depressed during therapy; appropriate hematologic tests should be performed during administration. (Note: Some degree of immunosuppression must exist for clinical response to occur.)

No longer available as intravenous formulation.

SPECIAL GROUPS

Children: No information.
Elderly: May have age-related renal impairment requiring dosage adjustment.
Renal impairment: May require dosage adjustment.
Hepatic impairment: Observe for possible adverse effects.
Pregnancy: Adequate human studies not performed; teratogenic in small animals and produces maternal toxicity. Use only when benefits outweigh risk.
Breast-feeding: Not known whether excreted. Decision to discontinue nursing or discontinue drug, with consideration of importance of drug to mother, must be made.

DOSAGE

No longer available for parenteral therapy of HSV encephalitis or herpes zoster.

OVERDOSAGE

No serious effects seen after acute massive overdose. Acute fluid overloading has greater potential danger for patient than vidarabine (due to its low solubility). Doses over 20 mg/kg/d may produce bone marrow depression with thrombocytopenia and leukopenia. Monitor hematologic, liver, and renal functions in the event of overdose.

PATIENT INFORMATION

No information

AVAILABILITY

Ophthalmic prep

The information here is provided as guidance only. Prescribers should always consult the manufacturer's current prescribing information.

ZALCITABINE (Hivid®)

Zalcitabine, as illustrated in Fig. 12-11, is a dideoxynucleoside analogue licensed for the treatment of HIV infection. Currently, it is used in combination with zidovudine for patients with advanced AIDS. The structure of zalcitabine indicates that the compound requires phosphorylation in order to function as a reverse transcriptase inhibitor. Potential toxicity of the compound has limited its routine deployment. The drug is not currently licensed as monotherapy for HIV infection.

Zalcitabine is a synthetic pyrimidine nucleoside analogue of the naturally occurring nucleoside 2'-hydroxyl group is replaced by hydrogen. The full safety and efficacy profile for zalcitabine, alone or in combination with zidovudine, has yet to be completely defined, especially for prolonged use and in patients with less-advanced HIV disease.

Zalcitabine in combination with zidovudine may be used for the see treatment of adult patients with advanced HIV infection (CD4 cell count $\leq 300/mm^3$) who have demonstrated significant clinical or immunologic deterioration. This indication is based on very limited data from two small studies in which zidovudine-naive patients with a CD4 cell count of $300/mm^3$ or less who were treated with zalcitabine plus zidovudine had a greater CD4 response than patients treated with zidovudine alone. Neither study included a concurrent control group taking the currently recommended zidovudine dose of 100 mg every 4 hours, and these studies were not designed to measure the clinical efficacy of the combination. No data are available on the combined use of zalcitabine and zidovudine in patients who have previously received zidovudine monotherapy, although controlled studies are ongoing. Results are also unavailable from controlled studies evaluating the effect of combined use on the clinical progression of HIV infection (such as survival or incidence of opportunistic infections).

Because zidovudine prolongs survival and decreases the incidence of opportunistic infections in patients with advanced HIV disease, consider zidovudine as initial therapy for adult patients with HIV infection who have evidence of impaired immunity (CD4 cell counts of $\leq 500/mm^3$).

The major clinical toxicities of zalcitabine are peripheral neuropathy and, much less frequently, pancreatitis. Moderate or severe peripheral neuropathy, which for some patients was clinically disabling, occurred in 17% to 31% of patients treated with zalcitabine monotherapy. It is unknown whether the risk of peripheral neuropathy is increased with combination therapy versus monotherapy. There are no data regarding the use of zalcitabine in patients with preexisting peripheral neuropathy because these patients were excluded from clinical trials; therefore, use with extreme caution in these patients. The occurrence of peripheral neuropathy in patients treated with zalcitabine was greater in patients with more advanced HIV disease (*see* Special Precautions).

Documented fatal pancreatitis has been observed with the administration of zalcitabine alone or in combination with zidovudine. Suspend the use of both agents immediately in patients who develop any symptoms suggestive of pancreatitis until this diagnosis is excluded. Overall, pancreatitis is an uncommon complication of zalcitabine monotherapy, occurring in less than 1% of patients.

Toxicities previously associated with zidovudine monotherapy are likely to occur in patients treated with combined therapy. Refer to the zidovudine product information before using combination therapy.

FIGURE 12-11.
The chemical structure of zalcitabine.

INDICATIONS

For use in combination therapy with zidovudine for treatment of advanced HIV infection in adult patients (CD4 cell count $\leq 300/mm^3$) who have demonstrated significant clinical or immunologic deterioration

CONTRAINDICATIONS

Allergy or hypersensitivity to zalcitabine or any product components

INTERACTIONS

Agents with potential to cause peripheral neuropathy: chloramphenicol, cisplatin, dapsone, didanosine (concurrent therapy not recommended), disulfiram, ethionamide, glutethimide, gold, hydralazine, iodoquinol, isoniazid, metronidazole, nitrofurantoin, phenytoin, ribavirin, vincristine, amphotericin, foscarnet, aminoglycosides

Agents with potential to cause pancreatitis: intravenous pentamidine (Note: If intravenous pentamidine is necessary for treatment of *Pneumocystis carinii* pneumonia, interrupt zalcitabine treatment.)

Drug and food interaction: Absorption is reduced with food by 14% and mean plasma concentrations by 39%.

ADVERSE EFFECTS

Body as a whole: pain, malaise, asthenia, fatigue, pharyngitis, fever, rigors, weight decrease, generalized edema (< 1%)

Cardiovascular: hypertension, palpitation, syncope, chest pain, atrial fibrillation, tachycardia, heart racing (< 1%)

Central or peripheral nervous system: headache, dizziness, seizures, ataxia, abnormal coordination, Bell's palsy, dysphonia, hyperkinesia, hypokinesia, migraine, neuralgia, neuritis, stupor, tremor, vertigo, hypertonia, hand tremor, twitching (< 1%)

Dermatologic: rash (erythematous, maculopapular, follicular) pruritus, night sweats, dermatitis (1.3%), skin lesions, acne, alopecia, bullous eruptions, flushing, increased sweating, urticaria, erythematous papules (< 1%)

Endocrine: diabetes mellitus, hyperglycemia, hypocalcemia, impotence, hot flashes (< 1%)

Gastrointestinal: oral ulcers, nausea, vomiting, constipation, ulcerative stomatitis, aphthous stomatitis, diarrhea, dry mouth, esophageal ulcers (1.6%), dyspepsia, glossitis (1.3%), rectal hemorrhage, hemorrhoids, enlarged abdomen, gum disorders, increased amylase, flatulence, anorexia, stomatitis, tongue ulceration, dysphagis, eructation, gastritis, gastrointestinal hemorrhage, pancreatitis (*see* Special Precautions), left quadrant pain, salivary gland enlargement, jaundice, esophageal pain, esophagitis, rectal ulcers (< 1%)

Hematologic: epistaxis (< 1%)

Hepatic: abnormal hepatic function, hepatitis, jaundice, hepatocellular damage (< 1%)

(Continued on next page)

The information here is provided as guidance only. Prescribers should always consult the manufacturer's current prescribing information.

ZALCITABINE (CONTINUED)

MICROBIOLOGY
Active against HIV.

SPECIAL PRECAUTIONS
Peripheral neuropathy (up to 30% of patients) is the major clinical toxicity of zalcitabine and is initially characterized by numbness and burning dysesthesia in the distal extremities. Sharp shooting pains or severe continuous burning pain may follow if the drug is not withdrawn. This neuropathy may progress to severe pain necessitating narcotic analgesics and is potentially irreversible, particularly if zalcitabine is not discontinued immediately. Symptoms may progress despite cessation of therapy in some patients; however, with prompt discontinuation, neuropathy is usually slowly reversible. Pancreatitis, including fatal pancreatitis, has occurred with zalcitabine monotherapy and with combination therapy with zidovudine. It is an uncommon complication (< 1% of patients). Use caution in patients with histories of pancreatitis or with known risk factors for pancreatitis; monitor such patients closely during therapy. If rising serum amylase levels associated with dysglycemia, rising triglyceride level, decreasing serum calcium, or other parameters or symptoms (nausea, vomiting, abdominal pain) occur, interrupt treatment until a clinical diagnosis can be obtained. Reinstitute zalcitabine only if pancreatitis has been ruled out. If pancreatitis occurs, discontinue drug permanently.

Esophageal ulcers have occurred infrequently, and consideration of suspension of therapy should be made in patients who do not respond to specific treatment of opportunistic pathogens, in order to assess possible relationship to zalcitabine.

Cardiomyopathy or congestive heart failure has occurred in patients with AIDS receiving nucleoside antiretroviral agents, and infrequent cases have occurred in those receiving zalcitabine. Use caution in patients with baseline cardiomyopathy or history of congestive heart failure.

Anaphylactoid reaction has occurred in one instance in a patient receiving combination zalcitabine and zidovudine therapy. Additionally, several reports of urticaria have been made in absence of other anaphylactoid-like symptoms.

Severe adverse effects may be caused by either zalcitabine or zidovudine or to both in combination therapy; thorough consultation with all product information should be performed before reinstitution of either agent alone or in combination after an adverse reaction has occurred.

Renal function impairment presents an increased risk of toxicity due to decreased clearance of drug; a reduction in dosage should be considered.

Hepatic function impairment may be exacerbated by zalcitabine, especially in patients with preexisting liver disease or with a history of alcoholism or abuse. Such patients should be monitored closely, and a reduction or interruption of dosage should be considered if necessary.

Human peripheral blood lymphocytes exposed to zalcitabine, and dose-related (1.5 µg/mL and over) increases in chromosomal aberrations were noted.

ADVERSE EFFECTS *(CONTINUED)*
Laboratory test abnormalities: (Not necessarily in order of frequency, these values varied significantly in occurrence according to duration and history of prior treatment with zidovudine therapy.) anemia, leukopenia, neutropenia, eosinophilia, thrombocytopenia, ALT (>250 U/L), AST (>250 U/L), alkaline phosphatase (>625 U/L)

Musculoskeletal: myalgia, arthralgia, foot pain, arm pain, arthritis, arthropathy, cold feet, leg cramps, myositis, shoulder pain, wrist pain, cold extremities (< 1%)

Psychiatric: confusion, impaired concentration (1.3%), insomnia, agitation, depersonalization, hallucination, emotional lability, nervousness, anxiety, depression, euphoria, manic reaction, dementia, amnesia, somnolence, abnormal thinking (< 1%)

Special senses: abnormal vision, ear blockage, parosmia, loss of taste, taste perversion, burning or itching eyes, deafness, xerophthalmia, eye pain or abnormality, tinnitus (< 1%)

Urinary: gout, toxic nephropathy, polyuria, renal calculus, acute renal failure, hyperuricemia, micturition frequency, abnormal renal function, renal cyst (< 1%)

PHARMACOKINETICS AND PHARMACODYNAMICS
Peak serum levels: 25.2 ng/mL after a 1.5-mg oral dose (reduced significantly with food)

Serum half-life: 1 to 3 h

Bioavailability: > 80%

Protein binding: < 4%

Metabolism: has not been evaluated fully; phosphorylated intracellularly to zalcitabine triphosphate, the active substrate for HIV-reverse transcriptase; does not appear to undergo significant metabolism by the liver

Excretion: renal, 70% of oral dose within 24 h

Renal impairment: prolonged elimination

Hepatic impairment: no information

The information here is provided as guidance only. Prescribers should always consult the manufacturer's current prescribing information.

ZALCITABINE (CONTINUED)

SPECIAL GROUPS

Children: Safety and efficacy of zalcitabine plus zidovudine combination or zalcitabine monotherapy in children under 13 and infected with HIV have not been established.

Elderly: May have age-related renal impairment (*see* Special Precautions).

Renal Impairment: Dosage reduction may be necessary (*see* Special Precautions).

Hepatic impairment: Monitor function closely; dosage reduction may be necessary (*see* Special Precautions).

Pregnancy: Adequate human studies not performed; use only if benefits outweigh risk. Women of childbearing potential should not receive zalcitabine unless they use effective contraceptive measures during therapy.

Breast-feeding: Not known whether excreted in breast milk. Decision to discontinue nursing or discontinue therapy must be made, with consideration of the importance of the drug to the mother (current recommended practice in the United States is that HIV-infected women do not breast-feed infants, regardless of their use of antiretroviral agents).

DOSAGE

Adults: For combination therapy with zidovudine in advanced HIV infection, 0.75 mg given concomitantly with 200 mg zidovudine every 8 hours (total daily dose: 2.25 mg zalcitabine/d and 600 mg zidovudine/d). Dosage reduction not necessary for patients whose weight is down to 30 kg.

Dosage adjustments should be based on known toxicity profile of either drug; interruption or reduction of dose is usually necessary in the event of toxic symptoms. Frequent monitoring of patient is essential during therapy, especially in those with preexisting conditions (*see* Special Precautions).

Elderly: No information.

Children: Dosage not established for children under 13 years of age.

Renal impairment: The following guidelines should be considered: estimated creatinine clearance 10 to 40 mL/min, reduce dose to 0.75 mg every 12 hours; estimated creatinine clearance less than 10 mL/min, reduce dose to 0.75 mg every 24 hours.

OVERDOSAGE

In early phase I studies, all patients receiving zalcitabine at six times current total daily recommendations experienced peripheral neuropathy by week 10; 80% who received approximately two times the current total daily recommendations experienced peripheral neuropathy by week 12. Sequelae of acute zalcitabine overdose are unknown because little experience exists. It is unknown whether zalcitabine is dialyzable by hemodialysis or peritoneal dialysis.

PATIENT INFORMATION

Zalcitabine is not a cure for HIV infection, and patients may continue to develop associated illnesses. Any and all changes in physical condition should be reported to physician immediately. Use of zalcitabine or other antiretroviral agents does not preclude the ongoing need to maintain practices against HIV transmission.

Do not exceed prescribed dose. If symptoms of peripheral neuropathy or pancreatitis occur, contact physician immediately.

Women of childbearing potential should use effective contraceptive measures during therapy.

AVAILABILITY

Tablets—0.375 mg and 0.75 mg

The information here is provided as guidance only. Prescribers should always consult the manufacturer's current prescribing information.

ZIDOVUDINE (Retrovir®)

Zidovudine, as illustrated in Fig. 12-12, is the treatment of choice for HIV at this time. It was the first drug established to be of value in slowing progression of HIV disease and death. It is not a cure for HIV infection. The administration of zidovudine is not without toxicity. Bone marrow suppression is the most commonly encountered form of zidovudine toxicity. Only the oral formulation is licensed for administration. The currently recommended dosage is 100 mg five times per day or 200 mg three times per day.

Zidovudine is a thymidine analogue available for oral and intravenous administration.

FIGURE 12-12
The chemical structure of zidovudine.

MICROBIOLOGY

Inhibits *in vitro* replication of some retroviruses, including HIV-1 and -2 and human T-cell lymphotrophic virus-1.

SPECIAL PRECAUTIONS

Zidovudine is frequently associated with hematologic toxicity and disease including granulocytopenia and severe anemia, which is dose-dependent, requiring transfusions. Patients may continue to develop opportunistic infections and other complications of AIDS and AIDS-related complex (ARC) due to HIV; therefore, patients should be under careful clinical observation at all times by physicians experienced in treatment of HIV-associated diseases.

Bone marrow compromise (granulocyte count < 1000 mm^3 or hemoglobin < 9.5 g/dL) calls for the use of extreme caution. Anemia and granulocytopenia are the most significant adverse effects; reversible pancytopenia also has been reported. Sensitivity reactions, including anaphylaxis reaction in one patient, have occurred with zidovudine therapy. If a rash occurs, evaluate patient for hypersensitivity or toxicity.

Renal or hepatic impairment may present a greater risk of toxicity from zidovudine; however, no data are currently available regarding the use of zidovudine with these conditions.

Carcinogenesis occurred in mice given the highest dose of zidovudine.

Capsules and syrup must be stored away from light.

INDICATIONS

ORAL: Management of adult patients with HIV infection and evidence of impaired immunity (CD4 cell count of < 200/mm^3)

For treatment of children infected with HIV who have HIV-associated symptoms or who are asymptomatic with abnormal laboratory test values indicating significant HIV-related immunosuppression.

INTRAVENOUS: Management of certain adult patients (including pregnant women) with HIV infection who have symptomatic HIV infection (AIDS and advanced ARC) who have a history of cytologically confirmed *Pneumocystis carinii* pneumonia or an absolute CD4 (T4 helper-inducer) lymphocyte count of less than 200/mm^3 in peripheral blood before therapy is initiated.

ORAL and *INTRAVENOUS*: HIV-infected pregnant women.

CONTRAINDICATIONS

Life-threatening allergy or allergic reactions to any of the product components

INTERACTIONS

Dapsone, pentamidine, amphotericin B, flucytosine, vincristine, vinblastine, adriamycin, interferon, probenecid, acetaminophen, aspirin, indomethacin, experimental nucleoside analogues, trimethoprim-sulfamethoxazole, pyrimethamine, acyclovir

ADVERSE EFFECTS

Most frequent: anemia, granulocytopenia

Body as a whole: asthenia, diaphoresis, fever, malaise, body odor, chills, edema of the lip, flu syndrome, hyperalgesia, back pain, chest pain, lymphadenopathy

Cardiovascular: vasodilation

Central nervous system: headache, dizziness, insomnia, paresthesia, somnolence, anxiety, confusion, depression, emotional liability, nervousness, syncope, loss of mental acuity, vertigo

Dermatologic: acne, pruritus, urticaria

Gastrointestinal: constipation, dysphagia, edema of the tongue, eructation, flatulence, bleeding gums, rectal hemorrhage, mouth ulcer

Genitourinary: dysuria, polyuria, urinary frequency, urinary hesitancy

Musculoskeletal: arthralgia, muscle spasm, tremor, twitch

Respiratory: cough, epistaxis, pharyngitis, rhinitis, sinusitis, hoarseness

Special senses: amblyopia, hearing loss, photophobia

The information here is provided as guidance only. Prescribers should always consult the manufacturer's current prescribing information.

ZIDOVUDINE (CONTINUED)

SPECIAL GROUPS

Children: Dosing regimen not established for infants under 3 months of age (limited clinical experience). (Note: Positive tests for HIV antibody in children under 15 months of age may represent passively acquired maternal antibodies rather than active antibody response to infection in the child. Therefore, detection of HIV antibody in a child under 15 months of age should be interpreted with caution, particularly in asymptomatic patients. Confirmatory tests [*eg*, serum P_{24} antigen or viral culture] should be performed in such children.)

Elderly: May have age-related renal impairment (*see* Special Precautions).

Renal impairment: May increase risk of toxicity.

Hepatic impairment: May increase risk of toxicity.

Pregnancy: Not known whether zidovudine can cause fetal harm; use only if clearly indicated.

Breast-feeding: Not known whether excreted in breast milk. Because of the potential for serious adverse effects in the infant, decision must be made to discontinue nursing or discontinue zidovudine.

DOSAGE

(Note: Hematologic indices should be monitored every 2 to 4 weeks for serious anemia or granulocytopenia. Patients with hematologic toxicity may experience reduction in hemoglobin as early as 2 to 4 weeks; granulocytopenia usually occurs after 6 to 8 weeks. Dosage adjustment is indicated in significant anemia [hemoglobin of < 7.5 g/dL or reduction of > 50% from baseline] and may necessitate an interruption in dosing until bone marrow recovery is observed. Dose reduction may be sufficient in less severe anemia or granulocytopenia. In significant anemia, dose reduction does not necessarily eliminate need for transfusion. Gradual increases in dose may be appropriate after bone marrow recovery following dose adjustment, depending on hematologic indices and patient tolerance.)

Adults: *ORAL*: For patients with CD4 counts below 200/mm^3, initial dose is 100 mg five times per day (two 100-mg capsules or 4 teaspoons [20 mL] syrup), this dose corresponds to 2.9 mg/kg every 4 hours. Dose may be reduced after 1 month to 100 mg every 4 hours. (Note: The effectiveness of reduced dose in improving neurologic dysfunction associated with HIV disease is unknown.) Use intravenous infusion only until oral therapy is possible. Dosing regimen, equivalent to oral administration of 100 mg every 4 hours, is approximately 1 mg/kg intravenous every 4 hours. (Note: Admixture is not recommended with biologic or colloidal fluids [*eg*, blood products or protein solutions].)

Elderly: May have age-related renal impairment or potential increased risk of toxicity; otherwise, same as adults.

Children: *ORAL*: (3 months to 12 years of age), initial dose is 180 mg/m^2 every 6 hours (720 mg/m^2/d); do not exceed 200 mg every 6 hours.

Renal impairment: No special dosage given (*see* Special Precautions).

PHARMACOKINETICS AND PHARMACODYNAMICS

Peak serum levels: occur 0.5 to 1.5 h; mean steady-state concentrations with chronic oral use of 250 mg every 4 h predose and postdose were 0.16 µg/mL and 0.62 µg/mL

Serum half-life: 1 h

Bioavailability: 65%

Protein binding: 34% to 38%

Metabolism: liver, to inactive metabolite

Excretion: renal, glomerular filtration and tubular secretion; total urinary recovery averaged 90%

Renal impairment: prolonged elimination, increased risk of toxicity

Hepatic impairment: possible increased risk of toxicity

OVERDOSAGE

Acute overdose in both children and adults has occurred with doses as high as 50 g; no cases were fatal. The single most consistent effects were nausea and vomiting. Hematologic changes were transient and not severe. Hemodialysis has negligible effect, although elimination of its primary metabolite is enhanced.

PATIENT INFORMATION

Zidovudine is not a cure for HIV infections. Patients may continue to contract illnesses related to AIDS or ARC, including opportunistic infections. Contact physician immediately if any significant change in health condition occurs.

Blood counts must be monitored during therapy. Anemia and granulocytopenia are the major toxicities of zidovudine and can require transfusions or dose modifications. Do not use medications that may exacerbate the toxicity of zidovudine.

Zidovudine therapy does not reduce the risk of transmission of HIV to others.

ORAL ONLY: Take medication exactly as prescribed, every 4 hours around the clock, even though it may interrupt normal sleep (except asymptomatic patients whose dosing interval is every 4 hours while awake). Do not exceed recommended dosage. Do not share medication with others.

Long-term effects of zidovudine are not known.

AVAILABILITY

Capsules—100 mg

Syrup—50 mg/5 mL

Injection—10 mg/mL

The information here is provided as guidance only. Prescribers should always consult the manufacturer's current prescribing information.

INTRODUCTION

The antiparasitic agents that are covered in this section represent a diverse class of pharmaceutical agents directed against some of the most unfamiliar diseases health professionals are asked to consider in their clinical practices. Despite the fact that these diseases and the agents used to treat them seem so unfamiliar, antiparasitic agents are important drugs: physicians should become familiar with them over the next decade and into the 21st century. To ignore parasitic diseases and antiparasitic agents is to put oneself at a considerable disadvantage, given several long-term trends that are moving clinicians to familiarize themselves even more with both these infectious organisms and the pharmaceutical agents used to treat them.

Throughout the 20th century, much of the impetus for understanding antiparasitic drugs and their use has been influenced by the occurrence of war and social upheaval. In North America, for example, there were great flurries of activity around the use of antiparasitic agents, particularly antimalarial drugs, during World War II and the Vietnam conflict. During such times, medical schools and training programs were geared to produce physicians with considerable expertise in the use of antiparasitic agents because these agents would be needed almost immediately upon graduation.

The impetus for dealing with parasitic agents in one's clinical practice has changed. The major influences are not all that difficult to discern. Over the past 50 years, with the development of rapid air travel, it has become possible for individuals to live in an environment with intense exposure to parasitic organisms and, within 24 hours, to find themselves in a major, industrialized, urban area. Often, and well within the incubation time of diseases caused by such parasitic agents, individuals may have forgotten their previous travels, and often physicians do not request the necessary travel information that could provide the clue to diagnosing a somewhat exotic, yet all too familiar, infectious disease in the developing world.

Over the past three decades, it has become increasingly common for clinicians to encounter patients who have undergone iatrogenic immunosuppression of various forms. This not only includes the treatment of malignancies but also includes solid organ and bone marrow transplant recipients, who are markedly immunosuppressed by a variety of pharmaceutical agents that predispose to reactivation of viral and parasitic infections. These patients may also travel and continue to lead productive lives. During this process they may encounter parasitic agents, not only from their endogenous latent state but also in the developing world. Clinicians practicing in a travel clinic may be called to advise an immunocompromised patient with a solid organ transplant regarding a major trip into a developing world where parasitic agents are endemic.

Although each of these trends has been important, one of the major forces working toward the resurgence of interest in parasitic agents and the drugs used to treat them has been the AIDS pandemic. There has been a rapid emergence of newly appreciated gastrointestinal organisms producing chronic infection in these immunocompromised hosts and parasitic agents, such as *Toxoplasma gondii*. This organism can devastate the central nervous system when latent infection relapses; toxoplasmosis has really underscored the importance of understanding the use of antiparasitic drugs, as have the various intestinal opportunistic infections seen in patients with AIDS.

With that in mind, it must be understood that of all classes of pharmacologic agents, the use of antiparasitic drugs has been one of the most empiric in its evolution. Recall that the use of quinine for the treatment of malaria preceded our understanding of the pathogenesis of the disease by almost 300 years. In fact, during the 17th century it was suggested that the diagnosis of malaria, whatever that disease might be, could be made by observing the response of fever to the administration of cinchona bark (which contains cinchona alkaloids, including quinine). Often, the means by which an antiparasitic agent has been found effective for a given disease state has been through empiric observation and the occurrence of fortuitous circumstances, ultimately leading to controlled trials and the evolution of therapy for a parasitic infection. Although it is not easy to keep up with developments in this field, we strongly suggest that health professionals keep a copy of the *Medical Letter on Drugs and Therapeutics* issue, which is published every 2 years, entitled *Drugs for Parasitic Infections* [1]. In this brief summary, it is possible to obtain a clear understanding of the drugs of choice, both for adults and children, used in the treatment of parasitic infections and to have some idea of the adverse effects of these antiparasitic drugs. This monograph also is useful because it provides the means for obtaining those drugs that are not yet approved for use in the United States or Canada but are nevertheless available through pharmaceutical companies and the Centers for Disease Control and Prevention (CDC). If one keeps nothing else on one's desk for the treatment of parasitic infections, this would be a useful monograph to have available.

We also suggest that the physician have available the United States Pharmacopeia's most recent edition of *Drug Information for the Health Care Professional*. This is one of the few sources of information on antiparasitic agents that also includes some of those drugs not yet approved for use in the United States and Canada. It is exhaustive in its coverage and provides the next level of information beyond the current chapter.

Lastly, because many clinicians will have only a few critical opportunities to use these agents, they should avail themselves of the opportunity to consult with experts in the field whenever they are using an unfamiliar antiparasitic agent. This can be done by contacting the CDC, which maintains a drug service. (Telephone number: 404-639-6370.)

This chapter is only a synopsis or guide to current usage of antiparasitic agents. We strongly suggest that health-care providers consult the most current edition of the Drug Information for the Health Care Professional before using these agents.

REFERENCES

1. Drugs for parasitic infections. In *Medical Letter on Drugs and Therapeutics*. December 10, 1993, vol 35 (911).

2. The United States Pharmaceutical Convention: *Drug Information for the Health Care Professional*, 15th ed. Taunton, MA: Rand McNally; 1995.

The information here is provided as guidance only. Prescribers should always consult the manufacturer's current prescribing information.

ATOVAQUONE (Mepron®)

Atovaquone is an antiprotozoal agent that is currently used for the treatment of mild to moderate *Pneumocystis carinii* pneumonia. Structurally, it is a hydroxynaphthoquinone, but its mechanism of action against agents such as *P. carinii* is not completely understood. Its chemical structure makes it similar to ubiquinone, an agent that inhibits the mitochondrial electron transport chain. This could potentially lead to an inhibition of nucleic acid synthesis. The agent does not have significant antibacterial, antiviral, or antifungal activity but has been shown to have *in vitro* activity against *Toxoplasma gondii*.

The bioavailability of atovaquone is markedly influenced by administration with meals. Fatty meals significantly enhance the absorption of the drug. The most frequent side effects include fever, rash, nausea, and occasionally diarrhea.

ACTIVITY

Active against *P. carinii* and *Plasmodium* spp.

SPECIAL PRECAUTIONS

Severe *P. carinii* pneumonia has not been included in clinical experience to date; likewise, patients with mild to moderate *P. carinii* pneumonia who are failing therapy with trimethoprim-sulfamethoxazole have not been studied. Atovaquone has not been evaluated for *P. carinii* pneumonia prophylaxis.

Orally administered atovaquone has limited absorption; absorption increases if taken with food. Plasma concentrations correlate with potential of successful treatment and survival; therefore, for patients who have difficulty taking atovaquone with food, parenteral therapy with other agents should be considered.

Gastrointestinal disorders may limit absorption of orally administered agents. Concurrent pulmonary conditions (bacterial, viral, or fungal pneumonia or mycobacterial diseases) are not effectively treated with atovaquone; carefully evaluate all patients with acute *P. carinii* pneumonia for other possible causes of pulmonary disease and treat with additional drugs if necessary.

Plasma protein binding of atovaquone is high (> 99.9%); therefore, caution is necessary when administering concurrently with other highly plasma protein–bound agents with narrow therapeutic indices because competition for binding sites may occur (not affected by phenytoin or vice versa). Concurrent administration of rifampin, sulfamethoxazole, or trimethoprim may decrease atovaquone serum concentrations. Zidovudine may increase serum concentrations.

SPECIAL GROUPS

Children: Efficacy studies not performed; no children under 5 months of age participated in Phase I trial.

Elderly: Has not been evaluated systematically in patients aged 65 years and over; use caution in treating elderly patients because of frequency of age-related decreased hepatic, renal, and cardiac function in this group.

Renal impairment: No information.

Hepatic impairment: No information.

Pregnancy: Adequate human studies not performed; maternal toxicity and decreased mean fetal body lengths and weights (and other effects) have occurred in rabbits; use only if benefits outweigh risk to fetus.

Breast-feeding: Not known whether excreted; use with caution.

DOSAGE

Adults: 750 mg given with food three times a day for 21 days (total daily dose, 2250 mg). Atovaquone administered without food may result in lower plasma concentrations and may limit response to therapy.

Elderly: Use caution in administering adult dose.

Children: No dosage given.

Renal impairment: No information.

INDICATIONS

Acute oral treatment of mild to moderate *P. carinii* pneumonia in patients who are intolerant of trimethoprim-sulfamethoxazole

CONTRAINDICATIONS

History or development of potentially life-threatening allergic reaction to any product components; risk–benefit should be considered with presence of gastrointestinal disorders that may inhibit absorption

INTERACTIONS

Highly plasma protein–bound drugs (*see* Special Precautions)

ADVERSE EFFECTS

(Note: Due to the fact that patients who participated in clinical trials had complications of advanced HIV disease, adverse events caused by atovaquone were difficult to distinguish from those caused by underlying medical conditions. No life-threatening or fatal effects were attributed to atovaquone.)

Rash, nausea, diarrhea, headache, vomiting, fever, insomnia, cough, sweating, anxiety, anorexia, sinusitis, dyspepsia, rhinitis, taste perversion, hypoglycemia, hypotension, asthenia, pruritus, monilia (oral), abdominal pain, constipation, dizziness

Laboratory test abnormalities: elevated alkaline phosphatase, elevated amylase, hyponatremia, elevated ALT, anemia, elevated AST, neutropenia

PHARMACOKINETICS AND PHARMACODYNAMICS

Peak serum levels: approximately 13.9 μg/mL in AIDS patients taking 750 mg three times a day with food

Oral suspension: approximately 24 μg/mL in patients taking 750 mg two times a day with food

Serum half-life: 2.2 to 2.9 days in adult AIDS patients, healthy adult volunteers, and immunocompromised children

Bioavailability: low, variable; decreases significantly with single doses greater than 750 mg

Protein binding: > 99.9%

Metabolism: no evidence of metabolism

Excretion: > 94% of dose recovered in feces over 21 days; < 0.6% excreted in the urine

Renal impairment: no information

Hepatic impairment: no information

OVERDOSAGE

No information

PATIENT INFORMATION

Take prescribed dose with high-fat meals

AVAILABILITY

Tablets—250 mg, oral suspension recently approved (*See* peak serum levels under Pharmacokinetics and Pharmacodynamics)

The information here is provided as guidance only. Prescribers should always consult the manufacturer's current prescribing information.

CHLOROQUINE (Aralen®)

As an antiparasitic agent, *chloroquine's* major use is for the prevention and treatment of chloroquine-sensitive strains of malaria. It is useful for both the suppression and treatment of acute attacks of malaria caused by sensitive strains of *Plasmodium vivax*, *Plasmodium malariae*, *Plasmodium ovale*, and *Plasmodium falciparum*. So-called *radical cure* of infection caused by *P. vivax* and *P. ovale* requires the concurrent or subsequent administration of primaquine to destroy the exoerythrocytic liver phase of these organisms. Over the past 30 years, chloroquine-sensitive strains of *P. falciparum* have become common, requiring the development of additional antimalarial agents. *P. vivax* also has recently emerged as a resistant strain. The mechanism of antimalarial action for chloroquine is not really known. It is taken up by the acidic food vacuoles of the parasite and causes an increase in the pH of acid vesicles. Current inquiry is centered around the inhibition of heme polymerase and the accumulation of toxic hemoglobin metabolites within the parasite as a major mechanism of antiparasitic action.

Chloroquine still represents a safe and important prophylactic and therapeutic antimalarial agent for limited geographic areas and is generally free of major side effects. Rare and irreversible retinal injury can occur when the total dosage exceeds 100 g, but this is generally not a problem during antimalarial prophylaxis or treatment. More likely, gastrointestinal disturbances or pruritus will occur. Blurred vision, headache, or tinnitus will occur infrequently, and they are usually transient and reversible. Although there is a lack of clinical studies, historical evidence does not demonstrate evidence for teratogenic effects, and chloroquine can be used during pregnancy for either prevention or treatment of malaria. Animal studies have raised questions about ototoxicity in first-trimester use. In young children, parenteral chloroquine has been associated with hypotension, shock, and sudden death. Although safe as prophylaxis for children, chloroquine must be kept out of reach. Enteric-coated chloroquine tablets may be mistaken for candy by children, and overdosage, even by the oral route, can cause death.

MICROBIOLOGY

P. vivax, *P. malariae*, *P. ovale*, and susceptible strains of *P. falciparum* (not the gametocytes).

SPECIAL PRECAUTIONS

Resistance occurs in many strains of *P. falciparum* and some strains of *P. vivax*; treatment with quinine or other specific therapy is recommended in such infections. Retinopathy has been reported and is dose related; irreversible retinal damage has been observed with long-term therapy or high doses. Discontinue therapy immediately and observe for progression if any visual symptoms not explainable by difficulties of accommodation or corneal opacities occur. Perform baseline and periodic ophthalmic examinations when prolonged therapy is considered.

Muscle weakness may occur and necessitates discontinuation of therapy; question and examine patients periodically (including reflex tests). If weakness occurs, stop drug.

Psoriasis or porphyria may be exacerbated by use of chloroquine; do not use unless benefits outweigh risk.

Hepatic function impairment indicates use of caution (as does alcoholism or concurrent administration of other hepatotoxic agents).

Periodic complete blood counts should be performed during prolonged therapy. If any significant blood disorder occurs that is not attributable to the disease being treated, discontinue therapy. Measure glucose-6-phosphate dehydrogenase (G-6-PD) in susceptible patients before initiating follow-up primoquine therapy (may otherwise induce hemolysis in such individuals in presence of infection or stress).

INDICATIONS

Prophylaxis and treatment of acute attacks of malaria due to *P. vivax*, *P. malariae*, *P. ovale*, and susceptible strains of *P. falciparum* (*see* Special Precautions). Chloroquine phosphate is the drug of choice in these conditions. Chloroquine hydrochloride is indicated only when oral therapy is not possible. Radical cure of *P. vivax* and *P. ovale* malaria necessitates concomitant primaquine therapy.

CONTRAINDICATIONS

Hypersensitivity to chloroquine or hydroxychloroquine (Note: *Hydroxychoroquine* is not for long-term use in children.)

INTERACTIONS

Cimetidine, kaolin, or magnesium trisilicate

ADVERSE EFFECTS

Cardiovascular: hypotension, electrocardiogram changes (especially inversion or depression of the T-wave, widening of QRS complex)

Central nervous system: mild, transient headache; psychic stimulation

Gastrointestinal: anorexia, nausea, vomiting, diarrhea, abdominal cramps

Ophthalmic: irreversible retinal damage in patients receiving long-term or high-dosage therapy; visual disturbances, nyctalopia, scotomatous vision with field defects of paracentral, precentral ring types and typically temporal scotomas

Otologic: nerve-type deafness after prolonged high doses (few cases); tinnitus and reduced hearing in one patient with preexisting auditory damage after administration of 500 mg once a week for a few months

Other: agranulocytosis, pruritus, neuropathy, blood dyscrasias, lichen planus–like eruptions, skin and mucosal pigmentary changes, pleomorphic skin eruptions (prolonged therapy)

PHARMACOKINETICS AND PHARMACODYNAMICS

Peak serum levels: 300 mg (base) in healthy adult patients—73 to 76 μg/L (oral)

Serum half-life: terminal elimination half-life—1 to 2 months

Bioavailability: rate of absorption varies; tablets, 89%

Protein binding: 50% to 65%

Metabolism: hepatic, partially, to active de-ethylated metabolites

Excretion: up to 47% unchanged and up to 12% as metabolite in urine; elimination is very slow (renal excretion is enhanced by urinary acidification)

Renal impairment: no information

Hepatic impairment: no information

The information here is provided as guidance only. Prescribers should always consult the manufacturer's current prescribing information.

CHLOROQUINE (CONTINUED)

SPECIAL GROUPS

Children: Do not exceed single dose of 5 mg base/kg of chloroquine hydrochloride in infants or children. Children are particularly sensitive to 4-aminoquinoline compounds, and fatalities following accidental ingestion of relatively small doses and sudden deaths from parenteral chloroquine have been reported.
Elderly: No information is available on the relationship of age to the effects of chlorquine in geriatric patients.
Renal impairment: No information.
Hepatic impairment: Use with caution (*see* Special Precautions).
Pregnancy: Use only when clearly indicated and when benefits outweigh risk.
Breast-feeding: Safety not established; excreted in breast milk.

DOSAGE

Adults: *As amebicide*: ORAL: 250 mg (150 mg base) four times a day for 2 days, followed by 250 mg two times a day for a minimum of 2 to 3 weeks. Therapy is usually combined with an effective intestinal amebicide.
INTRAMUSCULARLY: 4 to 5 mL (200–250 mg; 160–200 mg base) intramuscularly daily for 10 to 12 days. Oral administration should be substituted or resumed as soon as possible.
As antimalarial: ORAL: For suppression, 300 mg (base) weekly on the same day each week; begin 1 to 2 weeks prior to exposure and continue for 4 weeks after leaving endemic area.
For acute attack, follow the dosing guidelines below:

Chloroquine Phosphate Dose in Acute Malarial Attack

Dose	Time	Dosage, *mg of base*	
		Adults	**Children, *mg/kg***
Initial	Day 1	600	10
Second	6–8 h later	300	5
Third	Day 2	300	5
Fourth	Day 3	300	5

Elderly: No information.
Children: As antimalarial: For suppression, 5 mg base/kg weekly, up to maximum adult dose of 300 mg base (do not exceed); give on same day each week, beginning 1 to 2 weeks prior to exposure and continuing for 4 weeks after leaving endemic area.

Chloroquine Dose for Children Based on Age

Age, *y*	Chloroquine base equivalent, *mg*
< 1	37.5
1–3	75
4–6	100
7–10	150
11–16	225

Renal impairment: No information.
(Note: Chloroquine may be used as an alternative regimen for patients in whom mefloquine or doxycycline is contraindicated, especially in pregnant women and in children under 15 kg.)

OVERDOSAGE

Symptoms may occur within 30 minutes of overdose (headache, drowsiness, visual disturbances, cardiovascular collapse, and convulsions followed by sudden and early respiratory and cardiac arrest). Overdose of parenteral chloroquine hydrochloride 1 has resulted in respiratory depression, cardiovascular collapse, shock, convulsions, and death, especially in infants and children. In a retrospective study it was determined that ingestion of more than 2.25 g of chloroquine was an accurate predictor of fatal outcome in adults; the amount could be as low as 2 g (250 mg) in children.
Treatment is symptomatic and supportive; stomach must be evacuated immediately by emesis or gastric lavage. Activated charcoal may inhibit further absorption after lavage if given within 30 minutes of ingestion. Convulsions must be controlled before gastric lavage can be performed. If due to cerebral stimulation, cautious administration of a short-acting anticonvulsant may be tried. Anoxia-induced convulsions should be treated with oxygen, mechanical ventilation, or (in shock with hypotension) by vasopressor therapy. Tracheal intubation or tracheostomy may be necessary. Peritoneal dialysis and exchange transfusions have been suggested. Observe asymptomatic patients who survive acute phases of overdose closely for at least 6 hours. Acidify urine and force fluids to promote excretion. One study reported the successful use of diazepam and epinephrine for several days with mechanical ventilation (10 of 11 patients).

PATIENT INFORMATION

Take with food. May cause stomach upset. Complete full course of therapy. Contact physician if visual disturbances, difficulty in hearing, or ringing of the ears occurs.
Keep out of reach of children; overdosage is particularly dangerous in children.
May cause diarrhea, loss of appetite, nausea, stomach pain, vomiting, muscle weakness, or rash; contact physician if these effects become pronounced or bothersome.

AVAILABILITY

Tablets—250 mg
Tablets—500 mg (equivalent to 300 mg base)
Injection—50 mg/mL (equivalent to 40 mg base) in 5-mL amps

The information here is provided as guidance only. Prescribers should always consult the manufacturer's current prescribing information.

DIETHYLCARBAMAZINE (Hetrazan®)

Diethylcarbamazine is a systemic anthelminthic agent that is largely used in the treatment of various forms of filariasis and tropical pulmonary eosinophilia. In onchocerciasis, this drug is considered microfilaricidal in that it is able to reduce the number of intrauterine microfilaria by inhibiting the rate of embryogenesis. It also increases the rate of loss of *Onchocerca volvulus* microfilaria from nodules. It is now considered a secondary agent for the treatment of this disease, having been supplanted by ivermectin, the primary agent for the treatment of onchocerciasis. It has been used for prophylaxis for people traveling long term into endemic onchocerciasis or *Loa loa* areas. Diethylcarbamazine is still indicated as a primary agent in the treatment of *Wuchereria bancrofti* and *Brugia malayi* infections, *Loa loa*, and tropical pulmonary eosinophilia.

The use of diethylcarbamazine frequently is associated with severe allergic or febrile reactions in patients who have numerous microfilaria in the blood or the skin. Antihistamines or corticosteroids may be required to decrease allergic reactions due to disintegration of microfilariae during treatment, particularly those caused by *Loa loa*. It may also cause gastrointestinal disturbances, and rarely, encephalopathy.

ACTIVITY

Effective against *W. bancrofti*, *O. volvulus*, and *Loa loa*.

SPECIAL PRECAUTIONS

Careful administration is essential to avoid or control allergic or other adverse effects.

SPECIAL GROUPS

Children: No pediatric-specific problems to date.
Elderly: No information.
Renal impairment: No information.
Hepatic impairment: No information.
Pregnancy: Defer treatment until after delivery.
Breast-feeding: No information.

DOSAGE

(Note: Check *Medical Letter* 1993, 35:113 before dosing in patients with microfilaremia.)
Adults: For Bancroft's filariasis: 2 to 3 mg/kg three times a day immediately after meals. In acute and chronic stages of disease, continue treatment for 2 to 4 weeks. Incidence of recurrence is higher with smaller doses.
For tropical eosinophilia: 6 mg/kg/d for 4 to 7 days. For loiasis: 9 mg/kg/d are required.
Elderly: No information.
Children: Similar dosing by weight.
Renal impairment: No information.

INDICATIONS

Treatment of Bancroft's filariasis, onchocerciasis, ascariasis, tropical eosinophilia, and loiasis

CONTRAINDICATIONS

Hypersensitivity to diethylcarbamazine; onchocerciasis, ocular
(Note: Demonstrates a low order of toxicity in animals.)

INTERACTIONS

No information

ADVERSE EFFECTS

Treatment of *W. bancrofti:* Mild reactions occur and are transient but frequent. Headache, lassitude, weakness, general malaise; nausea, vomiting, and skin rash are occasional. If severe allergic symptoms occur in conjunction with skin rash, it may be necessary to stop therapy.
Treatment of onchocerciasis: Facial edema, pruritus (especially of eyes); severe reactions may occur after a single dose in treatment of rampant infestations, in which case only one dose should be given on day 1, two doses on day 2, and then three daily doses thereafter for 30 days. If extremely severe reactions occur, interrupt treatment and administer antihistamines. Therapy may be resumed after 1 to 2 days but only with extreme caution.
Treatment of ascariasis: Giddiness, nausea, vomiting, and malaise occur most frequently in children who are malnourished or who suffer from various debilitating diseases.

PHARMACOKINETICS AND PHARMACODYNAMICS

Peak serum levels: 80 to 200 µg/mL after a single 50-mg dose
Serum half-life: 8 h
Bioavailability: readily absorbed after oral administration
Protein binding: no information
Metabolism: partially metabolized to diethylcarbamazine *N*-oxide
Excretion: metabolite excreted in urine; 4% to 5% eliminated in feces
Renal impairment: no information
Hepatic impairment: no information

OVERDOSAGE

No information

PATIENT INFORMATION

Take immediately after meals. Complete full course of therapy.

AVAILABILITY

Tablets—200 mg
Tablets—400 mg

The information here is provided as guidance only. Prescribers should always consult the manufacturer's current prescribing information.

EFLORNITHINE (Ornidyl®)

Eflornithine, commonly referred to as *alpha-difloromethyl ornithine*, or *DFMO*, is indicated for the treatment of the meningoencephalitic stage of *Trypanosoma brucei* infection (West African sleeping sickness). However, all species are not susceptible to eflornithine. The mechanism of action is as an enzyme-activated irreversible blocker of ornithine dicarboxylase, which is involved in the conversion of ornithine to polyamines. The polyamines are important for the growth, differentiation, and replication of cells. Eflornithine is considered a cytostatic rather than a cytolytic agent, and animal studies suggest that an intact immune response is necessary for complete elimination of the blood-borne parasites.

Eflornithine is frequently associated with anemia and leukopenia. It may be occasionally associated with diarrhea, thrombocytopenia, seizures, and, rarely, hearing loss.

ACTIVITY

Inhibits growth of *T. brucei*.
(Note: Active in treatment of African trypanosomal infections in various animal models, including *T. brucei gambiense* infection.)

SPECIAL PRECAUTIONS

Concentrate must be diluted before use.
Thorough knowledge of natural history of trypanosomiasis due to *T. brucei gambiense* and of condition of the patient are essential for safe and effective use.
Myelosuppression is the most serious toxic effect and may be unavoidable if successful treatment is to be completed. Decisions to modify dosage should be based on response to treatment, severity of observed adverse effects, and the availability of support facilities.
Anemia occurred in approximately 55% of monitored patients and was generally found to be reversible upon discontinuation of treatment (many of these patients were chronically anemic prior to initiation of therapy). Leukopenia occurred in about 37% of patients monitored, and thrombocytopenia occurred in approximately 14%; both conditions were reversible once therapy was stopped.
Seizures have been temporally associated with eflornithine and also can be caused by underlying disease; no etiology has been determined.
Hearing impairment has occurred occasionally; serial audiograms should be obtained if possible.
Relapse information for Stage II *gambiense* trypanosomiasis is limited; therefore, it is recommended that physicians follow patients for at least 24 months to assure further therapy should relapse occur.
Renal function impairment necessitates caution; approximately 80% of intravenous dose is normally eliminated unchanged in the urine.
Fertility impairment (decreased spermatogenetic effects) was seen in rats and rabbits at doses equivalent to one half the recommended human dose.

SPECIAL GROUPS

Children: Safety and efficacy not established.
Elderly: May have age-related renal impairment; use with caution.
Renal impairment: Use with caution. Adjust dosage based on creatinine clearance. Consult the *USP DI* recommendations.
Hepatic impairment: No information.
Pregnancy: Adequate human studies not performed. Use only if benefits outweigh potential risk to fetus. (Note: Contragestational in rats, rabbits, and mice. Retarded development occurred in rat pups at doses only slightly higher than those for humans.)
Breast-feeding: Not known whether excreted. Because of potential for serious adverse effects in infants, decision must be made to discontinue nursing or discontinue drug.

INDICATIONS

Treatment of meningoencephalitic stage of *T. brucei gambiense* infection (sleeping sickness). An extended follow-up of patients is necessary to assure adequate additional therapy should a relapse occur.

CONTRAINDICATIONS

Pre-existing hematologic abnormalities, or eighth-cranial nerve or renal function impairment

INTERACTIONS

No information

ADVERSE EFFECTS

Anemia, leukopenia, thrombocytopenia, diarrhea, seizures, hearing impairment, vomiting, nausea, alopecia, abdominal pain, anorexia, headache, asthenia, facial edema, hematologic abnormalities, dizziness
(Note: Four percent of patients died during therapy or soon after completion of therapy. It was not established whether the deaths were due to underlying disease or to the use of eflornithine.)

PHARMACOKINETICS AND PHARMACODYNAMICS

Peak serum levels: 196.6 to 317.9 µg/mL after 100 mg/kg of body weight every 6 h
Serum half-life: 3.2 to 3.6 h
Bioavailability: well absorbed after administration; approximately 50%
Protein binding: not significant
Metabolism: no information
Excretion: through kidney at approximately same rate as creatinine clearance; 80% unchanged in urine within 24 h
Renal impairment: dosage adjustment necessary; excretion significantly slowed
Hepatic impairment: no information

The information here is provided as guidance only. Prescribers should always consult the manufacturer's current prescribing information.

EFLORNITHINE (CONTINUED)

DOSAGE

(Note: Concentrate must be diluted before administration; eflornithine is hypertonic and must be diluted with Sterile Water for Injection, USP. Solutions within 10% of plasma tonicity can be produced using one part eflornithine concentrate to four parts Sterile Water for Injection, by volume as described here: Using strict aseptic technique, withdraw entire contents of each 100-mL vial. Inject 25 mL into each of the four intravenous diluent bags, each of which contains 100 mL of Sterile Water for Injection, USP. The eflornithine concentration after dilution will be 40 mg/mL [5000 mg of eflornithine in 125-mL total volume; use diluted drug within 24 hours of preparation].)

Adults: For *T. brucei gambiense* infection (sleeping sickness): 100 mg/kg every 6 hours by intravenous infusion for 14 days followed by oral treatment with 300 mg/kg/d for 3 to 4 weeks. Administer over minimum period of 45 minutes; do not administer other drugs intravenously during infection of eflornithine.

Elderly: May have age-related renal impairment requiring reduced dosage.

Children: Safety not established.

Renal impairment: Dosage adjustment necessary to compensate for slower excretion. Base adjustment on creatinine clearance. When serum creatinine is available only, the following formula may be used to estimate creatinine clearance (serum creatinine should represent a steady-state of renal function):

$$\text{Males:} \quad \frac{\text{weight (kg)} \times (140 - \text{age})}{72 \times \text{serum creatinine (mg/dL)}} = \text{creatinine clearance}$$

Females: $0.85 \times$ above amount

OVERDOSAGE

After intraperitoneal doses of 3 g/kg in mice and rats, moderate central nervous system depression was observed after 2 to 4 hours. Convulsions were observed in three of 10 rats, and two of the rats died within 3 hours of receiving the drug.

PATIENT INFORMATION

Complete full course of therapy. Consult physician if fever, chills, unusual bleeding, bruising, or blood in stool occurs.

AVAILABILITY

Injection concentrate—200 mg/mL (as monohydrate)

FURAZOLIDONE (Furoxone®)

Furazolidone is a broad-spectrum anti-infective agent that has both antibacterial and antiprotozoal activity. Its mechanism of action is interference with bacterial enzyme systems, with additional activity against the parasite *Giardia lamblia*. Although furazolidone is considered a secondary agent in the treatment of giardiasis, its liquid preparation has made it a useful drug for treatment of *G. lamblia* in children.

Furazolidone is frequently associated with nausea and vomiting and occasionally with allergic reactions, including pulmonary infiltrates, hypotension, urticaria, fever, rashes, hypoglycemia, and headaches. Rarely, hemolytic anemia in glucose-6-phosphate dehydrogenase (G-6-PD)–deficient patients may occur. A disulfiram-like reaction may occur with alcohol. Because furazolidone also acts as a monoamine oxidase inhibitor, norepinephrine may be released from sympathetic nerve terminals and produce sudden increases in blood pressure. Polyneuritis also has been reported.

ACTIVITY

Furazolidone has a broad antibacterial spectrum covering many gastrointestinal tract pathogens, including *Escherichia coli*, staphylococci, *Salmonella*, *Shigella*, and *Proteus* spp, *Vibrio cholerae*, and *Giardia lamblia*.

INDICATIONS

Treatment (specific and symptomatic) of cholera (secondary agent), or of bacterial or protozoal diarrhea and enteritis due to susceptible organisms, including *Gardia lamblia*

Unlabeled: In the treatment of acute infantile diarrhea (when fecal leukocytes were present) in children 3 to 73 months of age, the use of furazolidone 7.5 mg/kg plus oral rehydration therapy for 5 days was more effective than oral rehydration therapy alone

CONTRAINDICATIONS

Infants under 1 month of age
Known allergy or hypersensitivity to furazolidone

INTERACTIONS

Alcohol, levodopa, meperidine, sympathomimetics (indirect and mixed), tricyclic antidepressants
Drug and food interactions: Foods high in amine content consumed concurrent with or after therapy may result in marked elevation of blood pressure, hypertensive crisis, or hemorrhagic strokes

The information here is provided as guidance only. Prescribers should always consult the manufacturer's current prescribing information.

FURAZOLIDONE (CONTINUED)

SPECIAL PRECAUTIONS

Orthostatic hypotension and hypoglycemia may occur.
Hemolysis may occur in patients with G-6-PD deficiency.
Hypertensive crisis may possibly occur; consider this if considering dosages larger than those recommended.
Monoamine oxidase (MAO) inhibition occurs. Doses of 400 mg/d for 5 days increase tyramine and amphetamine sensitivity two- to threefold. Use caution in administering with other MAO inhibitors.

SPECIAL GROUPS

Children: Not recommended in infants younger than 1 month of age.
Elderly: No information.
Renal impairment: No information.
Hepatic impairment: No information.
Pregnancy: Safety not established; however, teratogenic effects have not been reported.
Breast-feeding: Safety not established; not recommended in infants up to 1 month of age.

DOSAGE

(Dosage is based on average dose of 5 mg/kg/d administered in four equally divided doses. Do not exceed 8.8 mg/kg/d because of the possibility of nausea and emesis. If these effects occur and are severe, reduce dosage. If adequate clinical response is not obtained within 7 days, the pathogen is refractory to furazolidone; discontinue drug. Adjunctive therapy with other antibacterial agents or bismuth salts is not contraindicated.)
Adults: 100 mg four times a day. For bacterial diarrhea: 5 to 7 days. For giardiasis: 7 to 10 days.
Elderly: No information.
Children: 5 years of age or older: 25 to 50 mg four times a day in tablet or liquid form; 1 to 4 years: 17 to 25 mg four times a day (liquid); 1 month to 1 year: 8 to 17 mg four times a day (liquid).
Renal impairment: No information.

ADVERSE EFFECTS

(Note: Most significant adverse effects are eliminated by withdrawal of furazolidone)
Allergic: hypotension, urticaria, fever, arthralgia, vesicular morbilliform rash
Central nervous system: headache, malaise
Disulfiram-like reaction: (rare; in conjunction with alcohol consumption) fever, dyspnea, chest tightness
Gastrointestinal: colitis, proctitis, anal pruritus, staphylococcal enteritis, nausea and emesis
Hematologic: mild, reversible, intravascular hemolysis in G-6-PD deficiency, leukopenia

PHARMACOKINETICS AND PHARMACODYNAMICS

Peak serum levels: no information
Serum half-life: no information
Bioavailability: no percentage given; significant absorption following oral administration
Protein binding: no information
Metabolism: rapid and extensive, possibly in intestine
Excretion: 65% of an oral dose recovered in urine; also found in feces
Renal impairment: no information
Hepatic impairment: no information

OVERDOSAGE

No information

PATIENT INFORMATION

Avoid alcoholic beverages during and for 4 days after furazolidone therapy (disulfiram-like reaction may occur)
Avoid foods containing tyramine, especially in prolonged (more than 5 days) therapy
Avoid over-the-counter or prescription medications containing sympathomimetic drugs (*eg,* cold and hay fever remedies, anorexiants)
Urine may be colored dark yellow to brown from medication
Nausea, vomiting, or headache may occur; contact physician if such effects become severe

AVAILABILITY

Tablets—100 mg
Liquid—50 mg/15 mL

The information here is provided as guidance only. Prescribers should always consult the manufacturer's current prescribing information.

IODOQUINOL (Yodoxin®)

Iodoquinol is classified as an antiprotozoal agent useful in the treatment of asymptomatic intestinal amebiasis (*ie*, for asymptomatic carriers or cyst passers of *Entamoeba histolytica*). Its exact mechanism of action is not known. It produces its amebicidal effect at the actual site of infection in the colon because it is poorly absorbed from the gastrointestinal tract. It is an alternative agent in the treatment of balantidiasis and *Blastocystis hominis* infections.

Iodoquinol will occasionally be associated with rash, acne, or slight enlargement of the thyroid gland. Nausea, diarrhea, cramps, and anal pruritus also have been associated with its use. Rarely, optic neuritis, optic atrophy, loss of vision, and peripheral neuropathy have occurred after prolonged usage at high dosage for several months. Iodine sensitivity reactions are also possible.

ACTIVITY

Effective against cysts of *E. histolytica* in the large intestine.

SPECIAL PRECAUTIONS

Optic neuritis, optic atrophy, and peripheral neuropathy have occurred after prolonged high-dose therapy. Avoid long-term therapy.
Use caution in presence of thyroid disease.

SPECIAL GROUPS

Children: May be more susceptible to side effects, especially with prolonged, high-dose therapy.
Elderly: No information.
Renal impairment: Use cautiously in patients with renal disease.
Hepatic impairment: Contraindicated in hepatic damage.
Pregnancy: Safety not established; do not use.
Breast-feeding: Safety not established; do not use or do not nurse during use.

DOSAGE

(Take after meals to improve tolerance.)
Adults: 630 to 650 mg three times a day, for 20 days. Do not exceed 2 g in 24 hours.
Elderly: No information.
Children: 10 to 13.3 mg/kg three times a day for 20 days. Do not exceed 1.95 g in 24 hours.
Renal impairment: No information.

INDICATIONS

Treatment of asymptomatic amebiasis
(Note: Not indicated for treatment of chronic diarrhea, especially in children, because of potential association with optic atrophy and permanent loss of vision.)

CONTRAINDICATIONS

Allergy or hypersensitivity to any 8-hydroxyquinoline (*eg*, iodoquinol, iodochlorhydroxyquin) or to iodine-containing preparations; hepatic damage; renal disease

INTERACTIONS

Laboratory test interactions: because protein-bound iodine levels may increase during treatment, they may interfere with results of certain thyroid function tests; these effects can persist for up to 6 months after therapy has been discontinued

ADVERSE EFFECTS

Dermatologic: various skin eruptions (acneform, papular, pustular, bullae, vegetating, or tuberous iododerma), urticaria, pruritus
Gastrointestinal: nausea, vomiting, abdominal cramps, diarrhea, pruritus ani
Other: fever, chills, headache, vertigo, enlargement of thyroid; optic neuritis, optic atrophy, and peripheral neuropathy have occurred in association with prolonged high-dose therapy

PHARMACOKINETICS AND PHARMACODYNAMICS

Peak serum levels: no information
Serum half-life: no information
Bioavailability: poorly absorbed
Protein binding: no information
Metabolism: no information
Excretion: fecal; less than 10% recovered in urine
Renal impairment: no information
Hepatic impairment: no information

OVERDOSAGE

No information

PATIENT INFORMATION

Complete full course of therapy; blurred vision or loss of vision, nausea, gastrointestinal upset, vomiting, or diarrhea may occur; take after meals to improve tolerance

AVAILABILITY

Tablets—210 mg and 650 mg

The information here is provided as guidance only. Prescribers should always consult the manufacturer's current prescribing information.

MEBENDAZOLE (Vermox®)

Mebendazole is one of the most commonly used antihelminthic agents for a variety of parasitic nematodes. Its mechanism of action is vermicidal because it causes degeneration of the parasite's cytoplasmic microtubules. Because of this effect, it blocks glucose uptake in susceptible, adult, intestinal-dwelling helminths and tissue-dwelling larvae. As with albendazole, glucose uptake is diminished, and the parasite's glycogen stores are depleted, resulting in reduced formation of ATP. This results in the death of the parasite. There is no effect on serum glucose concentrations in humans.

Mebendazole is remarkably free of side effects. Occasionally, diarrhea, abdominal pain, or migration of ascaris worms will occur. Rarely, leukopenia, agranulocytosis, or hypospermia has been observed.

ACTIVITY

Active against *Trichuris trichiura* (whipworm), *Enterobius vermicularis* (pinworm), *Ascaris lumbricoides* (roundworm), *Ancylostoma duodenale* (common hookworm), and *Necator americanus* (American hookworm).

SPECIAL PRECAUTIONS

No evidence exists to suggest efficacy for hydatid disease.
Parasite immobilization and death are slow; complete clearance from gastrointestinal tract may take up to 3 days after therapy has ended. Efficacy varies as a function of factors, such as preexisting diarrhea, gastrointestinal transit time, degree of infection, and helminth strains.

SPECIAL GROUPS

Children: Safety and efficacy for use in children under 2 years of age not established.
Elderly: No information.
Renal impairment: No information.
Hepatic impairment: No information.
Pregnancy: Do not use unless benefits clearly outweigh risk, especially in first trimester. Embryotoxic and teratogenic in pregnant rats at single low doses of 10 mg/kg.
Breast-feeding: Safety not established.

DOSAGE

(Note: Tablets may be chewed, swallowed, or crushed and mixed with food. Neither fasting nor purging is necessary.)
Adults: For trichuriasis, ascariasis, and hookworm infection: One tablet morning and evening for 3 consecutive days.
For enterobiasis: A single dose of 100 mg; repeat after 2 weeks.
Elderly: Same as adults.
Children: Same as adults.
Renal impairment: No information.

INDICATIONS

Treatment of *T. trichiura* (whipworm), *E. vermicularis* (pinworm), *A. lumbricoides* (roundworm), *A. duodenale* (common hookworm), or *N. americanus* (American hookworm) in single and mixed infestations

CONTRAINDICATIONS

Allergy or hypersensitivity to mebendazole; hepatic

INTERACTIONS

May lower serum concentrations. Consider alternative therapy with valproic acid. Consult the *USP DI* recommendations.
Carbamazepine; Crohn's ileitis or ulcerative colitis

ADVERSE EFFECTS

Transient abdominal pain and diarrhea have occurred in cases of massive infection and expulsion of worms; fever has occurred (possible response to drug-induced tissue necrosis); severe but reversible neutropenia (apparently due to bone marrow suppression) in two patients receiving high doses for echinococcosis

PHARMACOKINETICS AND PHARMACODYNAMICS

Peak serum levels: 2 to 4 h after administration, no values given; after 100 mg twice a day for 3 consecutive days, plasma levels did not exceed 0.03 µg/mL
Serum half-life: normal hepatic function, 2.5 to 5.5 h
Bioavailability: poorly absorbed after oral administration (5%–10%); absorption may increase when taken with fatty food
Protein binding: no information
Metabolism: primarily hepatic; metabolized to inactive amino, hydroxy, and hydroxyamino metabolites
Excretion: 2% to 5% excreted in urine during first 24 to 48 h; majority of dose excreted in feces as unchanged drug or primary metabolites
Renal impairment: no information
Hepatic impairment: no information

OVERDOSAGE

Gastrointestinal effects may occur; treatment includes supportive therapy; induce vomiting and purging

PATIENT INFORMATION

Chew or crush tablet and mix with food
Removal of parasites may be slow (up to 3 days after end of treatment)
A second treatment is recommended if no cure occurs after 3 weeks
Pinworm infections are very contagious; all members of a family who are in contact with the patient should be treated to reduce spreading of infection
Strict hygiene is essential to prevent reinfection; disinfect toilet facilities daily; change and launder undergarments, bed linens, towels, and nightclothes daily

AVAILABILITY

Tablets (chewable)—100 mg

The information here is provided as guidance only. Prescribers should always consult the manufacturer's current prescribing information.

MEFLOQUINE (Lariam®)

Mefloquine is the standard antimalarial agent, indicated for both the prophylaxis and treatment of malaria caused by chloroquine-resistant and multidrug-resistant strains of *Plasmodium falciparum*. Mefloquine is also an effective prophylactic agent against malaria caused by *P. vivax*, *P. ovale*, and *P. malariae*. Mefloquine, like quinine, does not eliminate the exoerythrocytic liver forms of *P. vivax* or *P. ovale* and must be followed by subsequent treatment with a drug such as primaquine to produce a radical cure and to prevent relapses of such infections. Mefloquine acts as a blood schizonticide. Its effects are on the asexual form of the erythrocytic parasites, with no effect on the gametocytes. It is well absorbed from the gastrointestinal tract and can be administered on a once-a-week basis for prophylaxis. (Attempts to use this agent, with its long half-life, as a biweekly prophylactic agent were not successful, and breakthrough cases of malaria occurred. Currently, loading doses of mefloquine are being studied.)

The adverse effects of mefloquine are similar to those of chloroquine. However, 25% of travelers using mefloquine prophylaxis temporarily experience mild side effects, such as insomnia, bad dreams and irritability, headache, gastrointestinal upset, and dizziness. A severe neuropsychiatric reaction, including seizures and psychosis, has been reported in approximately one of 10,000 individuals who used the drug for prophylaxis. There is a greater frequency of severe reactions, in about one of 1000 patients who use the higher doses of mefloquine required for treatment of malaria. Mefloquine is gradually achieving use during pregnancy, although it is still not indicated for prophylaxis during the first trimester. Women of childbearing age who take mefloquine as malaria prophylaxis should use contraception while on this agent and for 2 months after the last dose because it has such a long half-life. The recommendation that mefloquine not be taken when beta-blockers or calcium channel blockers are used to regulate cardiac rhythm has been better studied: this is no longer contraindicated.

ACTIVITY

May act by increasing intravesicular pH in parasite acid vesicles.

SPECIAL PRECAUTIONS

Life-threatening, severe, or overwhelming malaria infections due to *P. falciparum* should initially be treated with an intravenous antimalarial drug. Mefloquine may be given after intravenous therapy is complete to finish course of therapy.
Use caution when driving or performing other activities requiring coordination and alertness. Dizziness, disturbed sense of balance, and neuropsychiatric reactions have occurred with use.
With prophylactic use, if unexplained anxiety, depression, restlessness, or confusion occurs, discontinue drug. These effects should be considered prodromal to more serious events.
Periodic evaluation of renal, hepatic, and hematologic values should be performed if mefloquine is to be administered for a prolonged period.
Ocular lesions occurred in rats fed mefloquine daily for 2 years.

INDICATIONS

Treatment of acute malarial infections due to mefloquine-susceptible strains of *P. falciparum* (both chloroquine-resistant and multidrug–resistant strains)
Prevention of malaria or prophylaxis of *P. falciparum*, *P. ovale*, *P. malariae*, and *P. vivax* malaria infections, including chloroquine-resistant and multidrug–resistant strains of *P. falciparum*

CONTRAINDICATIONS

Allergy or hypersensitivity to mefloquine, quinidine, quinine, or related compounds; consider risk–benefit in cases of heart block, history of psychiatric disorders, epilepsy, history of seizure disorder

INTERACTIONS

Beta-adrenergic blocking agents, calcium channel blocking agents, divalproex, chloroquine, quinine or quinidine, valproic acid

ADVERSE EFFECTS

(Note: At doses used for treatment of malarial infection, symptoms possibly due to drug are indistinguishable from those usually attributable to disease itself.)
Prophylaxis malaria: vomiting, dizziness, syncope, extrasystoles (< 1%), encephalopathy of unknown etiology
Treatment of malaria: dizziness, myalgia, nausea, fever, headache, vomiting, chills, diarrhea, skin rash, abdominal pain, fatigue, loss of appetite, tinnitus
Effects occurring in < 1% of patients: bradycardia, alopecia, emotional problems, pruritus, asthenia, transient emotional disturbances, telogen effluvium (loss of resting hair), seizures
Postmarketing surveillance: visual disturbances, central nervous system disturbances (*eg*, vertigo, psychotic manifestations, hallucinations, confusion, anxiety, depression, convulsions, insomnia)
Laboratory test abnormalities: decreased hematocrit, transient elevation of transaminases, leukopenia, thrombocytopenia (all in patients with acute malaria who received treatment doses; effects attributed to disease itself); transient elevation of transaminases, leukocytosis, thrombocytopenia (all with prophylactic administration)

The information here is provided as guidance only. Prescribers should always consult the manufacturer's current prescribing information.

MEFLOQUINE (CONTINUED)

SPECIAL GROUPS

Elderly: No information.
Renal impairment: Monitor function in prolonged therapy.
Hepatic impairment: Monitor function in prolonged therapy.
Pregnancy: Adequate human studies not performed; use only if benefits outweigh risk. Women of childbearing potential traveling to areas where malaria is endemic should be warned against becoming pregnant and advised to take reliable contraceptive measures while taking mefloquine and for at least 2 months after the last dose of mefloquine.
Breast-feeding: Low concentrations are excreted; use with caution.

DOSAGE

(Note: Use same day of each week for administration. Do not take on empty stomach.)
Adults: For mild to moderate malaria due to *P. vivax* or mefloquine-susceptible strains of *P. falciparum*: Use five tablets of mefloquine (1250 mg) as a single dose. Do not take on an empty stomach; take with at least 240 mL (8 oz) water. (Note: Patients with acute *P. vivax* malaria treated with mefloquine alone are at high risk of relapse because mefloquine does not eliminate exoerythrocytic [hepatic phase] parasites. Subsequent treatment with an 8-aminoquinolone [*eg*, primaquine] is necessary to avoid relapse.)
For malaria prophylaxis: The Centers for Disease Control and Prevention (CDC) recommends a single 250-mg dose taken weekly beginning 1 week before travel, continuing weekly during travel, and for 4 weeks after leaving endemic areas.
Elderly: May have age-related renal impairment; monitor function. Same as adults.
Children: For malaria prophylaxis, the CDC recommends the following doses to be taken weekly, beginning 1 week before travel, continuing weekly during travel, and for 4 weeks after leaving endemic areas: (15–19 kg of body weight) 1/4 tablet; (20–30 kg of body weight) 1/2 tablet; (31–45 kg of body weight) 3/4 tablet; (> 45 kg of body weight) 1 tablet.
Renal impairment: No dose reduction generally required because urinary clearance is very low.

PHARMACOKINETICS AND PHARMACODYNAMICS

Peak serum levels: no values given; greater concentration for longer periods of administration
Serum half-life: 13 to 33 days (median 20 days)
Bioavailability: absorption greater than 85%
Protein binding: very high (98%–99%)
Metabolism: hepatic (partial)
Excretion: approximately 5% is excreted in urine; fecal elimination very slow
Renal impairment: monitor function in prolonged therapy
Hepatic impairment: monitor function in prolonged therapy

OVERDOSAGE

No known specific antidote; treatment should include standard gastric decontamination procedures, and symptomatic and supportive treatments

PATIENT INFORMATION

Do not give to children under 2 years of age. Take with full glass of water and with food. Continue medication while staying in area and for 4 weeks after leaving area.

AVAILABILITY

Tablets—250 mg

The information here is provided as guidance only. Prescribers should always consult the manufacturer's current prescribing information.

NICLOSAMIDE (Niclocide®)

Niclosamide is an alternative drug for the treatment of various tapeworm infections, including those due to the fish, beef, pork, dog, and dwarf tapeworms. However, niclosamide is not considered effective treatment for cysticercosis. The mechanism of action includes its inhibition of oxidative metabolism within the mitochondria of cestodes. The scolex head is destroyed and loosened from its attachment to the intestinal wall, after which it can be digested. Niclosamide could release viable eggs from *Taenia solium* into the intestinal lumen, potentially allowing development of cysticercosis. This may no longer be an important issue because praziquantel has replaced niclosamide in the treatment of many of these tapeworm infections.

Niclosamide has occasionally been associated with nausea and abdominal pain. Nausea, vomiting, diarrhea, and abdominal discomfort may be expected in less than 4% of patients. Occasional headache, skin rash, urticaria, pruritus ani, and vertigo have been reported. There are no adequate studies with regard to the use of niclosamide during pregnancy. Alcohol consumption should be avoided on the day of therapy and for 1 day afterward.

ACTIVITY

Inhibits phosphorylation in the mitochondria of cestodes; scolex and proximal segments are killed on contact with the drug.

SPECIAL PRECAUTIONS

Niclosamide affects the cestodes of the intestine only; it does not affect cysticercosis.

SPECIAL GROUPS

Elderly: No information.
Renal impairment: No information.
Hepatic impairment: No information.
Pregnancy: Safety not established; use only when benefits outweigh risk.
Breast-feeding: Safety for use not established.

DOSAGE

(Note: Chew tablets thoroughly, then swallow with small amount of water. For young children, tablets may be crushed and mixed with small amount of water to form a paste. Dietary restrictions are not necessary; should preferably be taken after a light meal. Constipated patients may need a mild laxative.)
Adults: For *Taenia saginata*, *Taenia solium* and *Diphyllobothrium latum* (beef, pork and fish tapeworm), four tablets (2 g) as single dose. For *Hymenolepis nana* (dwarf tapeworm), four tablets (2 g) as single dose then two tablets (1g) daily for 6 days; strict personal hygiene must be observed to avoid autoinfection.
Elderly: No information.
Children: For *T. saginata*, *D. latum*, and *T. solium*: 11 to 34 kg of body weight, two tablets (1 g) as single dose; > 34 kg, three tablets (1.5 g) as single dose. For *H. nana* and *H. diminuta*: 11 to 34 kg, two tablets (1 g) on 1st day, then one tablet (0.5 g) daily for the following 6 days; > 34 kg, three tablets (1.5 g) on 1st day, then two tablets (1 g) daily for the following 6 days. Strict personal hygiene must be observed and enforced to avoid autoinfection.
Renal impairment: No information.

INDICATIONS

Treatment of *T. saginata* (beef tapeworm), *T. solium* (pork tapeworm), *D. latum* (fish tapeworm), and *H. nana* (dwarf tapeworm)

CONTRAINDICATIONS

Allergy or hypersensitivity to niclosamide or any product components

INTERACTIONS

No information

ADVERSE EFFECTS

Central nervous system: drowsiness, dizziness, headache, weakness
Dermatologic: skin rash (including pruritus ani), alopecia; two cases of urticaria were reported and may have been due to tapeworm breakdown products
Gastrointestinal: nausea and vomiting, abdominal discomfort, loss of appetite, diarrhea, constipation, rectal bleeding, oral irritation, bad taste in mouth
Miscellaneous: fever, sweating, palpitations, edema of an arm, backache, irritability; one report of transient rise in aspartate aminotransferase in an intravenous narcotic addict (all side effects were mild to moderate, transitory, and did not require discontinuation of treatment)

PHARMACOKINETICS AND PHARMACODYNAMICS

Peak serum levels: no information
Serum half-life: no information
Bioavailability: no significant absorption from gastrointestinal tract
Protein binding: no information
Metabolism: no information
Excretion: fecal
Renal impairment: no information
Hepatic impairment: no information

OVERDOSAGE

Administer fast-acting laxative and enema; do not induce vomiting

PATIENT INFORMATION

Chew tablets thoroughly and then swallow with small amount of water, take with food after a light meal (*eg*, breakfast); may cause stomach upset, mild laxatives may be used to relieve constipation
Comply with full course of therapy; second course may be required

AVAILABILITY

Tablets (chewable)—500 mg

The information here is provided as guidance only. Prescribers should always consult the manufacturer's current prescribing information.

OXAMNIQUINE (Vansil®)

Oxamniquine is an alternative agent for the treatment of *Schistosoma mansoni* infections. It has been replaced by praziquantel as the drug of choice for this infection. When praziquantel is not available, oxamniquine can be used for the treatment of all stages of *S. mansoni* infection, including the chronic phase with hepatosplenic involvement.

If oxamniquine is administered to patients with schistosomiasis, the adult worms move from the mesenteric veins to the liver. Both mature and immature worms are destroyed; male worms are more susceptible than the females. In the absence of the males, any female worms that remain may fail to lay eggs.

Oxamniquine may cause neuropsychiatric disturbances and seizures in some patients. Usually, headache, fever, dizziness, and somnolence are its side effects. Occasional side effects are nausea, diarrhea, rash, insomnia, hepatic enzyme changes, or even electrocardiogram changes. The drug can produce changes in the electrocardiogram and will turn the urine orange. Seizures and neuropsychiatric disturbances appear to be rare.

ACTIVITY

More effective against male schistosomes than females; however, after treatment, residual female schistosomes cease to lay eggs and thus lose their parasitologic significance.

SPECIAL PRECAUTIONS

Convulsions have rarely occurred within the first few hours after ingestion, most often in patients with a history of seizures. Caution should be exercised in these patients, and medical supervision and appropriate facilities should be present during treatment.

SPECIAL GROUPS

Children: No pediatric-specific problems have been documented.
Elderly: No information.
Renal impairment: No information.
Hepatic impairment: No information.
Pregnancy: Adequate human studies not performed; oxamniquine crosses the placenta; use only when clearly indicated and when benefits outweigh risk.
Breast-feeding: Distributed into breast milk; use with caution.

DOSAGE

Adults: 15 mg/kg as a single dose in patients with western hemisphere strains of *Schistosoma mansoni*. Dosage guidelines based on weight are as follows:

Recommended Dosage Guidelines for Oxamniquine

Weight, *kg*	Dose, *mg*
30–40	500
41–60	750
61–80	1000
81–100	1250

Elderly: No information.
Children: (< 30 kg) give 20 mg/kg in two divided doses of 10 mg/kg with 2 to 8 hours between doses.
Renal impairment: No information.

INDICATIONS

Alternative treatment of all stages of *S. mansoni* infection, including acute and chronic phase with hepatosplenic involvement
(Unlabeled): Successful low-dose, concurrent administration of oxamniquine with praziquantel has been used as single-dose treatment of neurocysticercosis

CONTRAINDICATIONS

Epilepsy or other seizure disorders; hypersensitivity to oxamniquine

INTERACTIONS

No information

ADVERSE EFFECTS

Central nervous system: transitory dizziness and drowsiness (33%), headache, epileptiform convulsions (rare; *see* Special Precautions), electroencephalogram abnormalities
Gastrointestinal: nausea, vomiting, abdominal pain, diarrhea, anorexia
Laboratory abnormalities: (not drug related and of no significance) mild to moderate liver enzyme elevations with no evidence of hepatotoxicity, even in patients with severe hepatosplenic involvement
Other: urticaria

PHARMACOKINETICS AND PHARMACODYNAMICS

Peak serum levels: no information
Serum half-life: 1 to 2.5 h
Bioavailability: no percentage given; well absorbed orally
Protein binding: no information
Metabolism: probably hepatic; extensively to inactive acidic metabolites
Excretion: approximately 40% to 70% excreted as 6-carboxy metabolites in urine
Renal impairment: no information
Hepatic impairment: no effect

OVERDOSAGE

No information

PATIENT INFORMATION

Take with food to improve tolerance
May cause dizziness or drowsiness

AVAILABILITY

Capsules—250 mg

The information here is provided as guidance only. Prescribers should always consult the manufacturer's current prescribing information.

PAROMOMYCIN (Humatin®, Aminosidine®)

Paromomycin is an amebicidal and antibacterial aminoglycoside agent derived from *Streptomyces rimosus* and available for oral administration. This drug is related to neomycin, kanamycin, and streptomycin, which are also aminoglycoside antibacterial agents. It has achieved considerable use for the treatment of giardiasis in women who are pregnant because it is essentially nonabsorbable. With the current AIDS pandemic and intestinal cryptosporidiosis, paromomycin is one of the few agents that has actually proved efficacious in the treatment of chronic diarrhea. Paromomycin has a direct amebicidal action. Because it is not significantly absorbed via the gastrointestinal tract, it has very little, if any, activity against extraintestinal infection. It also has been useful in *Blastocystis hominis* heavy infestation. Some accumulation of the drug still can occur, particularly in patients who have renal insufficiency, and it may reach toxic levels. For this reason, paromomycin is contraindicated in those patients who have impaired renal function or enough ulcerative bowel lesions from intestinal amebiasis and intestinal obstruction to cause increased absorption of the drug. The most frequent side effects are gastrointestinal disturbances, but occasionally eighth nerve damage, mainly auditory, will occur.

ACTIVITY

Active in intestinal amebiasis and has *in vitro* and *in vivo* antibacterial activity similar to neomycin. Also effective against the enteric bacteria *Salmonella* and *Shigella*.

SPECIAL PRECAUTIONS

Ototoxicity and renal damage may occur as a result of inadvertent absorption through ulcerative bowel lesions.

Antibiotic use (especially prolonged or repeated therapy) may result in superinfection due to bacterial or fungal overgrowth of nonsusceptible organisms. Appropriate measures should be taken if such superinfection or secondary infection occurs.

SPECIAL GROUPS

Children: Safe for use.
Elderly: No information.
Renal impairment: No specific information (*see* Special Precautions).
Hepatic impairment: No information.
Pregnancy: No information.
Breast-feeding: No information.

DOSAGE

Adults: For intestinal amebiasis, 25 to 35 mg/kg/d in three divided doses with meals for 5 to 10 days.
Elderly: Same as adults.
Children: For intestinal amebiasis, same as adults.
Renal impairment: No information.

INDICATIONS

Treatment of acute and chronic intestinal amebiasis, adjunctive therapy in management of hepatic coma (Unlabeled):

Useful in other parasitic infections such as *Dientamoeba fragilis* (25–30 mg/kg/d in three doses for 7 days), *Diphyllobothrium latum, Taenia saginata, Taenia solium, Dipylidium caninum* (adults: 1 g every 15 minutes for four doses; children: 11 mg/kg every 15 minutes for four doses), *Hymenolepis nana* (45 mg/kg/d for 5–7 days)

CONTRAINDICATIONS

Allergy or hypersensitivity to paromomycin, intestinal obstruction

INTERACTIONS

Because paromomycin is an aminoglycoside, interactions that may occur with other oral aminoglycosides may potentially occur with paromomycin

ADVERSE EFFECTS

Gastrointestinal: nausea, abdominal cramps, and diarrhea have been reported to occur with doses greater than 3 g/d

PHARMACOKINETICS AND PHARMACODYNAMICS

Peak serum levels: no information
Serum half-life: no information
Bioavailability: no information
Protein binding: no information
Metabolism: no information
Excretion: 100% recovered in feces
Renal impairment: no information
Hepatic impairment: no information

OVERDOSAGE

No information

PATIENT INFORMATION

Complete full course of therapy. Nausea, vomiting, or diarrhea may occur; if ringing of ears, hearing impairment, or dizziness occurs, contact physician

AVAILABILITY

Capsules—250 mg (as sulfate)

The information here is provided as guidance only. Prescribers should always consult the manufacturer's current prescribing information.

PENTAMIDINE (NebuPent®, Pentacarinat®, Pentam300®)

Pentamidine is an antiprotozoal agent whose mechanism of action is not clearly defined. It is thought to interfere with the incorporation of nucleotides into RNA and DNA. It inhibits oxidative phosphorylation and biosynthesis of DNA, RNA protein, and phospholipids and may also interfere with folate transformation. The major use for pentamidine is in the treatment and prophylaxis of *Pneumocystis carinii* pneumonia in immunocompromised patients, including those with AIDS (HIV-related). Although folic-acid antagonists are the drugs of choice for the treatment of this infection, they often result in allergic reactions, such as fever and skin rash. Thus, pentamidine has an important place in the treatment of these infections.

Pentamidine also has a role as a secondary agent for the treatment of visceral leishmaniasis and cutaneous leishmaniasis in addition to the treatment of African trypanosomiasis. Clinicians should be aware of the frequent occurrence of hypotension and hypoglycemia, sometimes followed by diabetes mellitus, and the potential for renal damage in patients receiving pentamidine. In addition, vomiting, blood dyscrasias, and gastrointestinal disturbances occur. Pentamidine may aggravate diabetes mellitus and has been associated with occasional shock, hypocalcemia, liver damage, cardiotoxicity, delirium, and rash. Acute pancreatitis occurring either during or following pentamidine administration has been a significant problem in patients being treated with the drug for *P. carinii* infections.

ACTIVITY

Active against *Pneumocystis carinii*.

SPECIAL PRECAUTIONS

Development of acute *P. carinii* pneumonia can still occur in patients receiving pentamidine prophylaxis. Any patient demonstrating symptoms suggestive of pulmonary infection should be thoroughly evaluated and tested for possible acute *P. carinii* pneumonia and other opportunistic and nonopportunistic pathogens. (Note: Aerosolized pentamidine may alter the clinical and radiographic features of *P. carinii* pneumonia and may cause an atypical or extrapulmonary presentation.) Fatalities have occurred because of severe hypotension, hypoglycemia, and cardiac arrhythmias with both intravenous and intramuscular administration. Severe hypotension may occur after a single dose. Pentamidine use should be limited to patients in whom *P. carinii* infection has been confirmed. Patients should be monitored closely for adverse effects.

Patients with hypertension, hypotension, hypoglycemia, hyperglycemia, hypocalcemia, leukopenia, thrombocytopenia, anemia, hepatic or renal dysfunction, ventricular tachycardia, pancreatitis, or Stevens-Johnson syndrome should be given pentamidine with caution.

Hypotension (severe and sudden) may occur after a single intravenous or intramuscular dose. Patients receiving this agent should be supine, and blood pressure should be monitored closely during administration and several times thereafter until it is stable. Emergency resuscitation equipment should be readily available. Infuse intravenously over 60-minute period.

Hypoglycemia induced by pentamidine has been associated with pancreatic islet cell necrosis and inappropriately high plasma insulin concentrations.

Hyperglycemia and diabetes mellitus (with or without preceding hypoglycemia) have occurred also, even several months after therapy. Blood glucose levels should be monitored daily during therapy and several times after it is complete.

Inhalation of pentamidine isethionate may cause bronchospasm or cough, especially in patients with a history of smoking or asthma. In those who experience these effects, administration of an inhaled bronchodilator before each pentamidine dose may minimize recurrence.

INDICATIONS

Treatment of *P. carinii* pneumonia
Prevention of *P. carinii* pneumonia in high-risk patients infected with HIV and defined by one or both of the following criteria: history of one or more episodes of *P. carinii* pneumonia or a peripheral CD4 (T_4 helper-inducer) lymphocyte count ≤ 200 mm^3
(Unlabeled): Treatment of trypanosomiasis and visceral leishmaniasis

CONTRAINDICATIONS

Allergic reaction to pentamidine, bleeding disorders, bone marrow depression, cardiac disease arrhythmias, hepatic or renal function impairment, diabetes mellitus, pregnancy

INTERACTIONS

Bone marrow depressants, radiation therapy, didanosine, erythromycin, foscarnet, nephrotoxic medications

ADVERSE EFFECTS

INJECTION: (Note: Most patients treated were infected with AIDS.)
Severe: Leukopenia, hypoglycemia, thrombocytopenia, hypotension, nephrotoxicity, hypocalcemia, Stevens-Johnson syndrome, ventricular tachycardia; fatalities due to severe hypotension, hypoglycemia, and cardiac arrhythmias
Moderate: Elevated serum creatinine, sterile abscess, pain or induration at intramuscular injection site, elevated liver function tests, leukopenia, nausea, anorexia, hypotension, fever, hypoglycemia, rash, bad taste in mouth, confusion or hallucinations, anemia, neuralgia, thrombocytopenia, hyperkalemia, phlebitis, dizziness without hypotension, increased thirst, increased urination
AEROSOL:
Most frequent: Fatigue, metallic taste, shortness of breath, decreased appetite, dizziness, rash, cough, nausea, pharyngitis, chest pain or congestion, night sweats, chills, vomiting, bronchospasm
Less frequent: Pneumothorax, diarrhea, headache, anemia (generally associated with zidovudine use), myalgia, abdominal pain, edema

The information here is provided as guidance only. Prescribers should always consult the manufacturer's current prescribing information.

PENTAMIDINE (CONTINUED)

SPECIAL PRECAUTIONS (CONTINUED)

Extrapulmonary infection due to *P. carinii* has been reported infrequently with inhalation use, most commonly in patients with a history of *P. carinii* pneumonia. When evaluating patients with unexplained signs and symptoms, consider presence of extrapulmonary pneumocystosis.

The following laboratory tests should be performed before, during, and after therapy with intravenous pentamidine: daily blood urea nitrogen, serum creatinine, and blood glucose; complete blood count and platelet counts; liver function test, including bilirubin, alkaline phosphatase, AST, and ALT; serum calcium; electrocardiogram at regular intervals.

SPECIAL GROUPS

Children: Side effects are similar to those seen in adults; no pediatric-specific problems have been documented.

Elderly: No information.

Renal impairment: Reduced dosage may be necessary.

Hepatic impairment: Pentamidine may cause increase in AST, ALT, bilirubin, and alkaline phosphatase.

Pregnancy: Safety and efficacy not established; use only when clearly needed and when benefits outweigh risk.

Breast-feeding: Not known whether excreted in breast milk; because of potential for serious adverse effects to fetus, breast-feeding is not recommended.

DOSAGE

Adults: (*P. carinii*) 4 mg/kg/d for 14 to 21 days administered intramuscularly or intravenously only. (Note: Benefits and risk for therapy exceeding 14 days are not defined.) Infuse intravenous solution over period of 1 hour. (Leishmaniasis) 2 to 4 mg/kg/d for up to 15 days, intravenously. Administer over 1 to 2 hours.

AEROSOL: For prevention of *P. carinii* pneumonia, 300 mg once every 4 weeks administered via the Respirgard II nebulizer (Marquest). Deliver until nebulizer chamber is empty, approximately 30 to 45 minutes. Flow rate should be 5 to 7 L/min from a 40 to 50 pounds per square inch air or oxygen source. Do not use low pressure compressors. To reconstitute, dissolve contents of one vial in 6 mL of sterile water for injection; it is essential that only sterile water for injection be used (saline will cause drug to precipitate). Place entire reconstituted contents of vial into nebulizer reservoir.

Elderly: No information.

Children: Same as adults.

Renal impairment: No dosage adjustment necessary.

ADVERSE EFFECTS (CONTINUED)

Cardiovascular: tachycardia, hypotension, hypertension, palpitations, syncope, cerebrovascular accident, vasodilation, vasculitis

Dermatologic: pruritus, erythema, dry skin, desquamation, urticaria

Gastrointestinal: gingivitis, dyspepsia, oral ulcer or abscess, gastritis, gastric ulcer, hypersalivation, dry mouth, splenomegaly, melena, hematochezia, esophagitis, colitis, pancreatitis, nausea and vomiting, diarrhea, loss of appetite

Hematologic: pancytopenia, neutropenia, eosinophilia

Hepatic: hepatitis, hepatomegaly, hepatic dysfunction

Metabolic: hypoglycemia, hyperglycemia, hypocalcemia

Miscellaneous: incontinence, miscarriage, arthralgia, allergic reactions, extrapulmonary pneumocystosis

Neurologic: tremors, confusion, anxiety, memory loss, seizure, neuropathy, paresthesia, hallucination, depression, unsteady gait

Renal: renal failure, nephritis

Respiratory: rhinitis, laryngitis, laryngospasm, hyperventilation, hemoptysis, eosinophilic or interstitial pneumonitis, pleuritis, cyanosis, tachypnea, rales

PHARMACOKINETICS AND PHARMACODYNAMICS

Peak serum levels: 0.5 to 3.4 μg/mL after 4 mg/kg intravenous dose; peak plasma levels were at or below lower limits of detection of the assay (2.3 ng/mL) after aerosolized 300 mg; 0.2 to 1.4 μg/mL after 4 mg/kg intramuscular dose

Serum half-life: 9.1 to 13.2 h, intramuscular; 6.5 h, intravenous

Bioavailability: poorly absorbed

Protein binding: high, 69% in humans

Metabolism: no information

Excretion: 4% to 17% of intramuscular dose excreted in urine over 24 h; 2.5% of intravenous dose excreted in urine in 24 h

Renal impairment: no information (excretion probably reduced)

Hepatic impairment: no information

OVERDOSAGE

Severe hypotension may occur; patient should lie down during administration; do not take if pentamidine; use caution in use of regular toothbrushes, dental floss, and toothpicks to reduce bleeding

PATIENT INFORMATION

Severe hypotension may occur; patient should lie down during administration; do not take if allergic to pentamidine; use caution in use of regular toothbrushes, dental floss, and toothpicks to reduce bleeding

AVAILABILITY

Injection—300 mg per vial
Aerosol—300 mg

The information here is provided as guidance only. Prescribers should always consult the manufacturer's current prescribing information.

PIPERAZINE CITRATE

Piperazine was accepted for treatment of ascaris and pinworm infections, but has recently been replaced by other agents. Piperazine causes paralysis of ascaris, and if the worm is paralyzed, it is readily discharged from the intestinal lumen and expelled from the body by normal peristalsis. Piperazine acts by blocking acetylcholine at the myoneural junction. It may have a similar myoneural blocking action on mammalian skeletal muscle, but this is not of any clinical significance. Nausea, vomiting, diarrhea, abdominal pain, and headache are generally mild if they occur. Neurotoxic side effects are rare. Patients with epilepsy have had exacerbation seizures and allergic reactions, including serum sickness. Piperazine has a somewhat limited usefulness in the current era of multiple alternative antiparasitic agents useful for the treatment of ascaris, including drugs such as mebendazole and albendazole.

ACTIVITY

Blocks response of *Ascaris lumbricoides* muscle to acetylcholine, resulting in flaccid paralysis of the worm. *A. lumbricoides* are then dislodged and expelled through peristalsis.

SPECIAL PRECAUTIONS

Prolonged, repeated, or excessive treatment should be avoided because of potential for neurotoxicity.
Take on empty stomach; surface contact between agent and parasite is diminished with presence of food.
Discontinue use if central nervous system, significant gastrointestinal, or hypersensitivity reactions occur.
Use with caution in patients with severe malnutrition or anemia.
Contraindicated in renal or hepatic impairment.

SPECIAL GROUPS

Children: Use cautiously; avoid prolonged or repeated treatment.
Elderly: No information.
Renal impairment: Contraindicated.
Hepatic impairment: Contraindicated.
Pregnancy: Safety not established; use only if benefits outweigh risks.
Breast-feeding: Safety not established; probably excreted in breast milk; women who are nursing should not take piperazine.

DOSAGE

(Note: All doses given in terms of hexahydrate equivalent.)
Adults: For ascariasis (roundworm), a single daily dose of 3.5 g for 2 consecutive days. For enterobiasis (pinworm), a single daily dose of 65 mg/kg for 7 consecutive days; maximum daily dose is 2.5 g.
Elderly: No information.
Children: For ascariasis (roundworm), a single daily dose of 75 mg/kg for 2 consecutive days with a maximum daily dose of 3.5 g. For enterobiasis (pinworm), same as adult. For severe infections, repeat treatment course after 1-week interval.
Renal impairment: Contraindicated.

INDICATIONS

Treatment of enterobiasis (pinworm) and ascariasis (roundworm) infections

CONTRAINDICATIONS

Renal or hepatic function impairment, convulsive disorders, hypersensitivity to piperazine

INTERACTIONS

No information

ADVERSE EFFECTS

Central nervous system: dizziness, drowsiness, headache, vertigo, ataxia, tremors, chorea, muscular weakness, hyporeflexia, paresthesia, seizures, electrocardiogram abnormalities, memory defect
Gastrointestinal: nausea, vomiting, abdominal cramps, diarrhea
Hypersensitivity: urticaria, erythema multiforme, purpura, fever, arthralgia, eczematous skin reactions, lacrimation, rhinorrhea, cough, bronchospasm
Ocular: cataracts, blurred vision, nystagmus, paralytic strabismus

PHARMACOKINETICS AND PHARMACODYNAMICS

Peak serum levels: no information
Serum half-life: no information
Bioavailability: no percentage given; readily absorbed from gastrointestinal tract
Protein binding: no information
Metabolism: 25% metabolized in liver
Excretion: variable; in urine, essentially unchanged within 24 h
Renal impairment: contraindicated
Hepatic impairment: contraindicated

OVERDOSAGE

Emesis or gastric lavage within a few hours of ingestion; supportive and symptomatic treatment

PATIENT INFORMATION

Take on full or empty stomach as directed by physician
If headache, vertigo, lack of coordination, muscle weakness, seizures, confusion, dizziness, nausea, vomiting, diarrhea, rash, or difficult breathing occurs, contact physician
Pinworm infections are very contagious; all family members in close contact with patient should be treated to decrease risk of spreading infection; severe infections require repeat of treatment 1 week after first course of therapy
Strict personal hygiene is essential to prevent reinfection; disinfect toilet facilities every day; change and launder undergarments, bed linens, towels, and nightclothes daily
For oral solution, dissolve in water, milk, or fruit juice

AVAILABILITY

Tablets—piperazine citrate equivalent to 250 mg piperazine hexahydrate
Syrup—piperazine citrate equivalent to 500 mg piperazine hexahydrate/5 mL

The information here is provided as guidance only. Prescribers should always consult the manufacturer's current prescribing information.

PRAZIQUANTEL (Biltricide®)

Praziquantel is one of the most exciting antiparasitic agents to be introduced into the therapeutic armamentarium over the past 20 years. This agent has a spectrum activity that is fairly wide, including schistosomes, tapeworms, and lung and liver flukes. Its most important recent use may have been in the treatment of neurocysticercosis, although it is currently being supplanted by the use of albendazole. In the treatment of neurocysticercosis, it is often necessary to consider the use of corticosteroids because the death of larvae may result in intense inflammatory reactions due to the action of praziquantel.

The precise mechanism of action is not known. Praziquantel is rapidly taken up by helminths. It decreases the permeability of the helminth cell membrane, leading to a loss of intracellular calcium. Rapid contraction and paralysis of the helminth's musculature occur. Vacuolization of the tegument appears in adult schistosomes.

Malaise, headache, and dizziness have been reported frequently. Occasionally, sedation, abdominal discomfort, fever, sweating, eosinophilia, or fatigue has been reported. Pruritus and rash are rare. Adequate and well-controlled studies in pregnancy have not yet been done, placing it in the Food and Drug Administration pregnancy Category B. Clinicians should familiarize themselves with the use of praziquantel because it has such wide application in the treatment of parasitic infections. Although it is a fairly expensive agent, it is anticipated that as price diminishes, praziquantel will have a long period of usefulness for the treatment of many parasitic infections.

ACTIVITY

Increases cell membrane permeability in susceptible worms, causing loss of intracellular calcium, massive contractions, and paralysis of their musculature. Also causes vacuolization and disintegration of schistosome tegument.

SPECIAL PRECAUTIONS

Use caution while driving or performing other tasks requiring alertness and coordination; praziquantel may produce drowsiness.
Minimal liver enzyme increases have occurred in some patients.
If schistosomiasis or fluke infection is found to be related to cerebral cysticercosis, patient should be hospitalized for duration of treatment.

SPECIAL GROUPS

Children: Safety for use in children under 4 years of age not established.
Elderly: No information.
Renal impairment: No information.
Hepatic impairment: No information.
Pregnancy: Adequate human studies not performed; increased abortion rate occurred in rats at three times normal human dosage; use only if benefits outweigh risk.
Breast-feeding: Excreted at concentrations 25% of maternal serum; do not nurse on day of treatment and for 72 hours thereafter.

DOSAGE

(Swallow tablets unchewed with some liquid at mealtime. Do not keep tablets in mouth; bitter taste may result in gagging or vomiting.)
Adults: Interval between doses should not be less than 4 hours and not greater than 6 hours. For clonorchiasis and opisthorchiasis, 25 mg/kg three times a day for 1 day. *S. hematobium* and *mansoni:* 20 mg/kg twice a day for 1 day. *S. japonicum* and *mekongi:* 20 mg/kg three times a day for 1 day. Neurocysticercosis: oral, 16.7 to 33 mg/kg three times a day for 15 to 30 days. May be repeated in 2 to 6 months. Diphyllobothriasis: oral, 10 to 20 mg/kg as a single dose. Paragonimiasis: 25 mg/kg three times a day for 2 days. Taeniasis (intestinal): 10 mg/kg as a single dose. Hymenolepiasis: 25 mg/kg as a single dose.
Elderly: No information.
Children: For children > 4 years of age, same as adults.
Renal impairment: No information.

INDICATIONS

Treatment of infections due to *Schistosoma mekongi*, *Schistosoma japonicum*, *Schistosoma mansoni*, and *Schistosoma haematobium;* infections due to liver flukes, *Clonorchis sinensis*, and *Opisthorchis viverrini* (unlabeled); infection due to lung fluke, *Paragonimus westermani;* infections due to *Taenia solium* (pork tapeworm) and *T. saginata* (beef tapeworm) (unlabeled)

CONTRAINDICATIONS

Previous hypersensitivity to praziquantel, pregnancy category B
(Note: Because parasite destruction within the eyes can cause irreparable lesions, do not treat ocular cysticercosis with praziquantel.)

INTERACTIONS

Carbamazepine, phenytoin

ADVERSE EFFECTS

Malaise, headache, dizziness, abdominal discomfort (with or without nausea), appetite loss, rising temperature, urticaria (rare)

PHARMACOKINETICS AND PHARMACODYNAMICS

Peak serum levels: normal liver function, 0.2 to 2.0 µg/mL
Serum half-life: 0.8 to 1.5 h for parent drug; 4 to 6 h for metabolites
Bioavailability: rapidly absorbed; however, undergoes extensive first-pass metabolism with only a small amount of drug likely to reach the systemic circulation
Protein binding: high, 80% to 85%
Metabolism: significant first-pass effect; completely metabolized to inactive mono- and polyhydroxylated derivatives
Excretion: metabolites (little or no activity) excreted primarily in urine; 72% excreted within 24 h
Renal impairment: no information
Hepatic impairment: no information

OVERDOSAGE

Administer a fast-acting laxative

PATIENT INFORMATION

Take with liquids at mealtime; do not chew tablets; do not double doses. Dizziness or drowsiness may occur; use caution when performing tasks requiring alertness or coordination (*eg*, driving).

AVAILABILITY

Tablets—600 mg (triple-scored for children)

The information here is provided as guidance only. Prescribers should always consult the manufacturer's current prescribing information.

PRIMAQUINE

Primaquine is an 8-aminoquinolone, and its major use is in the prevention of relapses of malaria caused by *Plasmodium vivax* and *Plasmodium ovale*. It is also used occasionally in combination with clindamycin for the treatment of *Pneumocystis carinii* infections. The mechanism of action is not clearly known, but primaquine is highly active against the exoerythrocytic states of *P. vivax* and *P. ovale*. It is usually administered to travelers after their return from areas endemic for *P. vivax* and *P. ovale* to prevent relapses, which may occur many months following exposure to mosquitoes infected with these species of plasmodia. Primaquine can cause hemolytic anemia in patients who are severely glucose-6-phosphate dehydrogenase (G-6-PD) deficient: this is its major side effect, and many travel consultants recommend that all patients who receive this drug be tested for G-6-PD deficiency. The use of primaquine is unfortunately often ignored by patients and their clinicians after return from a malarious area. The price to be paid is relapse of malarial infection in those who have had exposure to these two species of malaria. It should be anticipated that even 14-day courses of primaquine may fail to prevent relapses in about 25% of patients who have been heavily infected with *P. ovale*, and it may be necessary to double the dose from 15 mg/d of primaquine base to 30 mg/d for 14 days.

Primaquine has been used in combination with clindamycin for the treatment of *Pneumocystis carinii* pneumonia.

ACTIVITY

Primaquine is able to disrupt the parasite's mitochondria and bind to the native DNA, resulting in structural changes that cause a significant upset in the metabolic process. Gametocyte and exoerythrocyte forms are inhibited. The elimination of exoerythrocyte infection prevents development of blood forms that cause relapses of vivax malaria.

SPECIAL PRECAUTIONS

Hemolytic reactions can occur in the following cases during treatment with primaquine: patients with G-6-PD deficiency (most common in African, Asian, and Mediterranean peoples), idiosyncratic reactions (demonstrated by hemolytic anemia, methemoglobinemia, or leukopenia); nicotinamide adenine dinucleotide (NADH) methemoglobin reductase deficiency. Reactions may be moderate to severe. Stop treatment if significant darkening of the urine or sudden decrease in hemoglobin concentration or leukocyte count occurs. Do not exceed recommended dose.

Blood examinations (especially blood cell counts and hemoglobin determinations) should be done regularly.

SPECIAL GROUPS

Children: No pediatric-specific problems have been documented.
Elderly: No information.
Renal impairment: No information.
Hepatic impairment: No information.
Pregnancy: Safety not established; not recommended during pregnancy.
Breast-feeding: No information.

DOSAGE

Malaria (radical cure): (Note: Start treatment during last 2 weeks of, or following a course of, suppression with chloroquine or a comparable agent.)
Adults: 26.3 mg (15-mg base) per day for 14 days.
Elderly: No information.
Children: 680 µg/kg/d for 14 days.
Renal impairment: No information.
Unlabled pneumocytis pneumonia: (to be used with clindamycin) 15- to 30-mg base (26.3 to 52.6 mg) once a day for 21 days.

INDICATIONS

Exclusively for the radical cure of vivax malaria, the prevention of relapse in vivax malaria, infections caused by gametocytes of *P. falciparum*, or following the termination of chloroquine phosphate suppressive therapy in a geographic area in which vivax malaria is endemic
(Unlabled indication): In combination with clindamycin for *Pneumocystis carinii* pneumonia

CONTRAINDICATIONS

Concomitant administration of quinacrine and primaquine
Acutely ill patients suffering from systemic disease manifested by a tendency to granulocytopenia (*eg*, rheumatoid arthritis, lupus erythematosus)
Concurrent administration of other potentially hemolytic agents or bone marrow depressants

INTERACTIONS

Quinacrine, hemolytics

ADVERSE EFFECTS

Gastrointestinal: nausea, vomiting, epigastric distress, abdominal cramps
Hematologic: leukopenia, hemolytic anemia in patients with G-6-PD deficiency, methemoglobinemia in patients with nicotinamide-adenine dinucleotide methemoglobin reductase deficiency

PHARMACOKINETICS AND PHARMACODYNAMICS

Peak serum levels: 15 mg (base): 50 to 66 µg/mL
Serum half-life: mean, 5.8 h
Bioavailability: rapidly absorbed, 96%
Protein binding: no information
Metabolism: rapidly converted to carboxyprimaquine
Excretion: less than 2% excreted in urine in 24 h
Renal impairment: no information
Hepatic impairment: no information

OVERDOSAGE

No information

PATIENT INFORMATION

Finish full course of therapy
Stomach upset may occur and may be alleviated by taking medication with food; if nausea, vomiting, or abdominal pain continues, contact physician
Contact physician if urine becomes dark

AVAILABILITY

Tablets—26.3 mg (equivalent to 15-mg base)

The information here is provided as guidance only. Prescribers should always consult the manufacturer's current prescribing information.

PYRANTEL PAMOATE (Antiminth®, Cobantril®)

Pyrantel pamoate is an oral anthelminthic agent that is neither vermicidal nor ovicidal. It acts as a neuromuscular blocking agent, causing sudden contraction and paralysis of the helminths. It also acts as a cholinesterase inhibitor and ganglionic stimulant. The helminth is expelled from the body because it cannot maintain its position within the intestinal tract. Pyrantel pamoate has usefulness in the treatment of ascariasis and enterobiasis in addition to other helminth infections, including hookworm. It is less effective against *Necator americanus* than *Ancylostoma duodenale*. Pyrantel pamoate is a tetrahydropyrimidine derivative that is poorly absorbed in the gastrointestinal tract. Hence, it is effective against helminths within the gastrointestinal tract but not against migratory stages of the worms.

Side effects are fairly infrequent, and they include nausea, vomiting, diarrhea, and abdominal cramps, with occasional dizziness, headache, rash, or fever. A few patients have experienced an elevation in liver enzyme tests following administration. Usage in children under 2 years of age and safety during pregnancy have not been well evaluated.

ACTIVITY

Pyrantel causes spastic paralysis in the worm and also inhibits cholinesterases. It is active against *Enterobius vermicularis* (pinworm), *Ascaris lumbricoides* (roundworm), and hookworm.

SPECIAL PRECAUTIONS

Contraindicated in hepatic disease.
Contraindicated in pregnancy.
Safety and efficacy not established for use in children under 2 years of age.

SPECIAL GROUPS

Children: Safety and efficacy not established for use in children under 2 years of age.
Elderly: Because pyrantel is contraindicated in hepatic disease, hepatic function should be determined prior to administration.
Renal impairment: No information.
Hepatic impairment: Contraindicated.
Pregnancy: Contraindicated.
Breast-feeding: Maternal serum concentrations are low; unlikely that significant amounts are excreted in breast milk.

DOSAGE

(Note: Can be given without regard to meals, at any time of day. Taken with fruit juices or milk.)
Adults: One single dose of 11 mg/kg. Maximum single dose is 1 g. Repeat after 2 to 3 weeks if necessary.
Elderly: No information.
Children: For children > 2 years of age, same as adults.
Renal impairment: No information.

INDICATIONS

Treatment of ascariasis (roundworm), enterobiasis (pinworm), and multiple helminth infections

CONTRAINDICATIONS

Hypersensitivity to pyrantel, pregnancy

INTERACTIONS

Piperazine, theophylline

ADVERSE EFFECTS

Central nervous system: headache, dizziness, drowsiness, insomnia
Gastrointestinal (and hepatic): anorexia, nausea, vomiting, abdominal cramps, diarrhea
Skin: rash

PHARMACOKINETICS AND PHARMACODYNAMICS

Peak serum levels: no information
Serum half-life: no information
Bioavailability: poorly and incompletely absorbed from gastrointestinal tract
Protein binding: no information
Metabolism: no information
Excretion: over 50% excreted in feces as unchanged drug; 15% or less recovered in urine as parent drug and metabolites
Renal impairment: no information
Hepatic impairment: contraindicated

OVERDOSAGE

No information

PATIENT INFORMATION

One single dose is all that is necessary; dosage is based on body weight
Family members should be treated concurrently; wash all bedding and nightclothes after treatment to prevent reinfection
Laxative use is not necessary to facilitate removal of parasites
If anemia present before treatment, take iron supplement during and for up to 6 months after treatment

AVAILABILITY

Capsules—180 mg
Oral suspension—250 mg/5 mL
Liquid—144 mg/mL and 50 mg/mL

The information here is provided as guidance only. Prescribers should always consult the manufacturer's current prescribing information.

PYRIMETHAMINE-SULFADOXINE (Fansidar®)

This combination of agents is marketed under the name Fansidar® as a weekly prophylactic agent against malaria. Because of the potential for serious cutaneous side effects such as erythema multiforme and the Stevens-Johnson syndrome, its use is now limited to a single, three-tablet self-treatment dose for adult travelers who suspect malaria but are not within range of seeking medical treatment. This, in itself, may not always be successful because of the possibility of parasite resistance to this combination. In addition, this combination of agents should not be used in patients who have a history of allergy to sulfa drugs.

ACTIVITY

Pyrimethamine-sulfadoxine acts by reciprocal potentiation of its components and by a sequential blockade of two enzymes necessary in the biosynthesis of folinic acid within the parasites.

SPECIAL PRECAUTIONS

Fatalities have occurred because of severe reactions, including Stevens-Johnson syndrome and toxic epidermal necrolysis. Stop prophylaxis if skin rash occurs, if count of any formed blood elements is reduced, or if active bacterial or fungal infections occur.

Deaths associated with sulfonamide administration have occurred rarely and have happened because of severe reactions, including the following: fulminant hepatic necrosis, agranulocytosis, aplastic anemia, or other blood dyscrasias. The prophylactic regimen has caused leukopenia during treatment of 2 months or more; the condition has generally been mild and reversible.

Contraindicated in patients with severe renal impairment, liver parenchymal damage, or blood dyscrasias. Use with caution in patients with mild to moderate impairment. Urinalysis with microscopic examination and renal function tests should be performed in patients with renal impairment during therapy.

Pyrimethamine has been found to be mutagenic in laboratory animals and in human bone marrow.

Use with caution in patients with possible folate deficiency or severe allergy or bronchial asthma.

If folic acid deficiency or signs of folic acid deficiency occur, stop drug and give folinic acid (leucovorin) in doses of 5 to 15 mg intramuscularly per day for 3 days (longer if depressed platelet or leukocyte count recovery is too slow). Hemolysis can occur in patients with G-6-PD deficiency.

For prolonged administration, monitor blood counts and perform urinalysis for crystalluria.

SPECIAL GROUPS

Children: Do not administer to infants under 2 months of age because sulfonamides may cause kernicterus in neonates.

Elderly: No information.

Renal impairment: Contraindicated for prophylactic or repeated use when severe; use with caution if mild to moderate.

Hepatic impairment: Contraindicated for prophylactic or repeated use in cases of severe parenchymal damage; use with caution when mild to moderate.

Pregnancy: Contraindicated at term. Adequate human studies have not been performed; teratogenic effects have been observed in rats. Use only if potential benefits outweigh potential risks.

Breast-feeding: Both drugs are excreted in breast milk; do not nurse during treatment.

INDICATIONS

Treatment of *Plasmodium falciparum* malaria in patients for whom chloroquine resistance is suspected (Note: Chloroquine or mefloquine are the drugs of choice for travelers to malarious areas.)

Prophylaxis of malaria for travelers to areas where chloroquine-resistant *P. falciparum* malaria is endemic (resistant strains may be encountered nonetheless)

Isosporiasis (prophylaxis and treatment)

(Unlabeled): Prophylactic agent for prevention of *Pneumocystis carinii* pneumonia in patients with AIDS; most commonly as a second-line agent

CONTRAINDICATIONS

Allergy or hypersensitivity to sulfonamides, pyrimethamine, furosemide, thiazide diuretics, sulfonylureas, or carbonic anhydrase inhibitors

Patients with documented megaloblastic anemia due to folate deficiency

Infants under 2 months of age

Pregnancy at term

Nursing

Repeated (prophylactic) use in patients with severe renal insufficiency, marked liver parenchymal damage, or blood dyscrasias

Bone marrow depression or porphyria

INTERACTIONS

Anticoagulants, anticonvulsants, antidiabetic agents, bone marrow depressants, hemolytics, hepatotoxic medications

ADVERSE EFFECTS

(Note: The following are effects due to sulfonamides and pyrimethamine and may have not been reported with the combination. Sulfonamides have certain chemical similarities to some goitrogens, diuretics [acetazolamide and the thiazides] and oral hypoglycemic agents. Cross-sensitivity may exist with these agents, and diuresis and hypoglycemia have occurred rarely.)

Central nervous system: headache, peripheral neuritis, mental depression, convulsions, ataxia, hallucinations, tinnitus, vertigo, insomnia, apathy, fatigue, muscle weakness, nervousness

Gastrointestinal: glossitis, stomatitis, nausea, emesis, abdominal pains, hepatitis, hepatocellular necrosis, diarrhea, pancreatitis

Hematologic: agranulocytosis; aplastic, megaloblastic, or hemolytic anemia; thrombocytopenia, leukopenia, eosinophilia, hypoprothrombinemia, methemoglobinemia, blood dysrasias

Hypersensitivity: erythema multiforme (Stevens-Johnson syndrome), generalized skin eruptions, toxic epidermal necrolysis, urticaria, serum sickness, pruritus, exfoliative dermatitis, anaphylactoid reactions, periorbital edema, conjunctival and scleral infection, photosensitization, arthralgia, allergic myocarditis

Miscellaneous: drug fever, chills, toxic nephrosis with oliguria and anuria, polyarteritis nodosa LE phenomenon, pulmonary infiltrates

The information here is provided as guidance only. Prescribers should always consult the manufacturer's current prescribing information.

PYRIMETHAMINE-SULFADOXINE (CONTINUED)

DOSAGE

Adults: *See* table below for dosage guidelines.
Elderly: *See* table below for dosage guidelines.
Children: *See* table below for dosage guidelines.
Renal impairment: No special dosage given.

Presumptive Treatment Guidelines for Pyrimethamine-Sulfadoxine

	Treatment Dosages*
Adults	3 tablets (500 mg sulfadoxine/25 mg pyrimethamine) orally as a single dose
Children	
5–10 kg	0.5 tablet single dose
11–20 kg	1 tablet single dose
21–30 kg	1.5 tablets single dose
31–45 kg	2 tablets single dose
> 45 kg	3 tablets single dose

** Treatment should be used in combination with quinine if chloroquine-resistant P. falciparum is diagnosed.*

PHARMACOKINETICS AND PHARMACODYNAMICS

Peak serum levels: 51 to 76 µg/mL sulfadoxine in 2.5 to 6 h; 0.13 to 0.4 µg/mL pyrimethamine in 1.5 to 8 h
Serum half-life: 100 to 230 h (mean 169) for sulfadoxine; 54 to 148 h (mean 111) for pyrimethamine
Bioavailability: well absorbed after oral administration
Protein binding: pyrimethamine, high (87%), sulfadoxine, night (> 90%)
Metabolism: pyrimethamine, hepatic
Excretion: sulfadoxine, excreted primarily unchanged by kidneys; pyrimethamine, 20% to 30% excreted primarily unchanged by kidneys
Renal impairment: contraindicated for prophylactic or repeated use in severe impairment; use with caution in mild to moderate impairment
Hepatic impairment: contraindicated for prophylactic or repeated use in severe parenchymal damage; use with caution in mild to moderate impairment

OVERDOSAGE

Symptoms include anorexia, vomiting, and central nervous system stimulation (including convulsions); these effects can be followed by megaloblastic anemia, leukopenia, thrombocytopenia, glossitis, and crystalluria.

Treatment in acute intoxication may include emesis and gastric lavage followed by purges along with usual supportive measures. Patient should be adequately hydrated to prevent renal damage. Use of parenteral benzodiazepines or short-acting barbiturates is indicated for convulsions. Renal and hematopoietic systems should be monitored for a minimum of 1 month after overdose. If platelet or leukocyte counts are depressed, administer leucovorin in doses of 5 to 15 mg intramuscularly per day for 3 days or more.

PATIENT INFORMATION

Adequate fluid intake should be maintained to prevent crystalluria and stone formation

Contact physician immediately if any of the following occur: sore throat, fever, pallor, purpura, jaundice, glossitis, arthralgia, cough/shortness of breath, darkening of urine

If skin rash or symptoms of folic acid deficiency occur, stop taking drug and seek medical attention immediately

It is still possible to contract malaria regardless of the prophylactic regimen used; therefore, medical attention should be sought immediately if a febrile illness occurs

Do not give to children < 2 months of age

Delays in treating malaria may have serious or fatal consequences

Continue medication while in area and for 4 weeks after leaving area

Contraceptives should be used during therapy to avoid pregnancy

Breast-feeding should be avoided during therapy

AVAILABILITY

Tablets—500 mg sulfadoxine and 25 mg pyrimethamine

The information here is provided as guidance only. Prescribers should always consult the manufacturer's current prescribing information.

QUININE (Quinamm®)

Quinine has been the mainstay in the treatment of malarial infection for well over 300 years, even before our understanding of the pathogenesis of malaria. It still retains considerable usefulness in the treatment of chloroquine-resistant *Plasmodium falciparum* malaria, particularly in combination with the tetracyclines. Quinine also has a role in the treatment of severe babesiosis when used in combination with clindamycin.

Quinine has what is referred to as *schizonticidal activity*, and it can concentrate in parasitized red blood cells. It is therefore active against the erythrocytic stages of each of the malarial parasites, including those strains of *P. falciparum* that are resistant to chloroquine. Its precise mechanism of action is undetermined.

Clinicians should be aware of the frequent symptoms of cinchonism, which include tinnitus, headache, nausea, abdominal pain, and occasional vision disturbances. Occasionally, deafness, hemolytic anemia, and photosensitivity reactions have occurred. Hypoglycemia is important in the treatment of severe malarial infections, as are arrhythmias, hypotension, and drug fever. Rarely, blindness has been reported, as has sudden death if the agent is injected too rapidly. Intravenous quinine has been replaced by the use of intravenous quinidine in industrialized countries for the treatment of severe malarial infections.

ACTIVITY

Quinine acts primarily as a blood schizonticide; its antimalarial action is not clearly understood. It concentrates in parasitic vesicles causing an elevation of pH in in-intracellular organelles. This is thought to disrupt intracellular transport.

SPECIAL PRECAUTIONS

Cinchonism may be precipitated by repeated doses or overdosage of quinine. Less serious symptoms include tinnitus, headache, nausea, and disturbed vision, which rapidly subside when the drug is stopped. Large single doses or continuation of quinine therapy may result in other symptoms involving the gastrointestinal tact, nervous and cardiovascular systems, and the skin.

Tinnitus or impaired hearing may occur with plasma concentrations of more than 10 µg/mL, which is a level not normally reached with doses of 260 to 520 mg/d; however, patients who are hypersensitive may experience tinnitus with doses as small as 300 mg.

Hemolysis with the potential for hemolytic anemia has been associated with quinine therapy in patients with G-6-PD deficiency. Discontinue drug immediately if hemolysis occurs.

Quinine has a quinidine-like activity and should be used with caution in patients with cardiac arrhythmias or cardiac disease. For patients with atrial fibrillation, quinine requires the same precautions as quinidine. Quinine may cause cardiac toxicity.

Hypersensitivity (cutaneous flushing, pruritus, skin rash, fever, gastric distress, dyspnea, ringing in ears, and visual impairment) may occur, particularly with only small doses of quinine. Extreme flushing and intense generalized pruritus are most common. Hemoglobinuria and asthma are idiosyncratic. Discontinue drug if any signs of hypersensitivity occur.

INDICATIONS

Treatment of chloroquine-resistant malaria, concurrently with pyrimethamine and a sulfonamide, a tetracycline, or clindamycin

Alternative therapy for chloroquine-sensitive strains of *P. falciparum*, *P. malariae*, *P. ovale*, and *P. vivax* (Note: A parenteral preparation of quinine dihydrochloride is available from the Centers for Disease Control and Prevention only and may also be used.)

CONTRAINDICATIONS

Allergy or hypersensitivity to quinine, G-6-PD deficiency, optic neuritis, tinnitus, history of blackwater fever and thrombocytopenic purpura (associated with previous quinine therapy), pregnancy

Mefloquine concurrent use with quinine may result in increased incidence of seizures and electrocardiogram changes. It is recommended that mefloquine be administered at least 12 hours after quinine dose

If a patient is on mefloquine prophylaxis but has mefloquine-resistant malaria, it is recommended the patient be hospitalized and monitored for QT prolongation when given quinine

INTERACTIONS

Antacids (aluminum-containing), anticoagulants (oral), antimyasthenics, cimetidine, digoxin, mefloquine, neuromuscular blocking agents (depolarizing and nondepolarizing), urinary alkalinizers

Laboratory test interactions: elevated values for urinary 17 ketogenic steroids may occur with the Zimmerman method

ADVERSE EFFECTS

Cardiovascular: anginal symptoms

Cinchonism: may occur at therapeutic doses (*see* Special Precautions)

Central nervous system: tinnitus, deafness, vertigo, headache, fever, apprehension, restlessness, confusion, syncope, excitement, delirium, hypothermia, convulsions

Gastrointestinal: nausea, vomiting, epigastric pain, hepatitis

Hematologic: acute hemolysis, hemolytic anemia, thrombocytopenic purpura, agranulocytosis, hypoprothrombinemia

Hypersensitivity: cutaneous rashes (urticarial, papular, scarlatinal), pruritus, flushing, sweating, facial edema, asthmatic symptoms

Ophthalmic: visual disturbances (including color vision and perception), photophobia, blurred vision with scotomata, night blindness, amblyopia, diplopia, diminished visual fields, mydriasis, optic atrophy

The information here is provided as guidance only. Prescribers should always consult the manufacturer's current prescribing information.

QUININE (CONTINUED)

SPECIAL GROUPS

Children: Safety not established, although no pediatric-specific problems have been documented.
Elderly: No information.
Renal impairment: No information.
Hepatic impairment: No information.
Pregnancy: Contraindicated; studies in humans have shown congenital malformations, especially with large doses of quinine.
Breast-feeding: Small amounts excreted in breast milk; no problems documented.

DOSAGE

Adult: For chloroquine-resistant *P. falciparum* malaria: 600 to 650 mg every 8 hours for at least 3 days (7 days, Southeast Asia), concurrently with 250 mg of tetracycline every 6 hours for 7 days. Use concurrent tetracycline or doxycycline or sulfadoxine-pyrimethamine or clindamycin when administering quinine for malaria.
Babesiosis: Oral 650 mg three or four times a day with concurrent intravenous clindamycin (7 to 10 days)
Elderly: No information.
Children: For chloroquine-resistant *P. falciparum* malaria: 8.3 mg/kg every 8 hours for at least 3 days (7 days, Southeast Asia). Do not use quinine alone for treatment of malaria. Use concurrent clindamycin or pyrimethamine and sulfadoxine if child is under 8 years of age. Use concurrent tetracycline if child is over 8 years of age. Concurrent doses: clindamycin 6.7 to 13.3 mg/kg three times a day for 3 days; pyrimethamine (1.25 mg/kg) plus sulfadoxine (25 mg/kg) as a single dose; tetracycline 5 mg/kg every 6 hours for 1 week.
Renal impairment: No special dosage given.

PHARMACOKINETICS AND PHARMACODYNAMICS

Peak serum levels: chronic administration of 1 g/d gives an average concentration of 7 µg/mL
Serum half-life: cerebral malaria, 18 h; uncomplicated malaria, 16 h
Bioavailability: absorption is almost complete; approximately 80% in healthy subjects
Protein binding: 85% to 90% in uncomplicated malaria; > 90% in cerebral malaria
Metabolism: > 80% metabolized in the liver
Excretion: primarily renal, with about 20% excreted as unchanged drug
Renal impairment: no information
Hepatic impairment: no information

OVERDOSAGE

Use gastric lavage or induce emesis with ipecac syrup, administer supportive therapy, administer antiarrhythmics carefully

PATIENT INFORMATION

Take with food or following meals to prevent stomach upset

May cause diarrhea, nausea, stomach cramps or pain, vomiting, or ringing of ears; contact physician if these effects become serious

Use caution while driving or performing other tasks requiring alertness and coordination; may produce blurred vision, vertigo, restlessness, confusion, or dizziness

If any signs of allergy (flushing, itching, rash, fever, stomach pain, difficult breathing, ringing of ears, or vision disturbances) occur, stop drug and contact physician

AVAILABILITY

Capsules—64.8 mg (with 400 IU vitamin E [as d1-alpha tocopheryl acetate] and lecithin)
Tablets—162.5 mg (with calcium phosphate dibasic)
Capsules—200 mg
Tablets—260 mg
Capsules—300 mg
Capsules—325 mg
Tablets—325 mg

The information here is provided as guidance only. Prescribers should always consult the manufacturer's current prescribing information.

THIABENDAZOLE (Mintezol®)

Thiabendazole is an anthelminthic agent that has been useful in the treatment of certain nematode infections, including cutaneous larva migrans and strongyloidiasis. Its mechanism of action is not known, but it does inhibit a helminth-specific enzyme, fumarate reductase. Thiabendazole is largely being replaced by a new agent, ivermectin, for the treatment of cutaneous larva migrans and strongyloidiasis. It is anticipated that because of its frequent side effects of nausea, vomiting, and vertigo, thiabendazole use will decrease. The drug has occasionally been associated with leukopenia, crystalluria, rash, hallucination, olfactory disturbances, and erythema multiforme. Rarely, shock, intrahepatic cholestasis, convulsions, and angioneurotic edema, or Stevens-Johnson syndrome, have been reported.

ACTIVITY

Thiabendazole is vermicidal or vermifungal against *Enterobius vermicularis* (pinworm), *Ascaris lumbricoides* (roundworm), *Strongyloides stercoralis* (threadworm), *Necator americanus*, *Ancylostoma duodenale* (hookworm), *Trichuris trichiura* (whipworm), *Ancylostoma braziliense* (dog and cat hookworm), and *Toxocara canis* and *Toxocara cati* (ascarids).

SPECIAL PRECAUTIONS

Erythema multiforme has been associated with thiabendazole therapy, and in severe cases (*eg*, Stevens-Johnson syndrome), fatalities have occurred. Discontinue drug if hypersensitivity reaction occurs.

Central nervous system effects may occur; therefore, patients should be advised to avoid activities requiring alertness.

Supportive therapy is necessary for anemic, dehydrated, or malnourished patients before start of therapy. Patients with renal or hepatic impairment should be monitored carefully.

Not suitable for treatment of mixed infection with ascaris because it may cause the worms to migrate; use only in patients for whom susceptible worm infestation is diagnosed. Do not use prophylactically.

Transient elevations in AST have occurred rarely in patients receiving thiabendazole.

SPECIAL GROUPS

Children: Safety and efficacy not established for use in children weighing less than 13.6 kg.

Elderly: No information.

Renal impairment: Monitor function closely before and during therapy.

Hepatic impairment: Monitor function closely before and during therapy.

Pregnancy: Adequate human studies not performed; use only when benefits outweigh risk.

Breast-feeding: Not known whether excreted in breast milk; because of potential for serious adverse effects to fetus, decision must be made to discontinue nursing or discontinue drug.

INDICATIONS

Treatment of strongyloidiasis (threadworm) infection, cutaneous larva migrans (creeping eruption), and visceral larva migrans

(Note: Although thiabendazole is not indicated for primary treatment, when enterobiasis [pinworm] occurs with any of the above, additional therapy is not required for most patients. Thiabendazole should be used in the following infestations only if more specific therapy is unavailable or cannot be used or when further therapy with a second agent is desirable: uncinariasis [hookworm, *N. americanus* and *A. duodenale*], trichuriasis [whipworm], ascariasis [large roundworm].)

Alleviation of symptoms of trichinosis during invasive phase

CONTRAINDICATIONS

Allergy or hypersensitivity to thiabendazole, hepatic or renal function impairment

INTERACTIONS

Theophylline

ADVERSE EFFECTS

Central nervous system: dizziness, weariness, drowsiness, giddiness, headache, numbness, hyperirritability, convulsions, collapse

Gastrointestinal: anorexia, nausea, vomiting, diarrhea, epigastric distress, jaundice, cholestasis, parenchymal liver damage

Genitourinary: hematuria, enuresis, malodor of the urine, crystalluria

Hypersensitivity: pruritus, fever, facial flush, chills, conjunctival injections ("red eye"), angioedema, anaphylaxis, skin rashes (including perianal), erythema multiforme (including Stevens-Johnson syndrome), lymphadenopathy

Miscellaneous: appearance of live ascaris in the mouth and nose, hypotension, transient leukopenia

Special senses: tinnitus, abnormal sensation in eyes, xanthopsia, blurred vision, dry mucous membranes

PHARMACOKINETICS AND PHARMACODYNAMICS

Peak serum levels: 4.5 to 5.0 µg/mL after a single 25-mg/kg dose

Serum half-life: normal and anephric, 1.2 h

Bioavailability: rapidly absorbed

Protein binding: no information

Metabolism: hepatic; rapidly metabolized to inactive 5-hydroxythiabendazole

Excretion: of administered dose, 90% recovered in urine, most within 24 h, and 5% from feces in 48 h

Renal impairment: monitor function closely before and during therapy

Hepatic impairment: monitor function closely before and during therapy

The information here is provided as guidance only. Prescribers should always consult the manufacturer's current prescribing information.

THIABENDAZOLE (CONTINUED)

DOSAGE

(Note: Maximum daily dose is 3 g, after meals if possible.)
Adults: Weight less than 68 kg, 25 mg/kg/dose; weight 68 kg or more, 1.5 g/dose.
Elderly: *See* adult information above and table of indications below.
Children: For children weighing > 13.6 kg, *see* adult information above and table of indications below.
Renal impairment: No special dosage given.

Dosage of Thiabendazole

Indication	Regimen	Notes
Strongyloidiasis	Two doses/d for 2 consecutive days 25 mg/kg twice a day for 2 days	Can also use single dose of 44 mg/kg but with higher incidence of adverse effects
Cutaneous larva migrans (creeping eruption)	Two doses/d for 2 consecutive days 25 mg/kg twice a day for 2 days	If active lesions are still present 2 days after end of therapy, a second course is recommended
Trichinosis	Two doses/d for 2 to 4 consecutive days (individualize dosage) 25 mg/kg twice a day for 2–4 days	Optimal dosage not established
Visceral larva migrans	Two doses/d for 5–7 consecutive days 25 mg/kg twice a day	Safety and efficacy data on 7-day regimen are limited

OVERDOSAGE

There is no specific antidote for overdose. Care should be symptomatic and supportive; institute emesis or gastric lavage if necessary.

PATIENT INFORMATION

Take with food to reduce stomach upset
If using chewable tablets, chew or crush thoroughly before swallowing
Enemas are not necessary after drug therapy
Duration of therapy may be from 2 to 7 days depending on condition being treated
Pinworm infections are very contagious; all family members in close contact with patient should be treated to reduce risk of spread
Strict hygiene must be observed to prevent reinfection; disinfect toilet facilities daily, and change and launder undergarments, bed linens, towels, and nightclothes daily
Use caution when driving or performing other activities requiring alertness; may cause drowsiness or dizziness

AVAILABILITY

Tablets, chewable—500 mg
Oral suspension—500 mg/5 mL

The information here is provided as guidance only. Prescribers should always consult the manufacturer's current prescribing information.

Index

Index of Proprietary Names

Index of Indications